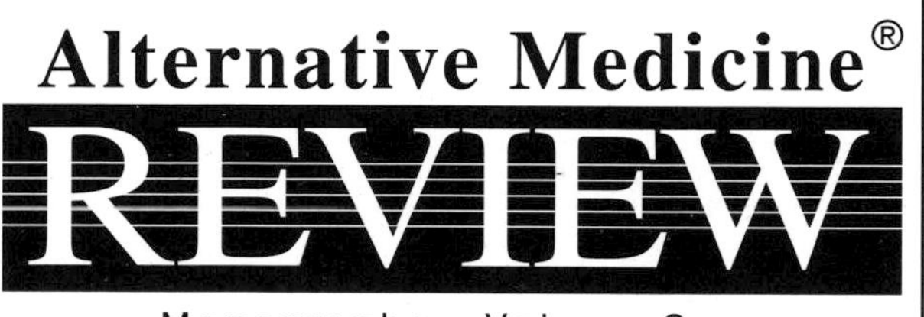

Monographs

Volume One

NOTICE

This book is intended for reference only. The authors of the monographs and the publisher believe the descriptions, pharmacokinetics, active constituents, mechanisms of action, clinical indications, therapeutic considerations, dosages, side effects, toxicity, and the drug, botanical, and nutrient interactions, as set forth in this book, are in accord with current knowledge, recommendations, and practice at the time of publication. The authors of the monographs and the publisher have utilized sources believed to be reliable in their effort to provide information that is complete and generally in accord with the standards accepted at the time of publication.

Because of ongoing research, development, clinical experience, and the rapid accumulation of information relating to the subject matter of this book, the reader is urged to carefully review and evaluate the information provided herein. Neither the authors of the monographs nor the publisher warrant that the information contained herein is in every respect accurate and complete, particularly as new research and clinical experience continue to expand and broaden knowledge pertaining to the subject matter of this book. Therefore, the authors of the monographs and the publisher must disclaim any responsibility and will not be responsible for any adverse effect resulting from the use or application of any of the information contained in this book. Any use or application of the information contained in this book is at the sole discretion and risk of the intended health-care professionals who read it.

The dosages in this book are suggested dosages for adults, not children, unless otherwise indicated.

Thorne Research, Inc.
P.O. Box 25
Dover, Idaho 83825

ISBN 0–9725815–0–2 (softcover)

Printed in the United States of America. First Edition

Library of Congress Cataloging-in-Publication Data: pending

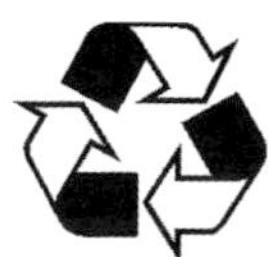

Table of Contents

This book is dedicated to a man who taught us that there is no greater personal satisfaction than to make a positive difference in someone's life just by doing your job well. To Dr. Allen Tyler, naturopath, chiropractor and medical doctor— a true healer, a true friend, and a great father.

Al and Kelly Czap

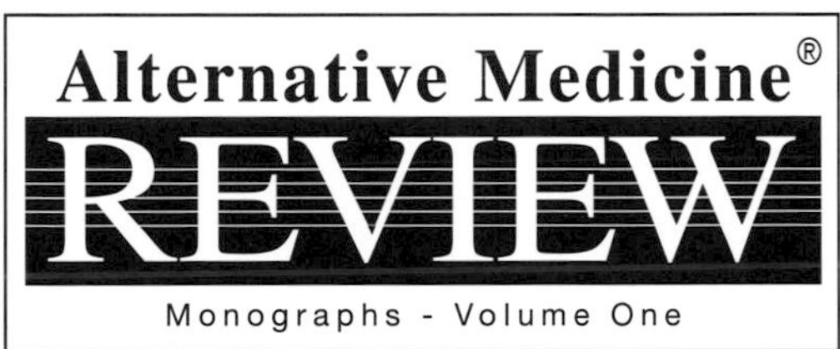
Alternative Medicine®
REVIEW
Monographs - Volume One

Jeremy Appleton, ND

Writer/educator in the field of complementary and alternative medicine. Department chair, National College of Naturopathic Medicine. Director of Scientific Affairs, Cardinal Nutrition. Co-author, *MSM: The Definitive Guide* (Freedom Press). Lecturer internationally on topics in clinical nutrition and botanical medicine.

Timothy Birdsall, ND

1985 graduate, Bastyr University. Technical Director, Thorne Research, 1989-1998 and the founding Editor-in-Chief of *Alternative Medicine Review*. National Director, Naturopathic Medicine and Research, Cancer Treatment Centers of America, 1998-present. Co-author, *How To Prevent and Treat Cancer With Natural Medicine* (Putnam, 2002).

Kerry Bone, BSc

Founder, Director of Research and Development, MediHerb, Warwick, Queensland, Australia (herbal manufacturer and exporter). Author, technical and clinical articles, phytotherapy text books. Lecturer in Australia, the United States, and other countries.

Patrick J.D. Bouic, PhD

Chair, Department of Immunology, University of Stellenbosch, South Africa. Research specialty (including clinical trials) on the impact of natural products on functioning of the immune system. Author of numerous international scientific publications and a book on the immune system. Holder of several international patents.

Matt Brignall, ND

Cancer Treatment and Wellness Center, Seattle, Washington. Instructor, Diet and Nutrient Therapy, Bastyr University. Product consultant, Thorne Research.

Donald Brown, ND

Practice specialty in evidence-based herbal medicine. Former assistant professor, Bastyr University. Founder and director, Natural Product Research Consultants. Advisory Board, American Botanical Council. President's Advisory Board, Bastyr University. Former advisor, Office of Dietary Supplements, National Institutes of Health. Contributing author, *HerbalGram*. Editor-in-chief, 1994-2000, *Healthnotes Review of Complementary and Integrative Medicine*. Author, *Herbal Prescriptions for Health and Healing* (Prima Publishing, 2000); co-author, *Natural Pharmacy* (Prima Publishing, 1999); co-author, *A-Z Guide to Drug-Herb-Vitamin Interactions* (Prima Publishing, 1999).

Michael Brown, ND

1998 graduate, Southwest College of Naturopathic Medicine. Private practice, Wellness Connection, Shawnee Mission, Kansas. Practice specialty in natural therapeutics, utilizing clinical nutrition, classical homeopathy, botanical medicine, and natural hormone replacement therapy.

Patrick Bufi, ND

1989 graduate, Bastyr University. Instructor at schools of naturopathic medicine and alternative medicine. Former chair, Western Clinical Medicine, Northwest Institute of Acupuncture and Oriental Medicine. Practice specialty in internal and pulmonary medicine and homeopathy. Contributing author, *Alternative Medicine Review.*

Walter Crinnion, ND

1982 graduate, Bastyr University. Former adjunct professor, Bastyr University. Former adjunct professor, Southwest College of Naturopathic Medicine. Professor, Environmental Medicine, and Director, Environmental Medicine Center for Excellence, Southwest College of Naturopathic Medicine. Product consultant, Thorne Research.

John Furlong, ND

1985 Graduate, Bastyr University. Medical Specialist, Nutrition and Metabolism, Great Smokies Diagnostic Laboratory. Practice specialty in novel approaches to diagnosis and treatment of cardiovascular and metabolic conditions. Community clinic participant, Mexico, botanical aspects of cross-cultural medicine and diabetes prevention.

Alan Gaby, MD

Past-president, American Holistic Medical Association. Author, *Preventing and Reversing Osteoporosis*. Co-author, *The Patient's Book of Natural Healing.* Contributing editor, *Alternative Medicine Review.*

Kathi Head, ND

1985 graduate, National College of Naturopathic Medicine. Technical Advisor, Thorne Research. Editor-in-Chief, *Alternative Medicine Review.* Contributing author, *Textbook of Natural Medicine*, 2nd Edition (Churchill Livingstone, 1999). Author, *The Natural Pharmacist: Complementary Treatments For Diabetes* (Random House, 2001)

Mark Janikula, ND Candidate 2003

Student representative, Thorne Research, Southwest College of Naturopathic Medicine. Contributing author, *Alternative Medicine Review.*

Julie S. Jurenka, MT(ASCP)

Research Assistant, Thorne Research. Contributor, *Alternative Medicine Review*. Graduated, Montana State University, 1982; BS, Microbiology. Former medical technologist, 1986-1997.

Gregory S. Kelly, ND

Co-founder, Body By Design, seminar series on weight regulation. Associate Editor, *Alternative Medicine Review*. Contributing editor, *Cook Right 4 Your Type* (Putnam, 1998). Contributing author, *Live Right 4 Your Type* (Putnam, 2001), *Textbook of Natural Medicine*, 2nd edition (Churchill Livingstone, 1999). Instructor, Advanced Nutrition, University of Bridgeport, College of Naturopathic Medicine.

Parris Kidd, PhD

University of California, Berkeley, PhD in cell biology. Contributing editor, *Alternative Medicine Review*. Health educator; biomedical consultant to the dietary supplement industry.

Duffy MacKay, ND

2001 graduate, National College of Naturopathic Medicine. Clinical practice, York, Maine. Student representative, Thorne Research, National College of Naturopathic Medicine, 1999-2001. Senior Editor, *Alternative Medicine Review*. Technical Advisor, Thorne Research.

Keri Marshall, MS, ND

1996 Master of Science Social and Preventive Medicine, State University of New York at Buffalo. 2001 graduate, National College of Naturopathic Medicine. Private practice, Sandpoint, Idaho.

Alan Miller, ND

1989 graduate, Bastyr University. Technical Advisor, Thorne Research. Senior Editor, *Alternative Medicine Review*. Contributing author, *Textbook of Natural Medicine*, 2nd Edition (Churchill Livingstone, 1999).

Lyn Patrick, ND

1984 graduate, Bastyr University. Associate Editor, *Alternative Medicine Review*. Private practice, Tucson, Arizona, 1984-2002.

Kendra Pearsall, ND

2001 graduate, Southwest College of Naturopathic Medicine. Private practice, Scottsdale, Arizona. Practice specialty in endocrinology and detoxification.

Gary Piscopo, ND, LAc
1999 graduate, Bastyr University. Co-founder, Healing Mountain Publishing (textbooks related to clinical natural medicine). Co-founder, vice-president, Alpine Valley Natural Health Clinic, Wenatchee, Washington. Consultant, MicroMedex (provider of computerized and printed medical information).

Ronald Reichert, ND
Private practice, Vancouver, British Columbia. Contributing author for articles on phytotherapy and applied nutrition to lay and professional publications in Canada and the United States.

Steve Sinclair, ND
1997 graduate, Southwest College of Naturopathic Medicine. Private practice, Frederick, Maryland. Practice specialty in clinical nutrition and integrative medicine.

Eric Yarnell, ND
Assistant professor of botanical medicine, Bastyr University. President, Botanical Medicine Academy, Seattle, Washington. Co-founder, president, Healing Mountain Publishing. Co-owner, Heron Botanicals, Inc. Former chair, botanical medicine, Southwest College of Naturopathic Medicine.

Image Credits

Photomicrograph of Phthalic Acid on the cover copyright © 2002 by Fredrick C. Skvara, MD. Used with permission.

A very special thanks to Laura Doerfler and Indena U.S.A for providing such great raw materials and allowing us access to such a variety of botanical photographs for this book.

Photographs of *Ananas comosus* and *Saccharum offinarum* by Harold St. John are used with permission. Carr Botanical Consultation Kaneohe, Hawaii

Photograph of *Piper methysticum* is used by permision of Kava Kauai. Kapaa, Hawaii

Photographs of *Camellia sinensis*, *Eleutherococcus senticosus*, *Gymnema sylvestre*, and *Withania somnifera* are copyright © 2002 Steven Foster. Used with permission. Steven Foster Group, Inc. Fayetteville, AR

Other botanical photographs were taken by the Thorne staff.

All the illustrations were done by Jared Johnston.

Preface

May 1996 marked the first date of publication of *Alternative Medicine Review* (*AMR*), a straightforward journal of clinical therapeutics for the complementary health care practitioner. With the publication of impartial, in-depth, cutting edge review and original research articles, the *AMR* quickly became the journal of choice for reference, clinical applications, and teaching. In June of 1998, the *AMR* was first indexed on Medline and quickly followed with acceptance by Cinahl, Index Medicus, and Embase.

In addition to the comprehensive articles, which comprise the backbone of each issue, the *AMR* has provided monographs on many compounds and extracts utilized by complementary health care practitioners worldwide.

In an effort to provide you with the most up-to-the minute information in a convenient form, the *AMR* now brings you volume one of *Alternative Medicine Review Monographs*, with both previously published but updated and never-before published monographs, written and updated by our editorial staff and numerous other physician contributors.

This exclusive book contains peer-reviewed monographs representing the most diverse assortment of botanicals and nutrients ever put into print. Each monograph provides a general description, active constituents and phamacokinetics, mechanisms of action, clinical indications, safety and dosage, as well as any currently identified drug interactions. Rather than just including basic vitamins and therapeutic plants, the *AMR* has included many of the more esoteric and cutting-edge substances that provide alternatives to the complementary practitioner.

I would personally like to extend a very heartfelt "thank you" to everyone for the enormous amount of work that has been put forth in the compilation of this body of work. Many long hours of research review, writing, editing and proof reading have resulted in what is certainly the most useful volume of its kind.

Al Czap
Publisher
Alternative Medicine Review

Forward

The practice of complementary and alternative medicine offers to the practitioner many choices of therapeutic regimens, including the use of a number of beneficial vitamins, minerals, amino acids, botanicals, hormones, and other substances. The use of these and other modalities is rapidly increasing among practitioners, as well as gaining widespread acceptance in venues previously antagonistic to their use. Hospitals are now offering acupuncture, yoga, and tai chi, and pharmacies are replete with herbal extracts and nutritional alternatives to pharmaceutical medications. If you are a health-care practitioner who is not utilizing nutritional supplements or herbs in your practice, it is guaranteed your patients will be asking you questions about them – if they are not doing so already. But, like most doctors, you may not have time to constantly review the scientific literature.

In the realm of herbal medicine, a number of publications offer information on sources, origins, constituents, and traditional indications for various botanicals. However, there has long been a need for a reference work that not only includes plant-source therapeutic substances, but also incorporates a well-rounded overview of the many necessary and useful alternative substances – from vitamins to life-improving compounds such as coenzyme Q-10, alpha lipoic acid, and acetyl L-carnitine.

The editors of *Alternative Medicine Review*, in addition to an impressive group of contributing authors, have compiled data from an exhaustive review of the technical literature and yielded a volume of monographs that addresses not only the basic information necessary to explain the "*what it is*," but also provides an impartial, peer-reviewed, in-depth discussion of "*what it's for.*" In addition to well-referenced information on biochemistry, pharmacokinetics, and clinical indications of more than 80 substances, also included are cautions, contraindications, and potential interactions.

Alternative Medicine Review – Monographs is that much needed reference source to assist the practitioner and subsequently help the patient in the quest for balanced good health.

Jonathan Collin, MD
Publisher
Townsend Letter for Doctors and Patients

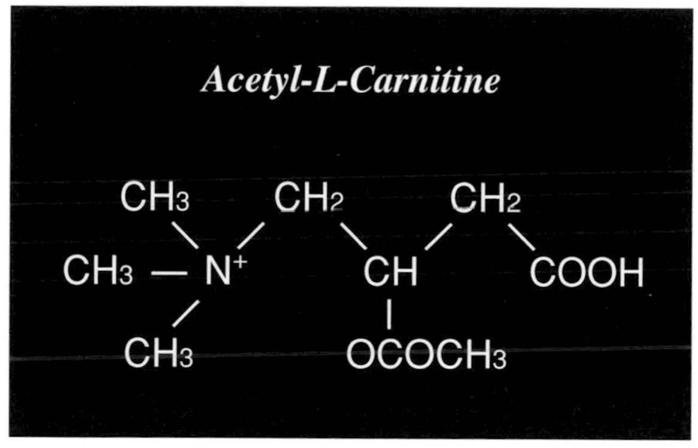

Acetyl-L-Carnitine

Introduction

Acetyl-L-carnitine (ALC) is an ester of the trimethylated amino acid, L-carnitine, and is synthesized in the human brain, liver, and kidney by the enzyme ALC-transferase. Acetyl-L-carnitine facilitates the uptake of acetyl CoA into the mitochondria for fatty acid oxidation, enhances acetylcholine production, and stimulates protein and membrane phospholipid synthesis. Similar in structure to acetylcholine, ALC exerts a cholinomimetic effect. Studies have shown ALC may be of benefit in treating Alzheimer's dementia, depression in the elderly, HIV infection, diabetic neuropathies, ischemia and reperfusion of the brain, and cognitive impairment of alcoholism.

Pharmacokinetics

L-carnitine and acetyl-L-carnitine are absorbed in the jejunum by simple diffusion. Transport into cellular tissue is via an active transport mechanism, with studies showing plasma concentrations of ALC and L-carnitine reaching equilibrium via carnitine acetyl-transferase activity. Both intravenous and oral administration result in a corresponding increase in cerebral spinal fluid concentrations of ALC, indicating it readily crosses the blood-brain barrier. L-carnitine and its esters undergo little metabolism and are subsequently excreted in the urine via renal tubular reabsorption. The rate of clearance increases with the plasma concentration of these substances.[1,2]

Mechanisms of Action

The exact mechanisms of action of acetyl-L-carnitine are unknown, but current research indicates they may be related to both ALC's cholinergic neural transmission activity and its ability to enhance neuronal metabolism in the mitochondria. Researchers have attributed the cholinergic effects of ALC to blocking of post-synaptic inhibition potentials,[3] while others have suggested it is due to direct stimulation of nerve cells.[4] Human studies have shown ALC has the ability to stabilize cell membrane fluidity via regulation of sphingomyelin levels. ALC can increase ATP levels in humans,[5] thereby preventing excessive neuronal cell death. Acetyl-L-carnitine has also been shown to increase hippocampal binding of glucocorticoids and nerve growth factor.[6]

Clinical Indications

Alzheimer's Dementia

Several studies have demonstrated the effectiveness of ALC in improving cognitive performance in patients with Alzheimer's dementia. These studies were three to six months in length and oral dosages ranged from 1-3 g ALC per day. Results varied, but generally, improvements were noted in spatial learning tasks, timed tasks of attention, discrimination-learning tasks, and tasks of personal recognition.[7-9] At a dosage of 2 g ALC daily, one study demonstrated a decrease in deterioration of reaction time, in addition to improvement in short-term memory related tasks.[7] Studies on the long-term effects of ALC administration are few, but Spagnoli et al demonstrated 1-2 g daily for one year resulted in decreased behavioral deterioration and an improvement in long-term memory performance.[10]

Depression

In cases of major depression it has been demonstrated that the circadian rhythm of cortisol secretion appears to be altered, with depressed patients having an increase in total cortisol secretion.[11] This is probably a result of an increased activation of the hypothalamo-pituitary-adrenocortical (HPA) system. Animal studies indicate ALC administration may have an inhibitory effect on HPA activity, resulting in a reduction of cortisol levels and thereby an improvement in depressive symptoms. No data is available on ALC's effectiveness in modulating HPA activity in humans.[12] In a two-month study of 24 depressed elderly patients it was demonstrated that ALC treatment was highly effective, particularly in patients with more serious depressive symptoms.[13] In another study of 28 elderly patients, Garzya et al demonstrated 500 mg ALC three times per day was effective in reducing symptoms of depression. Patients in both studies were evaluated using the Hamilton Rating Scale for Depression.[14]

HIV Infection

The main immunological abnormality of HIV-infected patients is decreased CD4 cell counts via lymphocyte apoptosis. In a small study of 11 asymptomatic HIV-infected patients, researchers investigated the effects of ALC (3 grams daily for five months) on CD4 and CD8 cell counts, apoptosis, and insulin-like growth factor-1 (IGF-1). Results indicated ALC administration substantially decreased lymphocyte apoptosis, possibly due to a reduction in ceramide generation and/or an increase in serum levels of IGF-1, a factor important to decreased apoptosis.[15]

Diabetic Neuropathy and Cataracts

Approximately one-third of diabetic patients are affected by peripheral neuropathy.[16] Animal studies have demonstrated a link between imbalances in carnitine metabolism and several metabolic and functional abnormalities associated with diabetic polyneuropathy,[17] although currently no human studies of oral ALC and its effects on diabetic neuropathy are available. Human studies using an injectable form of the supplement resulted in decreased neuropathy-associated pain and improved nerve function.[18,19] Patients with diabetes mellitus frequently develop cataracts as a result of the formation of advanced glycation end-products. Studies have shown a dramatic depletion of lenticular L-carnitine and acetyl-L-carnitine in experimentally-induced diabetic rats. An *in vitro* study of the effect of ALC and L-carnitine on calf lens tissue incubated with both of these substances for 15 days found L-carnitine had no effect on glycation, whereas acetyl-L-carnitine decreased crystallin glycation by 42 percent.[20]

Cerebral Ischemia and Reperfusion

The neuro-regenerative effects of ALC have been studied extensively in experimental animal models of post-ischemic cerebral injury. These studies demonstrate ALC administration improves neurological outcome,[21] prevents free radical-mediated protein oxidation, normalizes levels of brain energy metabolites,[22] and decreases lactic acid content during early post-ischemic reperfusion.[23] Rosadini et al investigated the effects of ALC on regional cerebral blood flow in 10 male patients with brain ischemia and observed beneficial effects in 8 of 10 patients one hour after intravenous administration of 1,500 mg ALC.[24]

Cardiovascular Applications

Like L-carnitine, acetyl-L-carnitine enhances fatty acid transport for ATP production in the mitochondria of both skeletal and heart muscle, thereby affording protection from free-radical damage.[25] Animal studies have also shown ALC administration reverses the age-associated decline in cardiolipin content of heart tissue mitochondria.[26]

Ethanol Ingestion

Animal studies have investigated the effects of both carnitine and ALC on hepatic detoxification of ethanol. Cha and Sachan demonstrated that administration of carnitine and ALC retarded ethanol oxidation, but that it required 100 times the concentration of carnitine to equal the maximal inhibition produced by acetyl-L-carnitine. They concluded acetyl-L-carnitine is the mediator of carnitine inhibition of ethanol oxidation and the inhibition is of a competitive nature with NAD^+.[27,28] In a 90-day study of 55 chronic alcoholics, ALC administration improved cognitive performance, suggesting acetyl-L-carnitine may be a useful therapeutic agent for treating cognitive disturbances in these individuals.[29]

Peyronie's Disease

An open trial compared ALC (1 g twice daily) with tamoxifen (20 mg twice daily) in the treatment of Peyronie's disease, a condition of unknown cause in which fibrosis of the cavernous sheaths of the penis leads to contracture, abnormal curvature, and painful erections. After three months, ALC was significantly more effective than tamoxifen in reducing penile curvature and pain, and inhibiting progression of the disease.[30]

Side Effects and Toxicity

ALC is considered safe at therapeutic dosages and without incidence of significant side effects, even with long-term (one year) administration. The most common adverse reactions noted have been agitation, nausea, and vomiting.[7,10]

Dosage

Acetyl-L-carnitine is usually given orally in dosages ranging from 1-3 grams daily. When administered intravenously the dosage is usually 1,500-2,000 mg.

References

1. Parnetti L, Gaiti A, Mecocci P, et al. Pharmacokinetics of IV and oral acetyl-L-carnitine in a multiple dose regimen in patients with senile dementia of Alzheimer type. *Eur J Clin Pharmacol* 1992;42:89-93.
2. Marcus R, Coulston AM. Water-soluble vitamins. In: Hardman JG, Limbird LE, eds. *The Pharmacological Basis of Therapeutics,* 9th ed. New York: McGraw-Hill; 1996.
3. Purpura DP, Girado M, Smith TG, et al. Structure activity determinants of pharmacological effects of amino acids and related compounds on central synapses. *J Neurochem* 1959;3:238.
4. Hayashi K. Action of carnitine on excitable tissues of vertebrates. In: Peeters H, ed. *Protides of the Biological Fluids.* Amsterdam: Elsevier; 1960:371-381.
5. Capecchi PL, Laghi Pasini F, Quartarolo E, Di Perri T. Carnitines increase plasma levels of adenosine and ATP in humans. *Vasc Med* 1997;2:77-81.
6. Perez Polo JR, Werrbach-Perez K, Ramacci MT, et al. Role of nerve growth factors in neurological disease. In: Agnoli A, Cahn J, Lassen N, et al. eds. *Senile dementias, 2nd International Symposium.* Paris: Libby; 1988:15-25.
7. Rai G, Wright G, Scott L, et al. Double-blind, placebo controlled study of acetyl-L-carnitine in patients with Alzheimer's dementia. *Curr Med Res Opin* 1990;11:638-647.
8. Bonavita E. Study of the efficacy and tolerability of L-acetylcarnitine therapy in the senile brain. *Int J Clin Pharm Ther Toxicol* 1986;24:511-516.
9. Sano M, Bell K, Cote L, et al. Double-blind parallel design pilot study of acetyl levocarnitine in patients with Alzheimer's disease. *Arch Neurol* 1992;49:1137-1141.
10. Spagnoli A, Lucca U, Menasce G, et al. Long-term acetyl-L-carnitine treatment in Alzheimer's disease. *Neurology* 1991;41:1726-1732.
11. Gecele M, Francesetti G, Meluzzi A. Acetyl-L-carnitine in aged subjects with major depression: clinical efficacy and effects on the circadian rhythm of cortisol. *Dementia* 1991;2:333-337.
12. Angelucci L, Ramacci MT. Hypothalamo-pituitary-adrenocortical functioning in aging: effects of acetyl-l-carnitine. In: DeSimone C, Martelli EA, eds. *Stress, Immunity and Aging, A Role for Acetyl-L-Carnitine.* Amsterdam: Elsevier; 1989.

13. Tempesta E, Casella L, Pirrongelli C, et al. L-acetylcarnitine in depressed elderly subjects. A cross-over study vs placebo. *Drugs Exp Clin Res* 1987;13:417-423.

14. Garzya G, Corallo D, Fiore A, et al. Evaluation of the effects of L-acetylcarnitine on senile patients suffering from depression. *Drugs Exp Clin Res* 1990;16:101-106.

15. Di Marzio L, Moretti S, D'Alo S, et al. Acetyl-L-carnitine administration increases insulin-like growth factor 1 levels in asymptomatic HIV-1-infected subjects: correlation with its suppressive effect on lymphocyte apoptosis and ceramide generation. *Clin Immunol* 1999;92:103-110.

16. Fedele D, Giugliano D. Peripheral diabetic neuropathy. Current recommendations and future prospects for its prevention and management. *Drugs* 1997;54:414-421.

17. Ido Y, McHowat J, Chang KC, et al. Neural dysfunction and metabolic imbalances in diabetic rats. Prevention by acetyl-L-carnitine. *Diabetes* 1994;43:1469-1477.

18. Onofrj M, Fulgente T, Melchionda D, et al. L-acetylcarnitine as a new therapeutic approach for peripheral neuropathies with pain. *Int J Clin Pharm Res* 1995;15:9-15.

19. Lowitt S, Malone JI, Salem AF, et al. Acetyl-L-carnitine corrects the altered peripheral nerve function of experimental diabetes. *Metabolism* 1995;44:677-680.

20. Swamy-Mruthinti S, Carter AL. Acetyl-L-carnitine decreases glycation of lens proteins: *in vitro* studies. *Exp Eye Res* 1999;69:109-115.

21. Calvani M, Arrigoni-Martelli E. Attenuation by acetyl-L-carnitine of neurological damage and biochemical derangement following brain ischemia and reperfusion. *Int J Tissue React* 1999;21:1-6.

22. Rosenthal RE, Williams R, Bogaert YE, et al. Prevention of postischemic canine neurological injury through potentiation of brain energy metabolism by acetyl-L-carnitine. *Stroke* 1992;23:1317-1318.

23. Aureli T, Miccheli A, Di Cocco ME, et al. Effect of acetyl-L-carnitine on recovery of brain phosphorus metabolites and lactic acid level during reperfusion after cerebral ischemia in the rat – study by 13P- and 1H-NMR spectroscopy. *Brain Res* 1994;18:92-99.

24. Rosadini G, Marenco S, Nobili F, et al. Acute effects of acetyl-L-carnitine on regional and cerebral blood flow in patients with brain ischaemia. *In J Clin Pharmacol Res* 1990;10:123-128.

25. Di Giacomo C, Latteri F, Fichera C, et al. Effect of acetyl-L-carnitine on lipid peroxidation and xanthine oxidase activity in rat skeletal muscle. *Neurochem Res* 1993;18:1157-1162.

26. Paradies G, Petrosillo G, Gadaleta MN, Ruggiero FM. The effect of aging and acetyl-L-carnitine on the pyruvate transport and oxidation in rat heart mitochondria. *FEBS Lett* 1999;454:207-209.

27. Cha YS, Sachan DS. Acetylcarnitine-mediated inhibition of ethanol oxidation in hepatocytes. *Alcohol* 1995;12:289-294.

28. Sachan DS, Cha YS. Acetylcarnitine inhibits alcohol dehydrogenase. *Biochem Biophys Res Commun* 1994;203:1496-1501.

29. Tempesta E, Troncon R, Janiri L, et al. Role of acetyl-L-carnitine in the treatment of cognitive deficit in chronic alcoholism. *Int J Clin Pharm Res* 1990;10:101-107.

30. Biagiotti G, Cavallini G. Acetyl-L-carnitine vs tamoxifen in the oral therapy of Peyronie's disease: a preliminary report. *BJU Int* 2001;88:63-67.

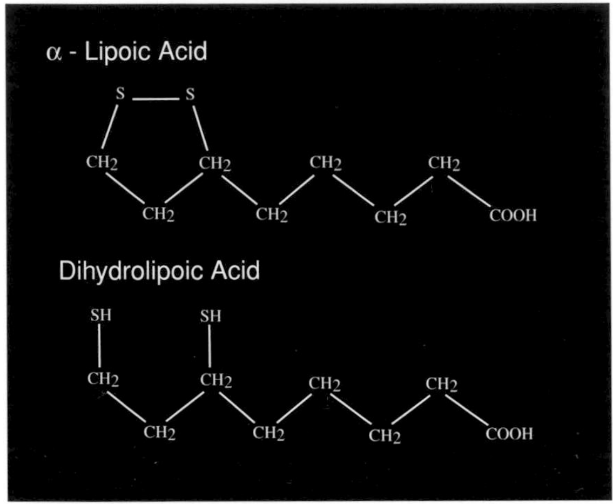

Alpha-lipoic Acid

Introduction

Alpha-lipoic acid (ALA – also known as thioctic acid) was discovered in 1951 as a molecule that assists in acyl-group transfer and as a coenzyme in the Krebs cycle. In the 1980s, the scientific community realized alpha-lipoic acid is a powerful antioxidant. Several qualities distinguish alpha-lipoic acid from other antioxidants: ALA can be synthesized by animals and humans;[1] it neutralizes free radicals in both the fatty and watery regions of cells, in contrast to vitamin C (water soluble) and vitamin E (fat soluble); and, ALA functions as an antioxidant in both its reduced and oxidized forms.[2]

Pharmacokinetics

ALA appears to be readily absorbed from an oral dose and converts easily to its reduced form, dihydrolipoic acid (DHLA), in many tissues of the body.[3] The effects of ALA and DHLA are present both intra- and extracellularly.

Mechanisms of Action

Alpha-lipoic acid is a potent antioxidant in both fat- and water-soluble mediums. Furthermore, its antioxidant activity extends to both its oxidized and reduced forms. DHLA is capable of directly regenerating ascorbic acid from dehydroascorbic acid and indirectly regenerating vitamin E.[4] Researchers have also found ALA increases intracellular glutathione[5] and coenzyme Q_{10}[6] levels.

Alpha-lipoic acid appears capable of chelating certain metals. It forms stable complexes with copper, manganese, and zinc.[7] In animal studies, it has been found to protect against arsenic poisoning,[8] and in both animal and *in vitro* studies ALA reduced cadmium-induced hepatotoxicity.[9] *In vitro*, ALA chelated mercury from renal slices.[10]

Mechanisms that may account for lipoic acid's benefit in preventing diabetic complications include prevention of protein glycosylation,[11] and inhibition of the enzyme aldose reductase, which subsequently inhibits conversion of glucose and galactose to sorbitol.[12,13] Accumulation of sorbitol in the lens of the eye stimulates diabetic cataract formation.

Clinical Indications

Diabetes

Lipoic acid has the potential to prevent diabetes (at least in animals), influence glucose control, and prevent chronic hyperglycemia-associated complications such as neuropathy.

Blood-sugar Management

Acting as a potent antioxidant, DHLA protected rat pancreatic islet cells from destruction by reactive oxygen species.[14] *In vitro*, lipoic acid stimulated glucose uptake by muscle cells in a manner similar to insulin.[15] Type 2 diabetics given 1,000 mg intravenously (IV) experienced a 50-percent improvement in insulin-stimulated glucose uptake.[16] In an uncontrolled pilot study, 20 type 2 diabetics were given 500 mg lipoic acid IV for 10 days. While there was an average of 30-percent increased uptake of glucose, there were no changes in fasting blood sugar or insulin levels.[17]

In a study examining the effect of lipoic acid as a co-factor of the pyruvate dehydrogenase complex on both lean and obese type 2 diabetics, insulin sensitivity, glucose effectiveness, serum lactate levels, and pyruvate levels were tested after oral glucose tolerance load. Treatment with 600 mg alpha-lipoic acid twice daily for four weeks increased insulin sensitivity and prevented serum lactate/pyruvate-induced hyperglycemia.[18]

Diabetic Neuropathy

Alpha-lipoic acid has been studied extensively in Europe for the treatment of diabetic neuropathy.[19-21] Three large-scale, double-blind, placebo-controlled trials have been conducted on the effect of ALA for neuropathy – the Alpha-Lipoic Acid in Diabetic Neuropathy (ALADIN) studies. The first ALADIN Study (n=328 type 2 diabetics) found three weeks of IV ALA at 600 mg daily was superior to placebo for reducing symptoms of neuropathy.[19] ALADIN II examined nerve conduction parameters in a two-year trial and found improvement in some nerve conduction parameters with ALA compared to placebo.[20] In the seven-month, ALADIN III trial, 509 subjects received either 600 mg IV ALA for three weeks, followed by 600 mg orally three times daily for six months; 600 mg IV ALA daily for three weeks, followed by placebo three times daily for six months; or double placebo. While no significant differences were noted in subjective symptom evaluation among the groups, treatment with ALA was associated with improvement in nerve function.[21]

Lipid peroxidation is believed to play a role in the development of neuropathy. In an *in vitro* study, lipoic acid decreased lipid peroxidation of nerve tissue.[22] ALA significantly reduced neuropathy symptoms in a group of 20 diabetics taking 600 mg per day for three months. It should be noted that two other groups of 20 each, one receiving vitamin E, the other selenium, also experienced significant improvement compared to the control group.[23]

ALA may be beneficial for diabetic cardiac autonomic neuropathy (CAN). A four-month trial of oral ALA at a dose of 800 mg daily (n=39) or placebo (n=34) demonstrated a trend toward improvement in measurements of CAN in the treatment group.[24]

Cataracts

The enzyme aldose reductase plays an important role in the development of cataracts in diabetes. Lipoic acid inhibited aldose reductase activity in the rat lens.[12] In another animal study, ALA inhibited cataract formation experimentally induced by buthionine sulfoxamine, an inhibitor of glutathione synthesis. ALA administration maintained levels of glutathione, ascorbic acid, and alpha-tocopherol in the lens.[25]

Glaucoma

Lipoic acid was administered to 75 subjects with open-angle glaucoma at dosages of either 75 mg daily for two months or 150 mg daily for one month. Thirty-one others served as controls and were given only local hypotensive therapy. The greatest improvements in the biochemical parameters of glaucoma and visual function were observed in the group receiving 150 mg lipoic acid.[26]

Ischemia-Reperfusion Injury

After an area of tissue has been deprived of blood for a period of time, such as occurs in the brain after a stroke or in the heart after clot dissolution, reperfusion of the tissues causes a burst of free radical formation. Several animal studies have demonstrated the effectiveness of DHLA in the prevention of reperfusion injury.[27-31]

Animal studies support the efficacy of alpha-lipoic acid in increasing perfusion and reperfusion.[32,33] One week after ischemia injury and reperfusion in rats, the amplitude of sensory action potential and sensory conduction velocity was significantly improved with ALA.[32]

Amanita Mushroom Poisoning

Alpha-lipoic acid infusions were used in the treatment of amanita mushroom poisoning in 75 patients between 1974 and 1978. Normally, up to 50 percent of patients recover without intervention; however, 89 percent (67 of 75) recovered after lipoic acid infusion.[34]

Alcoholic Liver Disease

Although preliminary studies have indicated possible benefit of lipoic acid in the treatment of alcoholic liver disease, the only controlled, double-blind, study found ALA had no significant influence on the course of the disease.[35]

Cognitive Function

Alpha-lipoic acid may have a positive effect on patients with Alzheimer's disease and other types of memory dysfunction secondary to trauma or cerebral vascular accident. By decreasing oxidative damage in the central nervous system, ALA may decrease the severity of central nervous system disorders.[2] Animal studies have shown supplementation with lipoic acid improved long-term memory in aged mice; however, it showed no effect in young mice. This lack of treatment effect in young mice suggests ALA does not improve memory from a general standpoint; instead, it appears ALA compensates for age-related memory deficits.[36] Alpha-lipoic acid also seems to protect brain cells from the damaging effects of some hazardous chemicals. Researchers at the University of Rochester reported neuron damage from excess N-methyl-D-aspartate was prevented by lipoic acid.[37]

Heavy Metal Toxicity

In vitro and animal studies suggest lipoic acid supplementation might be a beneficial component in the treatment of heavy metal toxicity, particularly toxicity involving lead, cadmium, and mercury. ALA appears to improve tissue redox status in metal toxicity, and during chelation with dithiol compounds, including dimercaptosuccinic acid (DMSA).[2,38-40] In addition, anecdotal reports note the use of lipoic acid may improve the clearance of toxic metals.

Other Indications

Other therapeutic uses for ALA or DHLA include protection from radiation injury, prevention of HIV viral replication by inhibition of reverse transcriptase and NF kappa-B (a protein that functions as a nuclear transcription factor and appears to play a role in inflammation),[41,42] and protection from the effects of cigarette smoke.

Side Effects and Toxicity

Alpha-lipoic acid appears to be safe in dosages generally prescribed clinically. The LD_{50} was 400-500 mg/kg after an oral dosage in dogs;[2] however, lower dosages (20 mg/kg) given intraperitoneally to severely thiamine-deficient rats proved fatal. These adverse effects were prevented when thiamine was administered with lipoic acid.[43] There have not been sufficient studies to guarantee safety for its use in pregnancy. Allergic skin conditions are among the few reported side effects of lipoic acid administration in humans.

Dosage

Recommended therapeutic dosage of alpha-lipoic acid is in the range of 300-800 mg taken orally. Larger doses, as much as 600 mg three times daily, have been used in some studies without apparent added benefit.

References

1. Carreau JP. Biosynthesis of lipoic acid via unsaturated fatty acids. *Methods Enzymol* 1979;62:152-158.
2. Packer L, Witt E, Tritschler HJ. Alpha-lipoic acid as a biological antioxidant. *Free Radic Biol Med* 1995;19:227-250.
3. Handelman GJ, Han D, Tritschler H, Packer L. Alpha-lipoic acid reduction by mammalian cells to the dithiol form and release into the culture medium. *Biochem Pharmacol* 1994;47:1725-1730.
4. Scholich H, Murphy ME, Sies H. Antioxidant activity of dihydrolipoate against microsomal lipid peroxidation and its dependence on alpha-tocopherol. *Biochem Biophys Acta* 1989;1001:256-261.
5. Busse E, Zimmer G, Schopohl B, et al. Influence of alpha-lipoic acid on intracellular glutathione *in vitro* and *in vivo*. *Arzneimittel-Forschung* 1992;42:829-831.
6. Kagan V, Serbinova E, Packer L. Antioxidant effects of ubiquinones in microsomes and mitochondria are mediated by tocopherol recycling. *Biochem Biophys Res Comm* 1990;169:851-857.
7. Sigel H, Prijs B, McCormick DB, Shih JCH. Stability and structure of binary and ternary complexes of alpha-lipoate and lipoate derivatives with $Mn2^+$, $Cu2^+$, and $Zn2^+$ in solution. *Arch Biochem Biophys* 1978;187:208-214.
8. Grunert RR. The effect of DL alpha-lipoic acid on heavy-metal intoxication in mice and dogs. *Arch Biochem Biophys* 1960;86:190-194.
9. Muller L, Menzel H. Studies on the efficacy of lipoate and dihydrolipoate in the alteration of cadmium toxicity in isolated hepatocytes. *Biochem Biophys Acta* 1990;1052:386-391.
10. Keith RL, Setiarahardjo I, Fernando Q, et al. Utilization of renal slices to evaluate the efficacy of chelating agents for removing mercury from the kidney. *Toxicology* 1997;116:67-75.
11. Schleicher ED, Wagner E, Nerlich AG. Increased accumulation of the glycoxidation product N(epsilon)-(carboxymethyl)lysine in human tissues in diabetes and aging. *J Clin Invest* 1997;99:457-468.
12. Ou P, Nourooz-Zadeh J, Tritschler HJ, Wolff S. Activation of aldose reductase in rat lens and metal-ion chelation by aldose reductase inhibitors and lipoic acid. *Free Radic Res* 1996;25:337-346.
13. Kishi Y, Schmelzer JD, Yao JK, et al. Alpha-lipoic acid: effect on glucose uptake, sorbitol pathway, and energy metabolism in experimental diabetic neuropathy. *Diabetes* 1999;48;2045-2051.
14. Heller B, Burkhart V, Lampeter E, Kolb H. Antioxidant therapy for the prevention of type 1 diabetes. *Adv Pharm* 1997;38:629-638.
15. Estrada DE, Ewart HS, Tsakiridis T, et al. Stimulation of glucose uptake by the natural coenzyme alpha-lipoic acid/thioctic acid: participation of elements of the insulin signaling pathway. *Diabetes* 1996;45:1798-1804.
16. Jacob S, Henriksen EJ, Schiemann AL, et al. Enhancement of glucose disposal in patients with type 2 diabetes by alpha-lipoic acid. *Arzneimittel-Forschung* 1995;45:872-874.
17. Jacob S, Henriksen EJ, Tritschler HJ, et al. Improvement of insulin-stimulated glucose-disposal in type 2 diabetes after repeated parenteral administration of thioctic acid. *Exp Clin Endocrinol Diabetes* 1996;104:284-288.
18. Konrad T, Vicini P, Kusterer K, et al. Alpha-lipoic acid treatment decreases serum lactate and pyruvate concentrations and improves glucose effectiveness in lean and obese patients with type 2 diabetes. *Diabetic Care* 1999;22:280-287.
19. Ziegler D, Hanefeld M, Ruhnau KJ, et al. Treatment of symptomatic diabetic peripheral neuropathy with the anti-oxidant alpha-lipoic acid. A 3-week multicentre randomized controlled trial (ALADIN Study). *Diabetologia* 1995;38:1425-1433.
20. Reljanovic M, Reichel G, Rett K, et al. Treatment of diabetic polyneuropathy with the antioxidant thioctic acid (alpha-lipoic acid): a two year multicenter randomized double-blind placebo-controlled trial (ALADIN II). Alpha Lipoic Acid In diabetic Neuropathy. *Free Radic Res* 1999;31:171-179.
21. Ziegler D, Hanefeld M, Ruhnau KJ, et al. Treatment of symptomatic diabetic polyneuropathy with the antioxidant alpha-lipoic acid: a 7-month multicenter randomized controlled trial (ALADIN III Study). ALADIN III Study Group. Alpha-Lipoic Acid in Diabetic Neuropathy. *Diabetes Care* 1999;22:1296-1301.

22. Nickander KK, McPhee BR, Low PA, Tritschler H. Alpha-lipoic acid: antioxidant potency against lipid peroxidation of neural tissues *in vitro* and implications for diabetic neuropathy. *Free Radic Biol Med* 1996;21:631-639.

23. Kahler W, Kuklinski B, Ruhlmann C, Plotz C. Diabetes mellitus: a free radical-associated disease. Results of adjuvant antioxidant supplementation. *Z Gesamte Inn Med* 1993;48:223-232. [Article in German]

24. Ziegler D, Schatz H, Contrad F, et al. Effects of treatment with the antioxidant alpha-lipoic acid on cardiac autonomic neuropathy in NIDDM patients. A 4-month randomized controlled multicenter trial (DEKAN Study). Deutsche Kardiale Autonome Neuropathie. *Diabetes Care* 1997;20:369-373.

25. Maitra, I., Serbinova E, Trischler H, Packer L. Alpha-lipoic acid prevents buthionine sulfoximine induced cataract formation in newborn rats. *Free Rad Biol Med* 1995;18:823-829.

26. Filina AA, Davydova NG, Endrikhovskii SN, et al. Lipoic acid as a means of metabolic therapy of open-angle glaucoma. *Vestn Oftalmol* 1995;111:6-8. [Article in Russian]

27. Scheer B, Zimmer G. Dihydrolipoic acid prevents hypoxic/reoxygenation and peroxidative damage in rat mitochondria. *Arch Biochem Biophys* 1993;302:385-390.

28. Assadnazari H, Zimmer G, Freisleben HJ, et al. Cardioprotective efficiency of dihydrolipoic acid in working rat hearts during hypoxia and reoxygenation. 31P nuclear magnetic resonance investigations. *Arzneimittel-Forschung* 1993;43:425-432.

29. Prehn JH, Karkoutly C, Nuglisch J, et al. Dihydrolipoate reduces neuronal injury after cerebral ischemia. *J Cereb Blood Flow Metab* 1992;12:78-87.

30. Panigrahi M, Sadguna Y, Shivakumar BR, et al. Alpha-lipoic acid protects against reperfusion injury following cerebral ischemia in rats. *Brain Res* 1996;717:184-188.

31. Cao X, Phillis JW. The free radical scavenger, alpha-lipoic acid, protects against cerebral ischemia-reperfusion injury in gerbils. *Free Rad Res* 1995;23:365-370.

32. Mitsui Y, Schmelzer JD, Zollman PJ, et al. Alpha-lipoic acid provides neuroprotection from ischemia-reperfusion injury of peripheral nerve. *J Neurol Sci* 1999;163:11-16.

33. Haramaki N, Assadnazari H, Zimmer G, et al. The influence of vitamin E and dihydrolipoic acid on cardiac energy and glutathione status under hypoxia-reoxygenation. *Biochem Mol Biol Int* 1995;37:591-597.

34. Bartter FC, Berkson BM, Gallelli J, et al. Thioctic acid in the treatment of poisoning with alpha-amanitin. In: Faulstich H, Kommerell B, Wieland T, eds. *Amanita Toxins and Poisoning*. Badan-Baden: Verlg Gerhard Witzstrock; 1980: 197-202.

35. Marshall AW, Graul RS, Morgan MY, Sherlock S. Treatment of alcohol-related liver disease with thioctic acid: A six month randomised double-blind trial. *Gut* 1982;23:1088-1093.

36. Stoll S, Hartmann H, Cohen SA, Muller WE. The potent free radical scavenger alpha-lipoic acid improves memory in aged mice: putative relationship to NMDA receptor deficits. *Pharmacol Biochem Behav* 1993;46:799-805.

37. Greenamyre JT, Garcia-Osuna M, Greene JG. The endogenous cofactors, thioctic acid and dihydrolipoic acid, are neuroprotective against NMDA and malonic acid lesions of striatum. *Neurosci Lett* 1994;171:17-20.

38. Gurer H, Ozgunes H, Oztezcan S, Ercal N. Antioxidant role of alpha-lipoic acid in lead toxicity. *Free Radic Biol Med* 1999;27:75-81.

39. Pande M, Flora SJ. Lead induced oxidative damage and its response to combined administration of alpha-lipoic acid and succimers in rats. *Toxicology* 2002;177:187-196.

40. Anuradha B, Varalakshmi P. Protective role of DL-alpha-lipoic acid against mercury-induced neural lipid peroxidation. *Pharmacol Res* 1999;39:67-80.

41. Baur A, Harrer T, Peukert M, et al. Alpha-lipoic acid is an effective inhibitor of human immuno-deficiency virus (HIV-1) replication. *Klin Wochenschr* 1991;69:722-724.

42. Suzuki YJ, Aggarwal BB, Packer L. Alpha-lipoic acid is a potent inhibitor of NF-kappa B activation in human T-cells. *Biochem Biophys Res Comm* 1992;189:1709-1715.

43. Gal EM. Reversal of selective toxicity of alpha-lipoic acid by thiamine in thiamine-deficient rats. *Nature* 1965;205:535.

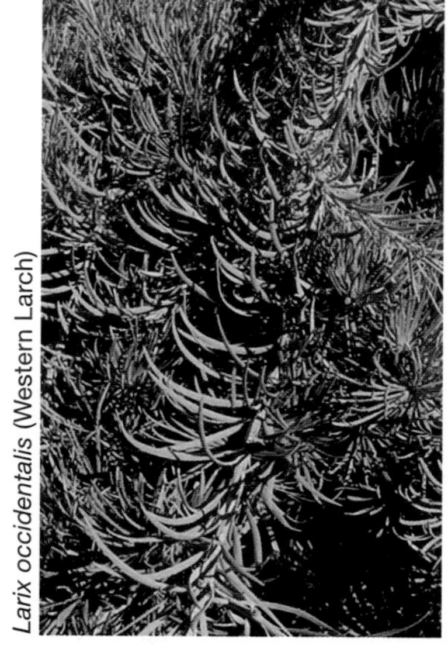
Larix occidentalis (Western Larch)

Larch Arabinogalactan

Description

Larch arabinogalactan is a polysaccharide powder derived from the wood of the larch tree (Larix species) and comprised of approximately 98 percent arabinogalactan. Arabinogalactans are found in a variety of plants but are more abundant in the Larix genus, primarily *Larix occidentalis* (Western Larch). The Western Larch is unique among pines in that it loses its needles in the fall. Western Larch is also known as Mountain Larch or Western Tamarack and is native to the Pacific and Inland Northwest United States as well as parts of British Columbia, Canada.[1] Larch arabinogalactan is approved by the U.S. Food and Drug Administration (FDA) as a source of dietary fiber, but also has potential therapeutic benefits as an immune stimulating agent and cancer protocol adjunct.

Pharmaceutical-grade larch arabinogalactan is a fine, dry, off-white powder with a slightly sweet taste and mild pine-like odor. It dissolves in water or juice and is low in viscosity; therefore easy to administer, even to children. It is composed of galactose and arabinose molecules in a 6:1 ratio, with a small amount of glucuronic acid. Arabinogalactans are long, densely branched polysaccharides of varying molecular weights (10,000-120,000).[2]

Pharmacokinetics

Human studies on the pharmacokinetics of larch arabinogalactan are few and the amount absorbed following an oral dose remains unclear. Animal studies indicate that intravenous injection of purified larch arabinogalactan results in 52.5 percent of the dose being present in the liver and 30 percent in the urine 90 minutes after dosing. Hepatic clearance occurred with a half-life of 3.42 days.[3] Non-absorbed larch arabinogalactan is actively fermented by intestinal microflora and is particularly effective at increasing beneficial anaerobes such as Bifidobacteria and Lactobacillus.[4]

Mechanism of Action

Lower molecular weight polysaccharides typically exhibit an anti-inflammatory, anti-complement, anti-allergy effect, while those of higher weights stimulate natural killer (NK) cell cytotoxicity and reticuloendothelial cells. In the case of larch arabinogalactan, molecular weights of the two major fractions are 16,000 and 100,000, perhaps accounting for its wide range of therapeutic properties.[2] The enhancement of NK cell activity appears to be mediated by a network of cytokines rather than by direct stimulation.[5] Larch arabinogalactan also stimulates the immune system by activating phagocytosis and potentiating the effect of the reticuloendothelial system.[1] One aspect of larch arabinogalactan's potential to enhance colon health is via its ability to increase concentrations of butyrate.[6]

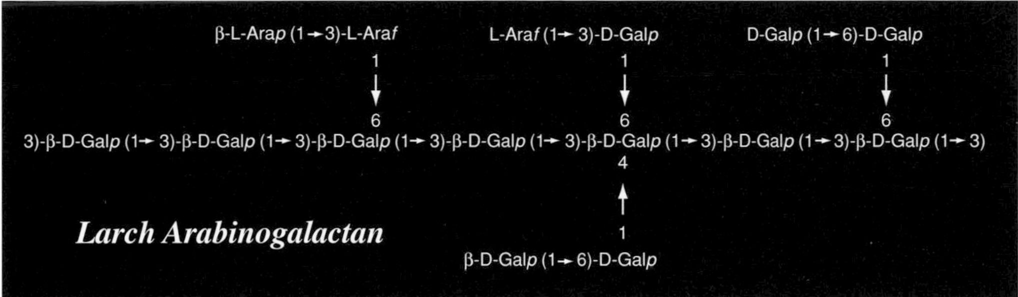

Larch Arabinogalactan

Clinical Indications

Dietary Fiber

Larch arabinogalactan is an excellent source of dietary fiber that is able to increase short-chain fatty acid production (primarily butyrate) via its vigorous fermentation by intestinal microflora.[2] It is well documented that butyrate is essential for proper colon health, as it is the preferred substrate for energy generation by colonic epithelial cells.[7] Butyrate also acts as a protectant for the intestinal mucosa against disease and cancer-promoting agents.[6] Arabinogalactan added to human fecal homogenates has also been shown to decrease ammonia generation, and therefore may be of clinical value in the treatment of portal-systemic encephalopathy, a disease characterized by ammonia build-up in the liver.[4] Larch arabinogalactan given to human subjects increased levels of beneficial intestinal anaerobes, particularly *Bifidobacterium longum*, via their fermentation specificity for arabinogalactan compared to other complex carbohydrates.[8,9]

Cancer Adjunct

Larch arabinogalactan may be an effective adjunct to cancer therapies due to its ability to stimulate NK cell cytotoxicity, stimulate the immune system, and block metastasis of tumor cells to the liver.[2] Tumor metastasis to the liver is more common than to other organ sites, probably due to tumor cell specificity for lectin-like receptor sites found in liver parenchyma. Animal studies have demonstrated arabinogalactan's ability to inhibit or block lectin receptor sites, thereby reducing tumor cell colonization of the liver and also increasing survival time of the subjects.[10-12] Pretreatment with larch arabinogalactan was found to stimulate NK cell cytotoxicity via potentiation of the cytokine network, primarily via an increase in the release of gamma interferon.[5]

Pediatric Otitis Media

Recurrent otitis media is common in pediatric populations and it appears that improving immune system function might lead to a decrease in both frequency and severity of this condition. Research has demonstrated larch and other arabinogalactans to be capable of enhancing the immune response to bacterial infection via stimulation of phagocytosis, competitive binding of bacterial fimbriae, or bacterial opsonization. This was found to be particularly true for infection by gram negative organisms such as *Escherichia coli* and Klebsiella species.[2,13] In addition, D'Adamo reports a decrease in occurrence and severity of otitis media in pediatric patients supplemented prophylactically with larch arabinogalactan.[2] Larch arabinogalactan's mild taste and excellent solubility in water and juice make it a relatively easy therapeutic tool to employ in pediatric populations.

Miscellaneous Chronic Diseases

A number of chronic diseases are characterized by decreased NK cell activity, including chronic fatigue syndrome,[14] viral hepatitis,[15,16] HIV/AIDS,[2] and autoimmune diseases such as multiple sclerosis.[17] Stimulation of NK cell activity by larch arabinogalactan has been associated with recovery in certain cases of chronic fatigue syndrome.[18] Viral hepatitis (hepatitis B and C) is also characterized by a decrease in NK cell cytotoxicity;[15,16] therefore, these patients may benefit from its stimulation by larch arabinogalactan. In the case of multiple sclerosis, a small two-year study of patients with the relapsing/remitting type concluded that disease severity was correlated with NK cell functional activity, supporting the hypothesis that NK cells play a role in the immunopathogenesis of this disease.[17] Consequently, stimulation of NK cell cytotoxicity might be of clinical benefit to these patients. Patients with HIV/AIDS develop low CD4 cell counts and often are plagued by opportunistic infections. By virtue of its immune-stimulating properties, larch arabinogalactan has been shown to effect a slight increase in CD4 cell counts, in addition to decreasing susceptibility to opportunistic pathogens.[2]

Side Effects and Toxicity

Larch arabinogalactan is a safe and effective immune-stimulating phytochemical. It is FDA-approved for use as a dietary fiber and in food applications. Both acute and long-term toxicity studies in rats and mice reveal no evidence of toxicity.[19] Human consumption is usually without side effects; however, a small percentage of people (<3%) experienced bloating and flatulence, possibly due to the vigorous fermentation of the arabinogalactan by intestinal microflora.[2] Because of its excellent safety profile and solubility in water and juice, larch arabinogalactan is considered a safe, effective immune-stimulating agent for pediatric use.

Dosage

Larch arabinogalactan in powder form is typically dosed in teaspoons or tablespoons at a concentration of approximately 4-5 grams per tablespoon. The typical adult dosage is one to three tablespoons per day in divided doses; the pediatric dose is one to three teaspoons per day. The powder is usually mixed with water or juice but can be added to food if desired.

References

1. Odonmazig P, Ebringerova A, Machova E, Alfoldi J. Structural and molecular properties of the arabinogalactan isolated from Mongolian larchwood (*Larix dahurica L.*). *Carbohydr Res* 1994;252:317-324.
2. D'Adamo P. Larch arabinogalactan. *J Naturopath Med* 1996;6:33-37.
3. Groman EV, Enriquez PM, Jung C, Josephson L. Arabinogalactan for hepatic drug delivery. *Bioconjug Chem* 1994;5:547-556.
4. Vince AJ, McNeil NI, Wager JD, Wrong OM. The effect of lactulose, pectin, arabinogalactan, and cellulose on the production of organic acids and metabolism of ammonia by intestinal bacteria in a faecal incubation system. *Br J Nutr* 1990;63:17-26.
5. Hauer J, Anderer FA. Mechanism of stimulation of human natural killer cytotoxicity by arabinogalactan from *Larix occidentalis*. *Cancer Immunol Immunother* 1993;36:237-244.
6. Tsao D, Shi Z, Wong A, Kim YS. Effect of sodium butyrate on carcinoembryonic antigen production by human colonic adenocarcinoma cells in culture. *Cancer Res* 1983;43:1217-1222.
7. Roediger WE. Utilization of nutrients by isolated epithelial cells of the rat colon. *Gastroenterology* 1989;83:424-429.
8. Crociani F, Alessandrini A, Mucci MM, Biavati B. Degradation of complex carbohydrates by *Bifidobacterium spp. Int J Food Microbiol* 1994;24:199-210.
9. Slavin J, Feirtag J, Robinson R, Causey J. Physiological effects of arabinogalactan (AG) in human subjects. Unpublished research.
10. Hagmar B, Ryd W, Skomedal H. Arabinogalactan blockade of experimental metastases to liver by murine hepatoma. *Invasion Metastasis* 1991;11:348-355.
11. Beuth J, Ko HL, Oette K, et al. Inhibition of liver metastasis in mice by blocking hepatocyte lectins with arabinogalactan infusions and D-galactose. *J Cancer Res Clin Oncol* 1987;113:51-55.
12. Beuth J, Ko HL, Schirrmacher V, et al. Inhibition of liver tumor cell colonization in two animal tumor models by lectin blocking with D-galactose or arabinogalactan. *Clin Exp Metastasis* 1988;6:115-120.

13. Reith FJ. Pharmaceuticals containing lactic acid derivatives and Echinacea. Bundesrepublik Deutsches Patentamt 27 21 014 11/16/78. [German Patent]
14. Levine PH, Whiteside TL, Friberg D, et al. Dysfunction of natural killer activity in a family with chronic fatigue syndrome. *Clin Immunol Immunopathol* 1998;88:96-104.
15. Corado J, Toro F, Rivera H, et al. Impairment of natural killer (NK) cytotoxicity activity in hepatitis C virus (HCV) infection. *Clin Exp Immunol* 1997;109:451-457.
16. Machado IV, Deibis L, Risquez E, et al. Immunoclinical, molecular and immunopathologic approach to chronic viral hepatitis. Therapeutic considerations. *GEN* 1994;48:124-132. [Article in Spanish]
17. Kastrukoff LF, Morgan NG, Zecchini D, et al. A role for natural killer cells in the immunopathogenesis of multiple sclerosis. *J Neuroimmunol* 1998;86:123-133.
18. Uchida A. Therapy of chronic fatigue syndrome. *Nippon Rinsho* 1992;50:2679-2683.
19. Wagner H. Low molecular weight polysaccharides from composite plants containing arabinogalactan, arabinoglucan, and arabinoxylan. Bundesrepublik Deutsches Patentamt DE 3042491 7/15/82. [German Patent]

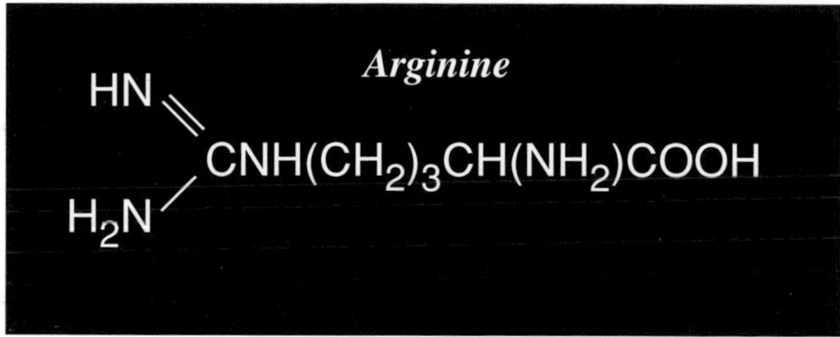

Arginine

Introduction

Arginine is a semi-essential amino acid involved in multiple areas of human physiology and metabolism. It is not considered essential because humans can synthesize it *de novo* from glutamine, glutamate, and proline. However, dietary intake remains the primary determinant of plasma arginine levels, since the rate of arginine biosynthesis does not increase to compensate for depletion or inadequate supply.[1,2]

Arginine contains four nitrogen atoms per molecule, making it the most abundant nitrogen carrier in humans and animals. Although it is not a major inter-organ shuttle of nitrogen, arginine nevertheless plays an important role in nitrogen metabolism as an intermediate in the urea cycle. It is essential for ammonia detoxification.[3]

Biochemistry and Pharmacokinetics

Arginine is synthesized in mammals from glutamine via pyrroline 5-carboxylate (P5C) synthetase and proline oxidase in a multi-step metabolic conversion.[4] In adults, most endogenous arginine is derived from citrulline, a by-product of glutamine metabolism in the gut or liver. Citrulline is released into the circulation and taken up primarily by the kidney for conversion into arginine.[5]

Supplemental arginine in enteral feeding is readily absorbed.[6] About half of ingested arginine is rapidly converted in the body to ornithine, primarily by the enzyme arginase.[7] Ornithine, in turn, can be metabolized to glutamate and proline, or through the enzyme ornithine decarboxylase into the polyamine pathway for degradation into compounds such as putrescine and other polyamines.

In addition to the above-mentioned metabolic activity, arginine is a precursor for the synthesis of proteins, as well as nitric oxide, urea, creatine, and agmatine.[8] Arginine that is not metabolized by arginase to ornithine is processed by one of four other enzymes: nitric oxide synthase (to become nitric oxide); arginine:glycine amidinotransferase (to become creatine); arginine decarboxylase (to become agmatine); or arginyl-tRNA synthetase (to become arginyl-tRNA, a precursor to protein synthesis). Arginine is also an allosteric activator of N-acetylglutamate synthase, which synthesizes N-acetylglutamate from glutamate and acetyl-CoA.[9]

Mechanisms of Action

Arginine has significant effects on endocrine function – particularly adrenal and pituitary secretion – in humans and animals. Arginine administration has long been known to stimulate the release of catecholamines,[10] insulin and glucagon,[11] prolactin,[12] and growth hormone (GH).[13,14] Little is known, however, about the exact mechanism by which arginine exerts these effects.

Arginine is the biologic precursor of nitric oxide (NO), an endogenous messenger molecule involved in a variety of endothelium-dependent physiological effects in the cardiovascular system.[15] As the precursor to nitric oxide, many of arginine's clinical effects are thought to be mediated by its effects on endothelial-derived relaxing factor. An immense quantity of research has explored the biologic roles and properties of nitric oxide,[16,17] which appear to be of critical importance in maintenance of normal blood pressure,[18] myocardial function,[19] inflammatory response,[20] apoptosis,[21] and protection against oxidative damage.[22] Arginine is also a critical component of vasopressin (anti-diuretic hormone).

Arginine is a potent immunomodulator. Supplemental arginine appears to up-regulate immune function and reduces the incidence of postoperative infection. A significant decrease in cell adhesion molecule and pro-inflammatory cytokine levels has also been observed. Arginine can positively influence aspects of immunity under some circumstances and influence cytokine balance. Arginine supplementation (30 g/day for 3 days) has been shown to significantly enhance natural killer (NK) cell activity, lymphokine-activated killer cell cytotoxicity, and lymphocyte mitogenic reactivity in patients with locally advanced breast cancer.[23,24]

Clinical Indications

Human Immunodeficiency Virus (HIV) and Acquired Immunodeficiency Syndrome (AIDS)

Arginine may be of benefit in individuals with HIV/AIDS. In a small pilot study of arginine supplementation in persons with HIV, 11 individuals were given 19.6 g/day arginine or placebo for 14 days. Natural killer cell cytotoxicity increased 18.9 lytic units, compared to +0.3 lytic units with placebo. This was not statistically significant, most likely due to the small number of patients.[25]

The combination of glutamine, arginine, and hydroxymethylbutyrate (HMB) may prevent loss of lean body mass in individuals with AIDS cachexia. In a double-blind trial, AIDS patients with documented weight loss of at least five percent in the previous three months received either placebo or a combination of 3 g HMB, 14 g L-glutamine, and 14 g arginine given in two divided doses daily for eight weeks. At eight weeks, subjects consuming the mixture gained 3.0 +/- 0.5 kg of body weight, while those supplemented with placebo gained only 0.37 +/- 0.84 kg (p = 0.009). The weight gain in the supplemented group was predominately lean muscle mass, while the placebo group lost lean mass.[26]

A six-month, randomized, double-blind trial of an arginine/essential fatty acid combination was undertaken in patients with HIV.[27] All patients received a daily oral nutritional supplement (606 kcal supplemented with vitamins, trace elements, and minerals). In addition, half of the patients were randomized to receive 7.4 g arginine plus 1.7 g omega-3 fatty acids per day. Body weight increased similarly in both groups, and there was no change in immunological parameters. Clinical trials evaluating the effect of arginine as monotherapy for AIDS patients have yet to be conducted.

Angina Pectoris

Arginine supplementation has been effective in the treatment of angina in some, but not all, clinical trials. In an uncontrolled trial, seven of ten people with intractable angina improved dramatically after taking 9 grams arginine per day for three months.[28] A significant decrease in cell adhesion molecule and pro-inflammatory cytokine levels was also observed. A double-blind trial in 22 patients with stable angina and healed myocardial infarction showed oral supplementation with 6 g arginine per day for three days increased exercise capacity.[29]

In men with stable angina, two-week oral supplementation with arginine (15 g/day) was not associated with improvement in endothelium-dependent vasodilation, oxidative stress, or exercise performance.[30] In patients with coronary artery disease, oral supplementation of arginine (6 g/day for 3 days) did not affect exercise-induced changes in QT interval duration, QT dispersion, or the magnitude of ST segment depression;[31] however, it did significantly increase exercise tolerance. The therapeutic effect of arginine in patients with microvascular angina is considered to be the result of improved endothelium-dependent coronary vasodilation.[32]

Athletic Performance

At high doses (approximately 250 mg/kg body weight), arginine aspartate has increased GH secretion,[33] an effect of interest to body builders wishing to take advantage of the anabolic properties of the hormone.[34] In a controlled clinical trial, arginine and ornithine (500 mg of each, twice per day, five times per week) produced a significant decrease in body fat when combined with exercise.[35] Acute, low-dose arginine (5 grams taken 30 minutes before exercise) did not increase GH secretion, and may have impaired release of GH in young adults.[36] Longer-term, low-dose supplementation of arginine and ornithine (1 g each, five days per week for five weeks) had higher gains in strength and enhancement of lean body mass when compared with controls receiving vitamin C and calcium.[37]

Growth hormone has been observed to be lower in older males than young men; however, data suggest oral arginine/lysine (3 g each per day) is not a practical means of enhancing long-term GH secretion in older men.[38]

Burns and Trauma

Burn injuries significantly increase arginine oxidation and fluctuations in arginine reserves. Total parenteral nutrition (TPN) increases conversion of arginine to ornithine and proportionally increases irreversible arginine oxidation. Elevated arginine oxidation, coupled with limited *de novo* synthesis from its immediate precursors, makes arginine conditionally essential in severely burned patients receiving TPN.[39] Several trials have demonstrated reduced length of hospital stay, fewer acquired infections, and improved immune function among burn patients[40] and trauma patients[41] supplemented with various combinations of fish or canola oil, nucleotides, and arginine.

Cancer

Animal research has shown large doses of arginine may interfere with tumor induction.[42] Short-term arginine supplementation may assist in maintenance of immune function during chemotherapy. Arginine supplementation (30 g/day for three days) reduced chemotherapy-induced suppression of natural killer (NK), lymphokine-activated killer cell cytotoxicity, and lymphocyte mitogenic reactivity in patients with locally advanced breast cancer.[23,24] In another study,[43] arginine supplementation (30 g/day for three days prior to surgery) significantly enhanced the activity of tumor-infiltrating lymphocytes in human colorectal cancers *in vivo*. Arginine, RNA, and fish oil have been combined to improve immune function in cancer patients.[44-46]

However, arginine has also promoted cancer growth in animal and human research.[47] Polyamines act as growth factors for cancers. In several types of cancer, drugs are being investigated to inhibit ornithine decarboxylase (ODC), and hence inhibit polyamine formation. The possibility of arginine stimulating polyamine formation might be a concern in chronic administration, since both arginase and ODC appear to be up-regulated in some cancers.

Congestive Heart Failure (CHF)

Patients with CHF have reduced peripheral blood flow at rest, during exercise, and in response to endothelium-dependent vasodilators. Nitric oxide formed from arginine metabolism in endothelial cells contributes to regulation of blood flow under these conditions. A randomized, double-blind trial[48] found six weeks of oral arginine supplementation (5.6-12.6 g/d) significantly improved blood flow, arterial compliance, and functional status compared to placebo. Another double-blind trial found arginine supplementation (5 grams three times per day) improved renal function in people with CHF.[49]

Coronary Heart Disease and Atherosclerosis

Impairment of the NO synthase pathway may be one of the earliest events in atherogenesis.[50] Animal studies have suggested anti-atherogenic effects of supplemental arginine, including improved endothelium-dependent vasodilation, inhibition of plaque formation,[51] and decreased thickening of the aortic tunica intima.[52] In humans, arginine supplementation normalized platelet aggregation in hypercholesterolemic adults.[53] However, increased dietary arginine has not been consistently associated with decreased mortality from coronary heart disease,[54] and arginine supplementation (a single intravenous dose of 16 g) failed to affect maximal working capacity, indices of myocardial ischemia, or blood flow in hypercholesterolemic patients.[55]

Diabetes

Endothelium-dependent relaxation is impaired in humans with both type 1 and type 2 diabetes mellitus (DM), as well as in animal models of diabetes. Endothelial nitric oxide deficiency is one likely explanation.[56] Diabetes is associated with reduced plasma levels of arginine,[57] and evidence suggests arginine supplementation may be an effective way to improve endothelial function in individuals with diabetes. An intravenous (IV) bolus of 3-5 g arginine reduced blood pressure and platelet aggregation in patients with type 1 diabetes.[58] Low-dose IV arginine improved insulin sensitivity in obese patients and type 2 DM patients as well as in healthy subjects.[59] Arginine may also counteract lipid peroxidation and thereby reduce microangiopathic long-term complications of DM.[60]

A double-blind trial found oral arginine supplementation (3 g three times per day) significantly improved, but did not completely normalize, peripheral and hepatic insulin sensitivity in patients with type 2 diabetes.[61] In young patients with type 1 DM, however, oral arginine (7 g twice per day for six weeks) failed to improve endothelial function.[62]

Erectile Dysfunction (ED)

In a small, uncontrolled trial, men with ED were given 2.8 g arginine per day for two weeks. Forty percent of the men in the treatment group experienced improvement, compared to none in the placebo group.[63] In a larger double-blind trial, men with ED were given 1,670 mg of arginine per day or a matching placebo for six weeks.[64] Arginine supplementation was effective at improving ED in men with abnormal nitric oxide metabolism. However, another double-blind trial of arginine for ED (500 mg three times per day for 17 days) found the amino acid no more effective than placebo.[65] Further double-blind research in large groups is needed to confirm the efficacy of arginine for ED.

Gastritis and Ulcer

Preliminary evidence suggests arginine accelerates ulcer healing due to its hyperemic, angiogenic, and growth-promoting actions, possibly involving NO, gastrin, and polyamines.[66,67] No clinical trials have yet explored the safety or efficacy of arginine supplementation as a treatment for gastritis or peptic ulcer in humans.

Gastroesophageal Reflux (GERD) and Sphincter Motility Disorders

A small, double-blind trial[68] found oral arginine supplementation significantly decreased the frequency and intensity of chest pain attacks, as well as the number of nitroglycerin tablets taken for analgesia, in patients with esophageal motility disorders. However, in another study,[69] arginine infusions (500 mg/kg body weight/120 min) failed to affect lower esophageal sphincter motility. No studies have yet explored the efficacy of arginine supplements for GERD.

Growth Hormone Deficiency

In rats, NO stimulates secretion of GH-releasing hormone (GHRH) and thereby increases secretion of GH. However, GHRH then increases production of NO in somatotroph cells, which subsequently inhibits GH secretion. In humans, arginine stimulates release of GH from the pituitary gland in some populations, but the mechanism is not well understood. Most studies suggest inhibition of somatostatin secretion is responsible for the effect.[70]

Hypertension

Administration of arginine prevented hypertension in salt-sensitive rats, but not in spontaneously hypertensive rats.[71] If arginine was provided early, hypertension and renal failure could be prevented. In healthy human subjects, IV administration of arginine had vasodilatory and antihypertensive effects.[72] In a small, controlled trial, hypertensive patients refractory to enalapril and hydrochlorothiazide responded favorably to the addition of oral arginine (2 grams three times per day).[73] Small, preliminary trials have found oral[74] and IV[75] arginine significantly lowers blood pressure in healthy volunteers.

Intravenous infusion of arginine (15 mg/kg body weight/min for 35 min) improved pulmonary vascular resistance index and cardiac output in infants with pulmonary hypertension.[76]

Preeclampsia

Endothelial dysfunction appears to be involved in the pathogenesis of preeclampsia.[77] In an animal model of experimental preeclampsia, IV administration of arginine (0.16 g/kg body weight/day) from gestational day 10 until term reversed hypertension, intrauterine growth retardation, proteinuria, and renal injury.[78] Intravenous infusion of arginine (30 g) in preeclamptic women has reportedly increased systemic NO production and reduced blood pressure.[79] Clinical trials are needed to validate the role of supplemental arginine in prevention and treatment of preeclampsia.

Infertility, Female

Supplementation with oral arginine (16 grams per day) in poor responders to *in vitro* fertilization improved ovarian response, endometrial receptivity and pregnancy rate in one study.[80]

Infertility, Male

Arginine is required for normal spermatogenesis. Over 50 years ago, researchers found that feeding an arginine-deficient diet to adult men for nine days decreased sperm counts by approximately 90 percent and increased the percentage of nonmotile sperm approximately 10-fold.[81] Oral administration of 500 mg arginine-HCl per day to infertile men for 6-8 weeks markedly increased sperm counts and motility in a majority of patients, and resulted in successful pregnancies.[82] Similar effects on oligospermia and conception rates have been reported in other preliminary trials.[83-86] However, when baseline sperm counts have been less than 10 million/ml, arginine supplementation produced little or no improvement.[87,88]

Intermittent Claudication

Intravenous arginine injections significantly improved symptoms of intermittent claudication in one double-blind trial. Eight grams of arginine, infused twice daily for three weeks, improved pain-free walking distance by 230 +/- 63 percent and the absolute walking distance by 155 +/- 48 percent (each $p < 0.05$) compared to no improvement with placebo.[89] To date, this is the only trial of arginine for intermittent claudication.

Interstitial Cystitis (IC)

In an uncontrolled trial,[90] 10 patients with IC took 1.5 g arginine orally daily for six months. Supplementation resulted in a significant decrease in urinary voiding discomfort, lower abdominal pain, and vaginal/urethral pain. Urinary frequency during the day and night also significantly decreased. In a five-week uncontrolled trial, however, arginine supplementation was not effective, even at higher doses of 3-10 grams per day.[91] In a randomized, double-blind trial of arginine for IC, patients took 1.5 g arginine per day for three months. Twenty-nine percent of patients in the arginine group and eight percent in the placebo group had clinical improvement (i.e., decreased pain and urgency) by the end of the trial ($p = 0.07$). The results fell short of statistical significance most likely because of the small sample size ($n = 53$).

Perioperative Nutrition

Arginine is a potent immunomodulator. Evidence is mounting for a beneficial effect of arginine supplementation in catabolic conditions such as sepsis and postoperative stress. Supplemental arginine appears to up-regulate immune function and reduce the incidence of postoperative infection.[92] Two controlled trials have demonstrated increased lymphocyte mitogenesis and improved wound healing in experimental surgical wounds in volunteers given 17-25 grams oral arginine per day.[93,94] Similar results have been obtained in healthy elderly volunteers.[95]

Preterm Labor and Delivery

Evidence from human and animal studies indicates nitric oxide inhibits uterine contractility and may help maintain uterine quiescence during pregnancy.[96] Intravenous arginine infusion (30 g over 30 min) in women with premature uterine contractions transiently reduced uterine contractility.[97] Further research is needed to confirm the efficacy and safety of arginine in prevention of preterm delivery.

Senile Dementia

Arginine (1.6 g/d) in 16 elderly patients with senile dementia reduced lipid peroxidation and increased cognitive function.[98]

Side Effects and Toxicity

Significant adverse effects have not been observed with arginine supplementation. However, long-term studies are needed to confirm its apparent safety. People with renal failure or hepatic disease may be unable to appropriately metabolize and excrete supplemental arginine and should be closely monitored when taking arginine supplements.

Dosage

Doses of arginine used in clinical research have varied considerably, from as little as 500 mg per day for oligospermia to as much as 30 g per day for cancer, preeclampsia and premature uterine contractions. Typical doses fall into either the 1-3 g per day range, or the 7-15 g per day range, depending on the condition being treated.

Warnings and Contraindications

It has been postulated, on the basis of older *in vitro* data[99] and anecdotal reporting, that arginine supplementation is contraindicated in persons with herpes infections (i.e., cold sores, genital herpes). The assumption is that arginine might stimulate replication of the virus and/or provoke an outbreak; however, this caution has not been validated by controlled clinical trials.

Bronchoconstriction is reportedly inhibited by the formation of NO in the airways of asthmatic patients, and a bronchoprotective effect of NO in asthma has been proposed.[100] Airway obstruction in asthma might be associated with endogenous NO deficiency caused by limited availability of NO synthase substrate (i.e., arginine). However, oral arginine (50 mg/kg body weight) in asthmatic patients triggered by a histamine challenge produced only a marginal, statistically insignificant improvement of airway hyper-responsiveness to histamine.[101] In fact, it is unclear whether NO acts as a protective or a stimulatory factor in airway hyper-responsiveness. Current data suggest modulating NO synthesis by giving oral arginine supplements has no significant benefit on airway response to exercise in asthmatic subjects,[102] and may even induce bronchoconstriction when nebulized and inhaled.[103] Until more is known, arginine should not be used to treat asthma.

Since polyamines act as growth factors for cancers, and arginine may stimulate polyamine synthesis, chronic administration of arginine in cancer patients should probably be avoided until information arises regarding the safety of this practice.

References

1. Castillo L, Chapman TE, Sanchez M, et al. Plasma arginine and citrulline kinetics in adults given adequate and arginine-free diets. *Proc Natl Acad Sci U S A* 1993;90:7749-7753.
2. Castillo L, Ajami A, Branch S, et al. Plasma arginine kinetics in adult man: response to an arginine-free diet. *Metabolism* 1994;43:114-122.
3. Abcouwer SF, Souba WW. Glutamine and arginine. In: Shils ME, Olson JA, Shike M, Ross AC, eds. *Modern Nutrition in Health and Disease*, 9th ed. Baltimore, MD: Williams & Wilkins; 1999:559-569.
4. Wu G, Davis PK, Flynn NE, et al. Endogenous synthesis of arginine plays an important role in maintaining arginine homeostasis in postweaning growing pigs. *J Nutr* 1997;127:2342-2349.
5. Dhanakoti SN, Brosnan JT, Herzberg GR, Brosnan ME. Renal arginine synthesis: studies *in vitro* and *in vivo*. *Am J Physiol* 1990;259:E437-E442.
6. Preiser JC, Berre PJ, Van Gossum A, et al. Metabolic effects of arginine addition to the enteral feeding of critically ill patients. *JPEN J Parenter Enteral Nutr* 2001;25:182-187.
7. Castillo L, Sanchez M, Vogt J, et al. Plasma arginine, citrulline, and ornithine kinetics in adults, with observations on nitric oxide synthesis. *Am J Physiol* 1995;268:E360-E367.
8. Wu G, Morris SM Jr. Arginine metabolism: nitric oxide and beyond. *Biochem J* 1998;336:1-17.
9. Meijer AJ, Lamers WH, Chamuleau RA. Nitrogen metabolism and ornithine cycle function. *Physiol Rev* 1990;70:701-748.
10. Imms FJ, London DR, Neame RL. The secretion of catecholamines from the adrenal gland following arginine infusion in the rat. *J Physiol* 1969;200:55P-56P.
11. Palmer JP, Walter RM, Ensinck JW. Arginine-stimulated acute phase of insulin and glucagon secretion. I. In normal man. *Diabetes* 1975;24:735-740.
12. Rakoff JS, Siler TM, Sinha YN, Yen SS. Prolactin and growth hormone release in response to sequential stimulation by arginine and synthetic TRF. *J Clin Endocrinol Metab* 1973;37:641-644.
13. Knopf RF, Conn JW, Fajans SS, et al. Plasma growth hormone response to intravenous administration of amino acids. *J Clin Endocrinol Metab* 1965;25:1140-1144.
14. Merimee TJ, Lillicrap DA, Rabinowitz D. Effect of arginine on serum-levels of human growth-hormone. *Lancet* 1965;2:668-670.

15. Wu G, Meininger CJ. Arginine nutrition and cardiovascular function. *J Nutr* 2000;130:2626-2629.
16. Gross SS, Wolin MS. Nitric oxide: pathophysiological mechanisms. *Annu Rev Physiol* 1995;57:737-769.
17. Wink DA, Hanbauer I, Grisham MB, et al. Chemical biology of nitric oxide: regulation and protective and toxic mechanisms. *Curr Top Cell Regul* 1996;34:159-187.
18. Umans JG, Levi R. Nitric oxide in the regulation of blood flow and arterial pressure. *Annu Rev Physiol* 1995;57:771-790.
19. Hare JM, Colucci WS. Role of nitric oxide in the regulation of myocardial function. *Prog Cardiovasc Dis* 1995;38:155-166.
20. Lyons CR. The role of nitric oxide in inflammation. *Adv Immunol* 1995;60:323-371.
21. Brune B, Messmer UK, Sandau K. The role of nitric oxide in cell injury. *Toxicol Lett* 1995;82-83:233-237.
22. Wink DA, Cook JA, Pacelli R, et al. Nitric oxide (NO) protects against cellular damage by reactive oxygen species. *Toxicol Lett* 1995;82-83:221-226.
23. Brittenden J, Heys SD, Ross J, et al. Natural cytotoxicity in breast cancer patients receiving neoadjuvant chemotherapy: effects of L-arginine supplementation. *Eur J Surg Oncol* 1994;20:467-472.
24. Brittenden J, Park KGM, Heys SD, et al. L-arginine stimulates host defenses in patients with breast cancer. *Surgery* 1994;115:205-212.
25. Swanson B, Keithley JK, Zeller JM, Sha BE. A pilot study of the safety and efficacy of supplemental arginine to enhance immune function in persons with HIV/AIDS. *Nutrition* 2002;18:688-690.
26. Clark RH, Feleke G, Din M, et al. Nutritional treatment for acquired immunodeficiency virus-associated wasting using beta-hydroxy beta-methylbutyrate, glutamine, and arginine: a randomized, double-blind, placebo-controlled study. *JPEN J Parenter Enteral Nutr* 2000;24:133-139.
27. Pichard C, Sudre P, Karsegard V, et al. A randomized double-blind controlled study of 6 months of oral nutritional supplementation with arginine and omega-3 fatty acids in HIV-infected patients. Swiss HIV Cohort Study. *AIDS* 1998;12:53-63.
28. Blum A, Porat R, Rosenschein U, et al. Clinical and inflammatory effects of dietary L-arginine in patients with intractable angina pectoris. *Am J Cardiol* 1999;83:1488-1490.
29. Ceremuzynski L, Chamiec T, Herbaczynska-Cedro K. Effect of supplemental oral L-arginine on exercise capacity in patients with stable angina pectoris. *Am J Cardiol* 1997;80:331-333.
30. Walker HA, McGing E, Fisher I, et al. Endothelium-dependent vasodilation is independent of the plasma L-arginine/ADMA ratio in men with stable angina: lack of effect of oral L-arginine on endothelial function, oxidative stress and exercise performance. *J Am Coll Cardiol* 2001;38:499-505.
31. Bednarz B, Wolk R, Chamiec T, et al. Effects of oral L-arginine supplementation on exercise-induced QT dispersion and exercise tolerance in stable angina pectoris. *Int J Cardiol* 2000;75:205-210.
32. Egashira K, Hirooka Y, Kuga T, et al. Effects of L-arginine supplementation on endothelium-dependent coronary vasodilation in patients with angina pectoris and normal coronary arteriograms. *Circulation* 1996;94:130-134.
33. Besset A, Bonardet A, Rondouin G, et al. Increase in sleep related GH and Prl secretion after chronic arginine aspartate administration in man. *Acta Endocrinol* 1982;99:18-23.
34. Macintyre JG. Growth hormone and athletes. *Sports Med* 1987;4:129-142.
35. Elam RP. Morphological changes in adult males from resistance exercise and amino acid supplementation. *J Sports Med Phys Fitness* 1988;28:35-39.
36. Marcell TJ, Taaffe DR, Hawkins SA, et al. Oral arginine does not stimulate basal or augment exercise-induced GH secretion in either young or old adults. *J Gerontol A Biol Sci Med Sci* 1999;54:M395-M399.
37. Elam RP. Effect of arginine and ornithine on strength, lean body mass and urinary hydroxyproline in adult males. *J Sports Nutr* 1989;29:52-56.
38. Corpas E, Blackman MR, Roberson, R, et al. Oral arginine-lysine does not increase growth hormone or insulin-like growth factor-I in old men. *J Gerontol* 1993;48:M128-M133.

39. Yu YM, Ryan CM, Castillo L, et al. Arginine and ornithine kinetics in severely burned patients: increased rate of arginine disposal. *Am J Physiol Endocrinol Metab* 2001;280:E509-E517.

40. Bower RH, Cerra FB, Bershadsky B, et al. Early enteral administration of a formula (Impact) supplemented with arginine, nucleotides, and fish oil in intensive care unit patients: results of a multicenter, prospective, randomized clinical trial. *Crit Care Med* 1995;23:436-439.

41. Weimann A, Bastian L, Bischoff WE, et al. Influence of arginine, omega-3 fatty acids and nucleotide-supplemented enteral support on systemic inflammatory response syndrome and multiple organ failure in patients after severe trauma. *Nutrition* 1998;14:165-172.

42. Takeda Y, Tominga T, Tei N, et al. Inhibitory effect of L-arginine on growth of rat mammary tumors induced by 7, 12, dimethlybenz(a)anthracine. *Cancer Res* 1975;35:390-393.

43. Heys SD, Segar A, Payne S, et al. Dietary supplementation with L-arginine: modulation of tumour-infiltrating lymphocytes in patients with colorectal cancer. *Br J Surg* 1997;84:238-241.

44. Kemen M, Senkal M, Homann HH, et al. Early postoperative enteral nutrition with arginine-omega-3 fatty acids and ribonucleic acid-supplemented diet versus placebo in cancer patients: an immunologic evaluation of Impact. *Crit Care Med* 1995;23:652-659.

45. Gianotti L, Braga M, Fortis C, et al. A prospective, randomized clinical trial on perioperative feeding with an arginine-, omega-3 fatty acid-, and RNA-enriched enteral diet: effect on host response and nutritional status. *JPEN J Parenter Enteral Nutr* 1999;23:314-320.

46. van Bokhorst-De Van Der Schueren MA, Quak JJ, von Blomberg-van der Flier BM, et al. Effect of perioperative nutrition, with and without arginine supplementation, on nutritional status, immune function, postoperative morbidity, and survival in severely malnourished head and neck cancer patients. *Am J Clin Nutr* 2001;73:323-332.

47. Park KGM. The Sir David Cuthbertson Medal Lecture 1992. The immunological and metabolic effects of L-arginine in human cancer. *Proc Nutr Soc* 1993;52:387-401.

48. Rector TS, Bank A, Mullen KA, et al. Randomized, double-blind, placebo controlled study of supplemental oral L-arginine in patients with heart failure. *Circulation* 1996;93:2135-2141.

49. Watanabe G, Tomiyama H, Doba N. Effects of oral administration of L-arginine on renal function in patients with heart failure. *J Hypertens* 2000;18:229-234.

50. Cooke JP. Is atherosclerosis an arginine deficiency disease? *J Investig Med* 1998;46:377-380.

51. Cooke JP, Singer AH, Tsao P, et al. Antiatherogenic effects of L-arginine in the hypercholesterolemic rabbit. *J Clin Invest* 1992;90:1168-1172.

52. Nakaki T, Kato R. Beneficial circulatory effect of L-arginine. *Jpn J Pharmacol* 1994;66:167-171.

53. Wolf A, Zalpour C, Theilmeier G, et al. Dietary L-arginine supplementation normalizes platelet aggregation in hypercholesterolemic humans. *J Am Coll Cardiol* 1997;29:479-485.

54. Oomen CM, van Erk MJ, Feskens EJ, et al. Arginine intake and risk of coronary heart disease mortality in elderly men. *Arterioscler Thromb Vasc Biol* 2000;20:2134-2139.

55. Wennmalm A, Edlund A, Granstrom EF, Wiklund O. Acute supplementation with the nitric oxide precursor L-arginine does not improve cardiovascular performance in patients with hypercholesterolemia. *Atherosclerosis* 1995;118:223-231.

56. Pieper GM. Review of alterations in endothelial nitric oxide production in diabetes. *Hypertension* 1998;31:1047-1060.

57. Pieper GM, Siebeneich W, Dondlinger LA. Short-term oral administration of L-arginine reverses defective endothelium-dependent relaxation and cGMP generation in diabetes. *Eur J Pharmacol* 1996;317:317-320.

58. Giugliano D, Marfella R, Verrazzo G, et al. L-arginine for testing endothelium-dependent vascular functions in health and disease. *Am J Physiol* 1997;273:E606-E612.

59. Wascher TC, Graier WF, Dittrich P, et al. Effects of low-dose L-arginine on insulin-mediated vasodilatation and insulin sensitivity. *Eur J Clin Invest* 1997;27:690-695.

60. Lubec B, Hayn M, Kitzmuller E, et al. L-arginine reduces lipid peroxidation in patients with diabetes mellitus. *Free Radic Biol Med* 1997;22:355-357.

61. Piatti PM, Monti LD, Valsecchi G, et al. Long-term oral L-arginine administration improves peripheral and hepatic insulin sensitivity in type 2 diabetic patients. *Diabetes Care* 2001;24:875-880.

62. Mullen MJ, Wright D, Donald AE, et al. Atorvastatin but not L-arginine improves endothelial function in type I diabetes mellitus: a double-blind study. *J Am Coll Cardiol* 2000;36:410-416.

63. Zorgniotti AW, Lizza EF. Effect of large doses of the nitric oxide precursor, L-arginine, on erectile dysfunction. *Int J Impot Res* 1994;6:33-36.

64. Chen J, Wollman Y, Chernichovsky T, et al. Effect of oral administration of high-dose nitric oxide donor L-arginine in men with organic erectile dysfunction: results of a double-blind, randomized study. *BJU Int* 1999;83:269-273.

65. Klotz T, Mathers MJ, Braun M, et al. Effectiveness of oral L-arginine in first-line treatment of erectile dysfunction in a controlled crossover study. *Urol Int* 1999;63:220-223.

66. Brzozowski T, Konturek SJ, Sliwowski Z, et al. Role of L-arginine, a substrate for nitric oxide-synthase, in gastroprotection and ulcer healing. *J Gastroenterol* 1997;32:442-452.

67. Brzozowski T, Konturek SJ, Drozdowicz D, et al. Healing of chronic gastric ulcerations by L-arginine. Role of nitric oxide, prostaglandins, gastrin and polyamines. *Digestion* 1995;56:463-471.

68. Bortolotti M, Brunelli F, Sarti P, Miglioli M. Clinical and manometric effects of L-arginine in patients with chest pain and oesophageal motor disorders. *Ital J Gastroenterol Hepatol* 1997;29:320-324.

69. Straathof JW, Adamse M, Onkenhout W, et al. Effect of L-arginine on lower oesophageal sphincter motility in man. *Eur J Gastroenterol Hepatol* 2000;12:419-424.

70. Fisker S, Nielsen S, Ebdrup L, et al. The role of nitric oxide in L-arginine-stimulated growth hormone release. *J Endocrinol Invest* 1999;22:S89-S93.

71. Sanders PW. Salt-sensitive hypertension: lessons from animal models. *Am J Kidney Dis* 1996;28:775-782.

72. Calver A, Collier J, Vallance P. Dilator actions of arginine in human peripheral vasculature. *Clin Sci* 1991;81:695-700.

73. Pezza V, Bernardini F, Pezza E, et al. Study of supplemental oral L-arginine in hypertensives treated with enalapril + hydrochlorothiazide. *Am J Hypertens* 1998;11:1267-1270.

74. Siani A, Pagano E, Iacone R, et al. Blood pressure and metabolic changes during dietary L-arginine supplementation in humans. *Am J Hypertens* 2000;13:547-551.

75. Maccario M, Oleandri SE, Procopio M, et al. Comparison among the effects of arginine, a nitric oxide precursor, isosorbide dinitrate and molsidomine, two nitric oxide donors, on hormonal secretions and blood pressure in man. *J Endocrinol Invest* 1997;20:488-492.

76. Schulze-Neick I, Penny DJ, Rigby ML, et al. L-arginine and substance P reverse the pulmonary endothelial dysfunction caused by congenital heart surgery. *Circulation* 1999;100:749-755.

77. Roberts JM. Objective evidence of endothelial dysfunction in preeclampsia. *Am J Kidney Dis* 1999;33:992-997.

78. Helmbrecht GD, Farhat MY, Lochbaum L, et al. L-arginine reverses the adverse pregnancy changes induced by nitric oxide synthase inhibition in the rat. *Am J Obstet Gynecol* 1996;175:800-805.

79. Facchinetti F, Longo M, Piccinini F, et al. L-arginine infusion reduces blood pressure in preeclamptic women through nitric oxide release. *J Soc Gynecol Invest* 1999;6:202-207.

80. Battaglia C, Salvatori M, Maxia N, et al. Adjuvant L-arginine treatment for *in-vitro* fertilization in poor responder patients. *Hum Reprod* 1999;14:1690-1697.

81. Holt LE Jr, Albanese AA. Observations on amino acid deficiencies in man. *Trans Assoc Am Physicians* 1944;58:143-156.

82. Tanimura J. Studies on arginine in human semen. Part II. The effects of medication with L-arginine-HCl on male infertility. *Bull Osaka Med School* 1967;13:84-89.

83. De Aloysio D, Mantuano R, Mauloni M, Nicoletti G. The clinical use of arginine aspartate in male infertility. *Acta Eur Fertil* 1982;13:133-167.

84. Scibona M, Meschini P, Capparelli S, et al. L-arginine and male infertility. *Minerva Urol Nefrol* 1994;46:251-253.

85. Schacter A, Goldman JA, Zukerman Z. Treatment of oligospermia with the amino acid arginine. *J Urol* 1973;110:311-313.

86. Schacter A, Friedman S, Goldman JA, Eckerling B. Treatment of oligospermia with the amino acid arginine. *Int J Gynaecol Obstet* 1973;11:206-209.

87. Pryor JP, Blandy JP, Evans P, et al. Controlled clinical trial of arginine for infertile men with oligozoospermia. *Br J Urol* 1978;50:47-50.

88. Mroueh A. Effect of arginine on oligospermia. *Fertil Steril* 1970:21:217-219.

89. Boger RH, Bode-Boger SM, Thiele W, et al. Restoring vascular nitric oxide formation by L-arginine improves the symptoms of intermittent claudication in patients with peripheral arterial occlusive disease. *J Am Coll Cardiol* 1998;32:1336-1344.

90. Smith SD, Wheeler MA, Foster HE Jr, Weiss RM. Improvement in interstitial cystitis symptom scores during treatment with oral L-arginine. *J Urol* 1997;158:703-708.

91. EhrÈn I, Lundberg JO, Adolfsson J. Effects of L-arginine treatment on symptoms and bladder nitric oxide levels in patients with interstitial cystitis. *Urology* 1998;52:1026-1029.

92. Evoy D, Lieberman MD, Fahey TJ 3rd, Daly JM. Immunonutrition: the role of arginine. *Nutrition* 1998;14:611-617.

93. Barbul A, Rettura G, Levenson SM, et al. Wound healing and thymotropic effects of arginine: a pituitary mechanism of action. *Am J Clin Nutr* 1983;37:786-794.

94. Barbul A, Lazarou SA, Efron DT, et al. Arginine enhances wound healing and lymphocyte immune responses in humans. *Surgery* 1990;108:331-337.

95. Kirk SJ, Hurson M, Regan MC, et al. Arginine stimulates wound healing and immune function in elderly human beings. *Surgery* 1993;114:155-160.

96. Buhimschi IA, Saade GR, Chwalisz K, Garfield RE. The nitric oxide pathway in pre-eclampsia: pathophysiological implications. *Human Reprod Update* 1998;4:25-42.

97. Facchinetti F, Neri I, Genazzani AR. L-arginine infusion reduces preterm uterine contractions. *J Perinat Med* 1996;24:283-285.

98. Ohtsuka Y, Nakaya J. Effect of oral administration of L-arginine on senile dementia. *Am J Med* 2000;108:439.

99. Tankersley RW. Amino acid requirements of herpes simplex virus in human cells. *J Bacteriol* 1964;87:609-613.

100. Ricciardolo FL, Geppetti P, Mistretta A, et al. Randomised double-blind placebo-controlled study of the effect of inhibition of nitric oxide synthesis in bradykinin-induced asthma. *Lancet* 1996;348:374-377.

101. de Gouw HW, Verbruggen MB, Twiss IM, Sterk PJ. Effect of oral L-arginine on airway hyperresponsiveness to histamine in asthma. *Thorax* 1999;54:1033-1035.

102. de Gouw HW, Marshall-Partridge SJ, Van Der Veen H, et al. Role of nitric oxide in the airway response to exercise in healthy and asthmatic subjects. *J Appl Physiol* 2001;90:586-592.

103. Chambers DC, Ayres JG. Effect of nebulised L- and D-arginine on exhaled nitric oxide in steroid naive asthma. *Thorax* 2001;56:602-606.

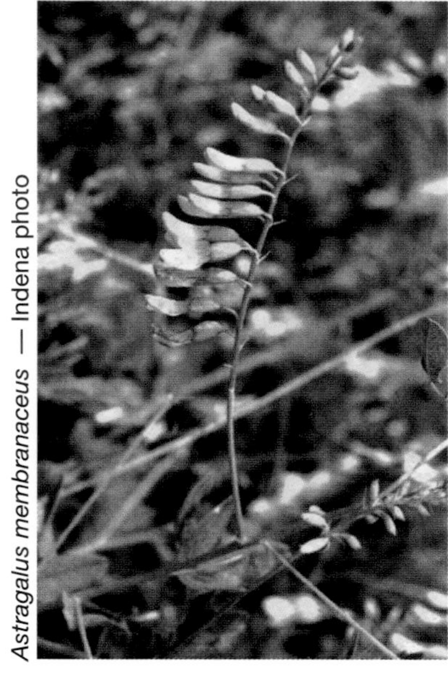
Astragalus membranaceus — Indena photo

Astragalus membranaceus

Description

Astragalus membranaceus is one of the important "Qi tonifying" adaptogenic herbs from the Chinese materia medica. It has been prescribed for centuries for general weakness, chronic illnesses, and to increase overall vitality. Currently, much of the pharmacological research on Astragalus is focused on its immune-stimulating polysaccharides and other active ingredients useful in treating immune deficiency conditions. Astragalus has demonstrated a wide range of potential therapeutic applications in immunodeficiency syndromes, as an adjunctive cancer therapy, and for its adaptogenic effect on the heart and kidneys.

Traditional Indications

In Traditional Chinese Medicine (TCM), Astragalus is indicated for symptoms of spleen deficiency such as diarrhea, fatigue, spontaneous sweating, and lack of appetite.[1] Astragalus tonifies the lungs and is used in cases of frequent colds and shortness of breath.[1] Other traditional indications include wasting disorders, night sweats,[2] chronic ulcerations and sores,[1] numbness and paralysis of the limbs, and edema.[1] Astragalus is classically prescribed in combination with other Chinese medicinal herbs depending on the desired therapeutic effect and the specific TCM diagnosis.

Clinical Indications

Immunotherapy

Astragalus has been shown to increase resistance to the immunosuppressive effects of chemotherapy drugs, while stimulating macrophages to produce interleukin-6 and tumor necrosis factor (TNF).[3] The use of recombinant interleukin-2 (rIL-2) in immunotherapy is limited by the toxicity associated with higher doses. Astragalus and 100 U/ml of rIL-2 was compared with 1,000 U/ml of rIL-2 alone in an *in vitro* study on murine renal carcinoma cells. The Astragalus/rIL-2 group had a tumor cell lysis rate of 88 percent, versus 86 percent in the group with 1000 U/ml rIL-2 alone. This suggests a 10-fold potentiation of the *in vitro* antitumor activity of rIL-2-generated lymphokine-activated killer (LAK) cells.[4] These results were confirmed in another study where Astragalus potentiated the LAK cell-inducing activity of rIL-2 against an Hs294T melanoma cell line.[5]

In viral myocarditis patients given an oral Astragalus extract, enhanced T3, T4 and T4/T8 cell ratios were demonstrated, suggesting improved immune response.[6] Patients with systemic lupus erythematosus have significantly decreased natural killer (NK) cell activity when compared to normal controls. Pre-incubation of their peripheral blood mononuclear cells with Astragalus stimulated NK cell cytotoxicity in SLE patients and in healthy controls.[7] Astragalus has also been shown to possess *in vitro* antibacterial activity against *Shigella dysenteriae, Streptococcus hemolyticus, Diplococcus pneumonia,* and *Staphylococcus aureus*.[2]

Adjunct Cancer Therapy

One-hundred-and-sixteen Chinese herbal formulas were screened and evaluated for their ability to ameliorate the toxic side effects of anticancer agents. A formula including both Astragalus and Ligusticum, Shi-Quan-Da-Bu-Tang, was selected as the most effective in stimulating hemopoietic factors and interleukin production. It was also shown to potentiate the activity of chemotherapeutic agents, inhibit recurrence of malignancies, prolong survival, and reduce the adverse toxicities of radiotherapy and antineoplastic agents such as mitomycin, cisplatin, cyclophosphamide, and 5-fluorouracil.[8]

Cardiovascular Disease

The saponins contained in Astragalus were found to have a positive effect on the function of the heart by inhibiting the formation of lipid peroxides in the myocardium and by decreasing blood coagulation.[9] Astragaloside IV was isolated and injected into 19 patients with congestive heart failure daily for two weeks. After two weeks, symptoms of chest pain and dyspnea were alleviated in 15 of 19 patients.[10]

Ninety-two patients with ischemic heart disease were treated with Astragalus. Not only did they have significant relief from angina, but also the effective rate of electrocardiogram improvement was 82.6 percent.[11] In another study on angina pectoris, 20 patients were given Astragalus for two weeks. Cardiac output was significantly increased and, unlike digitalis, adenosine triphosphatase activity was not inhibited with Astragalus.[12]

Infertility, Male

Water extracts of 18 herbs were tested for their effect on sperm motility. Only Astragalus demonstrated a significant stimulatory effect. Using a solution of 10 mg/ml, sperm motility was increased to 146.6 ± 22.6 percent of control.[13]

Dosage and Toxicity

Astragalus is safe, and doses as high as 100 g/kg of raw herb have been given by lavage to rats with no adverse effects.[1] Astragalus can be given in tincture form at 2-4 ml three times daily. The LD-50 of Astragalus is approximately 40 g/kg when administered by intraperitoneal injection.

References

1. Bensky D, Gamble A. *Chinese Herbal Medicine: Materia Medica, Revised Edition.* Seattle, WA: Eastland Press; 1993.
2. Hong YH. *Oriental Materia Medica: A Concise Guide.* Long Beach, CA: Oriental Healing Arts Institute; 1986.
3. Yoshida Y, Wang MQ, Shan BE, Yamashita U. Immunomodulating activity of Chinese medical herbs and *Oldenlandia diffusa* in particular. *Int J Immunopharmacol* 1997;19:359-370.
4. Wang Y, Qian XJ, Hadley HR, Lau BH. Phytochemicals potentiate interleukin-2 generated lymphokine-activated killer cell cytotoxicity against murine renal cell carcinoma. *Mol Biother* 1992;4:143-146.
5. Chu DT, Lin JR, Wong W. The in vitro potentiation of LAK cell cytotoxicity in cancer and AIDS patients induced by F3 – a fractionated extract of *Astragalus membranaceus. Zhonghua Zhong Liu Za Zhi* 1994;16:167-171. [article in Chinese]
6. Huang ZQ, Qin NP, Ye W. Effect of *Astragalus membranaceus* on T-lymphocyte subsets in patients with viral myocarditis. *Zhongguo Zhong Xi Yi Jie He Za Zhi* 1995;15:328-330. [article in Chinese]
7. Zhao XZ. Effects of *Astragalus membranaceus* and *Tripterygium hypoglancum* on natural killer cell activity of peripheral blood mononuclear in systemic lupus erythematosus. *Zhongguo Zhong Xi Yi Jie He Za Zhi* 1992;12:669-671. [article in Chinese]
8. Zee-Cheng RK. Shi-quan-da-bu-tang (ten significant tonic decoction), SQT. A potent Chinese biological response modifier in cancer immunotherapy, potentiation and detoxification of anticancer drugs. *Methods Find Exp Clin Pharmacol* 1992;14:725-736.
9. Purmova J, Opletal L. Phytotherapeutic aspects of diseases of the cardiovascular system. 5. Saponins and possibilities of their use in prevention and therapy. *Ceska Slov Farm* 1995;44:246-251. [article in Czech]
10. Luo HM, Dai RH, Li Y. Nuclear cardiology study on effective ingredients of *Astragalus membranaceus* in treating heart failure. *Zhongguo Zhong Xi Yi Jie He Za Zhi* 1995;15:707-709. [article in Chinese]
11. Li SQ, Yuan RX, Gao H. Clinical observation on the treatment of ischemic heart disease with *Astragalus membranaceus. Zhongguo Zhong Xi Yi Jie He Za Zhi* 1995;15:77-80. [article in Chinese]
12. Lei ZY, Qin H, Liao JZ. Action of *Astragalus membranaceus* on left ventricular function of angina pectoris. *Zhongguo Zhong Xi Yi Jie He Za Zhi* 1994;14:199-202. [article in Chinese]
13. Hong CY, Ku J, Wu P. *Astragalus membranaceus* stimulates human sperm motility *in vitro. Am J Chin Med* 1992;20:289-294.

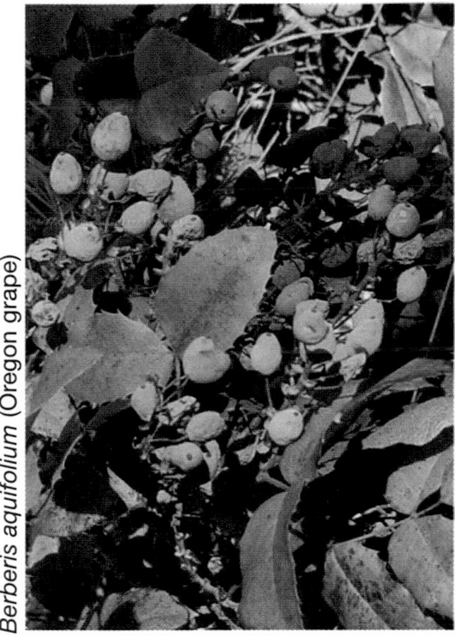

Berberis aquifolium (Oregon grape)

Berberine

Description

Berberine is a plant alkaloid with a long history of medicinal use in both Ayurvedic and Chinese medicine. It is present in many plants, including *Hydrastis canadensis* (goldenseal), *Coptis chinensis* (Coptis or goldenthread), *Berberis aquifolium* (Oregon grape), *Berberis vulgaris* (barberry), and *Berberis aristata* (tree turmeric). Berberine can be found in the root, rhizome, and stem bark of the plants. Berberine extracts and decoctions have demonstrated significant antimicrobial activity against a variety of organisms, including bacteria, viruses, fungi, protozoans, helminths, and chlamydia. Currently, the predominant clinical uses of berberine include bacterial diarrhea, intestinal parasite infections, and ocular trachoma infections.[1]

Mechanisms of Action

The pharmacologic actions of berberine include metabolic inhibition of certain organisms, inhibition of bacterial enterotoxin formation, inhibition of intestinal fluid accumulation and ion secretion, inhibition of smooth muscle contraction, reduction of inflammation, platelet aggregation inhibition, platelet count elevation in certain types of thrombocytopenia, stimulation of bile and bilirubin secretion, and inhibition of ventricular tachyarrhythmias.[1,2]

In vitro studies utilizing human cell lines demonstrate berberine inhibits activator protein 1 (AP-1), a key transcription factor in inflammation and carcinogenesis.[3] In another study utilizing human peripheral lymphocytes, berberine exerted a significant inhibitory effect on lymphocyte transformation; the authors concluded berberine's anti-inflammatory action might be due to inhibition of DNA synthesis in activated lymphocytes.[4] A third study noted that during platelet activation in response to tissue injury, berberine had a direct effect on several aspects of the inflammatory process, which include dose-dependent inhibition of arachidonic acid release from cell membrane phospholipids, inhibition of thromboxane A2 from platelets,[5] and inhibition of thrombus formation.[6]

Berberine has demonstrated a number of other beneficial effects, including immunostimulation via increased blood flow to the spleen, macrophage activation, elevation of platelet counts in cases of primary and secondary thrombocytopenia, and increased excretion of conjugated bilirubin in experimental hyperbilirubinemia.[1] In addition, berberine may possess anti-tumor properties as evidenced by inhibition of COX-2 transcription and N-acetyltransferase activity in colon and bladder cancer cell lines,[7,8] and transient, but marked, inhibitory action on the growth of mouse sarcoma cells in culture.[9]

Clinical Applications

Bacterial Diarrhea

Diarrhea caused by *Vibrio cholera* and *Escherichia coli* has been the focus of numerous berberine studies, and results indicate several mechanisms that may explain its ability to inhibit bacterial diarrhea. An animal study found berberine reduced the intestinal secretion of water and electrolytes induced by cholera toxin.[10] Other studies have shown berberine directly inhibits some *V. cholera* and *E. coli* enterotoxins,[11] significantly reduces smooth muscle contraction and intestinal motility,[2] and delays intestinal transit time in humans.[12] Berberine sulfate has also been found to be directly bacteriocidal to *V. cholera*.[13] In the case of *E. coli*, *in vitro* research indicates berberine sulfate inhibits bacterial adherence to mucosal or epithelial surfaces, the first step in the infective process. This may be a result of berberine's inhibitory effect on fimbrial structure formation on the surface of the bacteria.[14]

Intestinal Parasites

Berberine extracts and salts have demonstrated growth inhibition of *Giardia lamblia, Entamoeba histolytica, Trichomonas vaginalis*,[15] and *Leishmania donovani*,[16] with crude extracts being more effective than berberine salts.[17]

In tropical climates *Giardia lamblia* infestation (giardiasis) is a common occurrence, particularly in pediatric populations.[18] In clinical trials conducted in India, berberine administration improved gastrointestinal symptoms and resulted in a marked reduction in Giardia-positive stools. In comparison to metronidazole (Flagyl®), a popular giardiasis medication, berberine was nearly as effective at half the dose.[19]

Both *in vivo* and *in vitro* studies of berberine's effects on *E. histolytica* indicated berberine sulfate was amoebicidal and caused encystation, degeneration, and eventual lysis of the trophozoite forms.[20] Berberine sulfate inhibited the growth of *Trichomonas vaginalis* via formation of large autophagic vacuoles that eventually result in lysis of the trophozoite forms.[15]

Studies show berberine markedly decreases parasitic load and rapidly improves hematologic parameters in infected animals. *In vitro* results indicate berberine inhibits multiplication, respiration, and macromolecular biosynthesis of amastigote forms of the parasite, interferes with nuclear DNA of the promastigote form, and inhibits organism maturation.[16]

Ocular Trachoma Infections

A clinical study of aqueous berberine versus sulfacetamide for the treatment of *Chlamydia trachomatis* infection was conducted on 51 subjects in an outpatient eye clinic. It was determined that while sulfacetamide eye drops produced slightly better clinical results, conjunctival scrapings of these patients remained positive for the infective agent, and relapses occurred. In contrast, the conjunctival scrapings of patients receiving berberine chloride eye drops were negative for *C. trachomatis* and there were no relapses, even one year after treatment. It was also concluded that, while berberine chloride had no direct anti-chlamydial properties, it seemed to cure the infection by stimulating some protective mechanism in the host.[21] A second clinical study found berberine chloride superior to sulfacetamide in both the clinical course of trachoma and in achieving a drop in serum antibody titers against *C. trachomatis*.[22]

Hypertension and Arrhythmias

Clinical trials and animal research indicate berberine administration prevents ischemia-induced ventricular tachyarrhythmia, stimulates cardiac contractility, and lowers peripheral vascular resistance and blood pressure.[23,24] The mechanism for berberine's antiarrhythmic effect is unclear, but an animal study indicated it might be due to suppression of delayed after-depolarization in the ventricular muscle.[25] An animal study suggested, in addition to affecting several other parameters of cardiac performance, berberine might have a vasodilatory/hypotensive effect attributable to its potentiation of acetylcholine.[23]

Side Effects and Toxicity

Berberine is not considered toxic at doses used in clinical situations, nor has it been shown to be cytotoxic or mutagenic. Side effects can result from high dosages and may include gastrointestinal discomfort, dyspnea, lowered blood pressure, flu-like symptoms, and cardiac damage.

Dosage

The therapeutic dosage for most clinical situations is 200 mg orally two to four times daily.[1]

Warnings and Contraindications

Berberine usage should be avoided in pregnancy, due to potential for causing uterine contractions and miscarriage, and in jaundiced neonates because of its bilirubin displacement properties.

References

1. Birdsall TC, Kelly GS. Berberine: Therapeutic potential of an alkaloid found in several medicinal plants. *Altern Med Rev* 1997;2:94-103.
2. Akhter MH, Sabir M, Bhide NK. Possible mechanism of antidiarrhoel effect of berberine. *Indian J Med Res* 1979;70:233-241.
3. Fukuda K, Hibiya Y, Mutoh M, et al. Inhibition of activator protein 1 activity by berberine in human hepatoma cells. *Planta Med* 1999;65:381-383.
4. Ckless K, Schlottfeldt JL, Pasqual M, et al. Inhibition of *in vitro* lymphocyte transformation by the isoquinoline alkaloid berberine. *J Pharm Pharmacol* 1995;47:1029-1031.
5. Huang CG, Chu ZL, Yang ZM. Effects of berberine on synthesis of platelet TXA2 and plasma PGI2 in rabbits. *Chung Kuo Yao Li Hsueh Pao* 1991;12:526-528.
6. Wu JF, Liu TP. Effects of berberine on platelet aggregation and plasma levels of TXB2 and 6-keto-PGF1 alpha in rats with reversible middle cerebral artery occlusion. *Yao Hsueh Hsueh Pao* 1995;30:98-102.
7. Lin JG, Chung JG, Wu LT, et al. Effects of berberine on arylamine N-acetyltransferase activity in human colon tumor cells. *Am J Chin Med* 1999;27:265-275.
8. Fukuda K, Hibiya Y, Mutoh M, et al. Inhibition by berberine of cyclooxygenase-2 transcriptional activity in human colon cancer cells. *J Ethnopharmacol* 1999;66:227-233.
9. Creasey WA. Biochemical effects of berberine. *Biochem Pharmacol* 1979;28:1081-1084.
10. Swabb EA, Tai YH, Jordan L. Reversal of cholera toxin-induced secretion in rat ileum by luminal berberine. *Am J Physiol* 1981;241:G248-G252.
11. Sack RB, Froelich JL. Berberine inhibits intestinal secretory response of *Vibrio cholera* and *Escherichia coli* enteroxins. *Infect Immun* 1982;35:471-475.
12. Yuan J, Shen XZ, Zhu XS. Effect of berberine on transit time of human small intestine. *Chung Kuo Chung His I Chieh Ho Tsa Chih* 1994;14:718-720.
13. Amin AH, Subbaiah TV, Abbasi KM. Berberine sulfate: antimicrobial activity, bioassay, and mode of action. *Can J Microbiol* 1969;15:1067-1076.
14. Sun D, Abraham SN, Beachey EH. Influence of berberine sulfate on synthesis and expression of Pap fimbrial adhesin in uropathogenic *Escherichia coli*. *Antimicrob Agents Chemother* 1988;32:1274-1277.
15. Kaneda Y, Torii M, Tanaka T, Aikawa M. *In vitro* effects of berberine sulfate on the growth and structure of *Entamoeba histolytica*, *Giardia lamblia*, and *Trichomonas vaginalis*. *Ann Trop Med Parasitol* 1991;85:417-425.
16. Ghosh AK, Bhattacharyya FK, Ghosh DK. *Leismania donovani*: amastigote inhibition and mode of action of berberine. *Exp Parasitol* 1985;60:404-413.
17. Kaneda Y, Tanaka T, Saw T. Effects of berberine, a plant alkaloid, on the growth of anaerobic protozoa in axenic culture. *Tokai J Exp Clin Med* 1990;15:417-423.

18. Nair KP. Giardiasis in children. *Pediatric Clinics India* 1970;5:45.

19. Choudhry VP, Sabir M, Bhide VN. *Indian Pediatrics* 1972;9:143-146.

20. Subbaiah TV, Amin AH. Effect of berberine sulphate on *Entamoeba histolytica. Nature* 1967;215:527-528.

21. Babbar OP, Chhatwal VK, Ray IB, Mehra MK. Effect of berberine chloride eye drops on clinically positive trachoma patients. *Indian J Med Res* 1982;76:S83-S82.

22. Khosla PK, Neeraj VI, Gupta SK, Satpathy G. Berberine, a potential drug for trachoma. *Rev Int Trach Pathol Ocul Trop Subtrop Sante Publique* 1992;69:147-165.

23. Chun YT, Yip TT, Lau KL, Kong YC. A biochemical study on the hypotensive effect of berberine in rats. *Gen Pharmac* 1978;10:177-182.

24. Marin-Neto JA, Maciel BC, Secches AL, Gallo L. Cardiovascular effects of berberine in patients with severe congestive heart failure. *Clin Cardiol* 1988;11:253-260.

25. Wang YX, Yao XJ, Tan YH. Effects of berberine on delayed afterdepolarizations in ventricular muscles *in vitro* and *in vivo*. *J Cardiovasc Pharmacol* 1994;23:716-722.

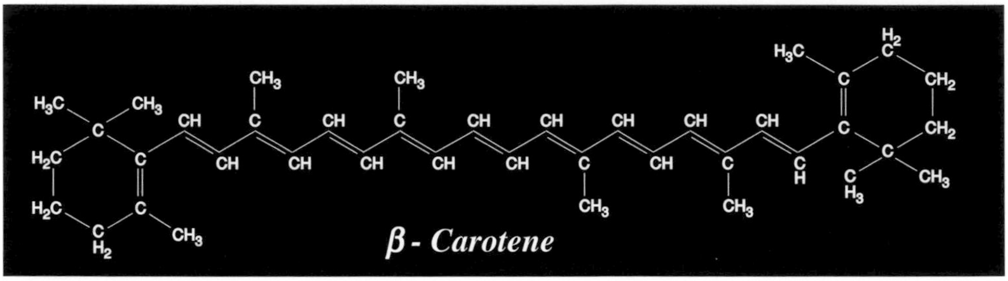

β - Carotene

Natural (Mixed cis/trans) Beta-Carotene

Introduction

Carotenes are a class of pigment molecules synthesized by plants. The human diet contains significant amounts of as many as 40 different carotenoid molecules, including alpha- and beta-carotene, lycopene, lutein, and zeaxanthin.

Mixed carotenes are a source of beta-carotene in a naturally occurring isomeric combination. Carotenes from an algal source (*Dunaliella bardawil*) contain 50-percent all-trans beta-carotene, with the other 50 percent consisting of 9-, 13-, 15-, and assorted di-cis forms.[1] Vegetable source mixed carotenes are slightly different, containing only 30 percent cis-isomers. Most dietary supplements contain a synthetic form of beta-carotene in the all-trans configuration.

Pharmacokinetics

Beta-carotene is readily absorbed in the small intestine. From there beta-carotene is either cleaved into two vitamin A molecules or it travels via the lymphatic system to the liver. Beta-carotene then travels in the serum to different target tissues. Levels of beta-carotene tend to be particularly high in specific tissues, including the liver, adrenals, and testes.[2]

The serum half-life of beta-carotene is thought to be quite long, estimated at 37 days in one study.[3] The major route of elimination of beta-carotene is the feces, although some appears to be eliminated in the urine as well.[4]

A 1989 absorption study indicated beta-carotene absorption varies three- to fourfold among healthy adults.[5] This study also found beta-carotene absorption was greater from a synthetic supplement than from carrots containing a similar amount of beta-carotene.

Because the serum concentrations of the cis-isomers of beta-carotene are less than five percent of the circulating pool,[2] the trans-isomer has been historically thought to be physiologically the most important isomer. However, the 9-, 13-, and 15-cis-isomers have been shown to make up 10-20 percent of beta-carotene at the tissue level.[2]

It is not entirely clear whether the cis- and trans-isomers of beta-carotene have different biochemical functions. One clinical trial concluded 9-cis beta-carotene was a more effective lipophilic antioxidant *in vivo*.[1]

Mechanisms of Action

There are several proposed mechanisms of action for beta-carotene. These include provitamin A activity, modulation of enzymes controlling inflammatory pathways, antioxidant activity, and modulation of genetic expression.[6]

As a fat-soluble antioxidant, beta-carotene scavenges singlet oxygen[7] and decreases lipid peroxidation.[8] As an immune modulator it has been found to increase CD4 counts, CD4/CD8 ratios, and total WBC counts.[9]

Beta-carotene may also act as a pro-oxidant, due to its long chain of double bonds that are susceptible to free radical attack. Its pro-oxidant effect may provide at least one of the mechanisms by which smokers taking beta-carotene (synthetic, all-trans) have a greater risk of developing lung cancer. Whether this same effect would occur with natural cis/trans beta-carotene supplementation is not known. One benefit of beta-carotene as a pro-oxidant may be its effect on tumor cells. Carotenes appear to act selectively as oxidizing agents on tumor cells by increasing production of heat shock proteins, ultimately enhancing tumor cytotoxicity.[10]

Clinical Indications

Asthma

Administration of 64 mg mixed carotenes from algae for one week reduced symptoms of exercise-induced asthma in 20 of 38 participants in a double-blind trial.[11] The algal preparation was well tolerated in this trial.

Cardiovascular Disease Prevention

Twenty patients with type 2 diabetes mellitus were supplemented for three weeks with 60 mg per day beta-carotene from algae. Compared to age- and sex-matched controls, supplementation with beta-carotene reduced the susceptibility of LDL to oxidation.[12] The authors of this study concluded natural source beta-carotene supplementation can delay development of atherosclerosis in the diabetic population.

Prevention of Vitamin A Deficiency Syndromes

The provitamin A activity of mixed carotenes from palm oil was compared to all-trans beta-carotene in a recent clinical trial.[13] Equivalent doses of the two carotene preparations led to similar increases in serum retinol levels. The authors concluded that given the other antioxidants in palm oil, together with its fatty acid profile, mixed carotenes from palm oil provide a good source of vitamin A fortification in foods.

Precancerous Conditions

In a clinical trial only reported in abstract form, 28 patients with premalignant changes in the gastric mucosa were randomized to receive either 30 mg natural mixed isomer beta-carotene, 30 mg of all-trans beta-carotene, or placebo for 180 days.[14] On repeat biopsy, significantly less inflammation was seen in patients taking the natural source beta-carotene compared to baseline. No significant benefit was seen with all-trans beta-carotene or placebo.

Miscellaneous Conditions

Most of the clinical trials using beta-carotene have used the all-trans form. With the notable exception of provitamin A activity, mixed isomeric beta-carotene has not been compared to all-trans beta-carotene as a suitable replacement. Mixed carotenes may, however, be useful for some of the conditions shown to respond to all-trans carotenes. These include oral leukoplakia,[15] photosensitivity,[16] and HIV[17] and other instances of compromised immune function.[18]

Drug-Nutrient Interactions

Cholesterol-lowering medications, such as cholestyramine and colestipol, and weight-loss medications that interfere with fat absorption, such as orlistat, may interfere with absorption of beta-carotene.[19]

Mineral oil, olestra, and pectin may also interfere with beta-carotene absorption.[19]

Side Effects and Toxicity

The acute and chronic toxicity of supplementation with carotenoids is generally considered to be quite low.[20] A benign and transient orange-yellowing of the skin, known as carotenemia, is sometimes seen in patients taking high doses of natural or synthetic beta-carotene.

Animal studies indicate a possible potentiation of the hepatotoxicity of alcohol by high doses of beta-carotene.[21] This has not been confirmed by human trials.

Dosage

Recommended dosages range from 15,000 IU to as high as 300,000 IU daily. Some studies report beta-carotene dosages in mgs rather than IUs (5,000 IU = 3 mg).

Warnings and Contraindications

The all-trans form of beta-carotene has been shown to increase the risk of lung cancer in two separate clinical trials.[22,23] This adverse effect appears to be confined to smokers.[24] The reason for this research finding is as yet unclear. It is also currently unknown if this effect would be seen with a natural source mixed-carotene supplement.

References

1. Ben-Amotz A, Levy Y. Bioavailability of a natural isomer mixture compared with synthetic all-trans beta-carotene in human serum. *Am J Clin Nutr* 1996;63:729-734.
2. Stahl W, Schwarz W, Sundquist AR, Sies H. Cis-trans isomers of lycopene and beta-carotene in human serum and tissues. *Arch Biochem Biophys* 1992;294:173-177.
3. Burri BJ, Neidlinger TR, Clifford AJ. Serum carotenoid depletion follows first-order kinetics in healthy adult women fed naturally low carotenoid diets. *J Nutr* 2001;131:2096-2100.
4. Dueker SR, Lin Y, Buchholz BA, et al. Long-term kinetic study of beta-carotene, using accelerator mass spectrometry in an adult volunteer. *J Lipid Res* 2000;41:1790-1800.
5. Brown ED, Micozzi MS, Craft NE, et al. Plasma carotenoids in normal men after a single ingestion of vegetables or purified beta-carotene. *Am J Clin Nutr* 1989;49:1258-1265.
6. Paiva SA, Russell RM. Beta-carotene and other carotenoids as antioxidants. *J Am Coll Nutr* 1999;18:426-433.
7. Bendich A, Olson JA. Biological actions of carotenoids. *FASEB J* 1989;3:1927-1932.
8. Favier A, Sappey C, Leclerc P, et al. Antioxidant status and lipid peroxidation in patients infected with HIV. *Chem Biol Interact* 1994;91:165-180.
9. Coodley GO, Nelson HD, Loveless MO, Folk C. Beta-carotene in HIV infection. *J Acquir Immune Defic Syndr* 1993;6:272-276.
10. Schwartz JL, Singh RP, Teicher B, et al. Induction of a 70 kD protein associated with the selective cytotoxicity of beta-carotene in human epidermal carcinoma. *Biochem Biophys Res Commun* 1990;169:941-946.
11. Neuman I, Nahum H, Ben-Amotz A. Prevention of exercise-induced asthma by a natural isomer mixture of beta-carotene. *Ann Allergy Asthma Immunol* 1999;82:549-553.
12. Levy Y, Zaltsberg H, Ben-Amotz A, et al. Dietary supplementation of a natural isomer mixture of beta-carotene inhibits oxidation of LDL derived from patients with diabetes mellitus. *Ann Nutr Metab* 2000;44:54-60.
13. van Stuijvenberg ME, Dhansay MA, Lombard CJ, et al. The effect of a biscuit with red palm oil as a source of beta-carotene on the vitamin A status of primary school children: a comparison with beta-carotene from a synthetic source in a randomised controlled trial. *Eur J Clin Nutr* 2001;55:657-662.
14. Yeum KJ, Zhu S, Xiao S, et al. Beta-carotene intervention trial in premalignant gastric lesions. *J Am Coll Nutr* 1995;14:536.
15. Garewal HS, Katz RV, Meyskens F, et al. Beta-carotene produces sustained remissions in patients with oral leukoplakia: results of a multicenter prospective trial. *Arch Otolaryngol Head Neck Surg* 1999;125:1305-1310.
16. Mathews-Roth MM. Carotenoids in erythropoietic protoporphyria and other photosensitivity diseases. *Ann N Y Acad Sci* 1993;691:127-138.
17. Patrick L. Nutrients and HIV: Part one – beta carotene and selenium. *Altern Med Rev* 1999;4:403-413.
18. Kazi N, Radvany R, Oldham T, et al. Immunomodulatory effect of beta-carotene on T lymphocyte subsets in patients with resected colonic polyps and cancer. *Nutr Cancer* 1997;28:140-145.
19. Hendler SS, Rorvik D. *PDR for Nutritional Supplements*, 1st ed. Des Moines, IA: Medical Economics – Thompson Healthcare; 2001.
20. Bendich A. The safety of beta-carotene. *Nutr Cancer* 1988;11:207-214.
21. Leo MA, Lieber CS. Alcohol, vitamin A, and beta-carotene: adverse interactions, including hepatotoxicity and carcinogenicity. *Am J Clin Nutr* 1999;69:1071-1085.
22. No authors listed. The effect of vitamin E and beta-carotene on the incidence of lung cancer and other cancers in male smokers. The Alpha-Tocopherol, Beta-Carotene Cancer Prevention Study Group. *N Engl J Med* 1994;330:1029-1035.
23. Omenn GS, Goodman GE, Thornquist MD, et al. Effects of a combination of beta-carotene and vitamin A on lung cancer and cardiovascular disease. *N Engl J Med* 1996;334:1150-1155.
24. Hennekens CH, Buring JE, Manson JE, et al. Lack of effect of long-term supplementation with beta carotene on the incidence of malignant neoplasms and cardiovascular disease. *N Engl J Med* 1996;334:1145-1149.

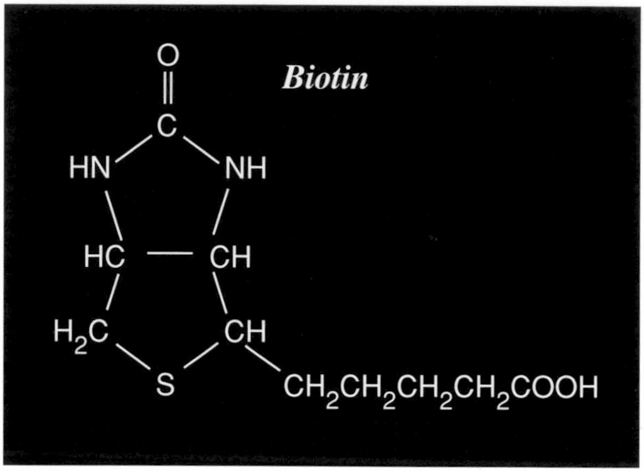

Biotin

Biotin

Introduction

Biotin is a water-soluble B-vitamin that is an essential cofactor for four carboxylase enzymes, each of which catalyzes an essential step in intermediary metabolism. Biotin is a bicyclic compound, one ring containing a ureido group (-N-CO-N-) and the other containing sulfur (a tetrahydrothiophene ring). Biotin was originally recognized when rats that were fed protein derived from egg whites developed severe dermatitis, hair loss, and neuromuscular dysfunction. A growth factor found in liver, then called "Protective Factor X," cured the condition. This growth factor is now known as biotin. It was later discovered that uncooked egg whites contain a glycoprotein called avidin, which binds to biotin and prevents its absorption, regardless of whether the biotin is from the diet or from intestinal bacteria synthesis.[1]

Biochemistry

The chemical structure of biotin was first elucidated in the early 1940s. Only one of eight possible stereoisomers of biotin is found in nature and is enzymatically active – d-(+)-biotin (or simply "D-biotin"). Mammals cannot synthesize biotin; thus, humans must derive biotin from dietary sources and *de novo* synthesis by intestinal bacteria. Biotin deficiency in humans is rare and generally associated with extended parenteral nutrition, consumption of large quantities of raw egg whites, severe malnutrition, or inborn errors of metabolism (e.g., biotinidase deficiency, multiple carboxylase deficiency). Studies of biotin status during pregnancy suggest marginal biotin deficiency occurs in a significant number of otherwise normal pregnancies, and that such a deficiency may be teratogenic.[2]

Pharmacokinetics

Oral biotin is completely absorbed, even at pharmacologic doses. Urinary excretion of biotin plus its metabolites is similar for oral supplementation at high doses and intravenous dosing, suggesting 100-percent bioavailability of orally administered biotin.[3] Percutaneous absorption of biotin from a biotin-containing ointment has been demonstrated in healthy subjects and in patients with atopic dermatitis.[4]

After transport from the intestines to the peripheral circulation biotin is taken up by the liver and eventually taken up into the central nervous system, across the blood-brain barrier by a saturable system.[5] In normal adults and children who are not receiving biotin supplements, the kidneys clear biotin and creatinine in a ratio of approximately 0.4.[1] Specific systems for transport of biotin from mother to fetus,[6-8] and from mother to infant via breastmilk,[9,10] have been described.

Mechanisms of Action

In humans, biotin is required as a prosthetic group for four major carboxylase enzymes involved in several critical metabolic pathways, including gluconeogenesis, fatty acid synthesis, and amino acid catabolism. All four carboxylase enzymes catalyze the incorporation of bicarbonate into a substrate as a carboxyl group. Three of these carboxylase enzymes are located in mitochondria; the fourth (acetyl-CoA carboxylase; ACC) is found in both cytosol and mitochondria. ACC catalyzes incorporation of bicarbonate into acetyl-CoA, and from there into malonyl Co-A. Malonyl Co-A subsequently acts as a substrate for fatty acid synthesis, with the effect of elongating the fatty acid chain. Other carboxylases, decarboxylases, and a transcarboxylase are also dependent on biotin as an enzyme cofactor.

Clinical Indications

Brittle Nails (onychoschizia)

Biotin has been used in veterinary medicine as a treatment for hoof disorders.[11] Although the mechanism is unknown, it is thought that biotin supplementation in humans improves brittle nails. In an uncontrolled trial,[12] 45 patients with brittle nails were treated with oral supplementation of 2.5 mg biotin per day for 1.5 to 7 months. Ninety-one percent showed "definite improvement," exhibiting firmer, harder nails after an average of two months of treatment. Another uncontrolled trial[13] reported a 63-percent response rate to biotin supplementation for brittle nails. In a controlled trial,[14] women with brittle nails who took 2.5 mg biotin per day for 6-15 months had increased nail thickness of 25 percent; nail splitting was also reduced.

Dermatitis

Deficiency of biotin causes alopecia and a characteristic scaly, erythematous dermatitis distributed around body orifices. The rash is similar to that of zinc deficiency. *Candida albicans* can often be cultured from the skin lesions. Reduced activities of the biotin-dependent carboxylases (particularly ACC) impair fatty acid metabolism and probably play an etiologic role in the dermatologic manifestations of biotin deficiency.[15] Dermatitis is a common feature among children with inherited biotinidase deficiency.[16] Seborrheic dermatitis in children with phenylketonuria has been associated with an impairment of biotin recycling.[17] However, although biotin deficiency can cause seborrheic dermatitis-like signs and symptoms, common infantile seborrheic dermatitis does not necessarily suggest biotin deficiency[18] or respond to biotin supplementation.[19] Further research is needed to demonstrate clinical efficacy of biotin supplements for non-deficiency related dermatitis.

Dyslipidemia

Animal[20,21] and human[22] data suggest poor biotin status adversely affects plasma lipid levels. In a double-blind trial,[23] healthy volunteers were given 900 mcg biotin per day for 71 days. Small, but statistically significant, positive changes in the lipid profile were observed for biotin-treated patients, as was an inverse association between biotin levels and total plasma lipids. Further clinical trials are needed to evaluate whether supplemental biotin can normalize cholesterol and lipoproteins in patients with dyslipidemia.

Diabetes

Biotin is thought to improve abnormal glucose metabolism by stimulating glucose-induced insulin secretion in pancreatic beta cells and by accelerating glycolysis in the liver and pancreas.[24] Administration of high-dose biotin has improved glycemic control in several diabetic animal models.[25] A Japanese study[26] found biotin levels to be lower in patients with non-insulin dependent diabetes than in healthy controls. Three milligrams of biotin three times per day orally for one month lowered fasting glucose levels by 45 percent; no effect on blood glucose levels was observed in those taking placebo. In another study,[27] patients with type 1 diabetes given 16 mg biotin per day for one week experienced reductions of 50 percent in fasting glucose levels. Biotin in high doses (10 mg/day intramuscularly for six weeks, followed by 5 mg per day orally for 64-130 weeks) was given to three diabetic patients suffering from severe diabetic peripheral neuropathy.[28] Within eight weeks a marked improvement in paresthesias and muscle cramps was observed, along with a disappearance of restless legs syndrome. There is also preliminary evidence that intravenous biotin (50 mg postdialysis) may normalize oral glucose tolerance tests in normoglycemic hemodialysis patients.[29]

Multiple Carboxylase Deficiency

Acquired biotin deficiency and the two known congenital disorders of biotin metabolism – biotinidase deficiency and holocarboxylase synthetase deficiency (HCS) – lead to deficiency of the four biotin-dependent carboxylase enzymes (i.e., to multiple carboxylase deficiency). The two inherited disorders of biotin metabolism, both discovered in the early 1980s, respond clinically and biochemically to oral biotin therapy. Ten milligrams of biotin per day is usually sufficient to treat severe biotinidase deficiency. The optimal biotin dose for patients with HCS deficiency is assessed on a case-by-case basis. If biotin therapy is initiated early and continued throughout life, the prognosis for both conditions is generally good. However, a delay in initiating therapy in biotinidase deficiency can cause irreversible neurological damage. In HCS deficiency, some patients respond only partially, even at doses of up to 100 mg biotin per day.[30]

Biotin-Responsive Basal Ganglia Disease

This novel condition has been described in 10 patients,[31] and presents with subacute encephalopathy and multiple neurologic symptoms. The etiology may be related to a defect in biotin transport across the blood-brain barrier. Biotin-responsive basal ganglia disease is reportedly responsive to biotin therapy.

Chronic Vaginal Candidiasis

A single case has been reported[32] of a 38-year-old female carrier of biotinidase deficiency who presented with a 14-month history of persistent vaginal candidiasis, despite therapy. After three months of pharmacologic doses of biotin, her symptoms resolved completely. The authors suggest, since one in every 123 people is thought to be a carrier of biotinidase deficiency, other women with chronic vaginal candidiasis might respond to biotin administration.

Sudden Infant Death Syndrome (SIDS)

Animal studies first suggested biotin deficiency might be a contributing factor in SIDS. On autopsy, levels of biotin in livers of 204 infants who had died of SIDS were significantly lower than those in livers of infants of similar age who had died of known causes.[33] No research has explored the effects of maternal or infant biotin supplementation on the incidence of the condition.

Uremic Neurologic Disorders

Encephalopathy and peripheral neuropathy commonly develop in uremic patients on hemodialysis. Nine such patients were treated with biotin (10 mg per day orally). Within three months, all nine patients experienced marked improvements that were maintained in six of the nine patients in the ensuing 15-25 months of follow-up (the other three died of renal failure).[34] Hemodialysis is thought to deplete biotin, which may in turn be responsible for neurologic symptoms that accompany severe uremia.

Drug-Nutrient Interactions

At least four studies have shown long-term therapy with anticonvulsants (e.g., phenobarbital, phenytoin, carbemazepine, primidone) depletes plasma concentrations of biotin.[35-38] This depletion is demonstrated by increased urinary 3-hydroxyisovaleric acid. Isotretinoin therapy impairs biotinidase activity, but the effect on biotin levels is unclear.[39] Since biotin is known to affect glucose regulation, theoretical drug interactions exist with glyburide, insulin or any other drug used to control blood glucose levels.

Side Effects and Toxicity

No toxicity of biotin has been reported in individuals who have received as much as 200 mg orally or 20 mg intravenously per day.[1]

Dosage

For brittle nails, 2.5 mg per day has been used successfully. For dyslipidemia, 900 mcg per day has been suggested, but no data exist to confirm the effectiveness of that dose in hyperlipidemic individuals. For type 2 diabetes, 9 mg per day has been used; for type 1 diabetes, 16 mg per day has been used. These are massive doses and may not be necessary to achieve the desired effects on glucose metabolism. However, no other data exist to suggest an alternative dose. For uremic neurologic disorders, 10 mg per day has been used with good results. For biotinidase deficiency, 10 mg per day has been used with success, but the supplement must be continued lifelong. Optimal daily intake of biotin remains speculative.[1]

References

1. Mock DM. Biotin. In: Ziegler EE, Filer LJ, eds. *Present Knowledge in Nutrition*, 7th ed. Washington, DC: ILSI Press; 1996:220-235.
2. Zempleni J, Mock DM. Marginal biotin deficiency is teratogenic. *Proc Soc Exp Biol Med* 2000;223:14-21.
3. Zempleni J, Mock DM. Bioavailability of biotin given orally to humans in pharmacologic doses. *Am J Clin Nutr* 1999;69:504-508.
4. Makino Y, Osada K, Sone H, et al. Percutaneous absorption of biotin in healthy subjects and in atopic dermatitis patients. *J Nutr Sci Vitaminol (Tokyo)* 1999;45:347-352.
5. Spector R, Mock DM. Biotin transport through the blood-brain barrier. *J Neurochem* 1987;48:400-404.
6. Karl PI, Fisher SE. Biotin transport in microvillous membrane vesicles, cultured trophoblasts, and isolated perfused human placenta. *Am J Physiol* 1992;262:C302-C308.
7. Schenker S, Hu ZQ, Johnson RF, et al. Human placental biotin transport: normal characteristics and effect of ethanol. *Alcohol Clin Exp Res* 1993;17:566-575.
8. Hu ZQ, Henderson GI, Mock DM, Schenker S. Biotin uptake by basolateral membrane vesicles of human placenta: normal characteristics and role of ethanol. *Proc Soc Exp Biol Med* 1994;206:404-408.
9. Mock DM, Mock NI, Dankle JA. Secretory patterns of biotin in human milk. *J Nutr* 1992;122:546-552.
10. Stratton S, Mock NI, Mock DM. Biotin and biotin metabolites in human milk: the metabolites are not negligible. *J Invest Med* 1996;44:58A.

11. Campbell JR, Greenough PR, Petrie L. The effects of dietary biotin supplementation on vertical fissures of the claw wall in beef cattle. *Can Vet J* 2000;41:690-694.

12. Floersheim GL. Treatment of brittle fingernails with biotin. *Z Hautkr* 1989;64:41-48. [Article in German]

13. Hochman LG, Scher RK, Meyerson MS. Brittle nails: response to daily biotin supplementation. *Cutis* 1993;51:303-305.

14. Colombo VE, Gerber F, Bronhofer M, Floersheim GL. Treatment of brittle fingernails and onychoschizia with biotin: scanning electron microscopy. *J Am Acad Dermatol* 1990;23:1127-1132.

15. Mock DM. Skin manifestations of biotin deficiency. *Semin Dermatol* 1991;10:296-302.

16. Coskun T, Tokatli A, Ozalp I. Inborn errors of biotin metabolism. Clinical and laboratory features of eight cases. *Turk J Pediatr* 1994;36:267-278.

17. Schulpis KH, Nyalala JO, Papakonstantinou ED, et al. Biotin recycling impairment in phenylketonuric children with seborrheic dermatitis. *Int J Dermatol* 1998;37:918-921.

18. Erlichman M, Goldstein R, Levi E, et al. Infantile flexural seborrhoeic dermatitis. Neither biotin nor essential fatty acid deficiency. *Arch Dis Child* 1981;56:560-562.

19. Keipert JA. Oral use of biotin in seborrhoeic dermatitis of infancy: a controlled trial. *Med J Aust* 1976;1:584-585.

20. Suchy SF, Wolf B. Effect of biotin deficiency and supplementation on lipid metabolism in rats: cholesterol and lipoproteins. *Am J Clin Nutr* 1986;43:831-838.

21. Marshall MW, Haubrich M, Washington VA, et al. Biotin status and lipid metabolism in adult obese hypercholesterolemic inbred rats. *Nutr Metab* 1976;20:41-61.

22. Mock DM, Johnson SB, Holman RT. Effects of biotin deficiency on serum fatty acid composition: evidence for abnormalities in humans. *J Nutr* 1988;118:342-348.

23. Marshall MW, Kliman PG, Washington VA, et al. Effects of biotin on lipids and other constituents of plasma of healthy men and women. *Artery* 1980;7:330-351.

24. Furukawa Y. Enhancement of glucose-induced insulin secretion and modification of glucose metabolism by biotin. *Nippon Rinsho* 1999;57:2261-2269. [Article in Japanese]

25. Zhang H, Osada K, Sone H, Furukawa Y. Biotin administration improves the impaired glucose tolerance of streptozotocin-induced diabetic Wistar rats. *J Nutr Sci Vitaminol (Tokyo)* 1997;43:271-280.

26. Maebashi M, Makino Y, Furukawa Y, et al. Therapeutic evaluation of the effect of biotin on hyperglycemia in patients with non-insulin dependent diabetes mellitus. *J Clin Biochem Nutr* 1993;14:211-218.

27. Coggeshall JC, Heggers JP, Robson MC, Baker H. Biotin status and plasma glucose in diabetics. *Ann N Y Acad Sci* 1985;447:389-392.

28. Koutsikos D, Agroyannis B, Tzanatos-Exarchou H. Biotin for diabetic peripheral neuropathy. *Biomed Pharmacother* 1990;44:511-514.

29. Koutsikos D, Fourtounas C, Kapetanaki A, et al. Oral glucose tolerance test after high-dose i.v. biotin administration in normoglucemic hemodialysis patients. *Ren Fail* 1996;18:131-137.

30. Baumgartner ER, Suormala T. Multiple carboxylase deficiency: inherited and acquired disorders of biotin metabolism. *Int J Vitam Nutr Res* 1997;67:377-384.

31. Ozand PT, Gascon GG, Al Essa M, et al. Biotin-responsive basal ganglia disease: a novel entity. *Brain* 1998;121:1267-1279.

32. Strom CM, Levine EM. Chronic vaginal candidiasis responsive to biotin therapy in a carrier of biotinidase deficiency. *Obstet Gynecol* 1998;92:644-646.

33. Johnson AR, Hood RL, Emery JL. Biotin and the sudden infant death syndrome. *Nature* 1980;285:159-160.

34. Yatzidis H, Koutsicos D, Agroyannis B, et al. Biotin in the management of uremic neurologic disorders. *Nephron* 1984;36:183-186.

35. Krause KH, Bonjour JP, Berlit P, Kochen W. Biotin status of epileptics. *Ann N Y Acad Sci* 1985;447:297-313.

36. Krause KH, Bonjour JP, Berlit P, et al. Effect of long-term treatment with antiepileptic drugs on the vitamin status. *Drug Nutr Interact* 1988;5:317-343.

37. Mock DM, Dyken ME. Biotin catabolism is accelerated in adults receiving long-term therapy with anticonvulsants. *Neurology* 1997;49:1444-1447.

38. Mock DM, Mock NI, Nelson RP, Lombard KA. Disturbances in biotin metabolism in children undergoing long-term anticonvulsant therapy. *J Pediatr Gastroenterol Nutr* 1998;26:245-250.

39. Schulpis KH, Georgala S, Papakonstantinou ED, et al. The effect of isotretinoin on biotinidase activity. *Skin Pharmacol Appl Skin Physiol* 1999;12:28-33.

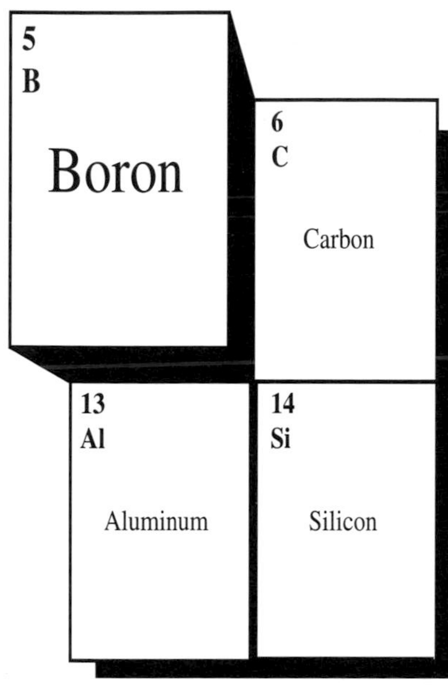

Boron

Introduction

Elemental boron was first isolated in 1808. Although it has yet to be recognized as an essential nutrient in humans, recent data from animal and human studies suggest boron may be important for mineral metabolism, brain function and performance, hormone regulation, and prevention of osteoporosis and osteoarthritis.

Daily intake of boron is dependent on concentration of boron in water supplies and food sources. Average daily intakes have been approximated at just over 2 mg per day in several population studies; however, chronic intakes of as much as 40 mg per day occur in some populations.[1,2]

Pharmacokinetics

Boron appears to be readily and completely absorbed in humans following an oral dose.[3] Following absorption, boron appears to concentrate to a higher degree in bone than in blood;[3] however, cessation of dietary boron results in a rapid drop in bone boron levels.[4]

There is no evidence for boron accumulation in tissue over time at normal dietary or supplemental levels. Tissue homeostasis is maintained by the rapid elimination of excess boron, primarily in the urine; with bile, sweat, and exhaled breath also routes of elimination.[5]

As dietary intake of boron increases, urinary excretion, and fecal excretion to a lesser degree, increase concomitantly, accounting for elimination of nearly 100 percent of boron intake. Urinary boron excretion rate changes rapidly subsequent to changes in boron intake, suggesting the kidney is the primary site of homeostatic regulation. At a dose of 10 g per day boron, 84 percent of the supplemented dose is recovered in the urine.[6] The half-life for elimination is approximately 21 hours, whether boron is administered orally or intravenously in healthy human subjects.[3]

Mechanism of Action

Boron complexes with organic compounds containing hydroxyl groups, sugars and polysaccharides, adenosine-5-phosphate, pyridoxine, riboflavin, dehydroascorbic acid, and pyridine nucleotides.[5]

Boron appears to have significant nutrient-nutrient metabolic interactions. Nutrients known to have some degree of interaction with boron under experimental conditions include vitamin D,[7-9] calcium,[9-12] magnesium,[4,10,12-14] phosphorous,[11,14] copper,[9,15] methionine,[16] and arginine.[16]

Boron impacts steroid hormone metabolism in humans, affecting the levels of estrogens and testosterone.[11] It has been hypothesized that boron interacts with steroid hormones by facilitating hydroxylation reactions and possibly by acting in some manner to protect steroid hormones from rapid degradation.[11]

Deficiency States

Information on boron deficiency in humans is minimal; however, it appears a deficiency in boron impacts mineral metabolism, cognitive function, growth, steroid hormone and vitamin levels, and bone integrity.[17]

Clinical Applications

Anemia

Boron supplementation to subjects who had previously followed a dietary regimen deficient in boron resulted in increases in blood hemoglobin concentrations, mean corpuscular hemoglobin and mean corpuscular hemoglobin concentration, and decreases in hematocrit, red cell count and platelet count.[18]

Osteo- and Rheumatoid Arthritis

In a double-blind, placebo-controlled trial of 20 subjects with osteoarthritis, half of the subjects receiving a daily supplement containing 6 mg boron noted subjective improvement in their condition.[19]

Clinical commentary suggests children with juvenile arthritis (Still's disease) improve with boron supplementation (6-9 mg per day).[20]

Individuals with rheumatoid arthritis might experience an aggravation of symptoms (Herxheimer response) for 1-3 weeks, but generally notice improvement within four weeks of beginning boron supplementation (6-9 mg per day).[20]

Cognitive Function

Collectively, data indicate that boron might play a role in human brain function, alertness, and cognitive performance. In humans, low boron intake has been shown to result in a decrease in the proportion of power in the alpha band and an increase in the proportion of power in the delta band.[21] These changes in brain electrical patterns are similar to those observed in nonspecific malnutrition.[22]

When contrasted with high boron intake, low dietary boron results in significantly poorer performance on tasks emphasizing manual dexterity, eye-hand coordination, attention, perception, encoding, and short- and long-term memory.[21]

Kidney Stones

Decreased total urinary oxalate has been noted following boron supplementation, leading some researchers to suggest a potential role in control of urolithiasis.[10]

Osteoporosis

There is evidence that compositional and functional properties of bone, as well as mineral status required for bone health, are affected by boron status with a worsening under circumstances of boron deprivation.[11,23] Animals with a magnesium deficiency appear to have an increased need for boron as well. In two human studies boron deprivation was associated with decreased plasma calcium and calcitonin and increased urinary calcium excretion.[23]

Steroid Hormone Regulation

The role of boron supplementation on sex hormone status is not completely understood; however, increased levels of sex steroids have been demonstrated in males and females after boron supplementation. Repletion of dietary boron by increasing intake from 0.25 to 3.25 mg per day has been reported to increase plasma 17 beta-estradiol by more than 50 percent and to more than double plasma testosterone levels in postmenopausal women.[11]

Supplementation with 10 mg boron per day for four weeks increased plasma estradiol concentrations significantly, with a trend for increased plasma testosterone levels, in healthy male subjects.[24]

Side Effects and Toxicity

Although boron is potentially toxic, and in the form of boric acid and borax has been used as a pesticide and food preservative, higher animals usually do not accumulate boron because of the ability to rapidly excrete it.[25]

A "No Observed Adverse Effect Level" and "Lowest Observed Adverse Effect Level" have been established based on animal models at 55 and 76 mg of boron (as boric acid) per kg body weight per day, respectively.[4] This is equivalent to an average-sized adult ingesting over 3 g boric acid (5 g borax) daily before reaching the "No Observed Adverse Effect Level" threshold.[26]

Subjects given 270 mg of boric acid orally reported no discomfort and showed no obvious signs of toxicity.[27] A fatal outcome has been reported following ingestion by a child of 1 g boric acid; however, adults have survived acute intakes of nearly 300 grams.[28]

Indications of acute boron toxicity include nausea, as well as vomiting and diarrhea blue-green in color.[28] Symptoms of chronic intoxication include anorexia, gastrointestinal disturbances, debility, confusion, dermatitis, menstrual disorders, anemia, convulsions, and alopecia.[29]

Dosage

No daily allowance for boron intake is established; however, the common supplemental dose of boron ranges from 3-9 mg per day.

References

1. Naghii MR, Lyons PM, Samman S. The boron content of selected foods and the estimation of its daily intake among free-living subjects. *J Amer Coll Nutr* 1996;15:614-619.
2. Samman S, Naghii MR, Lyons PM, Verus AP. The nutritional and metabolic effects of boron in humans and animals. *Biol Trace Elem Res* 1998;66:227-235.
3. Murray FJ. A comparative review of the pharmacokinetics of boric acid in rodents and humans. *Biol Trace Elem Res* 1998;66:331-341.
4. Moseman RF. Chemical disposition of boron in animals and humans. *Environ Health Perspect* 1994;102 Suppl 7:113-117.
5. Zittle CA. Reaction of borate with substances of biological interest. *Adv Enzymol* 1951;12:493-527.
6. Sutherland B, Strong P, King JC. Determining human dietary requirements for boron. *Biol Trace Elem Res* 1998;66:193-204.
7. Dupre JN, Keenan MJ, Hegsted M, et al. Effects of dietary boron in rats fed a vitamin D-deficient diet. *Environ Health Perspect* 1994;102 Suppl 7:55-58.
8. Hunt CD, Herbel JL, Idso JP. Dietary boron modifies the effects of vitamin D3 nutrition on indices of energy substrate utilization and mineral metabolism in the chick. *J Bone Miner Res* 1994;9:171-182.
9. Nielsen FH, Shuler TR, Gallagher SK. Effects of boron depletion and repletion on blood indicators of calcium status in humans fed a magnesium-low diet. *J Trace Elem Exp Med* 1990;3:45-54.
10. Hunt CD, Herbel JL, Nielsen FH. Metabolic responses of postmenopausal women to supplemental dietary boron and aluminum during usual and low magnesium intake: boron, calcium, and magnesium absorption and retention and blood mineral concentrations. *Am J Clin Nutr* 1997;65:803-813.
11. Nielsen FH, Hunt CD, Mullen LM, et al. Effect of dietary boron on mineral, estrogen, and testosterone metabolism in postmenopausal women. *FASEB J* 1987;1:394-397.
12. Beattie JH, Peace HS. The influence of a low-boron diet and boron supplementation on bone, major mineral and sex steroid metabolism in postmenopausal women. *Br J Nutr* 1993;69:871-884.
13. Hunt CD. Dietary boron modified the effects of magnesium and molybdenum on mineral metabolism in the cholecalciferol-deficient chick. *Biol Trace Elem Res* 1989;22:201-220.
14. Meacham SL, Taper LJ, Volpe SL. Effects of boron supplementation on bone mineral density and dietary, blood, and urinary calcium, phosphorus, magnesium, and boron in female athletes. *Environ Health Perspect* 1994;102 Suppl 7:79-82.
15. Nielsen FH. Biochemical and physiologic consequences of boron deprivation in humans. *Environ Health Perspect* 1994;102 Suppl 7:59-63.
16. Nielsen FH, Shuler TR, Zimmerman TJ, et al. Magnesium and methionine deprivation affect the response of rats to boron deprivation. *Biol Trace Elem Res* 1988;17:91-107.

17. Nielsen FH. New essential trace elements for the life sciences. *Biol Trace Elem Res* 1990;26-27:599-611.

18. Nielsen FH, Mullen LM, Nielsen EJ. Dietary boron affects blood cell counts and hemoglobin concentrations in humans. *J Trace Elem Exp Med* 1991;4:211-223.

19. Travers RL, Rennie GC, Newnham RE. Boron and arthritis: the result of a double-blind pilot study. *J Nutr Med* 1990;1:127-132.

20. Newnham RE. The role of boron in human nutrition. *J Appl Nutr* 1994;46:81-85.

21. Penland JG. Dietary boron, brain function, and cognitive performance. *Environ Health Perspect* 1994;102 Suppl 7:65-72.

22. Penland JG. The importance of boron nutrition for brain and psychological function. *Biol Trace Elem Res* 1998;66:299-317.

23. Nielsen FH. Studies on the relationship between boron and magnesium which possibly affects the formation and maintenance of bones. *Mag Trace Elem* 1990;9:61-69.

24. Naghii MR, Samman S. The effect of boron supplementation on its urinary excretion and selected cardiovascular risk factors in healthy male subjects. *Biol Trace Elem Res* 1997;56:273-286.

25. Loomis WD, Durst RW. Chemistry and biology of boron. *Biofactors* 1992;3:229-239.

26. Hubbard SA. Comparative toxicology of borates. *Biol Trace Elem Res* 1998;66:343-357.

27. Jansen J, Schou JS, Aggerbeck B. Gastro-intestinal absorption and *in vitro* release of boric acid from water emulsifying agents. *Food Chem Toxicol* 1984;22:49-53.

28. Von Burg R. Boron, boric acid, and boron oxide. *J Appl Toxicol* 1992;12:149-152.

29. Nielsen FH. Ultratrace minerals: Boron. In: Shils ME, Young VR, eds. *Modern Nutrition in Health and Disease*. Philadelphia, PA: Lea & Febiger; 1988:281-283.

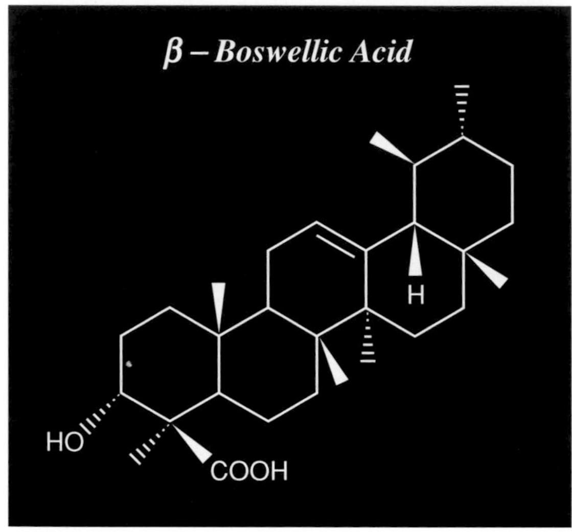

Boswellia serrata

Description

Boswellia serrata (also known as frankincense) is a moderate to large branching tree (growing to a height of about 12 feet) found in India, Northern Africa, and the Middle East. Strips of Boswellia bark are peeled away, yielding a gummy oleo-resin. Extracts of this gummy exudate have been traditionally used in the Ayurvedic system of medicine as an anti-arthritic, astringent, stimulant, expectorant, and antiseptic.

Active Constituents

Boswellia contains oils, terpenoids, sugars, and volatile oils. Up to 16 percent of the resin is essential oil, the majority being alpha-thujene and p-cymene. Four pentacyclic triterpene acids are also present, with beta-boswellic acid being the major constituent.

Mechanisms of Action

Animal studies performed in India showed ingestion of a defatted alcoholic extract of Boswellia decreased polymorphonuclear leukocyte infiltration and migration, decreased primary antibody synthesis,[1,2] and caused almost total inhibition of the classical complement pathway.[3] In an *in vitro* study of the effects of beta-boswellic acid on the complement system, the extract demonstrated a marked inhibitory effect on both the classical and alternate complement systems.[4] An investigation of Boswellia's analgesic and psychopharmacologic effects noted that it had marked sedative and analgesic effects in animal models.[5]

In vitro testing revealed Boswellia specifically, and in a dose-dependent manner, blocks the synthesis of pro-inflammatory 5-lipoxygenase products, including 5-hydroxyeicosatetraenoic acid (5-HETE) and leukotriene B4 (LTB4),[6] which cause bronchoconstriction, chemotaxis, and increased vascular permeability.[7] Other anti-inflammatory plant constituents, such as quercetin, also block this enzyme, but they do so in a more general fashion, as an antioxidant; whereas, Boswellia seems to be a specific inhibitor of 5-lipoxygenase.[8,9]

Boswellia has been observed to inhibit human leukocyte elastase (HLE), which may be involved in the pathogenesis of emphysema. HLE also stimulates mucus secretion and thus may play a role in cystic fibrosis, chronic bronchitis, and acute respiratory distress syndrome.[10,11] Boswellic acids from *Boswellia serrata* also have an inhibitory effect against the cellular growth of leukemia HL-60 cells.[12]

Non-steroidal anti-inflammatory drugs can cause a disruption of glycosaminoglycan synthesis, accelerating the articular damage in arthritic conditions.[13-16] A recent *in vivo* study examined Boswellia extract and ketoprofen for their effects on glycosaminoglycan metabolism. Boswellia significantly reduced the degradation of glycosaminoglycans compared to controls; whereas, ketoprofen caused a decrease in total tissue glycosaminoglycan content.[17]

Clinical Indications

Human clinical studies are minimal for this substance, and more need to be conducted to better elucidate its effects in humans, as well as to determine optimal dosing. Animal and *in vitro* studies suggest it is useful for a number of inflammatory and bronchoconstrictive conditions.

Ulcerative colitis

Leukotrienes are suggested to play a role in the inflammatory process of ulcerative colitis. Boswellia extract (350 mg three times daily) was compared to sulfasalazine (1 g three times daily) in ulcerative colitis patients. Patients on the Boswellia extract showed better improvements than patients on sulfasalazine; 82 percent of Boswellia patients went into remission, compared with 75 percent on sulfasalazine.[18]

A follow-up study of chronic colitis patients on gum resin of Boswellia (900 mg daily divided in three doses for six weeks) and sulfasalazine (3 g daily divided in three doses for six weeks) once again showed similar improvements. Furthermore, 14 of 20 patients (70%) treated with *Boswellia serrata* gum resin went into remission while only 4 of 10 patients (40%) treated with sulfasalazine went into remission.[19]

Crohn's Disease

Chemical mediators of inflammation were further addressed in a clinical trial comparing a *Boswellia serrata* extract with mesalazine in the treatment of acute Crohn's disease. The protocol population included 44 patients treated with Boswellia extract and 39 patients treated with mesalazine. Between enrollment and end of therapy, the Crohn's Disease Activity Index (CDAI) decreased significantly with both Boswellia extract and mesalazine. Although the difference between the two treatments was not statistically significant, the Boswellia extract proved to be as effective as the pharmaceutical.[20]

Asthma

In a 1998 study of Boswellia's effects on bronchial asthma, 40 patients took 300 mg of a Boswellia preparation three times daily for six weeks. Seventy percent of the asthma patients taking Boswellia had a significant improvement in their disease, measured by symptomatology as well as objective measures of lung and immune function. Only 27 percent of patients taking a placebo improved.[21]

Arthritis

While no studies on Boswellia alone have been conducted on osteoarthritis, a study on a combination formula provided positive results. A formula containing Boswellia, ashwagandha, turmeric, and zinc was evaluated in a double-blind, placebo-controlled, crossover study.[22] Forty-two patients received either the herbal-mineral formulation or placebo for three months; then switched to the other protocol after a 15-day washout period for another three months. The treatment group experienced significant decreases in pain severity ($p<0.001$) and disability scores ($p<0.05$). Radiological evaluation found no significant changes in either group.

A placebo (n=19) versus Boswellia (n=18) study in patients with rheumatoid arthritis found no significant differences between the two groups in any measured parameters. NSAID dosage decreased 5.8 percent in the treatment group and 3.1 percent in the placebo group.[23] The researchers concluded that controlled studies including a greater number of subjects are warranted.

Side Effects and Toxicity

Toxicity studies of Boswellia in rats and primates showed no pathological changes in hematological, biochemical, or histological parameters at doses of up to 1000 mg/kg. The LD_{50} was established at >2 g/kg.[24]

Dosage

For inflammatory or asthmatic conditions, 300-400 mg of a standardized extract (containing 60% boswellic acids) three times daily is suggested.

References

1. Sharma ML, Khajuria A, Kaul A, et al. Effect of salai guggal ex-*Boswellia serrata* on cellular and humoral immune responses and leukocyte migration. *Agents Actions* 1988;24:161-164.
2. Sharma ML, Bani S, Singh GB, et al. Anti-arthritic activity of boswellic acids in bovine serum albumin (BSA) - induced arthritis. *Int J Immunopharmacol* 1989;11:647-652.
3. Wagner H. Search for new plant constituents with potential antiphlogistic and antiallergic activity. *Planta Med* 1989;55:235-241.

4. Knaus U, Wagner H. Effects of boswellic acid of *Boswellia serrata* and other triterpenic acids on the complement system. *Phytomedicine* 1996;3:77-81.

5. Menon MK, Karr A. Analgesic and psychopharmacological effects of the gum resin of *Boswellia serrata*. *Planta Med* 1971;4:332-341.

6. Ammon HP, Mack T, Singh GB, Safayhi H. Inhibition of leukotriene B4 formation in rat peritoneal neutrophils by an ethanolic extract of the gum resin exudate of *Boswellia serrata*. *Planta Med* 1991;57:203-207.

7. Robertson RP. Arachidonic acid metabolites relevant to medicine. In: Braunwald E, Isselbacher KJ, Petersdorf RG, et al, eds. *Harrison's Principles of Internal Medicine*. 11th ed. New York. McGraw-Hill;1987:375.

8. Safayhi H, Mack T, Sabieral J, et al. Boswellic acids: novel, specific nonredox inhibitors of 5-lipoxygenase. *J Pharmacol Exp Ther* 1992;261:1143-1146.

9. Ammon HPT. Salai guggal – *Boswellia serrata*: from a herbal medicine to a specific inhibitor of leukotriene biosynthesis. *Phytomedicine* 1996;3:67-70.

10. Rall B, Ammon HPT, Safayhi H. Boswellic acids and protease activities. *Phytomedicine* 1996;3:75-76.

11. Safayhi H, Rall B, Sailer ER, Ammon HPT. Inhibition by boswellic acids of human leukocyte elastase. *J Pharmacol Exp Ther* 1997;281:460-463.

12. Shao Y, Ho CT, Chin CK, et al. Inhibitory activity of boswellic acids from *Boswellia serrata* against human leukemia HL-60 cells in culture. *Planta Med* 1998;64:328-331.

13. Lee KH, Spencer MR. Studies on mechanism of action of salicylates V: Effect of salicylic acid on enzymes involved in mucopolysaccharide synthesis. *J Pharmacol Sci* 1969;58:464-468.

14. Palmoski MJ, Brandt KD. Effect of salicylate on proteoglycan metabolism in normal canine articular cartilage *in vitro*. *Arthritis Rheum* 1979;22:746-754.

15. Dekel S, Falconer J, Francis MJO. The effect of anti-inflammatory drugs on glycosaminoglycan sulphation in pig cartilage. *Prostaglandins Med* 1980;4:133-140.

16. Brandt KD, Palmoski MJ. Effect of salicylates and other non-steroidal anti-inflammatory drugs on articular cartilage. *Am J Med* 1984;77:65-69.

17. Reddy GK, Chandraksan G, Dhar SC. Studies on the metabolism of glycosaminoglycans under the influence of new herbal anti-inflammatory agents. *Biochem Pharm* 1989;38:3527-3534.

18. Gupta I, Parihar A, Malhotra P, et al. Effects of *Boswellia serrata* gum resin in patients with ulcerative colitis. *Eur J Med Res* 1997;2:37-43.

19. Gupta I, Parihar A, Malhotra P, et al. Effects of gum resin of *Boswellia serrata* in patients with chronic colitis. *Planta Med* 2001;67:391-395.

20. Gerhardt H, Seifert F, Buvari P, et al.Therapy of active Crohn disease with *Boswellia serrata* extract H 15. *Z Gastroenterol* 2001;39:11-17.

21. Gupta I, Gupta V, Parihar A, et al. Effects of *Boswellia serrata* gum resin in patients with bronchial asthma: results of a double-blind, placebo-controlled, 6-week clinical study. *Eur J Med Res* 1998;3:511-514.

22. Kulkarni RR, Patki PS, Jog VP, et al. Treatment of osteoarthritis with a herbmineral formulation: a double-blind, placebo-controlled, cross-over study. *J Ethnopharmacol* 1991;33:91-95.

23. Sander O, Herborn G, Rau R. Is H15 (resin extract of *Boswellia serrata*, "incense") a useful supplement to established drug therapy of chronic polyarthritis? Results of a double-blind pilot study. *Z Rheumatol* 1998;57:11-16. [Article in German]

24. Singh GB, Atal CK. Pharmacology of an extract of salai guggal ex-*Boswellia serrata*, a new non-steroidal anti-inflammatory agent. *Agents Actions* 1986;18:407-412.

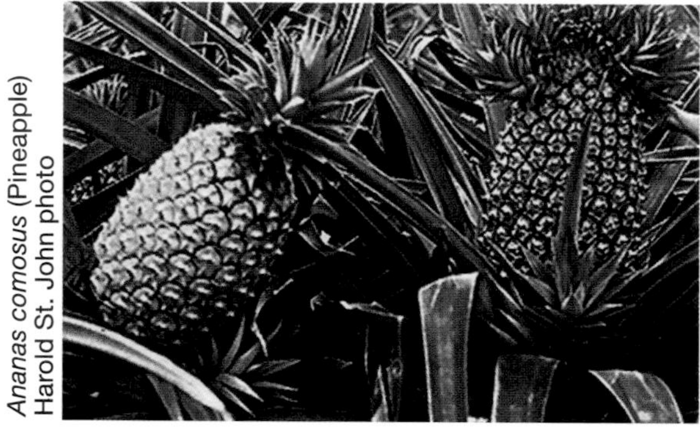
Ananas comosus (Pineapple)
Harold St. John photo

Bromelain

Description and Constituents

Bromelain is a general name for a family of sulfhydryl-containing proteolytic enzymes obtained from *Ananas comosus*, the pineapple plant. Bromelain's primary constituent is a sulfhydryl proteolytic fraction. Bromelain also contains peroxidase, acid phosphatase, several protease inhibitors, and organically-bound calcium. It appears a great deal of the physiological activity of bromelain cannot be accounted for by its proteolytic fraction and that the beneficial effects of bromelain are due to multiple constituents.

A variety of designations have been used to indicate the activity of bromelain, with published research varying in the designation utilized. Rorer units (r.u.), gelatin dissolving units (g.d.u.), and milk clotting units (m.c.u.) are the most commonly used measures of activity. One gram of bromelain standardized to 2,000 m.c.u would be approximately equal to one gram with 1,200 g.d.u. activity or eight grams with 100,000 r.u. activity.

Pharmacokinetics

In a rat study, bromelain was absorbed intact through the gastrointestinal tract, with up to 40 percent of the high molecular weight substances detected in the blood after oral administration. The highest concentration of bromelain was found in the blood one hour after administration; however, its proteolytic activity was rapidly deactivated.[1]

Mechanisms of Action

Bromelain's anti-inflammatory activity appears to be due to a variety of physiological actions. Evidence indicates bromelain's action is in part a result of inhibiting the generation of bradykinin at the inflammatory site via depletion of the plasma kallikrein system, as well as limiting the formation of fibrin by reduction of clotting cascade intermediates.[2-4] Bromelain has also been shown to stimulate conversion of plasminogen to plasmin, resulting in increased fibrinolysis.[4]

Bromelain might be capable of selectively modulating the biosynthesis of thromboxanes and prostacyclins, two groups of prostaglandins with opposite actions that ultimately influence activation of cyclic-3,5-adenosine, an important cell-growth modulating compound. It is hypothesized that bromelain therapy leads to a relative increase of the endogenous prostaglandins, PGI2 and PGE2, over thromboxane A2.[5]

Bromelain has been shown to decrease aggregation of blood platelets.[6] It is an effective fibrinolytic agent *in vitro* and *in vivo*; however, its effect is more evident in purified fibrinogen solutions than in plasma.[7]

Clinical Indications

Cancer

Several animal and human studies indicate bromelain might have some antimetastatic ability.[8-10] In doses over 1,000 mg daily, bromelain has been combined with chemotherapeutic agents such as 5-FU and vincristine, resulting in tumor regression.[8,11]

Immune Modulation

Bromelain can induce cytokine production in human peripheral blood mononuclear cells. Treatment leads to activation of natural killer cells and to the production of tumor necrosis factor-alpha, interleukin-1-beta, and interleukin-6 in a time- and dose-dependent manner.[12,13] Bromelain has also been shown to remove T-cell CD44 adhesion molecules from lymphocytes and to affect T-cell activation.[14]

Wound Debridement

Bromelain applied topically as a cream (35% bromelain in a lipid base) can be beneficial in the elimination of burn debris and in acceleration of healing.[15] A non-proteolytic component of bromelain is responsible for this effect. This component, referred to as escharase, has no hydrolytic enzyme activity against normal protein substrates or various glycosaminoglycan substrates, and its activity varies greatly from preparation to preparation.[16]

Antibiotic Potentiation

Antibiotic potentiation is one of the primary uses of bromelain in several foreign countries. In humans, bromelain has been documented to increase blood and urine levels of antibiotics.[17-19] Combined bromelain and antibiotic therapy has been shown to be more effective than antibiotics alone in a variety of conditions, including pneumonia, bronchitis, cutaneous Staphylococcus infection, thrombophlebitis, cellulitis, pyelonephritis, perirectal and rectal abscesses,[20] and sinusitis.[21]

Respiratory Conditions

In a clinical study of 124 patients hospitalized with chronic bronchitis, pneumonia, bronchopneumonia, bronchiectasis, or pulmonary abscess, those receiving bromelain orally showed a decrease in the volume and purulence of the sputum.[22]

Digestive Aid

Bromelain has been used successfully as a digestive enzyme following pancreatectomy, in cases of exocrine pancreas insufficiency, and in other intestinal disorders.[23] The combination of ox bile, pancreatin, and bromelain is effective in lowering stool fat excretion in patients with pancreatic steatorrhea, resulting in symptomatic improvements in pain, flatulence, and stool frequency.[24]

Ulcers

Bromelain has been reported to heal gastric ulcers in experimental animals. In an extensive study of the effect of bromelain on the gastric mucosa, bromelain increased the uptake of radioactive sulfur by 50 percent and glucosamine by 30-90 percent. Increased uptake of these substances may allow the gastric mucosa to heal more rapidly.[25]

Surgical Procedures and Musculoskeletal Injuries

Bromelain's most common application is in the treatment of inflammation and soft tissue injuries. It has been shown to speed healing from bruises and hematomas.[26] Treatment with bromelain following blunt injuries to the musculoskeletal system results in a clear reduction in swelling, pain at rest and during movement, and tenderness.[27] Administration of bromelain pre-surgically can reduce the average number of days for complete disappearance of pain and inflammation.[28,29]

Cardiovascular and Circulatory Applications

Research indicates bromelain prevents or minimizes the severity of angina pectoris.[30,31] A drastic reduction in the incidence of coronary infarct after administration of potassium and magnesium orotate along with 120-400 mg bromelain per day has been reported.[32] In a study involving 73 patients with acute thrombophlebitis, bromelain, in addition to analgesics, was shown to decrease symptoms of inflammation including pain, edema, tenderness, skin temperature, and disability.[33]

Side Effects and Toxicity

Bromelain is considered to have very low toxicity, with an LD_{50} greater than 10 g/kg. Toxicity tests on dogs, with increasing levels of bromelain up to 750 mg/kg administered daily, showed no toxic effects after six months. Dosages of 1.5 g/kg/day administered to rats showed no carcinogenic or teratogenic effects.[34]

In human clinical tests, side effects are generally not observed; however, caution is advised if administering bromelain to individuals with hypertension, since one report indicated individuals with pre-existing hypertension might experience tachycardia following high doses of bromelain.[35]

The allergenic potential of proteolytic enzymes should not be underestimated. They can cause IgE-mediated respiratory allergies of both the immediate type and the late-phase of immediate type.[36] Bromelain, due to its use as a meat tenderizer and to clarify beer, is considered a potential hidden dietary allergen.

Dosage

Bromelain has demonstrated therapeutic benefits in doses as small as 160 mg per day; however, it is thought for most conditions the best results occur at doses of 750-1,000 mg per day. Most research on bromelain has been performed utilizing four divided daily doses. Findings indicate results are dose-dependent.

References

1. White RR, Crawley FE, Vellini M, et al. Bioavailability of 125I bromelain after oral administration to rats. *Biopharm Drug Dispos* 1988;9:397-403.
2. Kumakura S, Yamashita M, Tsurufuji S. Effect of bromelain on kaolin-induced inflammation in rats. *Eur J Pharmacol* 1988;150:295-301.
3. Uchida Y, Katori M. Independent consumption of high and low molecular weight kininogens *in vivo*. *Adv Exp Med Biol* 1986;198:113-118.
4. Taussig SJ, Batkin S. Bromelain, the enzyme complex of pineapple (*Ananas comosus*) and its clinical application. An update. *J Ethnopharmacol* 1988;22:191-203.
5. Felton GE. Fibrinolytic and antithrombotic action of bromelain may eliminate thrombosis in heart patients. *Med Hypotheses* 1980;6:1123-1133.
6. Heinicke RM, Van der Wal M, Yokoyama MM. Effect of bromelain (Ananase) on human platelet aggregation. *Experientia* 1972;28:844-845.
7. De-Giuli M, Pirotta F. Bromelain: interaction with some protease inhibitors and rabbit specific antiserum. *Drugs Exp Clin Res* 1978;4:21-23.
8. Gerard G. Anti-cancer therapy with bromelain. *Agressologie* 1972;13:261-274.
9. Taussig SJ, Szekerezes J, Batkin S. Inhibition of tumor growth *in vitro* by bromelain, an extract of the pineapple plant (*Ananas comosus*). *Planta Med* 1985;6:538-539.
10. Batkin S, Taussig SJ, Szekerezes J. Antimetastatic effect of bromelain with or without its proteolytic and anticoagulant activity. *J Cancer Res Clin Oncol* 1988;114:507-508.
11. Nieper HA. A program for the treatment of cancer. *Krebs* 1974;6:124-127.
12. Desser L, Rehberger A, Paukovits W. Proteolytic enzymes and amylase induce cytokine production in human peripheral blood mononuclear cells *in vitro*. *Cancer Biother* 1994;9:253-263.
13. Engwerda CR, Andrew D, Murphy M, Mynott TL. Bromelain activates murine macrophages and natural killer cells in vitro. *Cell Immunol* 2001;210:5-10.
14. Munzig E, Eckert K, Harrach T, et al. Bromelain protease F9 reduces the CD44 mediated adhesion of human peripheral blood lymphocytes to human umbilical vein endothelial cells. *FEBS Lett* 1995;351:215-218.
15. Klaue P, Dilbert G, Hinke G, et al. Tier-experimentelle untersuchungen zur enzymatischen lokalbehandlung subdermaler verbrennungen mit bromelain. *Therapiewoche* 1979;29:796-799.
16. Houck JC, Chang CM, Klein G. Isolation of an effective debriding agent from the stems of pineapple plants. *Int J Tissue React* 1983;5:125-134.

17. Tinozzi S, Venegoni A. Effect of bromelain on serum and tissue levels of amoxicillin. *Drugs Exp Clin Res* 1978;4:39-44.
18. Luerti M, Vignali ML. Influence of bromelain on penetration of antibiotics in uterus, salpinx and ovary. *Drugs Exp Clin Res* 1978;4:45-48.
19. Renzini G, Varengo M. Absorption of tetracycline in presence of bromelain after oral administration. *Arzneimittelforschung* 1972;22:410-412. [Article in German]
20. Neubauer RA. A plant protease for potentiation of and possible replacement of antibiotics. *Exp Med Surg* 1961;19:143-160.
21. Ryan RE. A double-blind clinical evaluation of bromelains in the treatment of acute sinusits. *Headache* 1967;7:13-17.
22. Schafer A, Adelman B. Plasmin inhibition of platelet function and of arachidonic acid metabolism. *J Clin Invest* 1985;75:456-461.
23. Knill-Jones RP, Pearce H, Batten J, et al. Comparative trial of Nutrizym in chronic pancreatic insufficiency. *Brit Med J* 1970;4:21-24.
24. Balakrishnan V, Hareendran A, Sukumaran NC. Double-blind cross-over trial of an enzyme preparation in pancreatic steatorrhea. *J Assn Phys Ind* 1981;29:207-209.
25. Felton G. Does kinin released by pineapple stem bromelain stimulate production of prostaglandin E1-like compounds? *Hawaii Med J* 1976;2:39-47.
26. Blonstein JL. Control of swelling in boxing injuries. *Practitioner* 1960;185:78.
27. Masson M. Bromelain in blunt injuries of the locomotor system. A study of observed applications in general practice. *Fortschr Med* 1995;113:303-306.
28. Tassman GC, Zafran JN, Zayon GM. Evaluation of a plant proteolytic enzyme for the control of inflammation and pain. *J Dent Med* 1964;19:73-77.
29. Tassman GC, Zafran JN, Zayon GM. A double-blind crossover study of a plant proteolytic enzyme in oral surgery. *J Dent Med* 1965;20:51-54.
30. Nieper HA. Effect of bromelain on coronary heart disease and angina pectoris. *Acta Med Empirica* 1978;5:274-278.
31. Taussig SJ, Nieper HA. Bromelain: its use in prevention and treatment of cardiovascular disease, present status. *J IAPM* 1979;6:139-151.
32. Nieper HA. Decrease of the incidence of coronary heart infarct by Mg- and K-orotate and bromelain. *Acta Med Empirica* 1977;12:614-618.
33. Seligman B. Oral bromelains as adjuncts in the treatment of acute thrombophlebitis. *Angiology* 1969;20:22-26.
34. Taussig SJ, Yokoyama MM, Chinen N, et al. Bromelain: a proteolytic enzyme and its clinical application. *Hiroshima J Med Sci* 1975;24:185-193.
35. Gutfreund A, Taussig S, Morris A. Effect of oral bromelain on blood pressure and heart rate of hypertensive patients. *Hawaii Med J* 1978;37:143-146.
36. Gailhofer G, Wilders-Truschnig M, Smolle J, Ludvan M. Asthma caused by bromelain: an occupational allergy. *Clin Allergy* 1988;18:445-450.

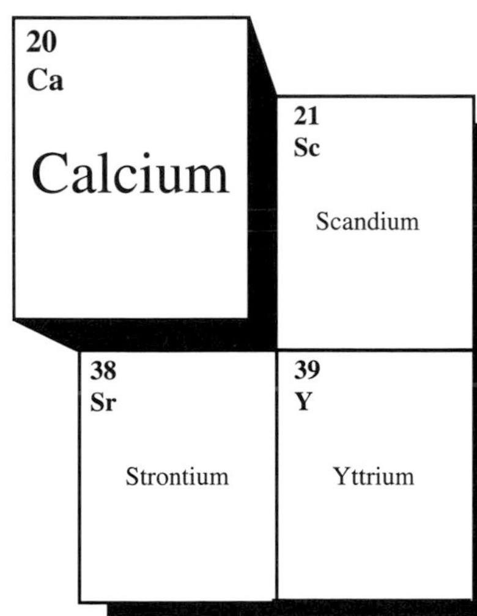

Calcium

Introduction

According to medical anthropologists, calcium intake among Paleolithic people (who ate no dairy products and little meat or fish) averaged 1,500 mg per day.[1] Actual current intakes of hunter-gatherer tribes have been calculated at 2,100-3,000 mg per day.[2] In contrast, the average daily calcium intake of the adult woman in the United States is 500 mg.[3] Several diseases, including osteoporosis, hypertension, and colon cancer have been linked to a drop in calcium intake and to increased dietary phosphorus from grains that has been occurring over the last several centuries.[4]

During the past 20 years, conflicting research in the area of calcium and osteoporosis prevention and treatment has created confusion in the scientific community. This confusion is partly due to the fact that calcium is a threshold nutrient,[5] which means that above a certain threshold there will be little, if any, improvement in response from increasing the dosage.

There are, however, several areas of clarity that have emerged from the burgeoning amount of research on calcium and bone loss. It now appears the source of calcium and its application in the female life cycle make a substantial difference. There are also indications for the use of calcium in specific types of hypertension, premenstrual syndrome, and prevention of colorectal cancer.

Pharmacokinetics

Absorption of calcium varies with age and the presence or absence of intestinal disease.[6] Although it has commonly been believed that solubility of a calcium source increases absorbability, absorption studies have not found a predictable linear relationship between solubility and absorption.[6] Absorption rates of commercially-available calcium supplements vary, with calcium carbonate as low as 22 percent[7] and calcium citrate malate (CCM) as high as 42 percent.[8] Studies looking at actual absorption of calcium supplements vary significantly based on the intra-individual differences in absorption capacity, including hydrochloric acid production.

Calcium research in the area of osteoporosis is difficult due to the complex nature of maintaining calcium balance. Twenty-five percent of the variance in calcium balance is a result of absorption differences, and absorption in menopausal women can vary as much as 61 percent. In some calcium trials, malabsorption of calcium was so common that 40 percent of women in the trials could not absorb enough calcium to stay in calcium balance even though they were ingesting 800 mg daily.[9]

Mechanisms of Action

Calcium has life-sustaining functions in all living cells, acting as a second messenger in transmitting signals between cellular plasma membranes and intracellular signal receptors. In the extracellular environment calcium is essential in promoting blood clotting and the production of cellular adhesion molecules. Recent evidence shows cell membranes in the kidney, parathyroid gland, and brain have specific receptors for calcium that initiate intracellular signals.[10]

In the kidney, calcium lowers dopaminergic activity, resulting in increased urinary volume and loss of sodium, a possible mechanism for calcium's blood pressure lowering effect.[11] Calcium supplementation also lowers levels of osteocalcin and parathormone (PTH), as well as 1,25-dihydroxy vitamin D. Both PTH and 1,25-dihydroxy vitamin D have hypertensive effects via increases in vascular tone.[12] Although the mechanism is not clear, calcium supplementation in subjects with essential hypertension appears to have an insulin-normalizing and insulin-sensitizing effect at levels of 2,000 mg daily.[13] Calcium also promotes normal histology of the colonic mucosa. It forms insoluble complexes with fatty acids and bile acids, preventing colonic hyperplasia induced by bile acids and dietary fats.[14] Calcium also appears to have direct effects on normal proliferation of colonic epithelium.[15]

Calcium, physical exercise, and gonadal hormones are the most important factors influencing bone mass and density.[16] By decreasing circulating levels of 1,25-dihydroxy vitamin D and PTH, calcium alters the remodeling rate of bone tissue by increasing osteoblast activity, thereby increasing bone density.[17]

Clinical Indications

Premenstrual Syndrome

At midcycle, levels of serum ionized calcium in menstruating women drop significantly with a simultaneous elevation of estradiol.[18] Women with premenstrual syndrome (PMS), however, have significantly lower levels of serum ionized calcium and 25-hydroxy vitamin D and higher levels of PTH at midcycle than age-matched women who are symptom free.[19] In women with PMS there is evidence that midcycle elevations of PTH and fluctuations of serum calcium and vitamin D occur more significantly than at other times in the cycle.[18]

A randomized, placebo-controlled, double-blind study of calcium in women with PMS showed a significant relationship between PMS symptoms and calcium intake. Supplementation of 1,200 mg/day calcium in 466 women with moderate-to-severe recurrent premenstrual syndrome resulted in a 48-percent reduction of PMS symptoms after three months of use ($p < 0.001$).[18] The mechanism for calcium's benefit for PMS is not known, although the vasoactive effects of low serum calcium and elevated PTH and 1,25-dihydroxy vitamin D may play a role.

Hypertension

The effect of calcium in hypertension is seen most clearly in those with low calcium intakes, indicating a role for calcium supplementation in treating hypertension, both in children and adults who have low dietary calcium levels.[20,21] Dietary calcium and magnesium were found to be independently associated with hypertension risk in 58,218 females in the Nurses' Health Study.[22] Those with dietary intakes of less than 700 mg calcium per day were at higher risk for hypertension than those with intakes higher than 700 mg per day.[23,24] Although a recent meta-analysis of calcium and hypertension revealed only small changes in blood pressure (-1.44 mm Hg systolic and -0.84 mm Hg),[25] studies using calcium along with vitamin D have resulted in significant results. In elderly women, 1,200 mg calcium plus 800 IU vitamin D resulted in a nine-percent decrease in systolic blood pressure.[26]

It appears that baseline dietary calcium levels are also a significant factor in pregnant women and their risk for hypertension and preeclampsia. Studies with lower calcium-intake populations demonstrated significant effects on risk for hypertension.[27] A supplemental dose of 1,800 mg calcium carbonate, taken from 24 weeks to term, reduced the relative risk of preeclampsia and risk for preterm birth – each by more than 50 percent.[28]

Colorectal Cancer

Low dietary intakes of both calcium and vitamin D have been associated with increased risk for colorectal cancers. Conversely, those with higher dietary intakes are at lower risk.[29,30] A three-year intervention trial found 1,600 mg elemental calcium (4.0 grams calcium carbonate) daily was effective in reducing both adenoma growth and rectal epithelial hyperplasia in those who were cancer free, and decreasing the occurrence of new adenomas in those with a history of polyps.[31] A similar intervention trial with 1,200 mg elemental calcium (3 grams calcium carbonate) daily lead to a significantly lower risk for recurrence of colorectal adenoma.[32]

Kidney Stones

Calcium restriction has been an accepted therapy for the prevention of recurrent nephrolithiasis. Epidemiological studies, however, have found an inverse relationship between dietary calcium levels and kidney stone formation.[33,34] Although increased urinary calcium is a risk factor for kidney stone formation,[35] calcium citrate or calcium citrate malate (CCM) supplementation actually reduces risk of oxalate stone formation. Trials with 800 mg elemental calcium as citrate increased urinary citrate and reduced calcium oxalate production, decreasing risk for oxalate stone formation.[36]

Calcium citrate malate, in doses of 300 mg elemental calcium, inhibits the absorption of oxalate from the gut and consequently decreases urinary oxalate levels.[37] When 600 mg CCM was given to patients with idiopathic hypercalciuria, the urine pH and urine citrate levels rose; both urine alkalinity and elevated citric acid levels have protective effects against stone formation.[38]

Age-related Osteoporosis

Emphasis on building peak bone mass is the most crucial step in osteoporosis prevention. More than 90 percent of bone mass is acquired before age 20 and acquisition of peak bone mass ends by age 30.[17] If peak bone density in young adults reaches one standard deviation above normal levels for that age group, a 15-percent loss of total bone mass during menopause will not result in negative consequences. Studies with adolescents given 500 mg calcium citrate malate per day in addition to approximately 1,000 mg calcium from dietary sources resulted in additional bone growth equal to 1.3 percent of the total skeleton per year.[39] If this growth was sustained through adulthood, the total gain would ensure protection against menopausal bone loss. Further studies in adolescents have repeated these findings and support the need for a re-evaluation of the National Institutes of Health (NIH) guidelines for calcium intake in this age group. Optimal gains in bone mass were achieved with total calcium intakes of an average of 1,600 mg daily.[40]

During the first 5-7 years of menopause, bone loss is under hormonal control and researchers in the field have agreed calcium supplementation alone is not able to alter the average of 15 percent bone loss that occurs, nor is calcium alone able to reduce risk of spinal fracture.[17] However, in three separate meta-analyses of calcium's effect in reducing bone loss prior to and after menopause in women and in men over 40, calcium had a significant effect in preventing bone loss. In postmenopausal populations calcium was effective in preventing the one-percent bone loss per year that occurs as the average postmenopausal bone-mass decline.[41-43]

Relative risk of fracture is the most sensitive and accurate way to assess the efficacy of treatments for osteoporosis. Studies with CCM in combination with vitamin D (500 mg CCM and 700 IU vitamin D) in menopausal women reduced non-vertebral fracture risk by 50 percent, equivalent to hormone replacement therapy.[44] Another large trial using a calcium triphosphate and vitamin D3 combination protocol has replicated this research.[45]

Glucocorticoid-induced Osteoporosis

Glucocorticoids have an immediate effect on bone metabolism by impeding formation and accelerating resorption of bone, inhibiting calcium absorption, suppressing circulating estrogen, and increasing urinary calcium levels. Glucocorticoid-induced osteoporosis is the most devastating side effect of long-term glucocorticoid therapy and the second most common form of osteoporosis seen in subspecialty clinics.[46] It is recommended that those receiving long-term (more than six months) treatment with glucocorticoids at doses over 7.5 mg/day be monitored every 6-12 months for bone loss.[47] Studies support the use of calcium and vitamin D in these patients as a means to maintain and increase bone density (in some trials). Dosages of 800-1,000 mg calcium carbonate and 250-500 IU vitamin D daily have stabilized lumbar and hip bone density in those on low-dose prednisone (11-15 mg).[48,49]

Drug-Nutrient Interactions

Inhibition of Drug Absorption

Calcium interferes with absorption of some drugs, including bisphosphonates for osteoporosis, quinilone antibiotics (ciprofloxacin, gatifloxacin, etc.), and tetracycline.[50] Calcium carbonate was found to decrease absorption of levothyroxine, while increasing serum thyrotropin levels.[50] Calcium supplements should be taken at a different time of day than these medications.

Inhibition of Calcium Absorption

Absorption of calcium can be inhibited by H_2 blockers (cimetidine, ranitidine, etc.), proton pump inhibitors, inositol hexaphosphate, sodium alginate, and oxalate- and phytic-acid rich foods.[50] Calcium may also be depleted by the use of thiazide diuretics.[51]

Enhancement of Calcium Absorption

Absorption of calcium is enhanced by consumption of vitamin D, vitamin D analogs (calcitriol, alfacalcidol), and fructooligosaccharides.[50]

Side Effects and Toxicity

Dosages up to 2,500 mg per day are considered safe in healthy adults.[2] People with idiopathic hypercalciuria, hyperparathyroidism, vitamin D intoxication, milk-alkali syndrome, and sarcoidosis may need special consideration.

Dosage

Dosages for calcium vary with individual age, gender, and condition. Federal guidelines for calcium intake are sex- and age-specific and vary from 1,000-1,300 mg per day.[17] As indicated by research in adolescent women, higher doses, in the range of 1,500 mg daily, may be a better recommendation.[40]

References

1. Eaton SB, Konner M. Paleolithic nutrition: a consideration of its nature and current implications. *New Engl J Med* 1985;312:283-289.
2. Heaney RP. Non-pharmacologic prevention of osteoporosis. In: Meunier PJ, ed. *Osteoporosis: Diagnosis and Management.* St. Louis, MO: Mosby; 1998:162-163.
3. Carroll MD, Abraham S, Dresser CM. Dietary Intake Source Data US, 1976-1980. *Vital Health Stat* 1983;11:1-483.
4. Heaney RJ, Barger-Lux MJ. ADSA Foundation Lecture. Low calcium intake: the culprit in many chronic diseases. *J Dairy Sci* 1994;77:1155-1160.
5. Matkovic V. Calcium balance during human growth: evidence for threshold behavior. *Am J Clin Nutr* 1992;55:992-996.
6. Heaney RP, Recker R, Weaver CM. Absorbability of calcium sources: the limited role of solubility. *Calcif Tissue Int* 1990;46:300-304.
7. Recker RR, Bammi A, Barger-Lux MJ, et al. Calcium absorbability from milk products, imitation milk, and calcium carbonate. *Am J Clin Nutr* 1998;47:93-95.
8. Andon M, Peacock M, Kanerva RL. Supplemental trials with calcium citrate malate: evidence in favor of increasing the calcium RDA during childhood and adolescence. *J Nutr* 1994;124:1412S-1417S.
9. Heaney R, Recker R. Distribution of calcium absorption in middle-aged women. A*m J Clin Nutr* 1986;43:299-305.
10. Brown EM, Gamba G, Riccardi D, et al. Cloning and characterization of an extracellular Ca2+ sensing receptor from bovine parathyroid. *Nature* 1993;366:575-580.
11. Dazai Y, Iwata T, Hiwada K. Augmentation of the renal tubular dopaminergic activity by oral calcium supplementation in patients with essential hypertension. *Am J Hypertens* 1993;6:933-937.
12. Sowers JR, Zemel MB, Zemel PC, et al. Calcium metabolism and dietary calcium in salt-sensitive hypertension. *Am J Hyperten* 1991;4:557-563.
13. Sanchez M, de la Sierra A, Coca A, et al. Oral calcium supplementation reduces intraplatelet free calcium concentration and insulin resistance in essential hypertensive patients. *Hypertension* 1997;29:531-536.
14. Garay CA, Engstrom PF. Chemoprevention of colorectal cancer: dietary and pharmacologic approaches. *Oncology (Huntingt)* 1999;13:89-97.
15. Bostick RM. Human studies of calcium supplementation and colorectal epithelial cell proliferation. *Cancer Epidemiol Biomarkers Prev* 1997;6:971-980.
16. Heaney RP. Nutritional factors in osteoporosis. *Annu Rev Nutr* 1993;13:287-316.
17. Power ML, Heaney RP, Kalwkarf JH. The role of calcium in health and disease. *Am J Obstet Gynecol* 1999;181:1560-1569.
18. Thys-Jacobs S, Alvir J. Calcium regulating hormones across the menstrual cycle: evidence of a secondary hyperparathyroidism in women with PMS. *J Clin Endocrinol Metab* 1995;80:2227-2232.
19. Penland JG, Johnson PE. Dietary calcium and manganese effects on menstrual cycle symptoms. *Am J Obstet Gynecol* 1993;168:1417-1423.

20. Repke JT, Robinson JN. The prevention and management of pre-eclampsia and eclampsia. *Int J Gynaecol Obstet* 1998;62:1-9.
21. Bukosski RD, Ishibahi K, Bian K. Vascular actions of the calcium-regulating hormones. *Semin Nephrol* 1995;15:536-549.
22. Witterman JCM, Willett WC, Stampfer MJ, et al. A prospective study of nutritional factors and hypertension among U.S. women. *Circulation* 1989;80:1320-1327.
23. McCarron DA, Morris CD, Young E, et al. Dietary calcium and blood pressure: modifying factors in specific populations. *Am J Clin Nutr* 1991;54:215S-219S.
24. Barger-Lux MJ, Heaney R. The role of calcium intake in preventing bone fragility, hypertension, and certain cancers. *J Nutr* 1994;124:1406S-1411S.
25. Griffith LE, Guyatt GH, Cook RJ, et al. The influence of dietary and nondietary calcium supplementation on blood pressure: an updated metaanalysis of randomized controlled trials. *Am J Hypertens* 1999;12:84-92.
26. Pfiefer M, Bergerow B, Minne HW, et al. Effects of a short-term vitamin D3 and calcium supplementation on blood pressure and parathyroid hormone levels in elderly women. *J Clin Endocrinol Metab* 2001;86:1633-1637.
27. Bucher HC, Guyatt GH, Cook RJ, et al. Effect of calcium supplementation on pregnancy-induced hypertension and preeclampsia: a meta-analysis of randomized controlled trials. *JAMA* 1996;275:1113-1117.
28. Crowther CA, Hiller JE, Pridmore B, et al. Calcium supplementation in nulliparous women for the prevention of pregnancy-induced hypertension, preeclampsia and preterm birth: an Australian randomized trial. FRACOG and the ACT Study Group. *Aust N Z J Obstet Gynaecol* 1999;39:12-18.
29. Garland CF, Garland FC, Gorham ED. Can colon cancer incidence and death rates be reduced with calcium and vitamin D? *Am J Clin Nutr* 1991;54:193S-201S.
30. Kampman E, Slattery ML, Caan B, et al. Calcium, vitamin D, sunshine exposure, dairy products and colon cancer risk. *Cancer Causes Control* 2000;11:459-466.
31. Hofstad B, Almendigen K, Vatn M, et al. Growth and recurrence of colorectal polyps: a double-blind 3-year intervention with calcium and antioxidants. *Digestion* 1998;59:148-156.
32. Baron JA, Beach M, Mandel JS, et al. Calcium supplements for the prevention of colorectal adenomas, *N Engl J Med* 1999;340:101-107.
33. Curhan GC, Willett WC, Rimm EB, et al. A prospective study of dietary calcium and other nutrients and the risk of symptomatic kidney stones. *N Engl J Med* 1993;328:880-882.
34. Curhan GC, Willett WC, Speizer FE, et al. Comparison of dietary calcium and supplemental calcium and other nutrients as factors affecting the risk of kidney stones in women. *Ann Intern Med* 1997;126:497-504.
35. Cappuio FP, Kalaitzidis R, Duneclift S, et al. Unraveling the links between calcium excretion, salt intake, hypertension, kidney stones, and bone metabolism. *J Nephrol* 2000;12:169-177.
36. Harvey JA, Zobitz MM, Pak CY. Calcium citrate: reduced propensity for the crystallization of calcium oxalate in urine resulting from induced hypercalciuria of calcium supplementation. *J Clin Endocrinol Metab* 1985;61:1223-1225.
37. Liebman M, Chai W. Effect of dietary calcium on urinary oxalate excretion after oxalate loads. *Am J Clin Nutr* 1997;65:1453-1459.
38. Coe FL, Parks JH, Webb DR. Stone-forming potential of milk or calcium-fortified orange juice in idiopathic hypercalciuric adults. *Kidney Int* 1992;41:139-142.
39. Lloyd T, Andon MB, Rollis N. Calcium supplementation and bone mineral density in adolescent girls. *JAMA* 1993;270:841-844.
40. Patrick L. Comparative absorption of calcium sources and calcium citrate malate for the prevention of osteoporosis. *Altern Med Rev* 1999;4:74-85.

41. Heaney R. Nutrition and risk for osteoporosis: In: Marcus R, Feldman D, Kelsey J, eds. *Osteoporosis*. San Diego, CA: Academic Press Inc.; 1996;498-499.

42. Cumming RG. Calcium intake and bone mass: a quantitative review of the evidence. *Calc Tissue Int* 1990;47:194-201.

43. Welten DC, Kemper HC, Post GB, et al. A meta-analysis of the effect of calcium on bone mass in young and middle aged females and males. *J Nutr* 1995;125:2802-2813.

44. Dawson-Hughes B, Harris S, Krall E, et al. Effect of calcium and vitamin D supplementation on bone density in men and women 65 years of age or older. *N Engl J Med* 1997;337:670-676.

45. Chapuy MC, Arlot M, Dunboeuf F. Vitamin D3 and calcium to prevent hip fractures in elderly women. *N Engl J Med* 1997;327:1637-1642.

46. Dempster D, Lindsay R. Pathogenesis of osteoporosis. *Lancet* 1993;341:797-801.

47. No authors listed. Recommendations for the prevention and treatment of glucocorticoid-induced osteoporosis: 2001 update. American College of Rheumatology Ad Hoc Committee of Glucocortocoid-Induced Osteoporosis. *Arthritis Rheum* 2001;44:1496-1503.

48. Buckley LM, Leib ES, Cartularo KS, et al. Calcium and vitamin D supplementation prevents bone loss in the spine secondary to low dose corticosteroids in patients with rheumatoid arthritis: a randomized, double-blind, placebo controlled trial. *Ann Intern Med* 1996;125:961-986.

49. Saag KG, Emkey R, Schnitzer TJ, et al. Alendronate for the treatment and prevention of glucocorticoid-induced osteoporosis. *N Engl J Med* 1998;339:292-299.

50. Hendler SS, Rorvik D. *PDR for Nutritional Supplements*, 1st ed. Des Moines, IA: Medical Economics – Thompson Healthcare; 2001.

51. Pelton R, LaValle JB, Hawkins EB, Krinsky DL. *Drug-induced Nutrient Depletion Handbook*, 2nd ed. Hudson, OH: Lexi-comp, Inc; 2001.

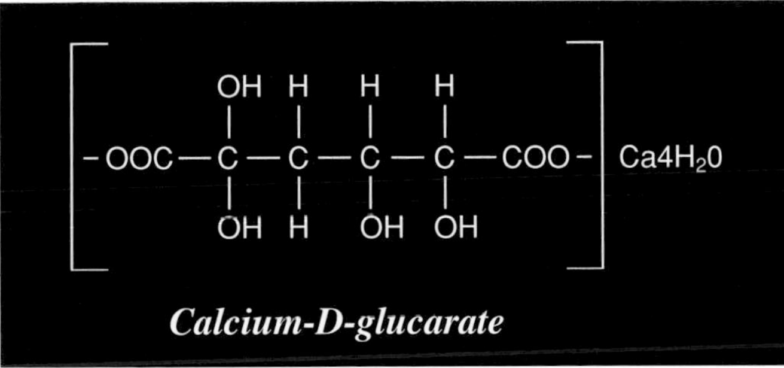

Calcium-D-glucarate

Calcium-D-Glucarate

Introduction

Calcium-D-glucarate is the calcium salt of D-glucaric acid, a substance produced naturally in small amounts by mammals, including humans. Glucaric acid is also found in many fruits and vegetables, with the highest concentrations found in oranges, apples, grapefruit, and cruciferous vegetables.[1] Oral supplementation of calcium-D-glucarate has been shown to inhibit beta-glucuronidase, an enzyme produced by colonic microflora. Elevated beta-glucuronidase activity is associated with an increased risk for various cancers, particularly hormone-dependent cancers such as breast, prostate, and colon cancers.[2] Potential clinical applications of oral calcium-D-glucarate include cancer prevention, regulation of estrogen metabolism, and as a lipid-lowering agent.

Pharmacokinetics

Upon ingestion and exposure to the acidic environment of the stomach, calcium-D-glucarate is metabolized to form D-glucaric acid. D-glucaric acid is further metabolized in the gastrointestinal tract into three compounds existing in equilibrium and comprised of approximately 40-percent D-glucaric acid, 30-percent D-glucaro-1,4-lactone, and 30-percent D-glucaro-6,3-lactone. These compounds are then transported to the blood and various internal organs, and are subsequently excreted in the urine and bile. Although D-glucaro-1,4-lactone seems to be the most pharmacologically active of the three, it is not commercially available. Additionally, in a rat study, oral ingestion of calcium-D-glucarate administration resulted in longer inhibition of beta-glucuronidase (five hours versus one hour) than D-glucaro-1,4-lactone.[3]

Mechanism of Action

Calcium-D-glucarate's detoxifying and anticarcinogenic properties are attributed to its ability to increase net glucuronidation and excretion of potentially toxic compounds. During hepatic phase II detoxification, chemical carcinogens, steroid hormones, and other lipid-soluble toxins are conjugated with glucuronic acid in the liver (glucuronidation), and excreted through the biliary tract. Beta-glucuronidase is capable of deconjugating these potential toxins, making it possible for them to be reabsorbed rather than excreted. D-glucaro-1,4-lactone, the active metabolite of calcium d-glucarate, inhibits beta-glucuronidase, resulting in increased excretion of conjugated xenobiotic compounds,[4,5] which may decrease the risk of carcinogenesis.[6] In addition, D-glucaric acid salts have been shown to lower cholesterol levels. It is theorized that D-glucaro-1,4-lactone acts systemically to regulate cholesterol synthesis and might also regulate steroidogenesis, DNA synthesis, and cell proliferation.[2,7]

Deficiency States

Since calcium-D-glucarate is not an essential nutrient, no actual deficiency state exists. However, since it is only produced in small amounts by humans, it is important that dietary intake be adequate. Diets low in fruits (particularly oranges, apples, and grapefruit) and cruciferous vegetables (broccoli, cabbage, and brussel sprouts) may result in a relative deficiency of calcium-D-glucarate and its metabolites. Research has shown a low level of D-glucaric acid correlates with a higher level of beta-glucuronidase, which in turn is associated with an increased risk for various cancers.[2]

Clinical Indications

Cancer

The anticarcinogenic properties of D-glucaric acid and its salts have been studied in various animal tumor models, including colon,[8,9] prostate,[2] lung,[10] liver,[11,12] skin,[13] and breast[14-19] cancer, with the mechanism of action for tumor inhibition being very similar in each. These studies demonstrated decreases in beta-glucuronidase activity, carcinogen levels, and tumorigenesis. The preponderance of research, however, has been conducted on mammary tumors in the rat, the animal model most frequently used for breast cancer research.

Breast Cancer

A number of studies have shown calcium-D-glucarate alone, and in combination with retinoids, inhibits mammary carcinogenesis in rats by as much as 70 percent.[19] Natural retinoids have been shown to be effective chemopreventive agents at high doses, but unfortunately the cumulative toxic effects of high doses have restricted their prolonged use. Several studies have demonstrated low-dose retinoids in combination with calcium-D-glucarate interact synergistically to inhibit mammary tumor growth in both animal models and human cell lines.[14-19] The mechanisms responsible for the chemopreventive effects of these two agents may be similar. Both retinoids and calcium-D-glucarate inhibit carcinogenesis during the promotion and initiation phases. Calcium-D-glucarate inhibits protein tyrosine kinase-C activity and induces transformation growth factor beta, possibly resulting in an increase in cellular differentiation and slower progression through the cell cycle.[15] Retinoids induce many of these same biochemical effects.[20] Additionally, calcium-D-glucarate enhances net glucuronidation by increasing excretion of carcinogens and other cancer-promoting agents.

Published human studies on calcium-D-glucarate and breast cancer are few but, due to encouraging results of animal studies, the National Cancer Institute has initiated a phase I trial in patients at high risk for breast cancer at Memorial Sloan Kettering Cancer Center. This trial is examining the use of calcium-D-glucarate as an alternative to tamoxifen's blocking of estrogen receptors. Preliminary results are encouraging and due to calcium-D-glucarate's excellent safety profile, it may be a more effective option than tamoxifen, which has numerous side effects.[19] Other human trials are being conducted at M.D. Anderson Cancer Center in Houston, Texas, and AMC Cancer Research Center in Denver, Colorado.

Colon Cancer

Studies in rats have shown D-glucarate salts inhibit colon carcinogenesis alone and in combination with 5-fluorouracil (5-FU). In one study, D-glucarate markedly inhibited azoxymethane-induced colon carcinogenesis, as evidenced by a 60-percent reduction in both tumor incidence and multiplicity. It was hypothesized that malignant cell proliferation was suppressed by inhibition of beta-glucuronidase. Another possible mechanism may involve alterations in cholesterol synthesis or its conversion to bile acids.[8] The second study demonstrated that salts of D-glucarate, in combination with 5-FU in rat colon tumor explants, resulted in a potentiation of 5-FU's antitumor activity. D-glucarate alone also showed antitumor activity.[9]

Liver Cancer

Hepatocarcinogenesis is thought to be preceded by premalignant hepatic foci subsequently transformed to malignant cells. Two separate rat studies by a group of researchers at Ohio State University have demonstrated calcium-D-glucarate delays the appearance of altered hepatic foci and significantly inhibits hepatocarcinogenesis, if given during both the initiation and promotion phases. Maximal inhibition was obtained when calcium-D-glucarate was administered by gavage prior to the carcinogenic agent, diethylnitrosamine.[11,12]

Lung Cancer

A study conducted on mice demonstrated calcium-D-glucarate inhibits benzo[a]pyrene's ability to bind DNA and induce pulmonary adenomas.[10] Another unpublished phase I clinical trial of 62 patients found D-glucaric acid levels were approximately 29-percent lower in smokers than non-smokers. Regardless of gender, K-ras (an oncogene linked to lung cancer) mutations were found to be present in 38 percent of subjects who smoked, while no K-ras mutations were found in the non-smoking control subjects. It was hypothesized that D-glucaric acid deficiency correlates with K-ras mutations and might be indicative of a higher risk for developing lung cancer.[21]

Skin Cancer

The efficacy of dietary calcium-D-glucarate as a chemopreventive agent has also been studied in the mouse skin tumorigenesis system. Mice were given 7,12-dimethylbenz[a]anthracene (DMBA) to induce skin tumorigenesis and were fed either a regular chow diet or a chow diet fortified with calcium-D-glucarate. When fed the calcium-D-glucarate chow through both the initiation and promotion phases, papilloma formation was inhibited by over 30 percent. The data indicate supplementation of calcium-D-glucarate results in a marked alteration in the retention, activity, and metabolism of carcinogenic substances.[13]

Estrogen Metabolism

Calcium-D-glucarate's inhibition of beta-glucuronidase activity allows the body to excrete hormones such as estrogen before they can become reabsorbed. Administration of large oral doses of calcium-D-glucarate lowers serum estrogen levels in rats by 23 percent.[22] Because many breast cancers are estrogen-dependent, calcium-D-glucarate's ability to affect estrogen and other hormone levels has led to phase I clinical trials at several major cancer centers in the United States. Results of these studies are pending.

Lipid Lowering

Side effects of currently available hypolipidemic agents present a need for safe and effective lipid-lowering agents. D-glucarates have been shown to significantly reduce total serum cholesterol in rats by as much as 12-15 percent and LDL-cholesterol by 30-35 percent. Preliminary results in humans show D-glucarate reduced total serum cholesterol up to 12 percent, LDL-cholesterol up to 28 percent, and triglycerides up to 43 percent. The lipid-lowering effect of calcium-D-glucarate may be attributed to the ability of D-glucaro-1,4-lactone to increase cholesterol excretion, as well as to regulate steroidogenesis and cholesterol biosynthesis.[7]

Drug-Nutrient Interactions

There are no known drug interactions with calcium-D-glucarate, but many drugs and hormones are metabolized in the liver via glucuronidation. Therefore, taking calcium-D-glucarate may increase elimination of these substances, possibly reducing their effectiveness.

Side Effects and Toxicity

No adverse effects have been observed after prolonged feeding to rats or mice at concentrations of 70, 140, or even 350 mmol/kg.[6] Preliminary results of clinical trials in humans have shown calcium-D-glucarate is without adverse effects.

Dosage

The recommended oral dosage of calcium-d-glucarate is generally in the range of 1,500-3,000 mg daily. Until human trials have been completed the optimal dosage remains elusive.

References

1. Dwivedi C, Heck WJ, Downie AA, et al. Effect of calcium glucarate on beta-glucuronidase activity and glucarate content of certain vegetables and fruits. *Biochem Med Metab Biol* 1990;43:83-92.
2. Walaszek Z, Szemraj J, Narog M, et al. Metabolism, uptake, and excretion of a D-glucaric acid salt and its potential use in cancer prevention. *Cancer Detect Prev* 1997;21:178-190.
3. Walaszek Z, Hanausek-Walaszek M, Webb TE. Repression by sustained-release beta-glucuronidase inhibitors of chemical carcinogen-mediated induction of a marker oncofetal protein in rodents. *J Toxicol Environ Health* 1988;23:15-27.
4. Horton D, Walaszek Z. Conformations of the D-glucarolactones and D-glucaric acid in solution. *Carbohydr Res* 1982;105:95-109.
5. Walaszek Z, Hanausek-Walaszek M. D-glucaro-1,4-lactone: its excretion in the bile and urine and effect on biliary excretion of beta-glucuronidase after oral administration in rats. *Hepatology* 1988;9:552-556.
6. Selkirk JK, Cohen GM, MacLeod MC. Glucuronic acid conjugation in the metabolism of chemical carcinogens by rodent cells. *Arch Toxicol* 1980;139:S171-S178.
7. Walaszek Z, Hanausek-Walaszek M, Adams AK, Sherman U. Cholesterol lowering effects of dietary D-glucarate. *FASEB J* 1991;5:A930.
8. Yoshimi N, Walaszek Z, Mori H, et al. Inhibition of azoxymethane-induced rat colon carcinogenesis by potassium hydrogen D-glucarate. *Int J Oncol* 2000;16:43-48.
9. Schmittgen TD, Koolemans-Beynen A, Webb TE, et al. Effects of 5-fluorouracil, leucovorin, and glucarate in rat colon-tumor explants. *Cancer Chemother Pharmacol* 1992;30:25-30.
10. Walaszek Z, Hanausek-Walaszek M, Webb TE. Dietary glucarate-mediated reduction of sensitivity of murine strains to chemical carcinogenesis. *Cancer Lett* 1986;33:25-32.
11. Oredipe OA, Barth RF, Hanausek-Walaszek M, et al. Effects of an inhibitor of beta-glucuronidase on hepatocarcinogenesis. *Proc Am Assoc Cancer Res* 1987;28:156.
12. Oredipe OA, Barth RF, Hanausek-Walaszek M, et al. Effects of calcium glucarate on the promotion of diethylnitrosamine-initiated altered hepatic loci in rats. *Cancer Lett* 1987;38:95-99.
13. Dwivedi C, Downie AA, Webb TE. Modulation of chemically initiated and promoted skin tumorigenesis in CD-1 mice by dietary glucarate. *J Environ Path Toxicol Oncol* 1989;9:253-259.
14. Abou-Issa H, Koolemans-Beynen A, Meredith TA, Webb TE. Antitumour synergism between non-toxic dietary combinations of isotretinoin and glucarate. *Eur J Cancer* 1992;28:784-788.
15. Webb TE, Abou-Issa H, Stromberg PC, et al. Mechanism of growth inhibition of mammary carcinomas by glucarate and the glucarate:retinoid combination. *Anticancer Res* 1993;13:2095-2100.
16. Bhatnagar R, Abou-Issa H, Curley RW, et al. Growth suppression of human breast carcinoma cells in culture by N-(4-hydroxyphenyl) retinamide and its glucuronide and through synergism with glucarate. *Biochem Pharmacol* 1991;41:1471-1477.
17. Curley RW, Humpries KA, Koolemans-Beynan A, et al. Activity of d-glucarate analogues: synergistic antiproliferative effect in cultured human mammary tumor cells appear to specifically require the d-glucarate structure. *Life Sci* 1994;54:1299-1303.
18. Abou-Issa H, Moeschberger M, Masry EI, et al. Relative efficacy of glucarate on the initiation and promotion phases of rat mammary carcinogenesis. *Cancer Res* 1995;15:805-810.
19. Heerdt AS, Young CW, Borgen PI. Calcium glucarate as a chemopreventive agent in breast cancer. *Isr J Med Sci* 1995;31:101-105.
20. DeLuca LM. Retinoids and their receptors in differentiation, embryogenesis and neoplasia. *FASEB J* 1991;5:2924-2933.
21. Walaszek Z, Raich PC, Hanausek M, et al. Role of D-glucaric acid in lung cancer prevention. Unpublished research. AMC Cancer Research Center, Denver, CO.
22. Walaszek Z, Hanausek-Walaszek M, Minto JP, Webb TE. Dietary glucarate as anti-promoter of 7,12-dimethylbenz[a]anthracene-induced mammary tumorigenesis. *Carcinogenesis* 1986;7:1463-1466.

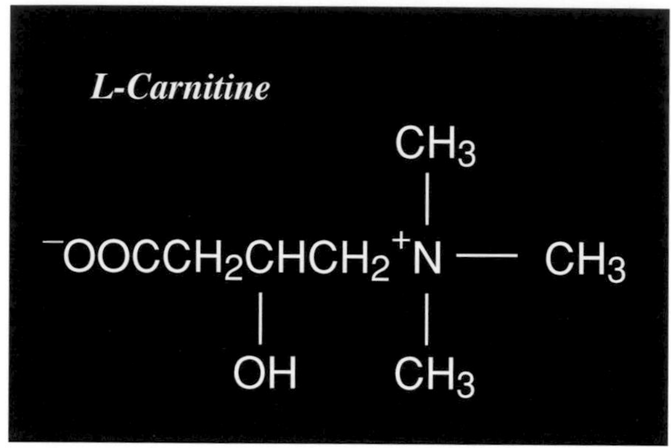

L-Carnitine

Introduction

A trimethylated amino acid, roughly similar in structure to choline, L-carnitine is a cofactor required for transformation of free long-chain fatty acids into acylcarnitines, and for their subsequent transport into the mitochondrial matrix, where they undergo beta-oxidation for cellular energy production. Conditions that appear to benefit from exogenous supplementation of L-carnitine include anorexia, chronic fatigue, cardiovascular disease, diphtheria, hypoglycemia, male infertility, muscular myopathies, and Rett syndrome. Preterm infants, dialysis patients, and HIV+ individuals seem to be prone to a deficiency of L-carnitine, and benefit from supplementation. Although originally discovered in 1905, its crucial role in metabolism was not elucidated until 1955, and primary L-carnitine deficiency was not described until 1972. The most significant source of L-carnitine in human nutrition is meat, although humans are also capable of synthesizing L-carnitine from dietary amino acids.

Biochemistry and Pharmacokinetics

Synthesis of carnitine begins with methylation of the amino acid L-lysine by S-adenosylmethionine (SAMe). Magnesium, vitamin C, iron, vitamins B3 and B6, and alpha-ketoglutarate, along with the cofactors responsible for creating SAMe (methionine, folic acid, vitamin B12, and betaine), are all required for endogenous carnitine synthesis.

Evidence indicates L-carnitine is absorbed in the intestine by a combination of active transport and passive diffusion.[1] Reports of bioavailability following an oral dose have varied substantially, with estimates as low as 16-18 percent[2,3] and as high as 54-87 percent.[4,5]

Oral supplementation of L-carnitine in amounts greater than 2 g appears to offer no advantage, since the mucosal absorption of carnitine appears to be saturated at about a 2 g dose.[2] Maximum blood concentrations are reached approximately 3.5 hours following an oral dose and slowly decrease, with a half-life of about 15 hours.[4] Elimination of carnitine occurs primarily through the kidneys.[4]

The heart, skeletal muscle, liver, kidneys, and epididymis have specific transport systems for carnitine that concentrate carnitine within these tissues. Despite evidence indicating increased levels of free carnitine and carnitine metabolites in the blood and urine following an oral dose, no significant change in red blood cell carnitine levels was noted in healthy subjects, suggesting either a slow repletion of tissue stores of carnitine following an oral dose or a low capability to transport carnitine into tissues under normal conditions.[6]

Mechanisms of Action

Carnitine's primary mechanism of action appears to be due to its role as a cofactor in the transformation of free long-chain fatty acids into acyl-carnitines for their subsequent transport into the mitochondrial matrix.

Carnitine is involved in the metabolism of ketones for energy and in the conversion of branched chain amino acids – valine, leucine, and isoleucine – into energy.

A carnitine-dependent pathway is a component of hepatic phase II detoxification.

Deficiency States and Symptoms

Although L-carnitine is supplied exogenously as a component of the diet and can also be synthesized endogenously, evidence suggests both primary and secondary deficiencies do occur. Carnitine deficiency can be acquired or a result of inborn errors of metabolism.

Infants fed carnitine-free formulas are in jeopardy of deficiency since endogenous synthesis is not adequate to cover systemic needs during the first few days of the postnatal period. Carnitine levels of vegetarians are reported to be below normal.

Deficiency can result in cardiomyopathy, congestive heart failure, encephalopathy, hepatomegaly, impaired growth and development in infants, and neuromuscular disorders.

Primary carnitine deficiency, although rare, is characterized by low plasma, red blood cell, and tissue levels of carnitine, and generally presents with symptoms such as muscle fatigue, cramps, and myoglobinemia following exercise.

Secondary carnitine deficiency is not as rare and is most commonly associated with dialysis, although intestinal resection, severe infection, and liver disease can also induce a secondary deficiency. Additional symptoms of chronic carnitine deficiency might include hypoglycemia, progressive myasthenia, hypotonia, or lethargy.

Pathological manifestations of chronic deficiency include accumulation of neutral lipid within skeletal muscle, cardiac muscle, and liver; a disruption of muscle fibers; and an accumulation of large aggregates of mitochondria within skeletal and smooth muscle.

Clinical Indications

Anorexia

Combined use of L-carnitine and adenosylcobalamin in patients with anorexia nervosa has been shown to accelerate body weight gain, normalize gastrointestinal function, decrease fatigue, and improve physical perfomance.[7,8] Children with infantile anorexia responded to a combination of carnitine and adenosylcobalamin with improved appetite.[9]

Athletic Performance

A clinical study reported improved running speed and decreased average oxygen consumption and heart rate following prolonged L-carnitine supplementation,[10] while other researchers reported increased maximal oxygen uptake and decreased plasma lactate when L-carnitine was supplemented acutely one hour prior to beginning exercise.[11] In contrast, other research has shown no ergogenic effects of either chronic or acute L-carnitine supplementation.[12-14] Its current role as an ergogenic substance capable of favorably impacting athletic performance is equivocal.

Cardiovascular Disease

Angina, Ischemia, and Peripheral Vascular Disease

L-carnitine (oral doses ranging from 900-3,000 mg daily) has been shown to moderately improve exercise tolerance and reduce ECG indices of ischemia in patients with stable angina. Estimates suggest as many as 22 percent of subjects might become angina-free during supplementation periods. Increasing benefits are often observed with longer supplementation.[15-18]

Angina patients receiving L-carnitine have experienced functional improvement, including a reduction in the number of premature ventricular contractions at rest, an increase in maximal systolic arterial blood pressure, and a reduction in ST-segment depression during maximal effort. In addition, a concomitant increase in the number of patients belonging to class I of the NYHA classification (as opposed to class II and III) and a reduction in the consumption of cardioactive drugs has been reported.[19]

In subjects with ischemia-induced NYHA II or III cardiac insufficiency, L-carnitine supplementation (1 g three times daily for 120 days), in addition to the usual medications (digitalis, beta-blockers, calcium antagonists, nitrates), resulted in improvements in exercise performance and hemodynamic parameters. Benefits were maintained beyond the L-carnitine supplementation period.[20]

In subjects with peripheral vascular disease, walking distance improved from an average of 174 minutes with placebo to 306 minutes with L-carnitine.[21]

Cardiogenic Shock

L-carnitine supplementation during cardiogenic shock improved metabolic acidosis and survival rate in hospitalized individuals.[22,23]

Cardiomyopathy

Long-term supplementation of L-carnitine (2 g daily) for the treatment of heart failure caused by dilated cardiomyopathy resulted in improvement in survival rate, ejection fraction, Weber classification, maximal time of cardiopulmonary exercise test, peak VO_2 consumption, arterial and pulmonary blood pressure, and cardiac output.[24,25]

Congestive Heart Failure and Myocardial Infarction

Following a recent myocardial infarction (MI), a marked reduction in mortality was observed with 12-month supplementation of 4 g daily L-carnitine (1.2%) when compared to controls (12.5%). Significant improvements were noted in heart rate and anginal attacks as well.[26] Additional research confirms a benefit in terms of reduced mortality in individuals given L-carnitine following MI.[27-29]

Hyperlipidemia

L-carnitine (2-3 g daily) resulted in improved lipid profiles in individuals with hyperlipidemia, with reductions in total and LDL-cholesterol and increased plasma apolipoprotein AI and B levels. Normalization of lipid levels occurred in many subjects with continued supplementation for one year.[30,31] L-carnitine supplementation (2 g daily) also resulted in a decrease in triglycerides in individuals with essential hypertension.[32]

L-carnitine (2 g daily) significantly reduced Lp(a) levels in 14 of 18 subjects. Reductions in Lp(a) were greater in individuals with more marked elevations prior to supplementation; in a significant number of subjects the reduction of Lp(a) resulted in a return to the normal range.[33]

Chronic Fatigue Syndrome

Administration of L-carnitine for two months resulted in improvement in 12 of 18 patients with chronic fatigue.[34]

Dialysis

Supplementation with L-carnitine, either orally or intravenously, mitigates some of the disorders associated with dialysis, including renal anemia, cardiac dysfunction, insulin resistance, lipid abnormalities, and oxidative stress.[35-38]

Hepatic Steatosis (Fatty Liver)

L-carnitine ameliorates ethanol-induced fatty liver in animals;[39] however, it has not been investigated in humans for this condition.

HIV and Immunity

Daily infusions of L-carnitine (6 g) for four months resulted in an increase in CD4 counts in HIV+ subjects who were not taking anti-retroviral therapy.[40] Administration of L-carnitine (6 g daily for two weeks) to AIDS patients treated with zidovudine (AZT) has been shown to result in improved immunity and a reduction in serum levels of tumor necrosis factor-alpha.[41]

Hyperthyroidism

L-carnitine is believed to be a peripheral antagonist of thyroid hormone action in some tissues. A randomized, double-blind, placebo-controlled, six-month trial reported both 2- and 4-g daily doses of L-carnitine were able to prevent and reverse hyperthyroidism-related symptoms, and provide a beneficial effect on bone mineralization.[42]

Male Infertility

Oral administration of L-carnitine (3 g daily for four months) resulted in significant improvements in sperm number, quality, and motility in patients with inadequate sperm.[43,44]

Respiratory Distress in Premature Infants

A combination of L-carnitine (4 g daily for five days) and betamethasone given to women in the prenatal period was found to reduce both the incidence of respiratory distress syndrome and the mortality of premature newborns.[45]

A case of siblings presenting with apnea and periodic breathing, along with biochemical defects consistent with a non-specific abnormality of beta-oxidation, suggests L-carnitine might prevent some cases of sudden infant death syndrome.[46]

Weight Loss

In a double-blind study, investigators found no effect of L-carnitine supplementation on weight loss or on any variable of body composition measured.[47]

Nutrient-Nutrient Interactions

A deficiency of ascorbic acid may decrease endogenous biosynthesis of carnitine.[48,49] In guinea pigs, supplementing the diet with ascorbic acid increased carnitine biosynthesis.[50]

A case report describes normalization of carnitine levels following administration with riboflavin.[51] In rats, administration of vitamin B12 increased carnitine biosynthesis.[52] Choline supplementation appears to decrease carnitine synthesis.[53]

Drug-Nutrient Interactions

- Anticonvulsant medications, including phenobarbital, valproic acid, phenytoin, and carbamazepine, have a significant lowering effect on carnitine levels.[54]
- Pivampicillin negatively impacts carnitine metabolism.[55]
- L-carnitine should be used cautiously, if at all, with pentylenetetrazol, since evidence suggests the combination might exacerbate the side effects of the drug.[56]
- Evidence suggests supplemental L-carnitine might prevent cardiac complications secondary to interleukin-2 immunotherapy in cancer patients[57] and cardiac toxicity secondary to adriamycin.[58]

- L-carnitine, when used concurrently with AZT, appears to prevent the drug-induced destruction of myotubes, preserve the structure and volume of mitochondria, and prevent the accumulation of lipids.[59]
- L-carnitine supplementation helps prevent elevation in liver enzymes, as well as the myalgia, weakness, and hypotension induced by isotretinoin.[60]
- Emetine (ipecac) appears to promote carnitine deficiency.[61] Another case report suggests carnitine deficiency was induced in a patient receiving sulfadiazine and pyrimethamine.[62]
- Evidence also suggests that L-carnitine potentiates the anti-arrhythmic effect of propafenone and mexiletine in patients with ischemia.[63]

Side Effects and Toxicity

A variety of mild gastrointestinal symptoms have been reported, including transient nausea and vomiting, abdominal cramps, and diarrhea. In mice, the LD50 is 19.2 g/kg. Mutagenicity data indicate no mutagenicity; however, experiments to determine long-term carcinogenicity have not been conducted.

Dosage

The average therapeutic dose is 1-2 g two to three times daily for a total of 2-6 g per day. No advantage appears to exist in giving an oral dose greater than 2 g at one time, since absorption studies indicate saturation at this dose.

Warnings and Contraindications

L-carnitine is listed as pregnancy category B, indicating animal studies have revealed no harm to the fetus but that no adequate studies in pregnant women have been conducted. L-carnitine has been given to pregnant women late in pregnancy with resulting positive outcomes.

The racemic mixture (D,L-carnitine) should be avoided. D-carnitine is not biologically active and might interfere with the proper utilization of the L isomer. In uremic patients, use of the racemic mixture has been correlated with myasthenia-like symptoms in some individuals.

References

1. Li B, Lloyd ML, Gudjonsson H, et al. The effect of enteral carnitine administration in humans. *Am J Clin Nutr* 1992;55:838-845.
2. Harper P, Elwin CE, Cederblad G. Pharmacokinetics of intravenous and oral bolus doses of L-carnitine in healthy subjects. *Eur J Clin Pharmacol* 1988;35:555-562.
3. Sahajwalla CG, Helton ED, Purich ED, et al. Multiple-dose pharmacokinetics and bioequivalence of L-carnitine 330-mg tablet versus 1-g chewable tablet versus enteral solution in healthy adult male volunteers. *J Pharm Sci* 1995;84:627-633.

4. Bach AC, Schirardin H, Sihr MO, Storck D. Free and total carnitine in human serum after oral ingestion of L-carnitine. *Diabete Metab* 1983;9:121-124.

5. Rebouche CJ, Chenard CA. Metabolic fate of dietary carnitine in human adults: identification and quantification of urinary and fecal metabolites. *J Nutr* 1991;121:539-546

6. Baker H, Frank O, DeAngelis B, Baker ER. Absorption and excretion of L-carnitine during single or multiple dosings in humans. *Int J Vitam Nutr Res* 1993;63:22-26.

7. Korkina MB, Korchak GM, Medvedev DI. Clinico-experimental substantiation of the use of carnitine and cobalamin in the treatment of anorexia nervosa. *Zh Nevropatol Psikhiatr* 1989;89:82-87. [article in Russian]

8. Korkina MV, Korchak GM, Kareva MA. Effects of carnitine and cobamamide on the dynamics of mental work capacity in patients with anorexia nervosa. *Zh Nevropatol Psikhiatr Im S S Korsakova* 1992;92:99-102. [article in Russian]

9. Giordano C, Perrotti G. Clinical studies of the effects of treatment with a combination of carnitine and cobamamide in infantile anorexia. *Clin Ter* 1979;88:51-60. [article in Italian]

10. Swart I, Rossouw J, Loots JM, Kruger MC. The effect of L-carnitine supplementation on plasma carnitine levels and various performance parameters of male marathon athletes. *Nutr Res* 1997;17:405-414.

11. Vecchiet L, Di Lisa F, Pieralisi G, et al. Influence of L-carnitine administration on maximal physical exercise. *Eur J Appl Physiol* 1990;61:486-490.

12. Vukovich MD, Costill DL, Fink WJ. Carnitine supplementation: effect on muscle carnitine and glycogen content during exercise. *Med Sci Sports Exerc* 1994;26:1122-1129.

13. Cooper MB, Jones DA, Edwards RH, et al. The effect of marathon running on carnitine metabolism and on some aspects of muscle mitochondrial activities and antioxidant mechanisms. *J Sports Sci* 1986;4:79-87.

14. Colombani P, Wenk C, Kunz I, et al. Effects of L-carnitine supplementation on physical performance and energy metabolism of endurance-trained athletes: a double-blind crossover field study. *Eur J Appl Physiol* 1996;73:434-439.

15. Kamikawa T, Suzuki Y, Kobayashi A, et al. Effects of L-carnitine on exercise tolerance in patients with stable angina pectoris. *Jpn Heart J* 1984;25:587-597.

16. Canale C, Terrachini V, Biagini A, et al. Bicycle ergometer and echocardiographic study in healthy subjects and patients with angina pectoris after administration of L-carnitine: semiautomatic computerized analysis of M-mode tracing. *Int J Clin Pharmacol Ther Toxicol* 1988;26:221-224.

17. Cherchi A, Lai C, Angelino F, et al. Effects of L-carnitine on exercise tolerance in chronic stable angina: a multicenter, double-blind, randomized, placebo controlled crossover study. *Int J Clin Pharmacol Ther Toxicol* 1985;23:569-572.

18. Iyer RN, Khan AA, Gupta A, et al. L-carnitine moderately improves the exercise tolerance in chronic stable angina. *J Assoc Physicians India* 2000;48:1050-1052.

19. Cacciatore L, Cerio R, Ciarimboli M, et al. The therapeutic effect of L-carnitine in patients with exercise-induced stable angina: a controlled study. *Drugs Exp Clin Res* 1991;17:225-235.

20. Loster H, Miehe K, Punzel M, et al. Prolonged oral L-carnitine substitution increases bicycle ergometer performance in patients with severe, ischemically induced cardiac insufficiency. *Cardiovasc Drugs Ther* 1999;13:537-546.

21. Brevetti G, Chiariello M, Ferulano G, et al. Increases in walking distance in patients with peripheral vascular disease treated with L-carnitine: a double-blind, cross-over study. *Circulation* 1988;77:767-773.

22. Corbucci GG, Lettieri B. Cardiogenic shock and L-carnitine: clinical data and therapeutic perspectives. *Int J Clin Pharmacol Res* 1991;11:283-293.

23. Corbucci GG, Loche F. L-carnitine in cardiogenic shock therapy: pharmacodynamic aspects and clinical data. *Int J Clin Pharmacol Res* 1993;13:87-91.

24. Rizos I. Three-year survival of patients with heart failure caused by dilated cardiomyopathy and L-carnitine administration. *Am Heart J* 2000;139:S120-S123.

25. Gurlek A, Tutar E, Akcil E, et al. The effects of L-carnitine treatment on left ventricular function and erythrocyte superoxide dismutase activity in patients with ischemic cardiomyopathy. *Eur J Heart Fail* 2000;2:189-193.

26. Davini P, Bigalli A, Lamanna F, Boem A. Controlled study on L-carnitine therapeutic efficacy in post-infarction. *Drugs Exp Clin Res* 1992;18:355-365.

27. De Pasquale B, Righetti G, Menotti A. L-carnitine for the treatment of acute myocardial infarct. *Cardiologia* 1990;35:591-596. [article in Italian]

28. Singh RB, Niaz MA, Agarwal P, et al. A randomised, double-blind, placebo-controlled trial of L-carnitine in suspected acute myocardial infarction. *Postgrad Med J* 1996;72:45-50.

29. Iliceto S, Scrutinio D, Bruzzi P, et al. Effects of L-carnitine administration on left ventricular remodeling after acute anterior myocardial infarction: the L-Carnitine Ecocardiografia Digitalizzata Infarto Miocardico (CEDIM) Trial. *J Am Coll Cardiol* 1995;26:380-387.

30. Stefanutti C, Vivenzio A, Lucani G, et al. Effect of L-carnitine on plasma lipoprotein fatty acids pattern in patients with primary hyperlipoproteinemia. *Clin Ter* 1998;149:115-119.

31. Fernandez C, Proto C. L-carnitine in the treatment of chronic myocardial ischemia. An analysis of 3 multicenter studies and a bibliographic review. *Clin Ter* 1992;140:353-377. [article in Italian]

32. Digiesi V, Cantini F, Bisi G, et al. L-carnitine adjuvant therapy in essential hypertension. *Clin Ter* 1994;144:391-395.

33. Sirtori CR, Calabresi L, Ferrara S, et al. L-carnitine reduces plasma lipoprotein(a) levels in patients with hyper Lp(a). *Nutr Metab Cardiovasc Dis* 2000;10:247-251.

34. Plioplys AV, Plioplys S. Amantadine and L-carnitine treatment of chronic fatigue syndrome. *Neuropsychobiology* 1997;35:16-23.

35. Gunal AI, Celiker H, Donder E, Gunal SY. The effect of L-carnitine on insulin resistance in hemodialysed patients with chronic renal failure. *J Nephrol* 1999;12:38-40.

36. Vesela E, Racek J, Trefil L, et al. Effect of L-carnitine supplementation in hemodialysis patients. *Nephron* 2001;88:218-223.

37. Matsumoto Y, Amano I, Hirose S, et al. Effects of L-carnitine supplementation on renal anemia in poor responders to erythropoietin. *Blood Purif* 2001;19:24-32.

38. Elisaf M, Bairaktari E, Katopodis K, et al. Effect of L-carnitine supplementation on lipid parameters in hemodialysis patients. *Am J Nephrol* 1998;18:416-421.

39. Sachan DS, Rhew TH, Ruark RA. Ameliorating effects of carnitine and its precursors on alcohol-induced fatty liver. *Am J Clin Nutr* 1984;39:738-744.

40. Moretti S, Alesse E, Di Marzio L, et al. Effect of L-carnitine on human immunodeficiency virus-1 infection-associated apoptosis: a pilot study. *Blood* 1998;91:3817-3824.

41. De Simone C, Tzantzoglou S, Famularo G, et al. High dose L-carnitine improves immunologic and metabolic parameters in AIDS patients. *Immunopharmacol Immunotoxicol* 1993;15:1-12.

42. Benvenga S, Ruggeri RM, Russo A, et al. Usefulness of L-carnitine, a naturally occurring peripheral antagonist of thyroid hormone action, in iatrogenic hyperthyroidism: a randomized, double-blind, placebo-controlled clinical trial. *J Clin Endocrinol Metab* 2001;86:3579-3594.

43. Costa M, Canale D, Filicori M, et al. L-carnitine in idiopathic asthenozoospermia: a multicenter study. Italian Study Group on Carnitine and Male Infertility. *Andrologia* 1994;26:155-159.

44. Vitali G, Parente R, Melotti C. Carnitine supplementation in human idiopathic asthenospermia: clinical results. *Drugs Exp Clin Res* 1995;21:157-159.

45. Kurz C, Arbeiter K, Obermair A, et al. L-carnitine-betamethasone combination therapy versus betamethasone therapy alone in prevention of respiratory distress syndrome. *Z Geburtshilfe Perinatol* 1993;197:215-219. [article in German]

46. Iafolla AK, Browning IB 3rd, Roe CR. Familial infantile apnea and immature beta oxidation. *Pediatr Pulmonol* 1995;20:167-171.

47. Villani RG, Gannon J, Self M, Rich PA. L-Carnitine supplementation combined with aerobic training does not promote weight loss in moderately obese women. *Int J Sport Nutr Exerc Metab* 2000;10:199-207.

48. Johnston CS, Solomon RE, Corte C. Vitamin C depletion is associated with alterations in blood histamine and plasma free carnitine in adults. *J Am Coll Nutr* 1996;15:586-591.

49. Ha TY, Otsuka M, Arakawa N. The effect of graded doses of ascorbic acid on the tissue carnitine and plasma lipid concentrations. *J Nutr Sci Vitaminol (Tokyo)* 1990;36:227-234.

50. Otsuka M, Matsuzawa M, Ha TY, Arakawa N. Contribution of a high dose of L-ascorbic acid to carnitine synthesis in guinea pigs fed high-fat diets. *J Nutr Sci Vitaminol (Tokyo)* 1999;45:163-171.

51. Triggs WJ, Roe CR, Rhead WJ, et al. Neuropsychiatric manifestations of defect in mitochondrial beta oxidation response to riboflavin. *J Neurol Neurosurg Psychiatry* 1992;55:209-211.

52. Podlepa EM, Gessler NN, Bykhovskii VIa. The effect of methylation on the carnitine synthesis. *Prikl Biokhim Mikrobiol* 1990;26:179-183. [article in Russian]

53. Dodson WL, Sachan DS. Choline supplementation reduces urinary carnitine excretion in humans. *Am J Clin Nutr* 1996;63:904-910.

54. Hug G, McGraw CA, Bates SR, Landrigan EA. Reduction of serum carnitine concentrations during anticonvulsant therapy with phenobarbital, valproic acid, phenytoin, and carbamazepine in children. *J Pediatr* 1991;119:799-802.

55. Melegh B, Pap M, Molnar D, et al. Carnitine administration ameliorates the changes in energy metabolism caused by short-term pivampicillin medication. *Eur J Pediatr* 1997;156:795-799.

56. Herink J. Enhancing effect of L-carnitine on some abnormal signs induced by pentylenetetrazol. *Acta Medica (Hradec Kralove)* 1996;39:63-66.

57. Lissoni P, Galli MA, Tancini G, Barni S. Prevention by L-carnitine of interleukin-2 related cardiac toxicity during cancer immunotherapy. *Tumori* 1993;79:202-204.

58. Kawasaki N, Lee JD, Shimizu H, Ueda T. Long-term L-carnitine treatment prolongs the survival in rats with adriamycin-induced heart failure. *J Card Fail* 1996;2:293-299.

59. Semino-Mora MC, Leon-Monzon ME, Dalakas MC. Effect of L-carnitine on the zidovudine-induced destruction of human myotubes. Part I: L-carnitine prevents the myotoxicity of AZT *in vitro*. *Lab Invest* 1994;71:102-112.

60. Georgala S, Schulpis KH, Georgala C, Michas T. L-carnitine supplementation in patients with cystic acne on isotretinoin therapy. *J Eur Acad Dermatol Venereol* 1999;13:205-209.

61. Kuntzer T, Reichmann H, Bogousslavsky J, Regli F. Emetine-induced myopathy and carnitine deficiency. *J Neurol* 1990;237:495-496.

62. Sekas G, Paul HS. Hyperammonemia and carnitine deficiency in a patient receiving sulfadiazine and pyrimethamine. *Am J Med* 1993;95:112-113.

63. Mondillo S, Faglia S, D'Aprile N, et al. Therapy of arrhythmia induced by myocardial ischemia. Association of L-carnitine, propafenone and mexiletine. *Clin Ter* 1995;146:769-774. [article in Italian]

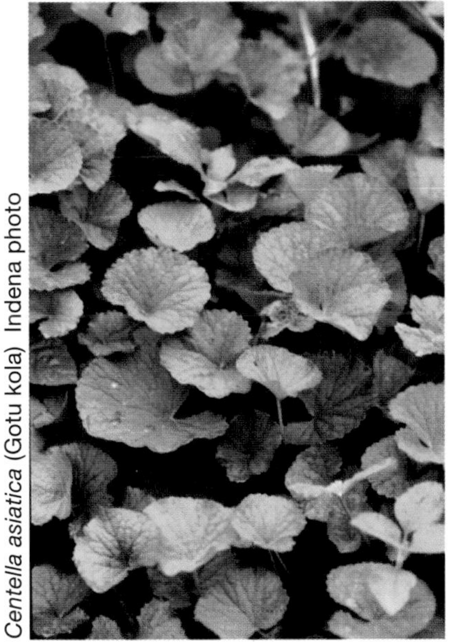

Centella asiatica (Gotu kola) Indena photo

Centella asiatica

Description

Centella asiatica (also known as Gotu kola and *Hydrocotyle asiatica*) is a slender, herbaceous creeper with kidney-shaped leaves, native to the countries of India, Sri Lanka, and Madagascar. It is typically found growing at an altitude of 600 to 2,000 meters.[1]

Active Constituents

Centella contains several active constituents, of which the most important are the triterpenoid saponins, including asiaticoside, centelloside, madecassoside, and asiatic acid. In addition, Gotu kola contains other components, including volatile oils, flavonoids, tannins, phytosterols, amino acids, and sugars.[2]

Mechanisms of Action

Gotu kola has several pharmacological actions, based primarily on *in vivo* experiments. A rat study found both oral and topical administration of gotu kola increased cellular hyperplasia and collagen production at the site of injury, as measured by increased granulation tissue levels of DNA, protein, total collagen, and hexosamine. Moreover, quicker maturation and cross-linking of collagen was seen in animals treated with the herbal extract, as evidenced by the elevated stability of acid-soluble collagen and an increase in aldehyde content and tensile strength. Compared to control wounds, rats treated with gotu kola had a higher degree of epithelialization and a significantly more rapid rate of wound contraction.[3]

In addition to improving wound healing, gotu kola may also have an effect on connective tissue of varicosities. After receiving 30 mg twice per day of total triterpenoid fraction of *Centella asiatica* (TTFCA) for three months, individuals with varicose veins had significant serum reductions in enzymes involved in mucopolysaccharide metabolism (beta glucuronidase, beta N acetylglucuronidase, and arylsulfatase) compared to baseline values ($p < 0.01$).[4]

In another *in vivo* study, intraperitoneal (i.p.) administration of 100 mg/kg body weight of gotu kola to male rats exposed to 2 Gy of ^{60}cobalt gamma irradiation helped protect the animals against both weight loss and conditioned taste aversion. The latter effects of gotu kola were comparable to the anti-nausea drug ondansetron.[5]

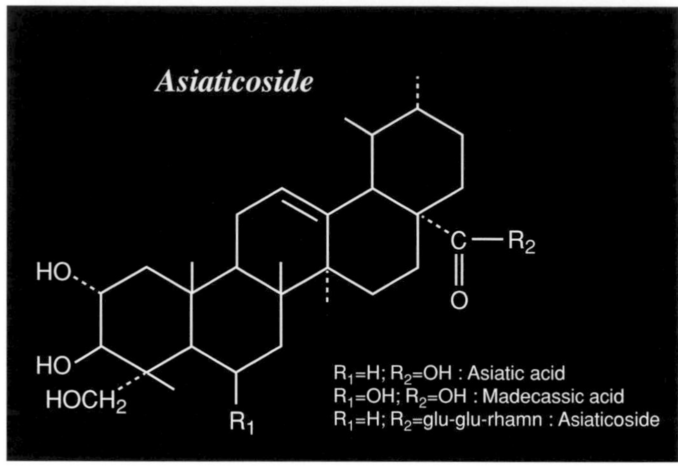

In addition to its radioprotective effects, the fresh juice extract of gotu kola at 200 and 600 mg/kg twice per day has not only proven to be protective against aspirin- and ethanol-induced gastric ulcers, but was similar in its effects to the medication sucralfate.[6] Gotu kola, the authors note, significantly induced gastric mucin secretion and mucosal cell glycoprotein production, markers of increased gastric mucosal defense factors.[6]

A pharmacokinetic study suggests the active ingredients in TTFCA are well absorbed in human volunteers.[7] After single oral administration of 30 and 60 mg of the extract, maximum plasma levels of asiatic acid were reached at 4.5 and 4.2 hours, respectively. Plasma half-lives were 2.2 hours in the 30 mg dose and 3.4 hours in the 60 mg dose, with no detectable levels of the saponin present 24 hours after single dosing. Seven-day treatment with the herb at the same dosing schedule resulted in higher peak plasma concentrations, longer half lives, and area-under-the-curve values.[7]

Clinical Indications

Venous Insufficiency

In a double-blind study, 94 patients (86 men, 8 women; age range 20 to 80 years) with venous insufficiency of the lower extremities for an average of 14 years, were randomized to one of three treatment groups and received a triterpenoid extract of *Centella asiatica* (TECA) at a daily dose of 60 mg, 120 mg, or placebo for three months. Individuals who took gotu kola at either dose had significant clinical improvements in limb heaviness ($p = 0.033$), edema ($p = 0.026$), and global evaluation of efficacy ($p = 0.05$). Venous distensibility as measured by plethysmography was significantly better in the active group at 40 mmHg ($p = 0.08$), 50 mmHg ($p = 0.055$) and 60 mmHg ($p = 0.09$), compared to deteriorating placebo values. Side effects included nausea and gastralgia.[8]

Venous Hypertensive Angiopathy

Forty patients (21 males, 19 females; mean age 47.6 to 48 years) with severe venous hypertension, with ankle swelling and lipodermatosclerosis, were randomized to receive TTFCA 60 mg twice per day or placebo for eight weeks. Patients in the study did not wear compression stockings. After conclusion of the trial, patients taking the herbal extract experienced a significant decrease in skin flux and rate of ankle swelling, compared to baseline values ($p < 0.05$). In addition, patients in the active group reported rapid clinical improvement, which was mirrored by a reduction in the analogue scale line score (e.g., symptoms of edema, pain, restless limbs, swelling, and change in skin condition/color) from 9.5 at baseline to 4.5 after eight weeks.[9] These improvements were confirmed in another study, in which patients took TTFCA at 60 mg twice per day for six weeks. Laser doppler evaluation demonstrated that patients who supplemented with gotu kola had a 29-percent decrease in resting flux ($p < 0.05$), 52-percent increase in venoarteriolar response ($p < 0.05$), and a 66-ml reduction in leg volume. Similarly, those utilizing gotu kola had a 7.2-percent increase in $P0_2$ and a 9.6-percent reduction in $PC0_2$ ($p < 0.05$).[10]

Airline Flight Microangiopathy

"Economy class syndrome" is a term widely employed by the media for the physical consequences of long-distance flights, ranging from simple swelling of the lower limbs to the formation of dangerous blood clots. In an evaluation of Centella's effectiveness in preventing these problems, 66 flight passengers (33 men; 33 women; mean ages 37.5 to 38.9 years) traveling in economy class from 3-12 hours were randomized to receive 60 mg TTFCA three times per day or a placebo two days before the flight, the day of the flight, and two days after the flight. Results showed significant improvements in microcirculatory function (transcutaneous PO_2 and PCO_2, laser doppler flowmetry, venoarteriolar response, rate of ankle swelling and edema) in those utilizing TTFCA ($p < 0.05$). In particular, the authors point out the reduction in edema and rate of ankle swelling approached normal values in those given TTFCA ($p < 0.025$).[11]

Echogenicity in Carotid and Femoral Plaques

Carotid artery plaques echolucent on ultrasound have greater amounts of certain physiological components (e.g., lipids, blood elements, limited amounts of collagen) that make plaque inherently weaker and increase the risk of embolization. This type of plaque is associated with a higher clinical risk of stroke and asymptomatic cerebral lesions.[12]

Asymptomatic patients (49 men; 38 women; mean ages 55.8 to 56 years) with higher risk echolucent carotid artery plaques were randomized to receive 60 mg TTFCA or placebo three times daily for one year. Patients also took platelet anti-aggregating medication throughout the trial. After 12 months, a significant increase in plaque echogenicity was noted, according to sonographic evaluation. Incidence of positive MRI images indicating cerebral ischemic lesions was 7 percent in the TTFCA group and 17 percent in the control group ($p < 0.05$).[12]

Employing a similar dose of gotu kola in patients with femoral plaques, another study also found an increase in plaque echogenicity after 12 months of therapy, compared to no change in the control group. Degree of stenosis and walking distance did not change in the two groups.[13]

Diabetic Microangiopathy

Forty-eight patients with diabetic microangiopathy were randomized into one of three treatment groups and received either 60 mg TTFCA twice per day, placebo, or no treatment for six months. Using laser doppler flowmetry measurements, the researchers concluded those taking TTFCA had significant reductions in skin blood flow at rest at three ($p < 0.05$) and six months ($p < 0.01$), compared to baseline numbers. In addition, VAR scores (decrease of skin blood flow on standing) increased significantly from 6.4 percent to 23.9 percent at three months, and 25.9 percent at six months ($p < 0.05$). During the investigation period $p0_2$ increased ($p < 0.05$) while $pC0_2$ values decreased ($p < 0.01$) significantly in those employing gotu kola. Fasting blood sugar and hemoglobin A1C values did not change.[14]

Keloid and Scar Management

Although gotu kola has long been recommended for the treatment of keloids and/or hypertrophic scars, few papers have addressed these topics. In one open clinical trial, 227 patients were divided into two groups and treated with oral gotu kola alone or surgical scar revision plus gotu kola at doses ranging from 60 to 150 mg daily for up to 18 months. In the *Centella asiatica*-only group 116/139 patients (82%) had relief of symptoms and disappearance of inflammation. In a controlled study of 35 of these patients, 22/27 (81%) improved, in contrast to only 9/19 (47%) in the placebo group ($p < 0.05$). Similarly, in 88 patients who combined surgery with the plant extract, 72 percent had an improvement in their condition.[15] In addition to its oral use, gotu kola has been employed as a cream topically as part of a comprehensive scar management program. Observationally, it was found to improve scar maturity from an average of six months without treatment to three months with treatment.[16]

Anxiety

Gotu kola has long been employed in Ayurvedic medicine for the treatment of anxiety. In a 2000 paper, Bradwin et al suggest this ancient claim may be therapeutically accurate. Following baseline measurements of acoustic startle response (ASR), mood self-rating scale, heart rate, and blood pressure, 40 healthy subjects (21 males, 19 females; age range 18 to 45 years) were randomized to receive 12 grams of non-standardized gotu kola dissolved in 300 ml grape juice or placebo. Evaluations were recorded at 30, 60, 90, and 120 minutes after beginning therapy. Use of gotu kola significantly decreased ASR amplitude, compared to placebo, at 30 ($p < 0.02$) and 60 minutes ($p < 0.001$). Heart rate, blood pressure, and mood did not change in the treated group.[17]

Other Indications

Several small clinical trails using Centella have provided preliminary data to support its use in the treatment of scleroderma,[18] alcohol-induced liver cirrhosis,[19] leg ulcers,[20] and as adjunctive treatment in leprosy.[21] More clinically-oriented research needs to be done in these areas to establish effective dosages and protocols.

Side Effects and Toxicity

Alcoholic extracts of gotu kola have shown no toxicity at doses of 350 mg/kg when given i.p. to rats.[1] Reported adverse effects include GI upset and nausea.[8] Topical use of the extract has led to reports of rash.[22]

Dosage

In adults, the recommended dose of TTFCA (or TECA) extracts standardized for asiaticoside, asiatic acid, and madecassic acid is 60 to 120 mg per day. The crude herb and 1:5 tincture dose is 0.5-6 grams and 10-20 ml, respectively, per day.[23]

Warnings and Contraindications

Gotu kola should be avoided during pregnancy, due to its emmenagogue action.[24]

References

1. Chemexcil. *Selected Medicinal Plants of India*. Bombay, India; Tata Press; 1992.
2. Leung AY, Foster S. *Encyclopedia of Common Natural Ingredients Used in Food, Drugs, and Cosmetics*, 2nd ed. New York: John Wiley & Son; 1998:284.
3. Suguna L, Sivakumar P, Chandrakasan G. Effects of *Centella asiatica* extract on dermal wound healing in rats. *Indian J Exp Biol* 1996;34:1208-1211.
4. Arpaia MR, Ferrone R, Amitrano M, et al. Effects of *Centella asiatica* extract on mucopolysaccharide metabolism in subjects with varicose veins. *Int J Clin Pharm Res* 1990;10:229-233.
5. Shobi V, Goel HC. Protection against radiation-induced conditioned taste aversion by *Centella asiatica*. *Physiol Behav* 2001;73:19-23.
6. Sairam K, Rao CV, Goel RK. Effect of *Centella asiatica* Linn on physical and chemical factors induced gastric ulceration and secretion in rats. *Indian J Exp Biol* 2001;39:137-142.
7. Grimaldi R, De Ponti F, D'angelo L, et al. Pharmacokinetics of the total triterpenic fraction of *Centella asiatica* after single and multiple administrations to healthy volunteers. A new assay for asiatic acid. *J Ethnopharmacol* 1990;28:235-241.
8. Pointel JP, Boccalon H, Cloarec M, et al. Titrated extract of *Centella asiatica* (TECA) in the treatment of venous insufficiency of the lower limbs. *Angiology* 1987;38:46-50.
9. Cesarone MR, Belcaro G, De Sanctis MT, et al. Effects of the total triterpenic fraction of *Centella asiatica* in venous hypertensive microangiopathy: a prospective, placebo-controlled, randomized trial. *Angiology* 2001;52:S15-S18.

10. Cesarone MR, Belcaro G, Rulo M, et al. Microcirculatory effects of total triterpenic fraction of *Centella asiatica* in chronic venous hypertension: measurement by laser doppler, $TcP0_2$-$C0_2$, and leg volumetry. *Angiology* 2001;52:S45-S48.
11. Cesarone MR, Incandela L, De Sanctis MT, et al. Flight microangiopathy in medium-to-long distance flights: prevention of edema and microcirculation alterations with total triterpenic fractions of *Centella asiatica*. *Angiology* 2001;52:S33-S37.
12. Cesarone MR, Belcaro G, Nicolaides N, et al. Increase in echogenicity of echolucent carotid plaques after treatment with total triterpenic fraction of *Centella asiatica*: a prospective placebo-controlled trial. *Angiology* 2001;52:S19-S25.
13. Incandela L, Belcaro G, Nicolaides AN, et al. Modification of the echogenicity of femoral plaques after treatment with total triterpenic fraction of *Centella asiatica*: a prospective, randomized, placebo-controlled trial. *Angiology* 2001;52:S69-S73.
14. Cesarone MR, Incandela L, De Sanctis MT, et al. Evaluation of treatment of diabetic microangiopathy with total triterpenic fraction of *Centella asiatica*: a clinical prospective randomized trial with a microcirculatory model. *Angiology* 2001;52:S49-S54.
15. Bosse JP, Papillon J, Frenette G, et al. Clinical study of a new anti-keloid agent. *Ann Plast Surg* 1979;3:13-21.
16. Widgerow AD, Chait LA, Stals R, et al. New innovations in scar management. *Aesth Plast Surg* 2000;24:227-234.
17. Bradwin J, Zhou Y, Koszycki D, et al. A double-blind, placebo-controlled study on the effects of gotu kola (*Centella asiatica*) on acoustic startle response in healthy subjects. *J Clin Psychopharmacol* 2000;20:680-684.
18. Sasaki S, Shinkai H, Akashi Y, et al. Studies on the mechanism of action of asiaticoside (Madecassol) on experimental granulation tissue and cultured fibroblasts and its clinical application in systemic scleroderma. *Acta Derm Venerol* 1972;52:141-150.
19. Darnis F, Orcel L, de Saint-Maur PP, et al. Use of a titrated extract of *Centella asiatica* in chronic hepatic disorders *Sem Hop* 1979;55:1749-1750. [article in French]
20. Huriez C. Action of titrated extract of *Centella asiatica* in the cicatrization of leg ulcers (10 mg tablets). Apropos of 50 cases. *Lille Med* 1971;17:S574-S579. [article in French]
21. Chaudhury S, Hazra S, Podder GC, et al. New multidrug regimen with indigenous drugs and dapsone in the treatment of lepromatous leprosy. *Indian J Dermatol* 1987;32:63-67.
22. Eun HC, Lee AY. Contact dermatitis due to Madecassol. *Contact Dermatitis* 1985;13:310-313.
23. Turton S. *Centella asiatica*. *Aust J Herbalism* 1993;5:60.
24. Brinker F. *Herb Contraindications and Drug Interactions* 2nd ed. Sandy, OR: Eclectic Medical Publications; 1998:78.

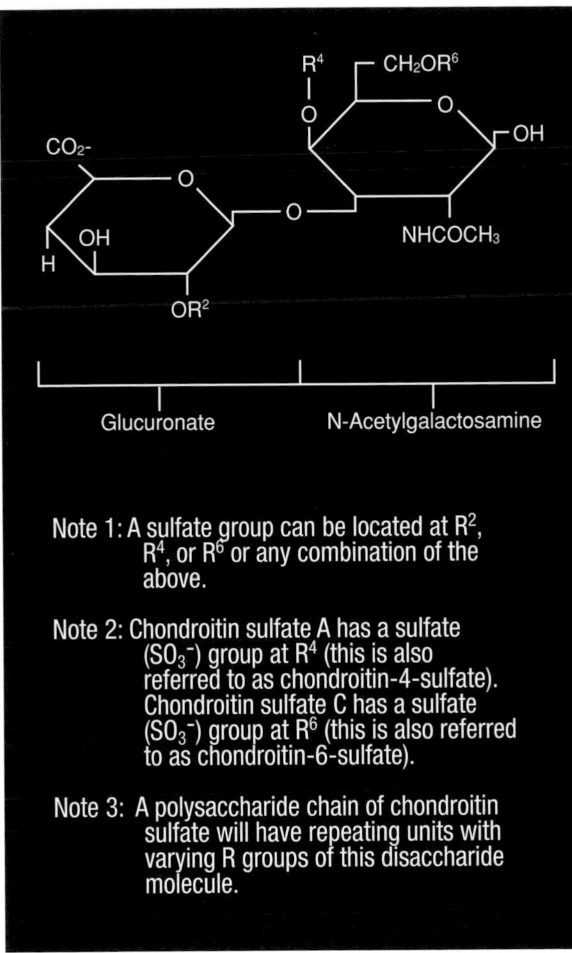

Chondroitin Sulfates

Introduction

Chondroitin sulfates, a class of glycosaminoglycans, are required for the formation of the proteoglycans found in joint cartilage. It is believed they improve joint function by both enhancing endogenous synthesis and preventing enzymatic degradation of joint glycosaminoglycans. Evidence supports oral administration of chondroitin sulfates for degenerative joint disease, both as an agent to slowly reduce symptoms and to decrease the need for non-steroidal anti-inflammatory drugs.

Biochemistry

Chondroitin sulfates are formed in the body from alternating sulfated and/or unsulfated residues of D-glucuronic acid and N-acetylgalactosamine, thus making a disaccharide. Sequences of these disaccharides are formed into polysaccharide chains. The most abundant of these disaccharides in joint tissue are chondroitin sulfate A (chondroitin-4-sulfate) and chondroitin sulfate C (chondroitin-6-sulfate).

Because of the potential biochemical variety of the disaccharides (based on the number and position of the sulfate groups and the percentage of similar disaccharides) comprising the primary structure of the polysaccharide chain, chondroitin sulfates are actually a heterogeneous group of compounds having different molecular masses and charge densities. Proprietary chondroitin sulfate products have been utilized in the majority of research on chondroitin sulfates and osteoarthritis.

Pharmacokinetics

The majority of an oral dose of chondroitin sulfate is hydrolyzed into monosaccharides during the digestive process. Smaller amounts of di-, oligo-, and polysaccharides survive the digestive processes intact. Because of this natural acid hydrolysis, absorption of intact chondroitin sulfate molecules is low following an oral dose, and is estimated to be zero percent for high molecular weight chondroitin sulfate polysaccharide chains and possibly between 8-12 percent for lower molecular weight and highly sulfated chondroitin sulfate polysaccharide chains.[1-3]

Despite this low absorption of intact chondroitin sulfate molecules, radio labeling in animals suggests as much as 70 percent of an oral dose of chondroitin sulfate is absorbed and subsequently found in urine and tissues.[1] The majority of the absorbed dose is in the form of the monosaccharides D-glucuronic acid and N-acetylgalactosamine. Lesser amounts of di-, oligo-, and polysaccharides, as well as intact chondroitin sulfates also appear in blood and tissues following an oral dose in humans.[3]

After absorption, the products of chondroitin sulfate hydrolysis concentrate in the small intestine, liver, and kidneys (tissues responsible for the absorption, metabolism, degradation, and elimination of the compound); however, a tropism for joints is also demonstrated, since relatively high amounts of chondroitin sulfate components also concentrate in tissues that utilize amino sugars; such as joint cartilage, synovial fluid, and the trachea.[1,3]

Mechanisms of Action

The primary mechanism of action is increased joint glycosaminoglycan concentration and a subsequent enhancement of synovial fluid viscosity. This improvement of joint structure and function appears to be a result of a combination of two factors: (1) increased endogenous synthesis of hyaluronic acid and sulfated glycosaminoglycans from chondroitin sulfate, and (2) reduced breakdown of joint glycosaminoglycans subsequent to decreased collagenolytic activity and inhibition of enzymes, such as phospholipase A2 and N-acetylglucosaminidase, which are capable of degrading existing joint glycosaminoglycans.[3-6]

Clinical Indications

Osteoarthritis

Current findings indicate oral administration of chondroitin sulfate is useful for the treatment of osteoarthritis, both as an agent to reduce symptomology and to decrease the need for non-steroidal anti-inflammatory drugs (NSAIDs).

Studies have shown oral administration of chondroitin sulfate to be superior to placebo in osteoarthritis of the knees and hands. An average improvement of 50 percent in parameters and variables assessed, such as pain, walking time, medicine use, and joint mobility has been consistently reported. Significant changes are produced after a minimum of 1-2 months of supplementation and appear to be both dose- and time-dependent, with better results often demonstrated when supplementation periods are extended over greater time periods. Long-term supplementation appears to protect against further erosive damage to joints as well as stabilizing joint width, thereby preventing further narrowing or destruction of the joint space.[7-15]

Co-administration of chondroitin sulfate with NSAIDs is reported to result in a significant reduction in the use of NSAIDS over time.[9,16] In one study, a 72-percent reduction in the effective dose of NSAIDs required to relieve pain was reported.[16]

A combination of chondroitin sulfate, glucosamine HCl, and manganese ascorbate demonstrated efficacy in osteoarthritis of the knee.[17,18] The design of these studies does not allow for any conclusions to be made with respect to additive effects or synergism, since the combination of nutrients was not compared to chondroitin sulfate as an exclusive therapy.

Inflammatory Bowel Disease

Oral administration of chondroitin sulfate decreased incidence of bloody stools and erosions, and enhanced certain aspects of immunity in dextran sulfate sodium-induced colitis in rats. Chondroitin sulfate's therapeutic effect was hypothesized to be secondary to protecting the integrity of the lining of the intestinal mucosa.[19] No evidence currently exists documenting efficacy in inflammatory conditions of the digestive tract in humans.

Surgery

A single intraperitoneal administration of chondroitin sulfate solution to rats has been shown to be effective in preventing post-operative adhesion formation following abdominal surgery. Both fibrin and collagen type I deposition were significantly reduced.[20]

Side Effects and Toxicity

Chondroitin sulfate is well tolerated following an oral dose, and no signs or symptoms of systemic toxicity have been reported.[1] Long-term tolerance after one year of treatment resulted in no side effects in more than 90 percent of subjects.[13] The most commonly occurring side effects of chondroitin sulfate administration are slight dyspepsia or nausea, which occur in about three percent of subjects.[21]

Dosage

The therapeutic oral dosage of chondroitin sulfate is 800-1,200 mg per day. A single daily dose appears to be as effective as two or three smaller doses per day.[1,15] Results obtained from administration of chondroitin sulfate are not permanent, so either chronic supplementation or repeated cycles of administration appear to be needed to produce optimal results.

Comment

The processing (degree of fractionation, range of particle size, and molecular mass), location and percentage of sulfation, and purity of chondroitin sulfate polysaccharides (based on the amount of other glycosaminoglycans such as keratan sulfate, dermatan sulfate, etc.) present in the preparation might dramatically alter the metabolic fate and the therapeutic results following oral or parenteral administration. The proprietary products utilized in the studies are extracted and purified to contain up to 97 percent chondroitin sulfate, primarily consisting of low molecular weight molecules with a high degree of sulfation. Until more information is available, using similar quality chondroitin sulfate products is prudent.

References

1. Conte A, Volpi N, Palmieri L, et al. Biochemical and pharmacokinetic aspects of oral treatment with chondroitin sulfate. *Arzneimittelforschung* 1995;45:918-925.
2. Morrison M. Therapeutic applications of chondroitin-4-sulfate, appraisal of biological properties. *Folia Angiol* 1977;25:225-232.
3. Ronca F, Palmieri L, Panicucci P, Ronca G. Anti-inflammatory activity of chondroitin sulfate. *Osteoarthritis Cartilage* 1998;6:S14-S21.
4. Glade MJ. Polysulfated glycosaminoglycan accelerates net synthesis of collagen and glycosaminoglycans by arthritic equine cartilage tissues and chondrocytes. *Am J Vet Res* 1990;51:779-785.
5. Johnson KA, Hulse DA, Hart RC, et al. Effects of an orally administered mixture of chondroitin sulfate, glucosamine hydrochloride and manganese ascorbate on synovial fluid chondroitin sulfate 3B3 and 7D4 epitope in a canine cruciate ligament transection model of osteoarthritis. *Osteoarthritis Cartilage* 2001;9:14-21.
6. Lippiello L, Woodward J, Karpman R, Hammad TA. *In vivo* chondroprotection and metabolic synergy of glucosamine and chondroitin sulfate. *Clin Orthop* 2000;381:229-240.
7. Rovetta G, Monteforte P. Galactosaminoglycuronglycan sulfate in erosive osteoarthritis of the hands: early diagnosis, early treatment. *Int J Tissue React* 1996;18:43-46.
8. Morreale P, Manopulo R, Galati M, et al. Comparison of the anti-inflammatory efficacy of chondroitin sulfate and diclofenac sodium in patients with knee osteoarthritis. *J Rheumatol* 1996;23:1385-1391.
9. Mazieres B, Loyau G, Menkes CJ, et al. Chondroitin sulfate in the treatment of gonarthrosis and coxarthrosis. 5-months result of a multicenter double-blind controlled prospective study using placebo. *Rev Rhum Mal Osteoartic* 1992;59:466-472. [Article in French]
10. Mazieres B, Combe B, Phan Van A, et al. Chondroitin sulfate in osteoarthritis of the knee: a prospective, double blind, placebo controlled multicenter clinical study. *J Rheumatol* 2001;28:173-181.
11. Bucsi L, Poor G. Efficacy and tolerability of oral chondroitin sulfate as a symptomatic slow-acting drug for osteoarthritis (SYSADOA) in the treatment of knee osteoarthritis. *Osteoarthritis Cartilage* 1998;6:S31-S36.
12. Verbruggen G, Goemaere S, Veys EM. Chondroitin sulfate: S/DMOAD (structure/disease modifying anti-osteoarthritis drug) in the treatment of finger joint OA. *Osteoarthritis Cartilage* 1998;6:S37-S38.
13. Conrozier T. Anti-arthrosis treatments: efficacy and tolerance of chondroitin sulfates (CS 4&6). *Presse Med* 1998;27:1862-1865. [Article in French]
14. Uebelhart D, Thonar EJ, Delmas PD, et al. Effects of oral chondroitin sulfate on the progression of knee osteoarthritis: a pilot study. *Osteoarthritis Cartilage* 1998;6:S39-S46.
15. Bourgeois P, Chales G, Dehais J, et al. Efficacy and tolerability of chondroitin sulfate 1200 mg/day vs chondroitin sulfate 3 x 400 mg/day vs placebo. *Osteoarthritis Cartilage* 1998;6:S25-S30.

16. Leeb BF, Petera P, Neumann K. Results of a multicenter study of chondroitin sulfate (Condrosulf) use in arthroses of the finger, knee and hip joints. *Wien Med Wochenschr* 1996;146:609-614. [Article in German]

17. Das A Jr, Hammad TA. Efficacy of a combination of FCHG49 glucosamine hydrochloride, TRH122 low molecular weight sodium chondroitin sulfate and manganese ascorbate in the management of knee osteoarthritis. *Osteoarthritis Cartilage* 2000;8:343-350.

18. Leffler CT, Philippi AF, Leffler SG, et al. Glucosamine, chondroitin, and manganese ascorbate for degenerative joint disease of the knee or low back: a randomized, double-blind, placebo-controlled pilot study. *Mil Med* 1999;164:85-91.

19. Hori Y, Hoshino J, Yamazaki C, et al. Effects of chondroitin sulfate on colitis induced by dextran sulfate sodium in rats. *Jpn J Pharmacol* 2001;85:155-160.

20. Tran HS, Chrzanowski FA Jr, Puc MM, et al. An *in vivo* evaluation of a chondroitin sulfate solution to prevent postoperative intraperitoneal adhesion formation. *J Surg Res* 2000;88:78-87.

21. Oliviero U, Sorrentino GP, De Paola P, et al. Effects of the treatment with matrix on elderly people with chronic articular degeneration. *Drugs Exp Clin Res* 1991;17:45-51.

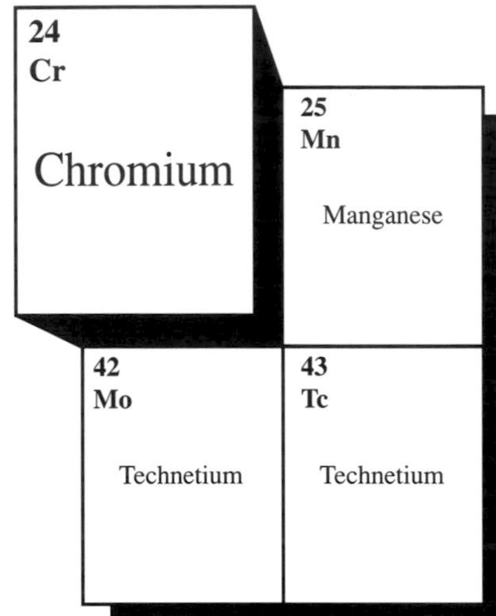

Chromium

Introduction

Chromium (Cr) is a transition element that can occur in several valence states (most commonly 0, +2, +3, and +6). Trivalent chromium (Cr^{+3}) is the most stable form in biological systems and the most abundant form found in the food supply.[1]

In early studies, an unknown factor was extracted from brewer's yeast that improved glucose tolerance in chromium-deficient rats.[1] Named Glucose Tolerance Factor (GTF), it was first identified in 1957. Chromium was later identified as the essential element of GTF that potentiates insulin action and restores normal glucose tolerance.[2] The GTF form of chromium was originally proposed as containing chromium bound to nicotinic acid, glycine, cysteine, and glutamic acid.[1] However, researchers have been unable to purify and isolate this compound to confirm its exact structure.

Chromium is widely distributed in foods, but in small quantities. Refining foods such as flour or sugar depletes them of chromium.[3] Stainless steel contains 11-30 percent chromium, which can be leached from containers when acidic foods (e.g., fruits and their juices) are stored or cooked in them.[4]

Pharmacokinetics

The bioavailability of chromium has been difficult to establish, owing to its rather low concentration in mammalian tissues. Intestinal absorption of chromium is low, with animal studies indicating rates in the range of less than 0.5-3 percent.[5]

Chromium is absorbed by an active transport mechanism and is transported to the liver bound to transferrin. It has been suggested iron interferes with the transport of chromium in patients with hemochromatosis.[6,7] This may partially explain the higher rate of diabetes seen in hemochromatosis patients. High-sugar diets increase chromium turnover and excretion in the urine.[8]

Mechanisms of Action

Chromium potentiates insulin by enhancing receptor binding, thereby stabilizing blood glucose levels. The chromium found in brewer's yeast was found in one study to be more effective than chromium chloride or torula yeast at stimulating glucose uptake.[9] In 12 of 15 controlled clinical trials, chromium supplementation improved the action of insulin or exerted beneficial effects on blood lipid balance.[10]

Chromium has been found to decrease C-reactive protein (a marker for inflammation) and increase insulin receptor number and binding.[11]

Animal studies indicate chromium may affect immune status by activating specific immune responses and immunoglobulins.[12-14]

Deficiency States and Symptoms

Chromium deficiency is rare and difficult to produce experimentally because chromium is ubiquitous in the environment. No Cr-dependent metabolic enzymes have been identified. Animal studies suggest inadequate dietary intake may produce insulin insensitivity and reduced sperm count. However, the long-term consequences of intakes less than 50 mcg per day have yet to be determined.

Chromium may be important for growth, based on animal studies[15] and on the observation that patients on Cr-deficient total parenteral nutrition (TPN) lost weight that was later regained after chromium supplementation.[16,17]

Metabolic stress, such as experienced by trauma patients or persons who exercise strenuously, increases the excretion of and possibly the need for chromium.[18] Chromium needs may also increase during pregnancy due to maternal depletion.[19,20]

No effective clinical test exists to identify chromium deficiency. Serum chromium is not easily detected and is a poor indicator of Cr status. Low levels of chromium in tissues and the potential for easy contamination of samples make testing a challenge. Moreover, tissue concentrations do not accurately reflect metabolic pools.

Clinical Indications

Diabetes

Chromium-rich brewer's yeast has been recognized since the mid-nineteenth century as a useful therapy for diabetes. Chromium supplementation improves glucose levels and potentiates the action of insulin in people with glucose intolerance, diabetes (types 1 and 2), gestational diabetes, and diabetes caused by corticosteroids.[21] More than 10 trials of chromium supplementation in patients with glucose intolerance and diabetes have demonstrated clinical efficacy of supplemental chromium.[22]

In a four-month, double-blind trial, 180 people with type 2 diabetes were supplemented with either 100 mcg chromium (picolinate), 500 mcg chromium (picolinate), or placebo, twice daily. A significant lowering of fasting blood sugar was experienced by the 500-mcg group, but not in the other two groups. Glycosylated hemoglobin was significantly decreased in both chromium groups (more so in the high-dose group), and cholesterol decreased significantly in the high-dose chromium group.[23]

In another study, 243 people with either type 1 or 2 diabetes took 200 mcg chromium daily. Subjects were asked to decrease oral hypoglycemic agents or insulin as needed to keep blood sugar within normal limits. Over one-half of the type 2 diabetics and one-third of the type 1 diabetics were able to decrease their medications significantly.[24]

Some studies have reported no therapeutic effect from chromium supplementation in diabetes;[25-27] however, these studies used daily doses of 200 mcg or less.

Hypoglycemia

In a double-blind, crossover study,[28] eight female patients with hypoglycemia were given supplemental chromium chloride (200 mcg per day elemental chromium) or placebo for three months. Chromium supplementation alleviated symptoms of hypoglycemia and raised the glucose nadir at 2-4 hours after a glucose load. In an uncontrolled trial,[29] chromium supplementation (125 mcg per day as a yeast supplement) produced improvement of chilliness in 47 percent of participants, with 15 percent indicating the chilliness disappeared entirely. Trembling, emotional instability, and disorientation improved as well. One case was reported of chromium supplementation inducing hypoglycemia.[30]

Hypercholesterolemia

Although one group of researchers found no beneficial effect of chromium supplementation on blood lipid levels,[27,31] several well-controlled clinical trials of chromium supplementation have demonstrated it can lower total[32,33] and LDL cholesterol,[34,35] and increase HDL cholesterol.[33,36] In one double-blind trial, 500 mcg chromium per day in combination with regular exercise reduced total cholesterol levels by 20 percent in 13 weeks.[37] It is impossible in this study to know which was more important, the chromium or the exercise. Supplementation with chromium-rich brewer's yeast has also lowered serum cholesterol.[38]

Dysthymia

After one patient reported a dramatic response to the addition of a chromium supplement to sertraline (Zoloft®) therapy for dysthymic disorder, a series of single-blind and open-label trials were undertaken to evaluate the effects of chromium picolinate or chromium polynicotinate on the treatment of antidepressant-refractory dysthymic disorder. In five patients, chromium supplementation led to remission of dysthymic symptoms. Single-blind substitution of other dietary supplements in each of the patients demonstrated specificity of response to chromium supplementation.[39]

Athletic Performance

Research in animals[40] and humans[41,42] have found chromium picolinate supplementation might increase fat loss and lean muscle gain when used in conjunction with a resistance-training program. These findings were validated by the results of two double-blind trials.[43,44]

However, more evidence exists that chromium supplementation has little or no effect on strength or body composition.[45-48] In one study, changes in body weight, a sum of three body circumferences, a sum of three skin folds, and the one-repetition maximum for the squat and bench press were examined in 59 college-age students over a 12-week weightlifting program. Half the students were given 200 mcg per day elemental chromium as picolinate, while the other half received a placebo. No treatment effects were seen for the strength measurements. The only significant treatment effect found was an increase in body weight observed in females supplementing with chromium.[48]

Several other studies using 200 mcg[49,50] or 400 mcg[51,52] chromium as picolinate found similar lack of effect on body composition or strength.

Weight Loss

Because chromium supplementation has been reported to increase lean body mass and decrease the percentage of body fat, chromium has been touted as a weight-loss product. The effect of chromium supplementation on body composition is controversial, although theoretically supported by animal studies.[47] According to one human study, chromium picolinate supplementation increased lean body mass in obese patients in the maintenance period after a very low-calorie diet without counteracting the weight loss achieved.[53] In another double-blind trial, 400 mcg per day of chromium as picolinate was ineffective in enhancing body fat reduction in healthy U.S. Navy personnel who exercised aerobically three times per week for at least 30 minutes.[51]

Drug-Nutrient Interactions

Chromium absorption is enhanced by vitamin C,[54] oxalates,[55] aspirin,[56] and indomethacin.[57] On the other hand, absorption of chromium is decreased by a high fiber meal, due to the presence of phytic acid.[58] It is therefore likely that dietary supplements containing phytic acid (i.e., inositol hexaphosphate; IP-6) would also chelate the mineral and decrease its absorption. Several antacids have been found to significantly reduce 51Cr in the blood and tissues compared to controls.[59]

Side Effects and Toxicity

Trivalent chromium is safe, not well absorbed, excreted rapidly with large exposures, and has low potential for toxicity. Trivalent chromium should not be confused with the toxic hexavalent chromium (Cr^{6+}), which is generated from the welding of stainless steel. Toxicity symptoms of Cr^{6+} include allergic dermatitis, skin and nasal septum lesions, and increased incidence of lung cancer and possibly other diseases.

Chromium picolinate supplementation has been linked with individual cases of systemic contact dermatitis[60] and acute, generalized, exanthematous pustulosis.[61] Another case was reported of a woman who took 1,200-2,400 mcg chromium per day for 4-5 months and suffered toxicity symptoms including weight loss, anemia, thrombocytopenia, hemolysis, and elevated liver enzymes.[62] Previous animal studies have shown, variously, that chromium picolinate produced chromosomal damage[63] or that is has no toxicity.[64] Toxicity of other supplemental forms of chromium (e.g., chromium polynicotinate) has not been reported.

Dosage

Mean chromium intake is 33 mcg per day in adult men, 25 mcg per day in women. The estimated safe and adequate daily dietary intake (ESADDI) is currently set at 50-200 mcg per day for adults; the ESADDI for infants (10-40 mcg per day) may not be attainable because human breast milk provides less than 1 mcg per day.[9]

In the studies cited above, effective doses range from 150-1,000 mcg per day. Typical dosage amounts used to treat diabetes and dysglycemia — conditions for which the strongest evidence exists in favor of chromium supplementation — are 200-1,000 mcg per day.

Warnings and Contraindications

Caution should be used in combining chromium supplements with any blood-sugar lowering medication, as the combination may induce hypoglycemia.

References

1. Mertz W. Chromium occurrence and function in biological systems. *Physiol Rev* 1969;49:163-239.
2. Schwarz K, Mertz W. Chromium(III) and the glucose tolerance factor. *Arch Biochem* 1959;85:292-295.
3. Anderson RA, Bryden NA, Polansky MM. Dietary chromium intake. Freely chosen diets, institutional diet, and individual foods. *Biol Trace Elem Res* 1992;32:117-121.
4. Offenbacher EG, Pi-Sunyer FX. Temperature and pH effects on the release of chromium from stainless steel into water and fruit juices. *J Agric Food Chem* 1983;31:89-92.
5. Sayato Y, Nakamuro K, Matsui S, Ando M. Metabolic fate of chromium compounds. I. Comparative behavior of chromium in rat administered with Na251CrO4 and 51CrCl3. *J Pharmacobiodyn* 1980;3:17-23.
6. Lim TH, Sargent T 3rd, Kusubov N. Kinetics of trace element chromium(III) in the human body. *Am J Physiol* 1983;244:R445-R454.
7. Sargent T 3rd, Lim TH, Jenson RL. Reduced chromium retention in patients with hemochromatosis, a possible basis of hemochromatotic diabetes. *Metabolism* 1979;28:70-79.
8. Kozlovsky AS, Moser PB, Reiser S, Anderson RA. Effects of diets high in simple sugars on urinary chromium losses. *Metabolism* 1986;35:515-518.
9. Stoecker BJ. Chromium. In: Ziegler EE, Filer LJ, eds. *Present Knowledge in Nutrition,* 7th ed. Washington DC: ILSI Press; 1996:344-352.

10. Mertz W. Chromium in human nutrition: a review. *J Nutr* 1993;123:626-633.
11. Anderson RA, Polansky MM, Bryden NA, et al. Effects of supplemental chromium on patients with symptoms of reactive hypoglycemia. *Metabolism* 1987;36:351-355.
12. Chang X, Mowat DN. Supplemental chromium for stressed and growing feeder calves. *J Anim Sci* 1992;70:559-565.
13. Moonsie-Shageer S, Mowat DN. Effect of level of supplemental chromium on performance, serum constituents, and immune status of stressed feeder calves. *J Anim Sci* 1993;71:232-238.
14. Burton JL, Mallard BA, Mowat DN. Effects of supplemental chromium on immune responses of periparturient and early lactation dairy cows. *J Anim Sci* 1993;71:1532-1539.
15. Gurson CT, Saner G. Effects of chromium supplementation on growth in marasmic protein-calorie malnutrition. *Am J Clin Nutr* 1973;26:988-991.
16. Jeejeebhoy KN, Chu RC, Marliss EB, et al. Chromium deficiency, glucose intolerance, and neuropathy reversed by chromium supplementation, in a patient receiving long-term total parenteral nutrition. *Am J Clin Nutr* 1977;30:531-538.
17. Freund H, Atamian S, Fischer JE. Chromium deficiency during total parenteral nutrition. *JAMA* 1979;241:496-498.
18. Nielsen FH. Nutritional significance of the ultratrace elements. *Nutr Rev* 1988;46:337-341.
19. Saner G. The effect of parity on maternal hair chromium concentration and the changes during pregnancy. *Am J Clin Nutr* 1981;34:853-855.
20. Wallach S, Verch RL. Placental transport of chromium. *J Am Coll Nutr* 1984;3:69-74.
21. Anderson RA. Chromium in the prevention and control of diabetes. *Diabetes Metab* 2000;26:22-27.
22. Anderson RA. Chromium, glucose intolerance and diabetes. *J Am Coll Nutr* 1998;17:548-555.
23. Anderson RA, Cheng N, Bryden NA, et al. Elevated intakes of supplemental chromium improve glucose and insulin variables in individuals with type 2 diabetes. *Diabetes* 1997;46:1786-1791.
24. Ravina A, Slezak L. Chromium in the treatment of clinical diabetes mellitus. *Harefuah* 1993;125:142-145. [article in Hebrew]
25. Sherman L, Glennon JA, Brech WJ, et al. Failure of trivalent chromium to improve hyperglycemia in diabetes mellitus. *Metabolism* 1968;17:439-442.
26. Rabinowitz MB, Gonick HC, Levin SR, Davidson MB. Effects of chromium and yeast supplements on carbohydrate and lipid metabolism in diabetic men. *Diabetes Care* 1983;6:319-327.
27. Uusitupa MI, Kumpulainen JT, Voutilainen E, et al. Effect of inorganic chromium supplementation on glucose tolerance, insulin response, and serum lipids in noninsulin-dependent diabetics. *Am J Clin Nutr* 1983;38:404-410.
28. Anderson RA, Polansky MM, Bryden NA, et al. Effects of supplemental chromium on patients with symptoms of reactive hypoglycemia. *Metabolism* 1987;36:351-355.
29. Clausen J. Chromium induced clinical improvement in symptomatic hypoglycemia. *Biol Trace Elem Res* 1988;17:229-236.
30. Bunner SP, McGinnis R. Chromium-induced hypoglycemia. *Psychosomatics* 1998;39:298-299.
31. Uusitupa MI, Mykkanen L, Siitonen O, et al. Chromium supplementation in impaired glucose tolerance of elderly: effects on blood glucose, plasma insulin, C-peptide and lipid levels. *Br J Nutr* 1992;68:209-216.
32. Offenbacher EG, Pi-Sunyer FX. Beneficial effect of chromium-rich yeast on glucose tolerance and blood lipids in elderly subjects. *Diabetes* 1980;29:919-925.
33. Press RI, Geller J, Evans GW. The effect of chromium picolinate on serum cholesterol and apolipoprotein fractions in human subjects. *West J Med* 1990;152:41-45.
34. Hermann J, Chung H, Arquitt A, et al. Effects of chromium or copper supplementation on plasma lipids, plasma glucose and serum insulin in adults over age fifty. *J Nutr Elderly* 1998;18:27-45.
35. Riales R, Albrink MJ. Effect of chromium chloride supplementation on glucose tolerance and serum lipids including high-density lipoprotein of adult men. *Am J Clin Nutr* 1981;34:2670-2678.
36. Roeback JR, Hla KM, Chambless LE, Fletcher RH. Effects of chromium supplementation on serum high-density lipoprotein cholesterol levels in men taking beta-blockers. *Ann Intern Med* 1991;115:917-924.

37. Boyd SG, Boone BE, Smith AR, et al. Combined dietary chromium picolinate supplementation and an exercise program leads to a reduction of serum cholesterol and insulin in college-aged subjects. *J Nutr Biochem* 1998;9:471-475.
38. Wang MM, Fox EA, Stoecker BJ, et al. Serum cholesterol of adults supplemented with brewer's yeast or chromium chloride. *Nutr Res* 1989;9:989-998.
39. McLeod MN, Gaynes BN, Golden RN. Chromium potentiation of antidepressant pharmacotherapy for dysthymic disorder in 5 patients. *J Clin Psychiatry* 1999;60:237-240.
40. Page TG, Ward TL, Southern LL. Effect of chromium picolinate on growth and carcass characteristics of growing-finishing pigs. *J Animal Sci* 1991;69:356.
41. Lefavi R, Anderson R, Keith R, et al. Efficacy of chromium supplementation in athletes: emphasis on anabolism. *Int J Sport Nutr* 1992;2:111-122.
42. McCarty MF. The case for supplemental chromium and a survey of clinical studies with chromium picolinate. *J Appl Nutr* 1991;43:59-66.
43. Kaats GR, Blum K, Fisher JA, Adelman JA. Effects of chromium picolinate supplementation on body composition: a randomized, double-masked, placebo-controlled study. *Curr Ther Res* 1996;57:747-756.
44. Kaats GR, Blum K, Pullin D, et al. A randomized, double-masked, placebo-controlled study of the effects of chromium picolinate supplementation on body composition: a replication and extension of a previous study. *Curr Ther Res* 1998;59:379-388.
45. Campbell WW, Joseph LJ, Davey SL, et al. Effects of resistance training and chromium picolinate on body composition and skeletal muscle in older men. *J Appl Physiol* 1999;86:29-39.
46. Walker LS, Bemben MG, Bemben DA, et al. Chromium picolinate effects on body composition and muscular performance in wrestlers. *Med Sci Sports Exerc* 1998;30:1730-1737.
47. Anderson RA. Effects of chromium on body composition and weight loss. *Nutr Rev* 1998;56:266-270.
48. Hasten DL, Rome EP, Franks BD, Hegsted M. Effects of chromium picolinate on beginning weight training students. *Int J Sports Nutr* 1992;2:343-350.
49. Clancy SP, Clarkson PM, DeCheke ME, et al. Effects of chromium picolinate supplementation on body composition, strength, and urinary chromium loss in football players. *Int J Sport Nutr* 1994;4:142-153.
50. Hallmark MA, Reynolds TH, DeSouza CA, et al. Effects of chromium and resistive training on muscle strength and body composition. *Med Sci Sports Exerc* 1996;28:139-144.
51. Trent LK, Thieding-Cancel D. Effects of chromium picolinate on body composition. *J Sports Med Phys Fitness* 1995;35:273-280.
52. Lukaski HC, Bolonchuk WW, Siders WA, et al. Chromium supplementation and resistance training: effects on body composition, strength, and trace element status of men. *Am J Clin Nutr* 1996;63:954-965.
53. Bahadori B, Wallner S, Schneider H, et al. Effect of chromium yeast and chromium picolinate on body composition of obese, non-diabetic patients during and after a formula diet. *Acta Med Austriaca* 1997;24:185-187. [article in German]
54. Offenbacher EG. Promotion of chromium absorption by ascorbic acid. *Trace Elem Electrolytes* 1994;11:178-181.
55. Chen NS, Tsai A, Dyer IA. Effect of chelating agents on chromium absorption in rats. *J Nutr* 1973;103:1182-1186.
56. Davis ML, Seaborn CD, Stoecker BJ. Effects of over-the-counter drugs on ^{51}chromium retention and urinary excretion in rats. *Nutr Res* 1995;15:202-210.
57. Kamath SM, Stoecker BJ, Whitenack MD, et al. Indomethacin and prostaglandin E_2 analogue effects on absorption, retention, and urinary excretion of ^{51}chromium. *FASEB J* 1995;9:A577.
58. Keim KS, Stoecker BJ, Henley S. Chromium status of the rat as affected by phytate. *Nutr Res* 1987;7:253-263.
59. Seaborn CD, Stoecker BJ. Effects of antacid or ascorbic acid on tissue accumulation and urinary excretion of ^{51}chromium. *Nutr Res* 1990;10:1401-1407.
60. Fowler JF Jr. Systemic contact dermatitis caused by oral chromium picolinate. *Cutis* 2000;65:116.
61. Young PC, Turiansky GW, Bonner MW, Benson PM. Acute generalized exanthematous pustulosis induced by chromium picolinate. *J Am Acad Dermatol* 1999;41:820-823.
62. Cerulli J, Grabe DW, Gauthier I, et al. Chromium picolinate toxicity. *Ann Pharmacother* 1998;32:428-431.
63. Stearns DM, Wise JP Sr, Patierno SR, Wetterhahn KE. Chromium(III) picolinate produces chromosome damage in Chinese hamster ovary cells. *FASEB J* 1995;9:1643-1648.
64. Anderson RA, Bryden NA, Polansky MM. Lack of toxicity of chromium chloride and chromium picolinate in rats. *J Am Coll Nutr* 1997;16:273-279.

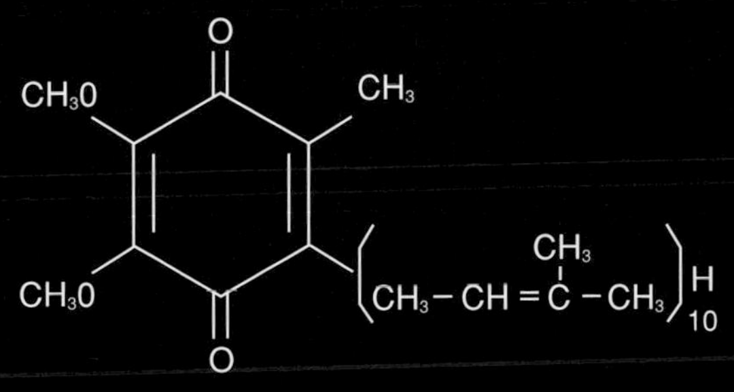

Coenzyme Q_{10}

Coenzyme Q_{10}

Introduction

Coenzyme Q_{10} (ubiquinone, CoQ_{10}) is a vital intermediate of the electron transport system in the mitochondria of every cell; thus, adequate amounts of CoQ_{10} are necessary for optimal production of ATP. CoQ_{10} also functions as an intercellular antioxidant. Overt deficiency states are rare; however, numerous disease processes have been linked to low levels of CoQ_{10}, and others have been shown to respond to CoQ_{10} supplementation.

Pharmacokinetics

CoQ_{10} can be synthesized *in vivo.* However, situations may arise when the need for CoQ_{10} surpasses the body's ability to synthesize it. CoQ_{10} is well absorbed by oral supplementation as evidenced by significant increases in serum CoQ_{10} levels after supplementation.[1] There is some evidence that CoQ_{10} in oil suspension has the highest bioavailability.[2]

Mechanisms of Action

Due to its involvement in ATP synthesis and as an essential antioxidant, CoQ_{10} affects the function of all cells in the body, making it crucial for the health of all human tissues and organs. CoQ_{10} particularly affects the most metabolically active cells: heart, immune system, gingiva, and gastric mucosa.

Clinical Indications

Immune Function

CoQ_{10} enhances phagocytic activity of macrophages and increases granulocyte proliferation in animals.[3-5] A dose-dependent increase in antibody titer is seen in healthy hepatitis B vaccine volunteers.[6] Its antioxidant activity helps prevent AIDS-related diseases caused by oxidative stress.[7,8] Blood levels of CoQ_{10} are lower in AIDS patients and 200 mg/day increased T-helper/suppresser ratios.[9]

Cancer

Decreased levels of CoQ_{10} were found in plasma of women with breast cancer, and in cancerous breast tissue, and low levels correlated with a worse prognosis.[10,11] Two small, uncontrolled clinical studies utilizing 390 mg/day noted tumor regression and decreased incidence of metastasis.[12,13] Mechanisms in cancer include immune system enhancement and antioxidant activity. CoQ_{10} can be depleted by the use of the cancer chemotherapeutic drug doxorubicin (Adriamycin), resulting in cardiotoxicity if a high enough cumulative dose is achieved. Supplemental CoQ_{10} (100-200 mg/day) can prevent cardiac damage, as well as diarrhea and stomatitis caused by this agent, without decreasing its chemotherapeutic effectiveness.[14-17]

Periodontal Disease

Gingival biopsies yield subnormal tissue levels of CoQ_{10} in patients with periodontal disease.[18-21] CoQ_{10} supplementation speeds healing after periodontal surgery.[22-24]

Gastric Ulcers

In an animal study, CoQ_{10} was protective of the gastric mucosa due to its antioxidant effects.[25] Production of protective mucus and rapid cell turnover of gastric mucosa are highly energy-dependent processes dependent on adequate CoQ_{10} levels.

Obesity

Individuals with a family history of obesity have a 50-percent reduction in thermogenic response to a meal and are often found to have low CoQ_{10} levels.[26] CoQ_{10}, being essential for energy production, may be of benefit.

Physical Performance

Supplementation may enhance aerobic capacity and muscle performance, especially in sedentary individuals.[27,28] In trained and elite athletes, little to no improvement in aerobic capacity was noted.[29,30]

Muscular Dystrophy

CoQ_{10} deficiency is found in cardiac and skeletal muscle in animals and humans with hereditary muscular dystrophy.[31-33]

Allergy

CoQ_{10} inhibits release of histamine and slow-reacting substance of anaphylaxis in antigen-challenged animals.[34]

Cardiovascular Disease

CoQ_{10} is especially indicated for myocardial function by enhancing energy production, improving contractility of the cardiac muscle, and providing potent antioxidant activity, particularly the prevention of LDL oxidation. Specific cardiac problems that may benefit from CoQ_{10} include:

- cardiomyopathy[35-38]
- congestive heart failure[39-42]
- angina[43,44]
- acute myocardial infarction[45]
- arrhythmias[46]
- prevention of adriamycin toxicity[14-16]
- protection during cardiac surgery[47,48]
- mitral valve prolapse[49]
- hypertension[50-53]

Male Infertility

CoQ_7 (a CoQ_{10} analog) at 10 mg/day resulted in significant increases in sperm count and motility.[54]

Diabetes Mellitus

The electron-transport chain is integrally involved in carbohydrate metabolism. CoQ_7 at a daily dose of 120 mg for 2-18 weeks reduced fasting blood sugar by 30 percent in 31 percent of patients.[55] Serum CoQ_{10} levels in type 2 diabetes patients are decreased and may be associated with subclinical diabetic cardiomyopathy reversible by CoQ_{10} supplementation.[56]

Parkinson's Disease

Data suggests CoQ_{10} may play a role in the cellular dysfunction found in Parkinson's disease and may be a potential protective agent for Parkinsonian patients.[57,58] A study published in 2002 found supplementation of 1,200 mg CoQ_{10} daily to early Parkinson's patients significantly decreases signs of disease progression compared to placebo.[59]

Drug-Nutrient Interactions

Cholesterol-lowering drugs such as lovastatin and pravastatin inhibit the enzyme 3-hydroxy-3-methyl glutaryl (HMG)-CoA reductase, required for synthesis of cholesterol as well as CoQ_{10}. These drugs decrease serum CoQ_{10} status.[60] Beta blockers propranolol and metaprolol inhibit CoQ_{10}-dependent enzymes. Phenothiazines and tri-cyclic antidepressants have also been shown to inhibit CoQ_{10}-dependent enzymes.

Side Effects and Toxicity

Occasional reports of nausea, anorexia, or skin eruptions have been reported with CoQ_{10} supplementation.

Dosage

Typical dose for most conditions is 30-60 mg twice daily; two studies on breast cancer used 390 mg daily.

References

1. Weber C, Bysted A, Holmer G. Intestinal absorption of coenzyme Q_{10} administered in a meal or as capsules to healthy subjects. *Nutr Res* 1997;17:941-945.
2. Weis M, Mortensent SA, Rassing MR, et al. Bioavailability of four oral coenzyme Q_{10} formulations in healthy volunteers. *Molec Aspects Med* 1994;15:S273-S280.
3. Mayer P, Hamberger H, Drews J. Differential effects of ubiquinone Q_7 and ubiquinone analogs on macrophage activation and experimental infections in granulocytopenic mice. *Infection* 1980;8:256-261.
4. Saiki I, Tokushima Y, Nishimura K, Azuma I. Macrophage activation with ubiquinones and their related compounds in mice. *Int J Vitam Nutr Res* 1983;53:312-320.
5. Bliznakov E, Casey A, Premuzic E. Coenzymes Q: stimulants of the phagocytic activity in rats and immune response in mice. *Experientia* 1970;26:953-954.
6. Barbieri B, Lund B, Lundstrom B, Scaglione F. Coenzyme Q_{10} administration increases antibody titer in hepatitis B vaccinated volunteers–a single blind placebo-controlled and randomized clinical study. *Biofactors* 1999;9:351-357.
7. Sugiyama S, Kitazawa M, Ozawa K. Anti-oxidative effect of coenzyme Q_{10}. *Experientia* 1980;36:1002-1003.
8. Batterham M, Gold J, Naidoo D, et al. A preliminary open label dose comparison using an antioxidant regimen to determine the effect on viral load and oxidative stress in men with HIV/AIDS. *Eur J Clin Nutr* 2001;55:107-114.
9. Folkers K, Langsjoen P, Nara Y, et al. Biochemical deficiencies of coenzyme Q_{10} in HIV-infection and exploratory treatment. *Biochem Biophys Res Commun* 1988;153:888-896.
10. Jolliet P, Simon N, Barre J, et al. Plasma coenzyme Q_{10} concentrations in breast cancer: prognosis and therapeutic consequences. *Int J Clin Pharmacol Ther* 1998;36:506-509.
11. Portakal O, Ozkaya O, Erden Inal M, et al. Coenzyme Q_{10} concentrations and antioxidant status in tissues of breast cancer patients. *Clin Biochem* 2000;33:279-284.
12. Lockwood K, Moesgaard S, Hanioka T, Folkers K. Apparent partial remission of breast cancer in 'high risk' patients supplemented with nutritional antioxidants, essential fatty acids and coenzyme Q_{10}. *Molec Aspects Med* 1994;15:S231-S240.
13. Lockwood K, Moesgaard S, Yamamoto T, Folkers K. Progress on therapy of breast cancer with vitamin Q10 and the regression of metastases. *Biochem Biophys Res Commun* 1995;212:172-177.
14. Domae N, Sawada H, Matsuyama E, et al. Cardiomyopathy and other chronic toxic effects induced in rabbits by doxorubicin and possible prevention by coenzyme Q_{10}. *Cancer Treat Rep* 1981;65:79-91.
15. Karlsson J, Folkers K, Astrum H, et al. Effect of adriamycin on heart and skeletal muscle coenzyme Q (CoQ_{10}) in man. In: Folkers K, Yamamura Y, eds. *Biomedical and Clinical Aspects of Coenzyme Q*, Vol. 5. Amsterdam: Elsevier/North-Holland Biomedical Press; 1986.
16. Judy WV, Hall JH, Dugan W, et al. Coenzyme Q_{10} reduction of adriamycin cardiotoxicity. In: Folkers K, Yamamura Y, eds. *Biomedical and Clinical Aspects of Coenzyme Q*, Vol. 4. Amsterdam: Elsevier/North-Holland Biomedical Press; 1984:231-241.

17. Iarussi D, Auricchio U, Agretto A, et al. Protective effect of coenzyme Q_{10} on anthracyclines cardiotoxicity: control study in children with acute lymphoblastic leukemia and non-Hodgkin's lymphoma. *Molec Aspects Med* 1994;15:S207-S212.

18. Nakamura R, Littarru GP, Folkers K, Wilkinson EG. Study of CoQ_{10}-enzymes in gingiva from patients with periodontal disease and evidence for a deficiency of coenzyme Q_{10}. *Proc Natl Acad Sci* 1974;71:1456-1460.

19. Hansen IL, Iwamoto Y, Kishi T, Folkers K. Bioenergetics in clinical medicine. IX. Gingival and leucocytic deficiencies of coenzyme Q_{10} in patients with periodontal disease. *Res Commun Chem Pathol Pharmacol* 1976;14:729 738.

20. Littarru GP, Nakamura R, Ho L, et al. Deficiency of coenzyme Q_{10} in gingival tissue from patients with periodontal disease. *Proc Natl Acad Sci* 1971;68:2332-2335.

21. Nakamura R, Littarru GP, Folkers K, Wilkinson EG. Deficiency of coenzyme Q in gingiva of patients with periodontal disease. *Int J Vitam Nutr Res* 1973;43:84-92.

22. Wilkinson EG, Arnold RM, Folkers K. Bioenergetics in clinical medicine. VI. Adjunctive treatment of periodontal disease with coenzyme Q_{10}. *Res Commun Chem Pathol Pharmacol* 1976;14:715-719.

23. Wilkinson EG, Arnold RM, Folkers K. Treatment of periodontal and other soft tissue diseases of the oral cavity with coenzyme Q. In: Folkers K, Yamamura Y, eds. *Biomedical and Clinical Aspects of Coenzyme Q*, Vol. 1. Amsterdam: Elsevier/North-Holland Biomedical Press; 1977:251-265.

24. Wilkinson EG, Arnold RM, Folkers K, et al. Bioenergetics in clinical medicine. II. Adjunctive treatment with coenzyme Q in periodontal therapy. *Res Commun Chem Pathol Pharmacol* 1975;12:111-124.

25. Kohli Y, Suto Y, Kodama T. Effect of hypoxia on acetic acid ulcer of the stomach in rats with or without coenzyme Q_{10}. *Jpn J Exp Med* 1981;51:105-108.

26. van Gaal L, de Leeuw ID, Vadhanavikit S, Folkers K. Exploratory study of coenzyme Q_{10} in obesity. In: Folkers K, Yamamura Y, eds. *Biomedical and Clinical Aspects of Coenzyme Q*, Vol. 4. Amsterdam: Elsevier/North-Holland Biomedical Press; 1984:369-373.

27. Vanfraecchem JHP, Folkers K. Coenzyme Q_{10} and physical performance. In: Folkers K, Yamamura Y, eds. *Biomedical and Clinical Aspects of Coenzyme Q*, Vol. 3. Amsterdam: Elsevier/North-Holland Biomedical Press; 1981:235-241.

28. Ylikoski T, Piirainen J, Hanninen O, Penttinen J. The effect of coenzyme Q_{10} on the exercise performance of cross-country skiers. *Mol Aspects Med* 1997;18:S283-S290.

29. Nielsen AN, Mizuno M, Ratkevicius A, et al. No effect of antioxidant supplementation in triathletes on maximal oxygen uptake, 31P-NMRS detected muscle energy metabolism and muscle fatigue. *Int J Sports Med* 1999;20:154-158.

30. Bonetti A, Solito F, Carmosino G, et al. Effect of ubidecarenone oral treatment on aerobic power in middle-aged trained subjects. *J Sports Med Phys Fitness* 2000;40:51-57.

31. Littarru GP, Jones D, Scholler J, Folkers K. Deficiency of coenzyme Q_{10} in mice having hereditary muscular dystrophy. *Biochem Biophys Res Commun* 1970;41:1306-1313.

32. Folkers K, Wolaniuk J, Simonsen R, et al. Biochemical rationale and the cardiac response of patients with muscle disease to therapy with coenzyme Q_{10}. *Proc Natl Acad Sci* 1985;82:4513-4516.

33. Tedeschi D, Lombardi V, Mancuso M, et al. Potential involvement of ubiquinone in myotonic dystrophy pathophysiology: new diagnostic approaches for new rationale therapeutics. *Neurol Sci* 2000;21:S979-S980.

34. Ishihara Y, Uchida Y, Kitamura S, Takaku F. Effect of coenzyme Q_{10}, a quinone derivative, on guinea pig lung and tracheal tissue. *Arzneimittelforschung* 1985;35:929-933.

35. Langsjoen PH, Langsjoen PH, Folkers K. Long-term efficacy and safety of coenzyme Q_{10} therapy for idiopathic dilated cardiomyopathy. *Am J Cardiol* 1990;65:521-523.

36. Langsjoen PH, Folkers K, Lyson K, et al. Effective and safe therapy with coenzyme Q_{10} for cardiomyopathy. *Klin Wochenschr* 1988;66:583-590.

37. Langsjoen PH, Vadhanavikit S, Folkers K. Effective treatment with coenzyme Q_{10} of patients with chronic myocardial disease. *Drugs Exptl Clin Res* 1985;11:577-579.

38. Keith ME, Ball A, Jeejeebhoy KN, et al. Conditioned nutritional deficiencies in the cardiomyopathic hamster heart. *Can J Cardiol* 2001;17:449-458.

39. Mortensen SA, Vadhanavikit S, Baandrup U, Folkers K. Long-term coenzyme Q_{10} therapy: a major advance in the management of resistant myocardial failure. *Drugs Exptl Clin Res* 1985;11:581-593.

40. Baggio E, Gandini R, Plancher AC, et al. Italian multicenter study on the safety and efficacy of coenzyme Q_{10} as adjunctive therapy in heart failure (interim analysis). *Clin Invest* 1993;71:S145-S149.

41. Morisco C, Trimarco B, Condorelli M. Effect of coenzyme Q_{10} in patients with congestive heart failure: a long-term multicenter randomized study. *Clin Invest* 1993;71:S134-S136.

42. Munkholm H, Hansen HH, Rasmussen K. Coenzyme Q_{10} treatment in serious heart failure. *Biofactors* 1999;9:285-289.

43. Kamikawa T, Kobayashi A, Yamashita T, et al. Effects of coenzyme Q_{10} on exercise tolerance in chronic stable angina pectoris. *Am J Cardiol* 1985;56:247-251.

44. Kogan AK, Syrkin AL, Drinitsina SV, Kokanova IV. The antioxidant protection of the heart by coenzyme Q_{10} in stable stenocardia of effort. *Patol Fiziol Eksp Ter* 1999;4:16-19. [Article in Russian]

45. Singh RB, Wander GS, Rastogi A, et al. Randomized, double-blind placebo-controlled trial of coenzyme Q_{10} in patients with acute myocardial infarction. *Cardiovasc Drugs Ther* 1998;12:347-353.

46. Fujioka T, Sakamoto Y, Mimura G. Clinical study of cardiac arrhythmias using a 24-hour continuous electrocardiographic recorder (5th report)–antiarrhythmic action of coenzyme Q_{10} in diabetics. *Tohoku J Exp Med* 1983;141:S453-S463.

47. Tanaka J, Tominaga R, Yoshitoshi M, et al. Coenzyme Q_{10}: the prophylactic effect on low cardiac output following cardiac valve replacement. *Ann Thorac Surg* 1982;33:145-151.

48. Zhou M, Zhi Q, Tang Y, et al. Effects of coenzyme Q_{10} on myocardial protection during cardiac valve replacement and scavenging free radical activity *in vitro*. *J Cardiovasc Surg (Torino)* 1999;40:355-361.

49. Oda T, Hamamoto K. Effect of coenzyme Q_{10} on the stress-induced decrease of cardiac performance in pediatric patients with mitral valve prolapse. *Jpn Circ J* 1984;48:1387.

50. Digiesi V, Cantini F, Oradei A, et al. Coenzyme Q_{10} in essential hypertension. *Molec Aspects Med* 1994;15:S257-S263.

51. Langsjoen PH, Langsjoen PH, Willis R, Folkers K. Treatment of essential hypertension with coenzyme Q_{10}. *Molec Aspects Med* 1994;15:S265-S272.

52. Digiesi V, Cantini F, Brodbeck B. Effect of coenzyme Q_{10} on essential hypertension. *Curr Ther Res* 1990;47:841-845.

53. Singh RB, Niaz MA, Rastogi SS, et al. Effect of hydrosoluble coenzyme Q_{10} on blood pressures and insulin resistance in hypertensive patients with coronary artery disease. *J Hum Hypertens* 1999;13:203-208.

54. Tanimura J. Studies on arginine in human semen. Part III. The influences of several drugs on male infertility. *Bull Osaka Med School* 1967;12:90-100.

55. Shigeta Y, Izumi K, Abe H. Effect of coenzyme Q_7 treatment on blood sugar and ketone bodies of diabetics. *J Vitaminol* 1966;12:293-298.

56. Miyake Y, Shouzu A, Nishikawa M, et al. Effect of treatment with 3-hydroxy-3-methylglutaryl coenzyme A reductase inhibitors on serum coenzyme Q_{10} in diabetic patients. *Arzneimittelforschung* 1999;49:324-329.

57. Shults CW, Haas RH, Beal MF. A possible role of coenzyme Q_{10} in the etiology and treatment of Parkinson's disease. *Biofactors* 1999;9:267-272.

58. Ebadi M, Govitrapong P, Sharma S, et al. Ubiquinone (coenzyme Q_{10}) and mitochondria in oxidative stress of Parkinson's disease. *Biol Signals Recept* 2001;10:224-253.

59. Shults CW, Oakes D, Kieburtz K, et al. Effects of coenzyme Q_{10} in early Parkinson disease: evidence of slowing functional decline. *Arch Neurol* 2002; 59:1541-1550.

60. Mortensen SA, Leth A, Agner E, Rohde M. Dose-related decrease of serum coenzyme Q_{10} during treatment with HMG-CoA reductase inhibitors. *Mol Aspects Med* 1997;18:S137-S144.

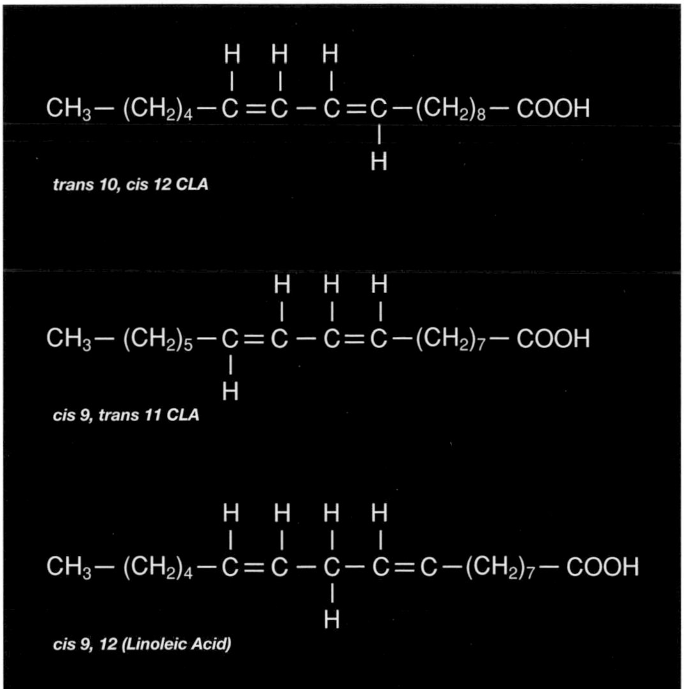

$CH_3-(CH_2)_4-CH=CH-CH=CH-(CH_2)_8-COOH$

trans 10, cis 12 CLA

$CH_3-(CH_2)_5-CH=CH-CH=CH-(CH_2)_7-COOH$

cis 9, trans 11 CLA

$CH_3-(CH_2)_4-CH=CH-CH_2-CH=CH-(CH_2)_7-COOH$

cis 9, 12 (Linoleic Acid)

Linoleic acid and Common CLA Isomers

Conjugated Linoleic Acid

Introduction

Conjugated linoleic acid (CLA) refers to a group of positional and geometric isomers of the omega-6 essential fatty acid linoleic acid (cis-9, cis-12, octadecadienoic acid). In humans, evidence is currently ambiguous whether CLA supplementation has a significant effect on body composition. Despite favorable changes in lipid levels in animal models, a beneficial effect in humans has not been established. While some of the changes reported are consistent with an improved lipid profile, declines in HDL and increases in lipoprotein(a) have also been observed in some subjects.

Exposure to dietary CLA is primarily a result of consumption of dairy products and beef fat, with the c-9, t-11 CLA isomer being the predominant form of CLA in the human diet.[1,2] Since the amount of CLA found in dairy and beef increases as animals are pasture-fed,[3] the quantity of CLA in an individual diet is variable and will depend on both the quantity of dairy and beef fat consumed as well as the feeding habits of the animals from which these products were derived.

Biochemistry

CLA is formed when reactions occur that shift the location of one or both of the double bonds of linoleic acid in such a manner the two double bonds are separated from each other by one single bond. Several dozen different CLA isomers are possible, depending on which double bonds are relocated and the resultant isomeric reconfigurations.

Commercially available CLA is a mixture of isomers with the cis-9, trans-11 octadecadienoic (c-9, t-11 CLA) and the trans-10, cis-12 octadecadienoic acid (t-10, c-12 CLA) isomers accounting for approximately 85-90 percent of the CLA. These two isomers are usually represented in about equal amounts, with 10 other minor CLA isomers representing the remaining 10-15 percent of the mixtures.[4]

Pharmacokinetics

Endogenous CLA production from linoleic acid does not appear to occur to any significant degree in humans.[5] Dietary CLA accumulates in tissues in a dose-dependent manner, with adipose and lung tissue containing the highest concentrations.[6] The primary isomer that accumulates in human tissue subsequent to dietary intake is c-9, t-11 CLA; however, since supplemental forms contain relatively equal quantities of both c-9, t-11 CLA and t-10, c-12 CLA, it is possible a different isomeric tissue distribution can occur following supplementation with CLA products.

In mice, tissue CLA levels decline steadily following withdrawal of CLA from the diet.[7] In rats, consumption of CLA-enriched butter results in greater accumulation of CLA in the mammary gland and other tissues compared to feeding CLA as free fatty acids.[8]

Mechanisms of Action

Effect on Body Composition

No definitive mechanism has been found to explain the changes in body composition found in animal studies. It is possible CLA might have slightly or even vastly different physiological actions, depending on the animal species, the genetic strain of a single species, and the specific CLA isomer added to the diet; thus, a consistent mechanism might not exist.

In vitro and *in vivo* evidence suggests different isomers of CLA might have different effects on body composition. The t-10, c-12 CLA isomer appeared to stimulate lipolysis and inhibit lipogenesis *in vitro*, and produce favorable changes in body composition, while the c-9, t-11 and t-9, t-11 CLA isomers appeared to be ineffective.[9,10]

In vivo human evidence currently does not adequately explain the acknowledged anti-obesity mechanism of action. Supplementation with CLA to female subjects did not appear to influence either energy expenditure[11] or the metabolism of fatty acids and glycerol.[12]

Anticancer Effects

It appears unlikely the anticancer mechanism of action is a result of increased lipid peroxidation in target tissue, despite suggestions to this effect based on *in vitro* animal research, since *in vivo* study found adding CLA to the diet of female rats exposed to carcinogens resulted in lower levels of mammary tissue malondialdehyde. This suggests the potential for some degree of *in vivo* antioxidant activity.[13]

Animal evidence suggests a degree of CLA's anticancer activity might be anti-inflammatory as a result of modifying eicosanoid production, since feeding CLA to mice resulted in a decrease in arachidonic acid production,[14,15] a reduction of synthesis and serum levels of PGE2, and a reduction in the release of leukotriene B4.[16]

CLA might have some effects on the estrogen-mediated mitogenic pathway. *In vitro* evidence found a higher percentage of estrogen receptor-positive MCF-7 cells treated with CLA remained in the G0/G1 phase as compared to control and those treated with linoleic acid.[17]

In vivo CLA induced apoptosis in rats, suggesting some of CLA's ability to decrease tumor mass might be a result of inducing programmed cell death.[18]

It is unlikely CLA's ability to protect rats and mice against cancer is directly related to immune system activation, since animal data has demonstrated protection against cancer formation and metastasis via mechanisms independent of the host immune system.[19,20]

Clinical Indications

Modulation of Body Composition

While a preponderance of data suggests CLA can modulate body composition in animal models, adding CLA to the diet does not produce identical body composition results in all animal models.[21,22] In fact, evidence indicates even within the species of Zucker rats, dietary CLA reduces fat pad weight in lean rats but increases fat pad weight in the obese genotype.[23]

With inconsistent findings from animal trials, it is no surprise available body composition information in humans is also not in agreement.

A six-month, placebo-controlled, randomized, double-blind study reported no changes in body composition variables among obese subjects given CLA (2.7 g per day).[24] No significant changes in body composition were observed in subjects fed CLA (3 g per day) for 64 days; however, a non-significant trend toward improved body composition was noted.[11]

In contrast to the two negative trials, a significant reduction in body fat mass was reported in obese male and female subjects receiving 3.4 and 6.8 grams per day,[25] and a double-blind trial reported that supplementation of CLA (4.2 g per day) for 12 weeks resulted in a significant reduction in the proportion of body fat.[26]

Additional research is required to clarify whether CLA supplementation has a role in improving body composition and to determine which subjects are likely to derive benefit.

Cardiovascular Disease

In animal studies, adding CLA to a diet that would be expected to produce atherosclerosis has resulted in mixed results depending on the type of animal, and, even within animals of the same species, the genetic strain being studied.[27-30] In pigs for example, CLA administration worsened lipid profiles.[31]

To further confuse the issue, in the C57BL/6 mouse atherosclerosis model, CLA addition to the diet resulted in a lipid profile considered less atherogenic (lower triglycerides and a higher serum HDL:total cholesterol ratio). Yet, despite the more favorable serum lipid profile, CLA-supplemented animals demonstrated a greater degree of fatty streak development in aortic tissue than did mice fed the control diet.

In humans, at doses of 3.9 g per day for 63 days and 4.2 g per day for 12 weeks, CLA resulted in no favorable changes to lipid and lipoprotein fractions measured.[26,32] Data also indicated an increase in lipoprotein(a) and a decline of HDL in one group of subjects supplementing CLA at doses at or above 3.4 g per day for 12 weeks.[25]

Contrary to assertions based on selected animal data, current evidence does not support a reduction in cardiovascular risk or a favorable impact on atherosclerosis, but instead indicates the potential for a worsening of some lipid parameters at high doses in some subjects.

Cancer

CLA appears to have direct anticancer activity in rodent models of prostate,[33] colon,[19] and mammary cancer.[8,13,34-36]

A critical time period of dietary exposure to CLA may exist, since feeding CLA in the time period prior to mammary gland maturation seems to provide a lasting degree of protection. If dietary CLA is not provided during this developmental time period, continuous administration of CLA post-carcinogen exposure appears to be required to provide a similar degree of protection against carcinogen-induced cancer formation.[20,35,36]

A role for CLA in cancer prevention or therapy in humans has yet to be established; however, epidemiological data suggest women with breast cancer consume lower quantities of CLA in their diet and have lower serum levels of CLA than matched controls.[37]

Side Effects and Toxicity

Rat toxicity data indicate CLA intake as 1.5 percent of the diet for 36 weeks results in no histopathological damage to organs and no hematological abnormalities.[38] However, in other studies, CLA at one percent of the diet has resulted in hepatomegaly in some mice.[39,40]

When CLA was added to the diet of autoimmune-prone NZB/W F1 mice, onset of proteinuria was accelerated and the CLA-fed mice had slightly earlier mortality than control-fed mice. No effect of dietary CLA was observed on anti-DNA antibody production.[41]

Data to support the safety of supplementing the diet with CLA in pregnant women or individuals with any pathological condition are currently unavailable.

Adverse effects reported after CLA administration in human subjects include gastrointestinal complaints and fatigue.

Dosage

While no conclusions on the efficacy of CLA can be drawn, research suggests a dose of at least 3.4 g per day might be required to influence body composition. Since most commercially available CLA is in the free fatty acid form (as opposed to the more expensive triglyceride-bound form), manufacturers of CLA products often recommend CLA be supplemented in conjunction with food containing milk fats. It is not currently known whether this recommendation influences CLA absorption and tissue distribution.

Warnings and Contraindications

In several animal studies CLA administration has increased insulin and glucose levels, suggesting an insulin-resistant state with impairment in the ability of insulin to dispose of glucose in tissues.[42]

In humans, 12 weeks of CLA (4.2 g/d) supplementation resulted in no impact on plasma insulin or blood glucose;[26] however, an insignificant trend toward increased mean insulin levels toward the end of the supplementation period was reported by other researchers at a dose of 3 grams per day CLA for three months.[43] Until more conclusive long-term data is available it seems prudent to monitor insulin and glucose levels in subjects supplementing with CLA.

References

1. Griinari JM, Corl BA, Lacy SH, et al. Conjugated linoleic acid is synthesized endogenously in lactating dairy cows by Delta(9)-desaturase. *J Nutr* 2000;130:2285-2291.
2. Bauman DE, Barbano DM, Dwyer DA, Griinari JM. Technical note: production of butter with enhanced conjugated linoleic acid for use in biomedical studies with animal models. *J Dairy Sci* 2000;83:2422-2425.
3. French P, Stanton C, Lawless F, et al. Fatty acid composition, including conjugated linoleic acid, of intramuscular fat from steers offered grazed grass, grass silage, or concentrate-based diets. *J Anim Sci* 2000;78:2849-2855.
4. Kritchevsky D. Antimutagenic and some other effects of conjugated linoleic acid. *Br J Nutr* 2000;83:459-465.
5. Herbel BK, McGuire MK, McGuire MA, Shultz TD. Safflower oil consumption does not increase plasma conjugated linoleic acid concentrations in humans. *Am J Clin Nutr* 1998;67:332-337.
6. Jiang J, Wolk A, Vessby B. Relation between the intake of milk fat and the occurrence of conjugated linoleic acid in human adipose tissue. *Am J Clin Nutr* 1999;70:21-27.
7. Park Y, Albright KJ, Storkson JM, et al. Changes in body composition in mice during feeding and withdrawal of conjugated linoleic acid. *Lipids* 1999;34:243-248.
8. Ip C, Banni S, Angioni E, et al. Conjugated linoleic acid-enriched butter fat alters mammary gland morphogenesis and reduces cancer risk in rats. *J Nutr* 1999;129:2135-2142.
9. Park Y, Storkson JM, Albright KJ, et al. Evidence that the trans-10, cis-12 isomer of conjugated linoleic acid induces body composition changes in mice. *Lipids* 1999;34:235-241.

10. Brown JM, Halvorsen YD, Lea-Currie YR, et al. Trans-10, cis-12, but not cis-9, trans-11, conjugated linoleic acid attenuates lipogenesis in primary cultures of stromal vascular cells from human adipose tissue. *J Nutr* 2001;131:2316-2321.
11. Zambell KL, Keim NL, Van Loan MD, et al. Conjugated linoleic acid supplementation in humans: effects on body composition and energy expenditure. *Lipids* 2000;35:777-782.
12. Zambell KL, Horn WF, Keim NL. Conjugated linoleic acid supplementation in humans: effects on fatty acid and glycerol kinetics. *Lipids* 2001;36:767-772.
13. Ip C, Briggs SP, Haegele AD, et al. The efficacy of conjugated linoleic acid in mammary cancer prevention is independent of the level or type of fat in the diet. *Carcinogenesis* 1996;17:1045-1050.
14. Banni S, Angioni E, Casu V, et al. Decrease in linoleic acid metabolites as a potential mechanism in cancer risk reduction by conjugated linoleic acid. *Carcinogenesis* 1999;20:1019-1024.
15. Belury MA, Kempa-Steczko A. Conjugated linoleic acid modulates hepatic lipid composition in mice. *Lipids* 1997;32:199-204.
16. Sugano M, Tsujita A, Yamasaki M, et al. Conjugated linoleic acid modulates tissue levels of chemical mediators and immunoglobulins in rats. *Lipids* 1998;33:521-527.
17. Durgam VR, Fernandes G. The growth inhibitory effect of conjugated linoleic acid on MCF-7 cells is related to estrogen response system. *Cancer Lett* 1997;116:121-130.
18. Ip C, Ip MM, Loftus T, et al. Induction of apoptosis by conjugated linoleic acid in cultured mammary tumor cells and premalignant lesions of the rat mammary gland. *Cancer Epidemiol Biomarkers Prev* 2000;9:689-696.
19. Liew C, Schut HAJ, Chin SF, et al. Protection of conjugated linoleic acids against 2-amino-3-methylimidazol[4,5-f]quinolone-induced colon carcinogenesis in the F344 rat: a study of inhibitory mechanisms. *Carcinogenesis* 1995;16:3037-3043.
20. Visonneau S, Cesano A, Tepper SA, et al. Conjugated linoleic acid suppresses the growth of human breast adenocarcinoma cells in SCID mice. *Anticancer Res* 1997;17:969-973.
21. West DB, Delany JP, Camet PM, et al. Effects of conjugated linoleic acid on body fat and energy metabolism in the mouse. *Am J Physiol* 1998;275:R667-R672.
22. Azain MJ, Hausman DB, Sisk MB, et al. Dietary conjugated linoleic acid reduces rat adipose tissue cell size rather than cell number. *J Nutr* 2000;130:1548-1554.
23. Sisk MB, Hausman DB, Martin RJ, Azain MJ. Dietary conjugated linoleic acid reduces adiposity in lean but not obese Zucker rats. *J Nutr* 2001;131:1668-1674.
24. Atkinson RL. Conjugated linoleic acid for altering body composition and treating obesity. In: Yurawecz MP, Mossoba MM, Kramer JKG, et al, eds. *Advances in Conjugated Linoleic Acid Research.* Champaign, IL: AOCS Press; 1999;1:328-353.
25. Blankson H, Stakkestad JA, Fagertun H, et al. Conjugated linoleic acid reduces body fat mass in overweight and obese humans. *J Nutr* 2000;130:2943-2948.
26. Smedman A, Vessby B. Conjugated linoleic acid supplementation in humans – metabolic effects. *Lipids* 2001;36:773-781.
27. Kritchevsky D, Tepper SA, Wright S, et al. Influence of conjugated linoleic acid (CLA) on establishment and progression of atherosclerosis in rabbits. *J Am Coll Nutr* 2000;19:S472-S477.
28. Lee KN, Kritchevsky D, Pariza MW. Conjugated linoleic acid and atherosclerosis in rabbits. *Atherosclerosis* 1994;108:19-25.
29. Nicolosi RJ, Rogers EJ, Kritchevsky D, et al. Dietary conjugated linoleic acid reduces plasma lipoproteins and early aortic atherosclerosis in hypercholesterolemic hamsters. *Artery* 1997;22:266-277.
30. Munday JS, Thompson KG, James KA. Dietary conjugated linoleic acids promote fatty streak formation in the C57BL/6 mouse atherosclerosis model. *Br J Nutr* 1999;81:251-255.

31. Stangl GI, Muller H, Kirchgessner M. Conjugated linoleic acid effects on circulating hormones, metabolites and lipoproteins, and its proportion in fasting serum and erythrocyte membranes of swine. *Eur J Nutr* 1999;38:271-277.

32. Benito P, Nelson GJ, Kelley DS, et al. The effect of conjugated linoleic acid on plasma lipoproteins and tissue fatty acid composition in humans. *Lipids* 2001;36:229-236.

33. Cesano A, Visonneau S, Scimeca JA, et al. Opposite effects of linoleic acid and conjugated linoleic acid on human prostatic cancer in SCID mice. *Anticancer Res* 1998;18:1429-1434.

34. Thompson H, Zhu Z, Banni S, et al. Morphological and biochemical status of the mammary gland as influenced by conjugated linoleic acid: implication for a reduction in mammary cancer risk. *Cancer Res* 1997;57:5067-5072.

35. Ip C, Jiang C, Thompson HJ, Scimeca JA. Retention of conjugated linoleic acid in the mammary gland is associated with tumor inhibition during the post-initiation phase of carcinogenesis. *Carcinogenesis* 1997;18:755-759.

36. Ip C, Scimeca JA, Thompson H. Effect of timing and duration of dietary conjugated linoleic acid on mammary cancer prevention. *Nutr Cancer* 1995;24:241-247.

37. Aro A, Mannisto S, Salminen I, et al. Inverse association between dietary and serum conjugated linoleic acid and risk of breast cancer in postmenopausal women. *Nutr Cancer* 2000;38:151-157.

38. Scimeca JA. Toxicological evaluation of dietary conjugated linoleic acid in male Fischer 344 rats. *Food Chem Toxicol* 1998;36:391-395.

39. DeLany JP, Blohm F, Truett AA, et al. Conjugated linoleic acid rapidly reduces body fat content in mice without affecting energy intake. *Am J Physiol* 1999;276:R1172-R1179.

40. Tsuboyama-Kasaoka N, Takahashi M, Tanemura K, et al. Conjugated linoleic acid supplementation reduces adipose tissue by apoptosis and develops lipodystrophy in mice. *Diabetes* 2000;49:1534-1542.

41. Yang M, Pariza MW, Cook ME. Dietary conjugated linoleic acid protects against end stage disease of systemic lupus erythematosus in the NZB/W F1 mouse. *Immunopharmacol Immunotoxicol* 2000;22:433-449.

42. West DB, Blohm FY, Truett AA, DeLany JP. Conjugated linoleic acid persistently increases total energy expenditure in AKR/J mice without increasing uncoupling protein gene expression. *J Nutr* 2000;130:2471-2477.

43. Medina EA, Horn WF, Keim NL, et al. Conjugated linoleic acid supplementation in humans: effects on circulating leptin concentrations and appetite. *Lipids* 2000;35:783-788.

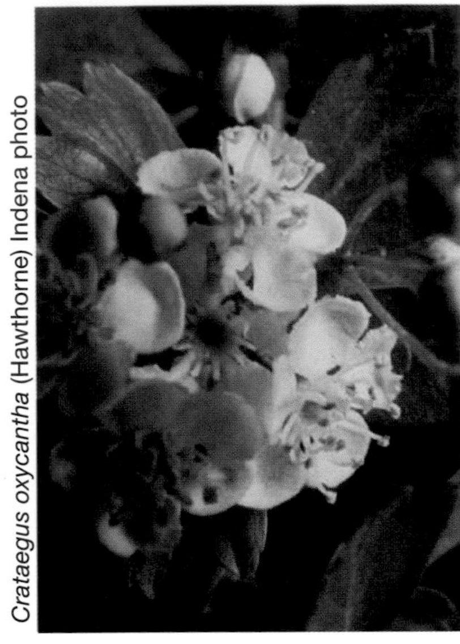
Crataegus oxycantha (Hawthorne) Indena photo

Crataegus oxycantha

Description

The berries and flowers of *Crataegus oxycantha*, also known as hawthorne, have been used traditionally as cardiac tonics and diuretics in a variety of functional heart disorders. Recent research shows Crataegus extracts exert a wide range of positive actions on heart function, supporting and validating historical observations.

Active Constituents

The main constituents of Crataegus are flavonoids, triterpene saponins, and a few cardioactive amines; however, the primary cardiovascular protective activity of the plant is generally attributed to its flavonoid content, particularly the oligomeric proanthocyanidins (OPCs). The OPCs are highly concentrated in the leaves, berries and flowers, and are responsible for providing the pigment that colors the berries. These flavonoids seem to work synergistically to enhance the activity of vitamin C and promote capillary stability.

Mechanisms of Action

Because of the high content of flavonoid compounds, particularly the OPCs, Crataegus has significant antioxidant activity.[1] In addition, it increases coronary blood flow,[2] enhancing oxygen flow and utilization by the heart. Crataegus extracts also have a positive inotropic effect on the contraction amplitude of myocytes.[3] Due to the flavonoid content, extracts of this herb exert considerable collagen-stabilizing effects, enhancing integrity of blood vessels.[4]

Crataegus extracts prevented elevation of plasma lipids, including total cholesterol, triglycerides, and LDL- and VLDL-fractions, in rats fed a hyperlipidemic diet.[5] Crataegus up-regulates hepatic LDL-receptors, resulting in greater influx of plasma LDL-cholesterol into the liver. It also prevents the accumulation of cholesterol in the liver by enhancing cholesterol degradation to bile acids, promoting bile flow, and suppressing cholesterol biosynthesis.[6] Additionally, it protects human LDL from oxidation and provides indirect protection via maintaining the concentration of alpha-tocopherol in LDL.[7]

Crataegus exerts a simultaneous cardiotropic and vasodilatory action. Because of these actions, it can be safely and effectively utilized for cardiac conditions for which digitalis is not yet indicated.[8]

Clinical Indications

Crataegus is an effective and low-risk phytotherapeutic for patients with coronary heart disease, atherosclerosis, hypertension, or hypercholesterolemia.

Congestive Heart Failure

Research indicates administration of Crataegus provides subjective and objective benefits in individuals with signs and symptoms of congestive heart failure. Over a period of eight weeks, supplementation with Crataegus resulted in a clear improvement in patients with congestive heart failure stage NYHA-II. Patients reported improvement in subjective symptoms, such as reduced performance, shortness of breath, and ankle edema.[9] Similar studies have shown oral Crataegus supplementation improves blood pressure, heart rate, dyspnea, exercise capacity, and change in heart rate in response to exercise under standardized loading on a bicycle ergometer.[10-12] A placebo-controlled, 16-week study of patients with NYHA class III congestive heart failure also revealed dose-dependent improvements in tolerated bicycle exercise workload.[13]

Hypertension

Crataegus exerts mild blood pressure-lowering activity, which appears to be a result of a number of diverse pharmacological effects. It dilates coronary vessels,[14] inhibits angiotensin converting enzyme,[15] acts as an inotropic agent,[3] and possesses mild diuretic activity.

Drug-Botanical Interactions

The root, leaves, and flowers of Crataegus all contain cardioactive compounds. Crataegus preparations may have a potentiating effect on digitalis, necessitating a reduction in the dosage of digitalis.[16]

Side Effects and Toxicity

Crataegus has been shown to have low toxicity. The German Commission E monograph states that mice and rats have been safely given a standardized extract at dosages up to 3 g/kg body weight.[17]

Dosage

Positive effects from supplementation will usually be observed within the first two weeks. In most instances, as a cardiac tonic, Crataegus is administered for prolonged intervals. Dosage will vary depending on the concentration of the extract. A typical therapeutic dose of an extract, standardized to contain 1.8-percent vitexin-4 rhamnoside, is 100-250 mg three times per day. A standardized extract containing 18-percent procyanidolic oligomers is dosed in the range of 250-500 mg daily.

References

1. Rakotoarison DA, Gressier B, Trotin F, et al. Antioxidant activities of polyphenolic extracts from flowers, *in vitro* callus and cell suspension cultures of *Crataegus monogyna*. *Pharmazie* 1997;52:60-64.
2. Schussler M, Holzl J, Fricke U. Myocardial effects of flavonoids from Crataegus species. *Arzneimittelforschung* 1995;45:842-845.
3. Popping S, Rose H, Ionescu I, et al. Effect of a hawthorn extract on contraction and energy turnover of isolated rat cardiomyocytes. *Arzneimittelforschung* 1995;45:1157-1161.
4. Gabor M. Pharmacological effects of flavonoids on blood vessels. *Angiologica* 1972;9:355-374.
5. Shanthi S, Parasakthy K, Deepalakshmi PD, Devaraj SN. Hypolipidemic activity of tincture of Crataegus in rats. *Indian J Biochem Biophys* 1994;31:143-146.
6. Rajendran S, Deepalakshmi PD, Parasakthy K, et al. Effect of tincture of Crataegus on the LDL-receptor activity of hepatic plasma membrane of rats fed an atherogenic diet. *Atherosclerosis* 1996;123:235-241.
7. Zhang Z, Chang Q, Zhu M, et al. Characterization of antioxidants present in hawthorn fruits. *J Nutr Biochem* 2001;12:144-152.
8. Blesken R. Crataegus in cardiology. *Fortschr Med* 1992;110:290-292. [Article in German]
9. Weikl A, Assmus KD, Neukum-Schmidt A, et al. Crataegus Special Extract WS 1442. Assessment of objective effectiveness in patients with heart failure. *Fortschr Med* 1996;114:291-296. [Article in German]
10. Leuchtgens H. Crataegus Special Extract WS 1442 in NYHA II heart failure. A placebo controlled randomized double-blind study. *Fortschr Med* 1993;111:352-354. [Article in German]
11. Rietbrock N, Hamel M, Hempel B, et al. Actions of standardized extracts of Crataegus berries on exercise tolerance and quality of life in patients with congestive heart failure. *Arzneimittelforschung* 2001;51:793-798. [Article in German]
12. Zapfejun G. Clinical efficacy of Crataegus extract WS 1442 in congestive heart failure NYHA class II. *Phytomedicine* 2001;8:262-266.
13. Tauchert M. Efficacy and safety of Crataegus extract WS1442 in comparison with placebo in patients with chronic stable New York Heart Association class-III heart failure. *Am Heart J* 2002;143:910-915.
14. Rewerski VW, Piechocki T, Tyalski M, Lewak S. Some pharmacological properties of oligomeric procyanadin isolated from hawthorn (*Crataegus oxycantha*). *Arzneimittelforschung* 1967;17:490-491.
15. Uchida S, Ikari N, Ohta H, et al. Inhibitory effects of condensed tannins on angiotensin converting enzyme. *Jpn J Pharmacol* 1987;43:242-246.
16. McGuffin M, Hobbs C, Upton R, Goldberg A, eds. *Botanical Safety Handbook*. New York: CRC Press; 1997:37.
17. Blumenthal M, Busse W, Goldberg A, et al., eds. *The Complete German Commission E Monographs*. Boston, MA: American Botanical Council; 1998:142-144.

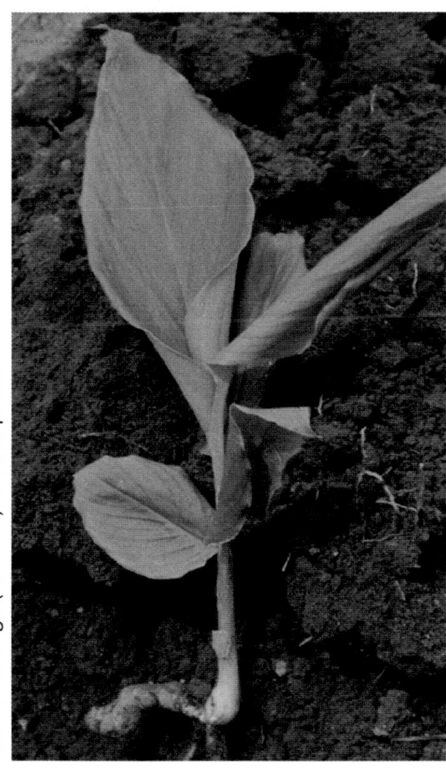
Curcuma longa (turmeric) Indena photo

Curcuma longa

Description

Curcuma longa, a perennial herb and member of the Zingiberaceae (ginger) family, grows to a height of three to five feet and is cultivated extensively in Asia, India, China, and other countries with a tropical climate. It has oblong, pointed leaves and funnel-shaped yellow flowers.[1] The rhizome, the portion of the plant used medicinally, is usually boiled, cleaned, and dried, yielding a yellow powder. Dried *Curcuma longa* is the source of the spice turmeric, the ingredient that gives curry powder its characteristic yellow color. Turmeric is used extensively in foods for both its flavor and color, as well as having a long tradition of use in the Chinese and Ayurvedic systems of medicine, particularly as an anti-inflammatory and for the treatment of flatulence, jaundice, menstrual difficulties, hematuria, hemorrhage, and colic. Turmeric can also be applied topically in poultices to relieve pain and inflammation.[2] Current research has focused on turmeric's antioxidant, hepatoprotective, anti-inflammatory, anticarcinogenic, and antimicrobial properties, in addition to its use in cardiovascular disease and gastrointestinal disorders.

Active Constituents

The active constituents of turmeric are the flavonoid curcumin (diferuloylmethane) and various volatile oils, including tumerone, atlantone, and zingiberone. Other constituents include sugars, proteins, and resins. The best-researched active constituent is curcumin, which comprises 0.3-5.4 percent of raw turmeric.[2]

Pharmacokinetics

Pharmacokinetic studies in animals have demonstrated that 40-85 percent of an oral dose of curcumin passes through the gastrointestinal tract unchanged, with most of the absorbed flavonoid being metabolized in the intestinal mucosa and liver.[3,4] Due to its low rate of absorption, curcumin is often formulated with bromelain for increased absorption and enhanced anti-inflammatory effect.

Mechanisms of Action

Antioxidant Effects

Water- and fat-soluble extracts of turmeric and its curcumin component exhibit strong antioxidant activity, comparable to vitamins C and E.[5] A study of ischemia in the feline heart demonstrated that curcumin pretreatment decreased ischemia-induced changes in the heart.[6] An *in vitro* study measuring the effect of curcumin on endothelial heme oxygenase-1, an inducible stress protein, was conducted utilizing bovine aortic endothelial cells. Incubation (18 hours) with curcumin resulted in enhanced cellular resistance to oxidative damage.[7]

Hepatoprotective Effects

Turmeric has been found to have a hepatoprotective characteristic similar to silymarin. Animal studies have demonstrated turmeric's hepatoprotective effects from a variety of hepatotoxic insults, including carbon tetrachloride (CCl_4),[8,9] galactosamine,[10] acetaminophen (paracetamol),[11] and Aspergillus aflatoxin.[12] Turmeric's hepatoprotective effect is mainly a result of its antioxidant properties, as well as its ability to decrease the formation of pro-inflammatory cytokines. In rats with CCl_4-induced acute and subacute liver injury, curcumin administration significantly decreased liver injury in test animals compared to controls.[9] Turmeric extract inhibited fungal aflatoxin production by 90 percent when given to ducklings infected with *Aspergillus parasiticus*. Turmeric and curcumin also reversed biliary hyperplasia, fatty changes, and necrosis induced by aflatoxin production.[12] Sodium curcuminate, a salt of curcumin, also exerts choleretic effects by increasing biliary excretion of bile salts, cholesterol, and bilirubin, as well as increasing bile solubility, therefore possibly preventing and treating cholelithiasis.[13]

Anti-inflammatory Effects

The volatile oils and curcumin of *Curcuma longa* exhibit potent anti-inflammatory effects.[14-16] Oral administration of curcumin in instances of acute inflammation was found to be as effective as cortisone or phenylbutazone, and one-half as effective in cases of chronic inflammation.[16] In rats with Freund's adjuvant-induced arthritis, oral administration of *Curcuma longa* significantly reduced inflammatory swelling compared to controls.[15] In monkeys, curcumin inhibited neutrophil aggregation associated with inflammation.[17] *C. longa's* anti-inflammatory properties may be attributed to its ability to inhibit both biosynthesis of inflammatory prostaglandins from arachidonic acid, and neutrophil function during inflammatory states. Curcumin may also be applied topically to counteract inflammation and irritation associated with inflammatory skin conditions and allergies, although care must be used to prevent staining of clothing from the yellow pigment.[16]

Anticarcinogenic Effects

Animal studies involving rats and mice, as well as *in vitro* studies utilizing human cell lines, have demonstrated curcumin's ability to inhibit carcinogenesis at three stages: tumor promotion,[18] angiogenesis,[19] and tumor growth.[20] In two studies of colon and prostate cancer, curcumin inhibited cell proliferation and tumor growth.[21,22] Turmeric and curcumin are also capable of suppressing the activity of several common mutagens and carcinogens in a variety of cell types in both *in vitro* and *in vivo* studies.[23-26] The anticarcinogenic effects of turmeric and curcumin are due to direct antioxidant and free-radical scavenging effects, as well as their ability to indirectly increase glutathione levels, thereby aiding in hepatic detoxification of mutagens and carcinogens, and inhibiting nitrosamine formation.[27]

Antimicrobial Effects

Turmeric extract and the essential oil of *Curcuma longa* inhibit the growth of a variety of bacteria, parasites, and pathogenic fungi. A study of chicks infected with the caccal parasite *Eimera maxima* demonstrated that diets supplemented with 1-percent turmeric resulted in a reduction in small intestinal lesion scores and improved weight gain.[28] Another animal study, in which guinea pigs were infected with either dermatophytes, pathogenic molds, or yeast, found that topically applied turmeric oil inhibited dermatophytes and pathogenic fungi, but neither curcumin nor turmeric oil affected the yeast isolates. Improvements in lesions were observed in the dermatophyte- and fungi-infected guinea pigs, and at seven days post-turmeric application the lesions disappeared.[29] Curcumin has also been found to have moderate activity against *Plasmodium falciparum* and *Leishmania major* organisms.[30]

Cardiovascular Effects

Turmeric's protective effects on the cardiovascular system include lowering cholesterol and triglyceride levels, decreasing susceptibility of low density lipoprotein (LDL) to lipid peroxidation,[31] and inhibiting platelet aggregation.[32] These effects have been noted even with low doses of turmeric. A study of 18 atherosclerotic rabbits given low-dose (1.6-3.2 mg/kg body weight daily) turmeric extract demonstrated decreased susceptibility of LDL to lipid peroxidation, in addition to lower plasma cholesterol and triglyceride levels. The higher dose did not decrease lipid peroxidation of LDL, but cholesterol and triglyceride level decreases were noted, although to a lesser degree than with the lower dose.[31] Turmeric extract's effect on cholesterol levels may be due to decreased cholesterol uptake in the intestines and increased conversion of cholesterol to bile acids in the liver.[13] Inhibition of platelet aggregation by *C. longa* constituents is thought to be via potentiation of prostacyclin synthesis and inhibition of thromboxane synthesis.[32]

Gastrointestinal Effects

Constituents of *Curcuma longa* exert several protective effects on the gastrointestinal tract. Sodium curcuminate inhibited intestinal spasm and p-tolymethylcarbinol, a turmeric component, increased gastrin, secretin, bicarbonate, and pancreatic enzyme secretion.[33] Turmeric has also been shown to inhibit ulcer formation caused by stress, alcohol, indomethacin, pyloric ligation, and reserpine, significantly increasing gastric wall mucus in rats subjected to these gastrointestinal insults.[34]

Clinical Indications

Hepatoprotection, Cholelithiasis, and Cholestasis

Turmeric's hepatoprotective effects, evidenced in a number of animal studies, suggest it may be used in cases of toxic insult due to exogenous toxins from lifestyle and environmental exposures. Curcumin has choleretic activity that increases bile output and solubility, which may be helpful in treating gallstones.[8-13]

Inflammation

Curcumin is a potent anti-inflammatory with specific lipoxygenase- and COX-2-inhibiting properties. Animal, *in vitro*, and *in vivo* studies demonstrate turmeric's effectiveness at decreasing both acute and chronic inflammation.[14-17] A double-blind, crossover, placebo-controlled human study of 42 patients with osteoarthritis used a combination product containing turmeric, *Boswellia serrata*, *Withania somnifera*, and zinc. After three months on the combination or placebo, patients noted a significant reduction in pain ($p<0.001$) and disability ($p<0.05$).[35]

Cancer

Numerous animal, *in vitro*, and *in vivo* studies have demonstrated the anticarcinogenic effects of turmeric and its flavonoid component curcumin against colon,[36,37] breast,[38-40] and prostate[22,41] cancers, as well as melanoma.[42] A human study of 25 individuals at high risk of neoplasia or with pre-malignant lesions noted histologic improvement in one of two patients with recently resected bladder cancer, two of seven patients with oral leukoplakia, one of six patients with intestinal metaplasia of the stomach, one of four patients with cervical intraepithelial neoplasm, and two of six patients with Bowen's disease. More clinical trials need to be performed to further elucidate the potential of this botanical in cancer prevention and treatment.[43]

Hyperlipidemia

Animal[31] and *in vitro* studies have shown the potential for turmeric to decrease blood lipids. Further clinical studies need to be performed in this area to discover optimal dosages for cardiovascular protection and lipid lowering.

Gastric Ulcer

An open, phase II trial was performed on 25 patients with endoscopically-diagnosed gastric ulcer. Participants were given 600 mg powdered turmeric five times daily. After four weeks, ulcers had completely healed in 48 percent of patients. The success rate increased over time, with 76 percent being ulcer free after 12 weeks of treatment. No significant adverse reactions or blood abnormalities were noted.[44]

Chronic Anterior Uveitis

Thirty-two patients with chronic anterior uveitis took 375 mg curcumin three times daily for 12 weeks. Curcumin was effective in 86 percent of individuals, and was as effective as corticosteroid therapy, the only available standard treatment.[45]

Side Effects and Toxicity

No significant toxicity has been reported following either acute or chronic administration of turmeric extracts at standard doses. At very high doses (100 mg/kg body weight), curcumin may be ulcerogenic in animals, as evidenced by one rat study.[33]

Dosage

Doses of 500-8,000 mg of powdered turmeric per day have been used in human studies. Standardized extracts are typically used in lower amounts, in the 250-2,000 mg range.

References

1. Dobelis IN, ed. *Magic and Medicine of Plants*. Pleasantville, NY: Reader's Digest Association, Inc. 1986.
2. Leung A. *Encyclopedia of Common Natural Ingredients Used in Food, Drugs, and Cosmetics*. New York, NY: John Wiley; 1980:313-314.
3. Wahlstrom B, Blennow G. A study on the fate of curcumin in the rat. *Acta Pharmacol Toxicol* 1978;43:86-92.
4. Ravindranath V, Chandrasekhara N. Absorption and tissue distribution of curcumin in rats. *Toxicol* 1980;16:259-265.
5. Toda S, Miyase T, Arich H, et al. Natural antioxidants. Antioxidative compounds isolated from rhizome of *Curcuma longa* L. *Chem Pharmacol Bull* 1985;33:1725-1728.
6. Dikshit M, Rastogi L, Shukla R, Srimal RC. Prevention of ischaemia-induced biochemical changes by curcumin and quinidine in the cat heart. *Indian J Med Res* 1995;101:31-35.

7. Mortellini R, Foresti R, Bassi R, Green CJ. Curcumin, an antioxidant and anti-inflammatory agent, induces heme oxygenase-1 and protects endothelial cells against oxidative stress. *Free Radic Biol Med* 2000;28:1303-1312.

8. Deshpande UR, Gadre SG, Raste AS, et al. Protective effect of turmeric (*Curcuma longa* L.) extract on carbon tetrachloride-induced liver damage in rats. *Indian J Exp Biol* 1998;36:573-577.

9. Park EJ, Jeon CH, Ko G, et al. Protective effect of curcumin in rat liver injury induced by carbon tetrachloride. *J Pharm Pharmacol* 2000;52:437-440.

10. Kiso Y, Suzuki Y, Watanabe N, et al. Antihepatotoxic principles of *Curcuma longa* rhizomes. *Planta Med* 1983;49:185-187.

11. Donatus IA, Sardjoko, Vermeulen NP. Cytotoxic and cytoprotective activities of curcumin. Effects on paracetamol-induced cytotoxicity, lipid peroxidation and glutathione depletion in rat hepatocytes. *Biochem Pharmacol* 1990;39:1869-1875.

12. Soni KB, Rajan A, Kuttan R. Reversal of aflatoxin induced liver damage by turmeric and curcumin. *Cancer Lett* 1992;66:115-121.

13. Ramprasad C, Sirsi M. *Curcuma longa* and bile secretion. Quantitative changes in the bile constituents induced by sodium curcuminate. *J Sci Indust Res* 1957;16C:108-110.

14. Chandra D, Gupta S. Anti-inflammatory and anti-arthritic activity of volatile oil of *Curcuma longa* (Haldi). *Indian J Med Res* 1972;60:138-142.

15. Arora R, Basu N, Kapoor V, et al. Anti-inflammatory studies on *Curcuma longa* (turmeric). *Indian J Med Res* 1971;59:1289-1295.

16. Mukhopadhyay A, Basu N, Ghatak N, et al. Anti-inflammatory and irritant activities of curcumin analogues in rats. *Agents Actions* 1982;12:508-515.

17. Srivastava R. Inhibition of neutrophil response by curcumin. *Agents Actions* 1989;28:298-303.

18. Kawamori T, Lubet R, Steele VE, et al. Chemopreventative effect of curcumin, a naturally occurring anti-inflammatory agent, during the promotion/progression stages of colon cancer. *Cancer Res* 1999;59:597-601.

19. Thaloor D, Singh AK, Sidhu GS, et al. Inhibition of angiogenic differentiation of human umbilical vein endothelial cells by curcumin. *Cell Growth Differ* 1998;9:305-312.

20. Limtrakul P, Lipigorngoson S, Namwong O, et al. Inhibitory effect of dietary curcumin on skin carcinogenesis in mice. *Cancer Lett* 1997;116:197-203.

21. Hanif R, Qiao L, Shiff SJ, Rigas B. Curcumin, a natural plant phenolic food additive, inhibits cell proliferation and induces cell cycle changes in colon adenocarcinoma cell lines by a prostaglandin-independent pathway. *J Lab Clin Med* 1997;130:576-584.

22. Dorai T, Cao YC, Dorai B, et al. Therapeutic potential of curcumin in human prostate cancer. III. Curcumin inhibits proliferation, induces apoptosis, and inhibits angiogenesis of LNCaP prostate cancer cells *in vivo*. *Prostate* 2001;47:293-303.

23. Mehta RG, Moon RC. Characterization of effective chemopreventive agents in mammary gland in vitro using an initiation-promotion protocol. *Anticancer Res* 1991;11:593-596.

24. Soudamini NK, Kuttan R. Inhibition of chemical carcinogenesis by curcumin. *J Ethnopharmacol* 1989;27:227-233.

25. Azuine M, Bhide S. Chemopreventive effect of turmeric against stomach and skin tumors induced by chemical carcinogens in Swiss mice. *Nutr Cancer* 1992;17:77-83.

26. Boone CW, Steele VE, Kelloff GJ. Screening of chemopreventive (anticarcinogenic) compounds in rodents. *Mut Res* 1992;267:251-255.

27. Pizorrno JE, Murray MT. *Textbook of Natural Medicine*, 2nd Ed. London: Churchill Livingstone; 1999;689-693.

28. Allen PC, Danforth HD, Augustine PC. Dietary modulation of avian coccidiosis. *Int J Parasitol* 1998;28:1131-1140.

29. Apisariyakul A, Vanittanakom N, Buddhasukh D. Antifungal activity of turmeric oil extracted from *Curcuma longa* (Zingiberaceae). *J Ethnopharmacol* 1995;49:163-169.

30. Rasmussen HB, Christensen SB, Kvist LP, Karazami A. A simple and efficient separation of the curcumins, the antiprotozoal constituents of *Curcuma longa. Planta Med* 2000;66:396-398.

31. Ramirez-Tortosa MC, Mesa MD, Aguilera MC, et al. Oral administration of a turmeric extract inhibits LDL oxidation and has hypocholesterolemic effects in rabbits with experimental atherosclerosis. *Atherosclerosis* 1999;147:371-378.

32. Srivastava R, Puri V, Srimal RC, Dhawan BN. Effect of curcumin on platelet aggregation and vascular prostacyclin synthesis. *Arzneimittelforschung* 1986;36:715-717.

33. Ammon HPT, Wahl MA. Pharmacology of *Curcuma longa. Planta Medica* 1991;57:1-7.

34. Rafatulla S, Tariq M, Alyahya MA, et al. Evaluation of turmeric (*Curcuma longa*) for gastric and duodenal antiulcer activity in rats. *J Ethnopharmacol* 1990;29:25-34.

35. Kulkarni RR, Patki PS, Jog VP, et al. Treatment of osteoarthritis with a herbomineral formulation: a double-blind, placebo-controlled, cross-over study. *J Ethnopharmacol* 1991;33:91-95.

36. Chauhan DP. Chemotherapeutic potential of curcumin for colorectal cancer. *Curr Pharm Des* 2002;8:1695-1706.

37. Reddy BS, Rao CV. Novel approaches for colon cancer prevention by cyclooxygenase-2 inhibitors. *J Environ Pathol Toxicol Onc*ol 2002;21:155-164.

38. Ramachandran C, Fonseca HB, Jhabvala P, et al. Curcumin inhibits telomerase activity through human telomerase reverse transcritpase in MCF-7 breast cancer cell line. *Cancer Lett* 2002;184:1-6.

39. Somasundaram S, Edmund NA, Moore DT, et al. Dietary curcumin inhibits chemotherapy-induced apoptosis in models of human breast cancer. *Cancer Res* 2002;62:3868-3875.

40. Shao ZM, Shen ZZ, Liu CH, et al. Curcumin exerts multiple suppressive effects on human breast carcinoma cells. *Int J Cancer* 2002;98:234-240.

41. Hour TC, Chen J, Huang CY, et al. Curcumin enhances cytotoxicity of chemotherapeutic agents in prostate cancer cells by inducing p21(WAF1/CIP1) and C/EBPbeta expressions and suppressing NF-kappaB activation. *Prostate* 2002;51:211-218.

42. Bush JA, Cheung KJ Jr, Li G. Curcumin induces apoptosis in human melanoma cells through a Fas receptor/caspase-8 pathway independent of p53. *Exp Cell Res* 2001;271:305-314.

43. Cheng AL, Hsu CH, Lin JK, et al. Phase I clinical trial of curcumin, a chemopreventive agent, in patients with high-risk or pre-malignant lesions. *Anticancer Res* 2001;21:2895-2900.

44. Prucksunand C, Indrasukhsri B, Leethochawalit M, Hungspreugs K. Phase II clinical trial on effect of the long turmeric (*Curcuma longa* Linn) on healing of peptic ulcer. *Southeast Asian J Trop Med Public Health* 2001;32:208-215.

45. Lal B, Kapoor AK, Asthana OP, et al. Efficacy of curcumin in the management of chronic anterior uveitis. *Phytother Res* 1999;13:318-322.

Dehydroepiandrosterone DHEA

Introduction

Dehydroepiandrosterone (DHEA) is a steroid hormone secreted primarily by the adrenal glands and to a lesser extent by the brain, skin, testes, and ovaries. It is the most abundant circulating steroid in humans and can be converted into other hormones, including estrogen and testosterone. It has been characterized as a pleiotropic "buffer hormone," with receptor sites in the liver, kidney, and testes, and has a key role in a wide range of physiological responses. Circulating levels of DHEA decline with age and a relationship has been suggested between lower DHEA levels and heart disease, cancer, diabetes, obesity, chronic fatigue syndrome, AIDS, and Alzheimer's disease. Other research suggests that autoimmune diseases such as systemic lupus erythematosus (SLE), rheumatoid arthritis, and multiple sclerosis might be associated with declining DHEA levels.[1]

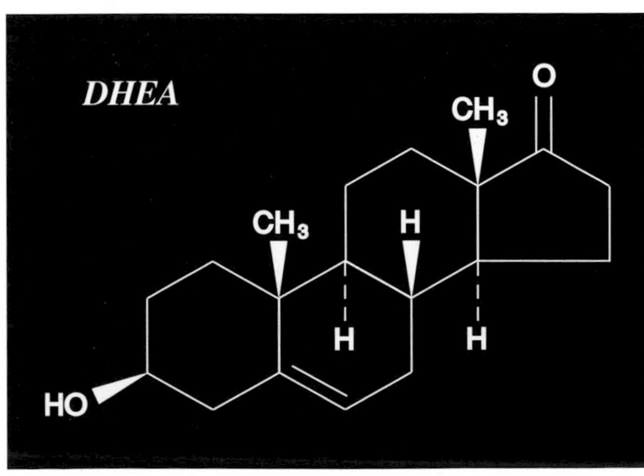

Biochemistry

DHEA is a 19-carbon steroid hormone, classified as an adrenal androgen. Plasma levels decline progressively with age beginning around age 40; therefore, the level of DHEA at age 70 is only about 20 percent as high as that in young adults.[2] DHEA is synthesized from pregnenolone and is rapidly sulfated to yield its ester, DHEA-S, the predominant form found circulating in the plasma.[1] DHEA is metabolized via two pathways — hepatic phase 1 and 2 detoxification, and a cutaneous pathway where it is metabolized by the skin and other tissues sensitive to sex steroids.[3,4] DHEA appears to act directly on targeted cells through specific receptor sites,[5] as well as indirectly to buffer corticosteroids, inhibiting stress-mediated tissue injury.[3]

Clinical Indications

Aging

Clinical evidence supporting DHEA's use as an anti-aging hormone is inconclusive; however, in one double-blind, cross-over study of 30 subjects, ages 40-70, supplementation with 50 mg/day DHEA or placebo for three months resulted in 67 percent of men and 84 percent of women in the DHEA group reporting a significant increase in physical and psychological well-being, with no side effects reported.[6] Supporting these results, mice treated with DHEA had glossier coats and less gray hair than control animals.[7] Anecdotal reports indicate treating elderly patients with 5-20 mg/day DHEA often results in improved mood, energy levels, memory, appetite, and skin condition.[8]

Cancer Prevention

Animal studies have shown DHEA administration to inhibit breast,[9] colon,[10] and liver cancers,[11] as well as skin papillomas.[12] In women with breast cancer, plasma DHEA levels vary significantly depending on whether the women are pre- or postmenopausal. Premenopausal women with breast cancer had lower levels than normal for age while postmenopausal women with breast cancer had higher levels than age-matched controls.[13] These studies suggest DHEA may have anti-carcinogenic properties; but further research is needed before DHEA can be used safely in cancer therapy, particularly in patients with, or at risk for developing, hormone-dependent cancers.

Immune Modulation

DHEA has several different effects on the immune system, some of which are likely to be a result of its anti-glucocorticoid action. Animal studies have shown DHEA to preserve immune competence and prevent immune suppression caused by viral infections.[14,15] Human studies of postmenopausal women given 50 mg/day DHEA demonstrated increased natural killer cell activity and a six-percent decrease in the proportion of T-helper cells.[16]

DHEA levels have also been found to be low in people infected with HIV. A study of 108 HIV-infected men found those with low DHEA levels were 2.3-times more likely to progress to AIDS.[17]

Autoimmune Diseases

Studies have shown DHEA to be of therapeutic value in systemic lupus erythematosus (SLE),[18] rheumatoid arthritis,[19] autoimmune hemolytic anemia,[20] and multiple sclerosis.[21] DHEA levels are often low in patients with these diseases, at least in part due to the use of adrenal suppressive drugs such as prednisone. A return to normal physiologic levels appears to reduce immune complex formation, inhibit lymphocyte proliferation, and increase stamina and sense of well-being.[1]

In a small clinical trial in which 10 women with mild to moderate SLE were given 200 mg/day DHEA for three to six months, eight of the 10 women reported improvement in fatigue, energy levels, and overall well-being.[22] Another double-blind, placebo-controlled, randomized, clinical trial of 21 patients with severe, active SLE demonstrated that 200 mg/day DHEA for six months, in addition to conventional SLE therapy, resulted in a protective effect with respect to corticosteroid-induced osteopenia.[23] An additional study was conducted in which 50 women with mild-to-moderate SLE were given 50-200 mg/day DHEA for six to 12 months. Thirty-four patients completed six months of treatment and 21 patients were treated for 12 months. Results demonstrated decreasing disease activity over the entire treatment period, as measured by the SLE Disease Activity Index. Benefits were sustained one year post-treatment, regardless of menopausal status.[24]

Allergic Disorders

Several clinical studies have demonstrated DHEA, given in doses of 10-74 mg/day, to be of benefit in treating food allergy, multiple chemical sensitivity, asthma, and hereditary angioedema. These studies reported a decrease in severity of symptoms regardless of whether patients were receiving corticosteroid therapy.[25,26]

Obesity

Animal studies demonstrated DHEA administration to genetically obese mice resulted in a significant weight decrease, without any change in diet or exercise.[1] DHEA's weight-loss properties are thought to be a result of its inhibition of glucose-6-phosphate dehydrogenase, an enzyme responsible for fat accumulation.[27] Human obesity studies with DHEA are few. One study of 659 fasting postmenopausal women, not on estrogen replacement therapy or antidiabetic drugs, demonstrated a positive association between elevated DHEA-S and central obesity, which contradicts the theory that DHEAS protects against obesity in postmenopausal females.[28]

Cardiovascular Disease

Low plasma DHEA-S levels and decreased insulin sensitivity have been associated with an increased risk of heart disease in men.[29] In women, the reverse has been found. Women with DHEA-S levels in the upper tertile had the highest cardiovascular death rate.[30] A recent clinical study of 1,167 men was conducted to determine whether serum DHEA and DHEA-S levels could predict ischemic heart disease over a nine-year interval. Men with serum DHEA and DHEA-S levels in the lowest quartile at baseline were significantly more likely to develop ischemic heart disease.[31]

Osteoporosis

Serum DHEA levels decline by more than 60 percent with onset of menopause, partially because ovarian DHEA production ceases. The subsequent loss of bone mineral density (BMD) has been shown to be significant, due at least in part to the rapid decline of DHEA. In a study of 457 women and 534 men the association between endogenous sex steroids and BMD was measured. Higher levels of circulating DHEA were positively associated with BMD of the radius, spine, and hip in women, but not in men.[32] DHEA's role in osteoporosis prevention may be attributed to three mechanisms: (1) inhibition of bone resorption; (2) DHEA and testosterone stimulation of bone formation and calcium absorption; and (3) conversion to estrogen or testosterone, providing extra protection against bone loss.[33]

Alzheimer's Disease/Dementia

DHEA status in Alzheimer's disease and dementia is unclear, with most studies having been conducted in animal models. An animal study using mice demonstrated DHEA's memory-enhancing effects, which may be due in part to its action on GABA neurotransmitters. One small, uncontrolled study of male Alzheimer's patients found DHEA administration resulted in modest improvements in cognition and behavior.[34]

Diabetes

Animal studies have demonstrated a correlation between diabetes and obesity that can be reversed by DHEA administration.[1,27] DHEA's anti-glucocorticoid activity may result in protection from diabetes, and insulin resistance appears to decrease when DHEA levels are returned to normal.[28,35]

Drug-Nutrient Interactions

Potential interactions between DHEA and pharmaceuticals include enhanced sedation seen in patients on benzodiazepines and related CNS active drugs,[21] as well as possible thyrotoxicosis in patients taking thyroid hormones.[36]

Side Effects and Toxicity

Despite being a steroid hormone, DHEA appears to be relatively safe if given at normal physiological doses. Among the few side effects noted with administration of physiological doses are breast tenderness, reversible hirsutism in women, and mild to moderate acne due to sebaceous secretion. Doses above 1,500 mg/day have been known to result in insulin resistance in humans[35] and pre-neoplastic pancreatic lesions in rats.[37] As the long-term effects of DHEA administration are not known, it should therefore be used with caution, particularly in patients at risk for developing hormone-dependent cancers.

Dosage

DHEA is usually administered as an encapsulated powder in two or three divided doses. Appropriate physiologic doses are not well defined and differ in men and women. Many of the clinical studies have been conducted using 50 mg/day for women and 100 mg/day for men, but it is possible these doses are supraphysiologic. Positive effects have been seen with doses as low as 5-10 mg/day for women and 10-20 mg/day for men. The one exception to this is in the treatment of SLE, which requires doses of 50-200 mg/day to show benefit. Studies of long-term DHEA administration are lacking.

References

1. Kalimi M, Regelson W, eds. *The Biologic Role of Dehydroepiandrosterone (DHEA).* New York: Walter de Gruyter, 1990.
2. Belanger A, Candas B, DuPont A, et al. Changes in serum concentrations of conjugated and unconjugated steroids in 40- to 80-year-old men. *J Clin Endocrinol Metab* 1994;79:1086-1090.
3. Regelson W, Kalimi M, Loria R. DHEA: Some thoughts as to its biologic and clinical action. In: Kalimi M, Regelson W, eds. *The Biologic Role of Dehydroepiandrosterone (DHEA).* New York: Walter de Gruyter; 1990:404-445.
4. Parker LN. *Adrenal Androgens in Clinical Medicine.* San Diego, CA: Academic Press; 1989:118-134.
5. Kalimi M, Opoku J, Sheng Lu Q, et al. Studies of the biochemical action and mechanism of dehydroepiandrosterone. In: Kalimi M, Regelson W, eds *The Biologic Role of Dehydroepiandrosterone (DHEA).* New York: Walter de Gruyter; 1990:397-404.
6. Yen SS, Morales AJ, Khorram O. Replacement of DHEA in aging men and women. Potential remedial effects. *Ann N Y Acad Sci* 1995;774:128-142.
7. No authors listed. Antiobesity drug may counter aging. *Science News* 1981;19:39.
8. Gaby AR. Dehydroepiandrosterone: biological and clinical significance. *Altern Med Rev* 1996;1:60-69.
9. Schwartz AG. Inhibition of spontaneous breast cancer formation in female C3H (Avy/a) mice by long-term treatment with dehydroepiandrosterone. *Cancer Res* 1979;39:1129-1132.
10. Nyce JW, Magee DN, Hard GC, Schwartz AG. Inhibition on 1,2-dimethylhydrazine-induced colon tumorigenesis in Balb/c mice by dehydroepiandrosterone. *Carcinogenesis* 1984;5:57-62.
11. Mayer D, et al. Modulation of liver carcinogenesis by dehydroepiandrosterone. In: Kalimi M, Regelson W, eds. *The Biologic Role of Dehydroepiandrosterone (DHEA).*: New York: Walter de Gruyter; 1990:361-385.
12. Pashko L, Rovito FJ, Williams JR, et al. Dehydroepiandrosterone (DHEA) and 3-beta-methylandrost-5-en-17-one: inhibitors of 7,12-dimethylbenz[a]anthracene (DMBA)-initiated and 12-O-tetradecanoylphorbol-13-acetate (TPA)-promoted skin papilloma formation in mice. *Carcinogenesis* 1984;5:463-466.
13. Zumoff B, Levin J, Rosenfeld RS, et al. Abnormal 24-hr mean plasma concentrations of dehydroisoandrosterone and dehydroisoandrosterone sulfate in women with primary operable breast cancer. *Cancer Res* 1981;41:3360-3363.
14. Araneo BA, Shelby J, Li GZ, et al. Administration of dehydroepiandrosterone to burned mice preserves normal immunologic competence. *Arch Surg* 1993;128:318-325.
15. Loria RM, Inge TH, Cook SS, et al. Protection against acute lethal viral infections with the native steroid dehydroepiandrosterone (DHEA). *J Med Virol* 1988;26:301-314.
16. Casson PR, Anderson RN, Herrod HG, et al. Oral dehydroepiandrosterone in physiologic doses modulates immune function in postmenopausal women. *Am J Obstet Gynecol* 1993;169:1536-1539.

17. Jacobson MA, Fusaro RE, Galmarini RM, Lang W. Decreased serum dehydroepiandrosterone is associated with an increased progression of human immunodeficiency virus in infected men with CD4 cell counts of 200-499. *J Infect Dis* 1991;164:864-868.

18. Hedman M, Nilsson E, de la Torre B. Low sulpho-conjugated steroid hormone levels in systemic lupus erythematosus (SLE). *Clin Exp Rheumatol* 1989;7:583-588.

19. de la Torre B, Hedman M, Nilsson E, et al. Relationship between blood and joint tissue DHEAS levels in rheumatoid arthritis and osteoarthritis. *Clin Exp Rheumatol* 1993;11:597-601.

20. Tannen RH, Schwartz AG. Reduced weight gain and delay of Coomb's positive hemolytic anemia in NZB mice treated with dehydroepiandrosterone (DHEA). *Fed Proc* 1982;41:463. [Abstract]

21. Calabrese VP, et al. Dehydroepiandrosterone in multiple sclerosis: positive effects on the fatigue syndrome in a non-randomized study. In: Kalimi M, Regelson W, eds. *The Biologic Role of Dehydroepiandrosterone (DHEA).* New York: Walter de Gruyter; 1990:95-100.

22. van Vollenhoven RF. Engleman EG, McGuire JL. An open study of dehydroepiandrosterone in systemic lupus erythematosus. *Arthritis Rheum* 1994;37:1305-1310.

23. van Vollenhoven RF, Park JL, Genovese MC, et al. A double-blind, placebo-controlled, clinical trial of dehydroepiandrosterone in severe systemic lupus erythematosus. *Lupus* 1999;8:181-187.

24. van Vollenhoven RF, Morabito LM, Engleman EG, McGuire JL. Treatment of systemic lupus erythematosus with dehydroepiandrosterone: 50 patients treated up to 12 months. *J Rheumatol* 1998;25:285-289.

25. Dunn PJ, Mahood CB, Speed JF, Jury DR. Dehydroepiandrosterone sulphate concentrations in asthmatic patients: pilot study. *NZ Med J* 1984;97:805-808.

26. Smith BJ, Buxton JR, Dickeson J, Heller RF. Does beclomethasone dipropionate suppress dehydroepiandrosterone sulphate in postmenopausal women? *Aust NZ J Med* 1994;24:396-401.

27. Cleary MP, Shepherd A, Jenks B. Effect of dehydroepiandrosterone on growth in lean and obese Zucker rats. *J Nutr* 1984;114:1242-1251.

28. Barrett-Connor E, Ferrara A. Dehydroepiandrosterone, dehydroepiandrosterone sulfate, obesity, waist-hip ratio, and non-insulin dependent diabetes in postmenopausal women: the Rancho Bernardo Study. *J Clin Endocrinol Metab* 1996;81:59-64.

29. Piedrola G, Novo E, Serrano-Gotarredona J, et al. Relationship between insulin sensitivity and dehydroepiandrosterone sulfate in patients with ischemic heart disease. *Horm Metab Res* 1997;29:566-571.

30. Barrett-Connor E, Khaw KT. Absence of an inverse relation of dehydroepiandrosterone sulfate with cardiovascular mortality in postmenopausal women. *N Engl J Med* 1987;317:711.

31. Feldman HA, Johannes CB, Araujo AB, et al. Low dehydroepiandrosterone and ischemic heart disease in middle-aged men: prospective results from the Massachusetts Male Aging Study. *Am J Epidemiol* 2001;153:79-89.

32. Greendale GA, Edelstein S, Barrett-Connor E. Endogenous sex steroids and bone mineral density in older women and men: the Rancho Bernardo Study. *J Bone Miner Res* 1997;11:1833-1843.

33. Taelman P, Kaufman JM, Janssens X, Vermeulen A. Persistence of increased bone resorption and possible role of dehydroepiandrosterone as a bone metabolism determinant in osteoporotic women in late post-menopause. *Maturitas* 1989;11:65-73.

34. Bonnet KA, Brown RP. Cognitive effects of DHEA replacement therapy. In: Kalimi M, Regelson W, eds.*The Biologic Role of Dehydroepiandrosterone (DHEA).* New York: Walter de Gruyter; 1990:65-79.

35. Nestler JE. Insulin and adrenal androgens. *Semin Reprod Endocrinol* 1994;12:1-5.

36. McIntosh MK, Berdanier CD. Influence of dehydroepiandrosterone (DHEA) on the thyroid hormone status of BHE/cdb rats. *J Nutr Biochem* 1992;3:194-199.

37. Tagliaferro AR, Roebuck BD, Ronan AM, Meeker LD. Enhancement of pancreatic carcinogenesis by dehydroepiandrosterone. *Adv Exp Med Biol* 1992;322:119-129.

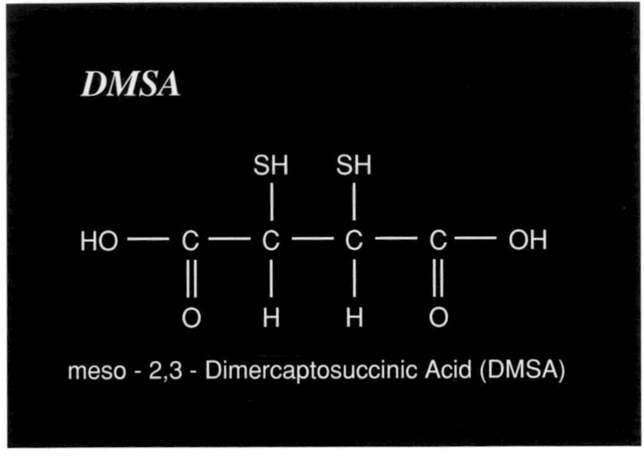

meso - 2,3 - Dimercaptosuccinic Acid (DMSA)

Meso 2,3-Dimercaptosuccinic Acid (DMSA)

Introduction

Contamination of water, air, and food by chemicals and heavy metals is an unfortunate consequence of our industrialized, high-tech society. The resultant accumulation of heavy metals in the human body poses a significant health risk, leading to a wide array of symptomatology and disease states. Although environmental lead levels have decreased in the United States since lead was eliminated from gasoline and lead-based paint, lead continues to be a significant problem, particularly in urban areas and areas of lead mining and smelting. In addition, mercury, cadmium, and arsenic toxicity from occupational and environmental exposure also continue to pose significant threats to public health. For these reasons, diagnostic testing for heavy metals and the subsequent decrease in the body's burden of these substances has become a necessity. Meso-2, 3-dimercaptosuccinic acid (DMSA) is a sulfhydryl-containing, water-soluble, non-toxic, orally administered, metal chelator[1] which has been in use as an antidote to heavy metal toxicity since the 1950s. DMSA's water solubility, oral dosing, large therapeutic window, and low toxicity[2,3] make it superior to other chelating agents available.

Pharmacokinetics and Mechanism of Action

The ability of sulfhydryl-containing compounds to chelate metals is well established. DMSA is a dithiol (containing two sulfhydryl, or S-H, groups) and an analogue of dimercaprol (BAL, British Anti-Lewisite), a lipid-soluble compound also used for metal chelation. Approximately 20 percent of an oral dose of DMSA is absorbed from the gastrointestinal tract of healthy individuals. Ninety-five percent of the DMSA that makes it to the bloodstream is bound to albumin. It is suggested that one of the sulfhydryls in DMSA binds to a cysteine residue on albumin, leaving the other S-H available to chelate metals.[4,5] DMSA and other dithiol agents have a binding affinity for lead, mercury, cadmium, arsenic, bismuth, tin, nickel, and thallium.[6] Studies indicate the half-life of oral DMSA is approximately three hours, with up to 70 percent of an oral dose eliminated in the first six hours.[7,8] Over 90 percent of DMSA found in urine is in a mixed disulfide form, in which one or two cysteine molecules are attached to each DMSA molecule.[5]

Clinical Indications

Lead Toxicity

Lead exposure continues to be a public health problem in the United States. Lead-containing paint is still found in millions of pre-1940s homes. Lead toxicity causes numerous malfunctions in calcium uptake and utilization, and also interferes with calcium-facilitated cellular metabolism. Lead is particularly toxic to the central nervous system (CNS), as evidenced by its particularly deleterious effects on mental development and intelligence in children with lead toxicity. In addition, neurobehavioral deficits resembling attention deficit disorder have been attributed to lead exposure.[9] In a child, blood lead concentrations of 20-25 mg/100 ml can cause irreversible CNS damage.[10] In adults, acute lead exposure leads to renal proximal tubular damage, while chronic exposure causes renal dysfunction characterized by hypertension, hyperuricemia, gout, and chronic renal failure.[11] DMSA has been shown to be successful in lowering blood lead levels in children[12,13] and adults[14,15] with lead toxicity, and is FDA approved for use in chelation of lead in children.

Mercury Toxicity

Human exposure to mercury is primarily in two forms: mercury vapor and methylmercury compounds. Mercury vapor in the atmosphere makes its way into fresh and salt water by falling in precipitation. Methylmercury compounds are created by bacterial conversion of inorganic mercury in water and soil, and are subsequently concentrated in seafood. Dietary fish intake has been found to have a direct correlation with methylmercury levels in blood and hair.[16,17] "Silver" amalgam dental fillings (which are approximately 50-percent mercury) are the major source of inorganic mercury exposure in humans.[18] Mercury vapor is released as the individual chews[19] or drinks hot beverages,[20] and is inhaled, resulting in increased blood mercury levels. Studies have shown a direct correlation between the number of amalgam fillings and concentration of blood[21] and urine mercury.[22]

DMSA is an effective mercury chelator,[23] and when compared to treatment with other chelating agents, results in the greatest urinary excretion of mercury,[24] It is the most effective at removing mercury from the blood, liver, brain, spleen, lungs, large intestine, skeletal muscle, and bone.[25] In animal studies following intravenous administration of methylmercury, DMSA was the "most efficient chelator for brain mercury,"[26] removing two-thirds of brain mercury deposits.

Cadmium and Arsenic Toxicity

Environmental cadmium exposure comes from pollutants discharged by industries utilizing it, including herbicide and battery manufacturers. It is also found in cigarette smoke. Cadmium, like lead and mercury, can interact metabolically with essential minerals. Cadmium interacts with calcium in the skeletal system to produce osteodystrophies, and competes with zinc for binding sites on metallothionein, which is important in the storage and transport of zinc during development. Cadmium poisoning can lead to rhinitis, nephropathy, and osteomalacia, and has a possible link to cardiomyopathy, hypertension, and hepatic and prostate disorders.[6,27]

Arsenic toxicity is also usually a result of exposure to industrial pollutants or cigarette smoke. Symptoms include eczema, dermatitis, malaise, muscle weakness, and "garlic breath."[14] The use of DMSA in arsenic chelation is more effective in cases of acute poisoning than in those of long-term exposure. This may be due, in part, to the possibility that DMSA is a more effective chelator of arsenic in the bloodstream than it is of the tissue-bound arsenic seen in long-term exposure.[14]

Side Effects and Toxicity

DMSA is very safe and generally well tolerated, with few side effects being noted. Some patients may experience slight gastrointestinal disturbances or urticaria, but it is not usually necessary to discontinue treatment.[28] Rare cases of a rash (which resolves upon discontinuation of DMSA) developing after two or three rounds of treatment have been reported. Any detoxification regimen requires the bowels to be fully functioning. If a patient is constipated, normal bowel function should be restored prior to DMSA chelation. DMSA can chelate other elements, including copper, manganese, molybdenum, and zinc, which might result in deficiencies. Although DMSA does not directly bind magnesium, cysteine, and glutathione, heavy metal detoxification can result in depletion of these nutrients as well.[6] Therefore, deficiencies of these essential elements should be screened for and corrected. Sulfhydryl compounds in DMSA can make urine smell very sulfurous, necessitating adequate communication with the patient regarding this issue.

Dosage

DMSA can be used, via an oral challenge and urinary analysis, to diagnose heavy metal toxicity. 500 mg is given per day, in divided doses between meals, for three days. During the third day the urine is collected for 24 hours. A sample is taken from the total amount and sent to a laboratory. An alternate method suggested by some labs is a 20-30 mg/kg body weight dosage, taken in one dose on an empty stomach, and urine is collected for six hours. A sample is then sent to the lab to be analyzed.

Dosing protocols for heavy metal toxicity treatment using DMSA vary depending on physician preference and individual patient need, but currently two protocols are most often used. In one protocol, 10-30 mg/kg body weight is given per day in three divided doses, using a three-days-on, 11-days-off cycle, with a minimum of eight cycles. A second protocol involves giving 500 mg per day (in two or three divided doses) every other day for a minimum of five weeks. DMSA appears to be absorbed best when taken between meals.[29]

References

1. Aposhian HV. DMSA and DMPS—Water-soluble antidotes for heavy metal poisoning. *Ann Rev Pharmacol Toxicol* 1983;23:193-215.
2. Muckter H, Liebl B, Reichl FX, et al. Are we ready to replace dimercaprol (BAL) as an arsenic antidote? *Hum Exp Toxicol* 1997;16:460-465.
3. Graziano JH. Role of 2,3-dimercaptosuccinic acid in the treatment of heavy metal poisoning. *Med Tox* 1986;1:155-162.
4. Aposhian HV, Maiorino RM, Rivera M, et al. Human studies with the chelating agents, DMPS and DMSA. *J Toxicol Clin Toxicol* 1992;30:505-528.
5. Maiorino RM, Bruce DC, Aposhian HV. Determination and metabolism of dithiol chelating agents. VI. Isolation and identification of the mixed disulfides of meso-2,3-dimercaptosuccinic acid with L-cysteine in human urine. *Toxicol Appl Pharmacol* 1989;97:338-349.
6. Quig D. Cysteine metabolism and metal toxicity. *Altern Med Rev* 1998;3:262-270.
7. Roels HA, Boeckx M, Ceulemans E, Lauwerys RR. Urinary excretion of mercury after occupational exposure to mercury vapour and influence of the chelating agent meso-2,3-dimercaptosuccinic acid (DMSA). *Br J Ind Med* 1991;48:247-253.
8. Dart RC, Hurlbut KM, Maiorino RM, et al. Pharmacokinetics of meso-2,3-dimercaptosuccinic acid in patients with lead poisoning and in healthy adults. *J Pediatr* 1994;125:309-316.
9. Winneke G, Kramer U. Neurobehavioral aspects of lead neurotoxicity in children. *Cent Eur J Public Health* 1997;5:65-69.
10. Landrigan PJ, Baker EL. Exposure of children to heavy metals from smelters: epidemiology and toxic consequences. *Environ Res* 1981;25:204-224.
11. Perazella MA. Lead and the kidney: nephropathy, hypertension, and gout. *Conn Med* 1996;60:521-526.
12. Farrar HC, McLeane LR, Wallace M, et al. A comparison of two dosing regimens of succimer in children with chronic lead poisoning. *J Clin Pharmacol* 1999;39:180-183.
13. Chisolm JJ Jr. Safety and efficacy of meso-2,3-dimercaptosuccinic acid (DMSA) in children with elevated blood lead concentrations. *J Toxicol Clin Toxicol* 2000;38:365-375.
14. Fournier L, Thomas G, Garnier R, et al. 2,3-Dimercaptosuccinic acid treatment of heavy metal poisoning in humans. *Med Toxicol Adverse Drug Exp* 1988;3:499-504.
15. Graziano JH, Siris ES, LoIacono N, et al. 2,3-Dimercaptosuccinic acid as an antidote for lead intoxication. *Clin Pharmacol Ther* 1985;37:431-438.
16. Turner MD, Marsh DO, Smith JC, et al. Methylmercury in populations eating large quantities of marine fish. *Arch Environ Health* 1980;35:367-377.
17. Wilhelm M, Muller F, Idel H. Biological monitoring of mercury vapour exposure by scalp hair analysis in comparison to blood and urine. *Toxicol Lett* 1996;88:221-226.
18. Sandborgh-Englund G, Elinder CG, Langworth S, et al. Mercury in biological fluids after amalgam removal. *J Dent Res* 1998;77:615-624.
19. Svare C, Peterson L, Reinhardt J, et al. The effect of dental amalgams on mercury levels in expired air. *J Dent Res* 1981;60:1668-1671.
20. Derand T. Mercury vapor from dental amalgams, an *in vitro* study. *Swed Dent J* 1989;13:169-175.
21. Snapp KR, Boyer DB, Peterson LC, Svare CW. The contribution of dental amalgam to mercury in blood. *J Dent Res* 1989;68:780-785.
22. Bjorkman L, Sandborgh-Englund G, Ekstrand J. Mercury in saliva and feces after removal of amalgam fillings. *Toxicol Appl Pharmacol* 1997;144:156-162.
23. Forman J, Moline J, Cernichiari E, et al. A cluster of pediatric metallic mercury exposure cases treated with meso-2,3-dimercaptosuccinic acid (DMSA). *Environ Health Perspect* 2000;108:575-577.

24. Bluhm RE, Bobbitt RG, Welch LG, et al. Elemental mercury vapour toxicity, treatment, and prognosis after acute, intensive exposure in chloralkali workers. Part I: History, neurophysical findings and chelator effects. *Hum Exp Toxicol* 1992;11:201-210.

25. Planas-Bohne F. The influence of chelating agents on the distribution and biotransformation of methylmercuric chloride in rats. *J Pharmacol Exp Ther* 1981;217:500-504.

26. Butterworth RF, Gonce M, Barbeau A. Accumulation and removal of Hg_2O_3 in different regions of the rat brain. *Can J Neurol Sci* 1978;5:397-400.

27. Chang LW. *Toxicology of Metals*. Boca Raton, FL: CRC Press; 1996.

28. Sandborgh-Englund G, Dahlqvist R, Lindelof B, et al. DMSA administration to patients with alleged mercury poisoning from dental amalgams: a placebo-controlled study. *J Dent Res* 1994;73:620-628.

29. Rozema TC. The protocol for the safe and effective administration of EDTA and other chelating agents for vascular disease, degenerative disease, and metal toxicity. *J Adv Med* 1997;10:95-100.

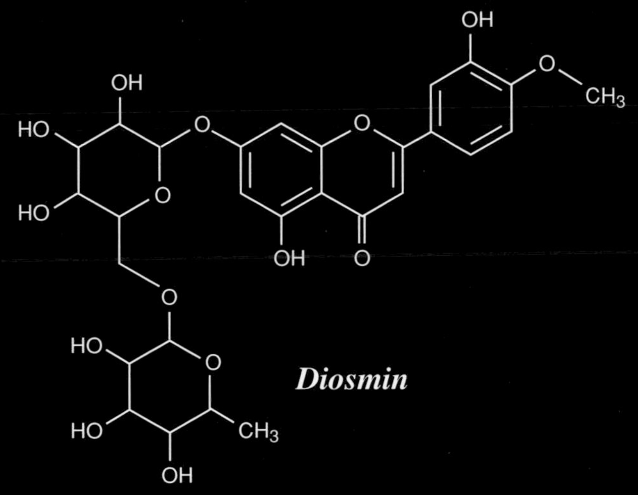

Diosmin

Diosmin

Introduction

Diosmin is a naturally occurring flavonoid glycoside that can be isolated from various plant sources or derived from the flavonoid hesperidin. Diosmin was first isolated in 1925 from *Scrophularia nodosa* and first introduced as a therapeutic agent in 1969. Diosmin is considered to be a vascular protecting agent used to treat chronic venous insufficiency, hemorrhoids, lymphedema, and varicose veins. As a flavonoid, diosmin also exhibits anti-inflammatory, free-radical scavenging, and antimutagenic properties.

Diosmin is molecularly different from hesperidin by the presence of a double bond between two carbon atoms in the central carbon ring of diosmin. Diosmin can be manufactured by extracting hesperidin from citrus rinds, followed by conversion of hesperidin into diosmin. Diosmin has been used for over 30 years as a phlebotonic and vascular protecting agent, and has recently begun to be investigated for other therapeutic purposes, including cancer, premenstrual syndrome, colitis, and diabetes.

Biochemistry and Pharmacokinetics

Flavonoids are a large group of plant pigments sharing the same basic chemical structure, a three-ringed molecule with hydroxyl (OH) groups attached. Diosmin ($C_{28}H_{32}O_{15}$) occurs naturally as a glycoside, meaning it has a sugar molecule attached to its three-ringed flavonoid structure.

Pharmacokinetic investigations have shown diosmin is rapidly absorbed and has a plasma half-life of 26-43 hours. Evidence suggests diosmin is rapidly converted into diosmetin, the aglycone derivative of diosmin, once it reaches the plasma. There appears to be no urinary elimination of diosmin or diosmetin; however, their metabolites are excreted through the urine.[1]

Mechanisms of Action

Diosmin's mechanisms of action include improvement of venous tone, increased lymphatic drainage, protection of capillary bed microcirculation, inhibition of inflammatory reactions, and reduced capillary permeability.[2-5] Certain flavonoids, including diosmin, are potent inhibitors of prostaglandin E2 (PGE2) and thromboxane A2 (TxA2)[6] as well as being inhibitors of leukocyte activation, migration, and adhesion. Diosmin causes a significant decrease in plasma levels of endothelial adhesion molecules and reduces neutrophil activation, thus providing protection against microcirculatory damage.[7,8]

Clinical Indications

Varicose Veins/Chronic Venous Insufficiency

Chronic venous insufficiency is characterized by pain, leg heaviness, a sensation of swelling, cramps, and is correlated with varicose veins. A multi-center international trial, carried out in 23 countries over two years, in which 5,052 symptomatic patients were enrolled, evaluated the efficacy of flavonoids in the treatment of chronic venous insufficiency. Patients were treated with 450 mg diosmin and 50 mg hesperidin daily for six months. Continuous clinical improvement was found throughout the study, as well as improvements in quality of life scores for participants.[9] Diosmin-containing flavonoid mixtures have also been effective in treating severe stages of chronic venous insufficiency, including venous ulceration and delayed healing.[2,4]

Hemorrhoids

Several large clinical trials have demonstrated diosmin to be effective in the treatment of acute and chronic symptoms of hemorrhoids. A double-blind, placebo-controlled study of 120 patients showed improvement of pain, pruritis, discharge, bleeding, edema, erythema, and bleeding on examination.[10] The treatment group was given a flavonoid mixture (90% diosmin and 10% hesperidin) at a dose of two 500 mg tablets daily for two months.

The use of diosmin in the treatment of hemorrhoids associated with pregnancy did not adversely affect pregnancy, fetal development, birth weight, infant growth, or infant feeding. Pregnant women suffering from acute hemorrhoids were treated eight weeks before delivery and four weeks after delivery. Over half of the women participating in the study reported relief from symptoms by the fourth day.[11] Diosmin is non-mutagenic and does not have any significant effect on reproductive function.[12]

Lymphedema

Diosmin acts on the lymphatic system by increasing lymph flow and lymph oncotic pressure.[13,14] A flavonoid mixture containing diosmin was used to treat upper limb lymphedema secondary to conventional therapy for breast cancer. Results showed improvement of symptoms and limb volume; the mean decrease in volume of the swollen limb reached 6.8 percent.[14] Additionally, lymphatic functional parameters assessed with scintigraphy were significantly improved. Animal studies of high-protein lymphedema, such as in burns and lung contusions, showed significant improvement with diosmin.[15]

Diabetes

Diosmin has been shown to improve factors associated with diabetic complications. Blood parameters of glycation and oxidative stress were measured in type 1 diabetic patients before and after intervention with a diosmin-containing flavonoid mixture. A decrease in hemoglobin A1c was accompanied by an increase in glutathione peroxidase,[16] demonstrating decreased long-term blood glucose levels and increased antioxidant activity.

Diosmin can normalize capillary filtration rate and prevent ischemia in diabetics. Rheological studies of type 1 diabetics show diosmin can facilitate hemorheological improvements due to decreased RBC aggregation, which decreases blood flow resistance, resulting in reduced stasis and ischemia.[17-19]

Cancer

Diosmin has been investigated in a number of animal models and human cancer cell lines, and has been found to be chemopreventive and antiproliferative.[20-24] More clinically-oriented research needs to be done in this area to discover effective dosages and protocols.

Other Clinical Indications

Studies have also investigated the use of diosmin for stasis dermatitis,[2] wound healing,[25] premenstrual syndrome,[26] mastodynia,[27,28] dermatofibrosclerosis,[2] viral infections,[29] and colitis.[30] More clinically-oriented research also needs to be done in these areas.

Drug-Nutrient Interactions

Diosmin can cause a decrease in RBC aggregation and decreased blood viscosity.[17] There are no documented cases of adverse interactions between diosmin and prescription medications, but caution should be taken when combining diosmin with aspirin or other blood-thinning medications.

Side Effects and Toxicity

In animal studies a flavonoid mixture containing 90-percent diosmin and 10-percent hesperidin had an LD50 of more than 3g/kg. Additionally, animal studies have shown the absence of any acute, subacute, or chronic toxicity after repeated oral dosing for 13 and 26 weeks using a dose representing 35 times the recommended daily dose.[12]

Diosmin is considered to have no mutagenic action, embryotoxicity, nor any significant effect on reproductive function. Transplacental migration and passage into breast milk are minimal.[12]

Dosage

The standard dose of diosmin is 500 mg twice per day. For acute dosing, a loading dose of 1,000 mg three times per day for four days is recommended, followed by 1,000 mg twice per day for three days, and a maintenance dose of 500 mg twice per day for two months.

References

1. Cova D, De Angelis L, Giavarini F, et al. Pharmacokinetics and metabolism of oral diosmin in healthy volunteers. *Int J Clin Pharmacol Ther Toxicol* 1992;30:29-33.
2. Ramelet AA. Clinical benefits of Daflon 500 mg in the most severe stages of chronic venous insufficiency. *Angiology* 2001;52:S49-S56.
3. Smith PD. Neutrophil activation and mediators of inflammation in chronic venous insufficiency. *J Vasc Res* 1999;36:24-36.
4. Bergan JJ, Schmid-Schonbein GW, Takase S. Therapeutic approach to chronic venous insufficiency and its complications: place of Daflon 500 mg. *Angiology* 2001;52:S43-S47.
5. Le Devehat C, Khodabandehlou T, Vimeux M, Kempf C. Evaluation of haemorheological and microcirculatory disturbances in chronic venous insufficiency: activity of Daflon 500 mg. *Int J Microcirc Clin Exp* 1997;17:27-33.
6. Labrid C. Pharmacologic properties of Daflon 500 mg. *Angiology* 1994;45:524-530.
7. Ramelet AA. Pharmacologic aspects of a phlebotropic drug in CVI-associated edema. *Angiology* 2000;51:19-23.
8. Manthey JA. Biological properties of flavonoids pertaining to inflammation. *Microcirculation* 2000;7:S29-S34.
9. Jantet G. Chronic venous insufficiency: worldwide results of the RELIEF study. Reflux assEssment and quaLity of lIfe improvEment with micronized Flavonoids. *Angiology* 2002;53:245-256.
10. Godeberge P. Daflon 500 mg in the treatment of hemorrhoidal disease: a demonstrated efficacy in comparison with placebo. *Angiology* 1994;45:574-578.
11. Buckshee K, Takkar D, Aggarwal N. Micronized flavonoid therapy in internal hemorrhoids of pregnancy. *Int J Gynaecol Obstet* 1997;57:145-151.
12. Meyer OC. Safety and security of Daflon 500 mg in venous insufficiency and in hemorrhoidal disease. *Angiology* 1994;45:579-584.
13. Pecking AP, Fevrier B, Wargon C, Pillion G. Efficacy of Daflon 500 mg in the treatment of lymphedema (secondary to conventional therapy of breast cancer). *Angiology* 1997;48:93-98.
14. Pecking AP. Evaluation by lymphoscintigraphy of the effect of a micronized flavonoid fraction (Daflon 500 mg) in the treatment of upper limb lymphedema. *Int Angiology* 1995;14:39-43.

15. Casley-Smith JR, Casley-Smith JR. The effects of diosmin (a benzo-pyrone) upon some high-protein oedemas: lung contusion, and burn and lymphoedema of rat legs. *Agents Actions* 1985;17:14-20.

16. Manuel Y, Keenoy B, Vertommen J, De Leeuw I. The effect of flavonoid treatment on the glycation and antioxidant status in Type 1 diabetic patients. *Diabetes Nutr Metab* 1999;12:256-263.

17. Lacombe C, Bucherer C, Lelievre JC. Hemorheological improvement after Daflon 500 mg treatment in diabetes. *Int Angiol* 1988;7:21-24.

18. Lacombe C, Lelievre JC, Bucherer C, Grimaldi A. Activity of Daflon 500 mg on the hemorheological disorders in diabetes. *Int Angiol* 1989;8:45-48.

19. Valensi PE, Behar A, de Champvallins MM, et al. Effects of a purified micronized flavonoid fraction on capillary filtration in diabetic patients. *Diabet Med* 1996;13:882-888.

20. Kuntz S, Wenzel U, Daniel H. Comparative analysis of the effects of flavonoids on proliferation, cytotoxicity, and apoptosis in human colon cancer cell lines. *Eur J Nutr* 1999;38:133-142.

21. Yang M, Tanaka T, Hirose Y, et al. Chemopreventive effects of diosmin and hesperidin on N-butyl-N-(4-hydroxybutyl) nitrosamine-induced urinary-bladder carcinogenesis in male ICR mice. *Int J Cancer* 1997;73:19-24.

22. Tanaka T, Makita H, Kawabata K, et al. Modulation of N-methyl-N-amylnitrosamine-induced rat oesophageal tumourigenesis by dietary feeding of diosmin and hesperidin, both alone and in combination. *Carcinogenesis* 1997;18:761-769.

23. Tanaka T, Makita H, Kawabata K, et al. Chemoprevention of azoxymethane-induced rat colon carcinogenesis by the naturally occurring flavonoids, diosmin and hesperidin. *Carcinogenesis* 1997;18:957-965.

24. Tanaka T, Makita H, Ohnishi M, et al. Chemoprevention of 4-nitroquinoline 1-oxide-induced oral carcinogenesis in rats by flavonoids diosmin and hesperidin, each alone and in combination. *Cancer Res* 1997;57:246-252.

25. Hasanoglu A, Ara C, Ozen S, et al. Efficacy of micronized flavonoid fraction in healing of clean and infected wounds. *Int J Angiol* 2001;10:41-44.

26. Serfaty D, Magneron AC. Premenstrual syndrome in France: epidemiology and therapeutic effectiveness of 1000 mg of micronized purified flavonoid fraction in 1,473 gynecological patients. *Contracept Fertil Sex* 1997;25:85-90. [Article in French]

27. Meggiorini ML, Cascialli GL, Luciani S, et al. Randomized study of the use of synthetic diosmin in premenstrual and vascular dysplastic mastodynia. *Minerva Ginecol* 1990;42:421-425. [Article in Italian]

28. Ciardetti P, Zucconi G, Ottanelli S, Casparis D. Treatment of mastodynia with synthetic diosmin. *Ann Ostet Ginecol Med Perinat* 1985;106:258-266. [Article in Italian]

29. Bae EA, Han MJ, Lee M, Kim DH. *In vitro* inhibitory effect of some flavonoids on rotavirus infectivity. *Biol Pharm Bull* 2000;23:1122-1124.

30. Crespo ME, Galvez J, Cruz T, et al. Anti-inflammatory activity of diosmin and hesperidin in rat colitis induced by TNBS. *Planta Med* 1999;65:651-653.

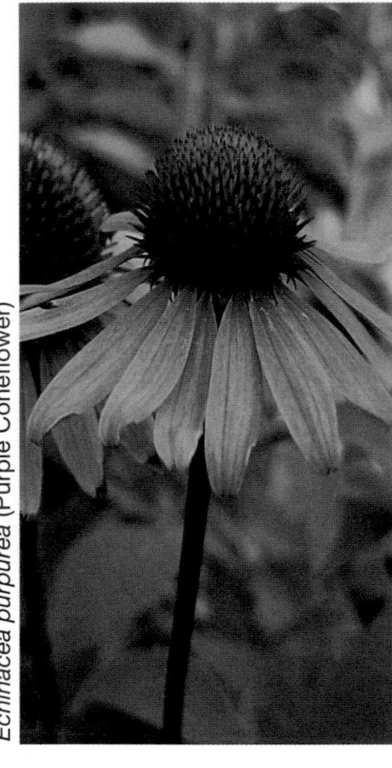
Echinacea purpurea (Purple Coneflower)

Echinacea

Description

Echinacea (also known as purple coneflower and Rudbeckia) is a member of the Compositae family; the three species of medicinal interest being *Echinacea angustifolia, Echinacea purpurea,* and *Echinacea pallida. Echinacea angustifolia* has been used therapeutically for centuries by Native Americans as a remedy for eye conditions, snake bites, insect stings, infected wounds, eczema, enlarged glands, mumps, and rabies. It was also used as a painkiller for a variety of conditions from stomach aches to epilepsy. In the early 20th century, Echinacea was used by a group of physicians known as the "Eclectics," whose medicinal practice relied primarily on the use of plants and their disease-healing properties. During the Eclectic era, Echinacea was used to treat a variety of kidney and urinary tract conditions, chronic bacterial infections, and syphilis.[1] From the 1930s-1970s, antibiotic development resulted in a sharp decline in Echinacea use, but due to a subsequent disenchantment with the medical establishment, an herbal medicine "renaissance" in the 1980s led to renewed interest in Echinacea's benefits. Echinacea research during the last 20 years has focused on its immune-stimulating properties. Currently, Echinacea is being used to combat bacterial, viral, protozoan, and fungal infections, as an anti-inflammatory agent, and as a possible chemopreventive agent.

Echinacea is native to much of the United States, with species varying by location, and is usually found in open meadows or damp locations such as woods, swamps, ditches, river banks, and low-lying thickets. It has a thick, black, pungent root, narrow leaves, and a stem growing to a height of three feet.[2] The flowering head is orange and cone-shaped, bearing purple, rose, or white petals from June to September.[3]

Active Constituents

Active constituents vary slightly according to species and include caffeic acid derivatives (primarily echinacoside), flavonoids, essential oils, polyacetylenes, alkylamides, and polysaccharides. No single constituent has been found to be primarily responsible for Echinacea's immune-stimulating effect; rather they appear to all work together to accomplish this. Therefore, extracts standardized to a specific echinacoside concentration may not be the most beneficial, as this standardization may be at the expense of other active constituents.[2]

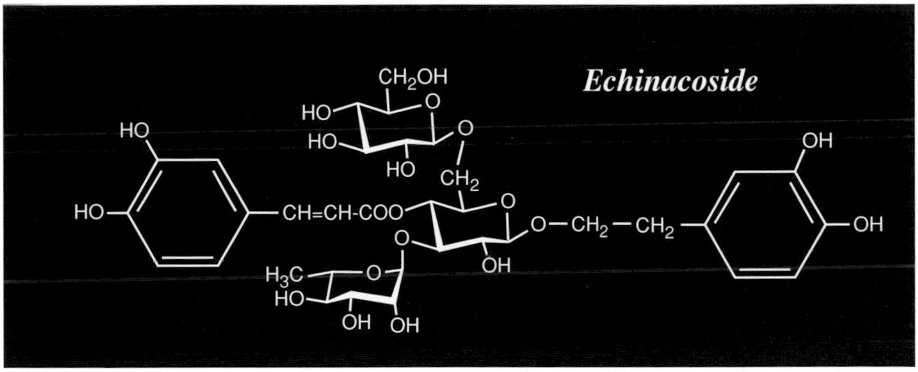

Echinacoside

Mechanisms of Action/Clinical Indications

Immune Stimulation

Echinacea's immune-stimulating properties are quite complex and are attributed to the combined effect of several of its constituents.[4] The Eclectic physicians discovered alcohol extracts of Echinacea directly stimulated white blood cell production and phagocytic activity.[5] Modern clinical and *in vitro* research has confirmed the Eclectics' observations regarding increased phagocytosis,[6] NK cell activity, and increased antibody-dependent cellular cytotoxicity, mediated by tumor necrosis factor-alpha (TNF-α). The latter study was conducted using peripheral blood mononuclear cells from normal individuals and patients with either chronic fatigue syndrome or AIDS.[7] Due to its potential to stimulate TNF-α and interleukins 1 and 6, it has been suggested that Echinacea should not be used by AIDS patients as it may speed the course of the disease, although this is not a universally held theory.[3,8]

Echinacea angustifolia also appears to have a mild antibiotic effect, probably attributable to its caffeic acid constituent, which is capable of directly inhibiting *Staphylococcus aureus*. In addition, certain polyacetylene constituents of Echinacea have been found to be bacteriostatic against *E.coli* and *Pseudomonas aeruginosa*.[4] *E. angustifolia* was also used by the Eclectics to treat fungal and protozoan infections, most notably malaria and *Trichomonas vaginalis*,[4] although current research in this area is lacking.

Echinacea research during the past few years has primarily focused on its therapeutic benefit in treating symptoms of the common cold. A review of several clinical studies, comprised of over 3,900 patients, demonstrates that Echinacea extracts decrease the frequency, symptoms, and severity of the common cold.[9-12] However, other similar studies (although fewer in number) have demonstrated Echinacea use to be of no significant benefit in lessening cold and flu symptoms.[13,14]

Inflammation

Native American and Eclectic uses of Echinacea as an anti-inflammatory agent were centered around poisonous snake bites and insect stings. Caffeic acid derivatives, high molecular weight polysaccharides, flavonoids, and essential oils found in Echinacea all possess anti-inflammatory properties.[4] Although current research on Echinacea's anti-inflammatory effect is minimal, animal studies using *E. angustifolia* have indicated the polysaccharide constituents of the extracts possess significant anti-inflammatory activity in attenuating paw and ear edema when applied topically to the skin of mice and rats.[15-17]

Cancer

Research on Echinacea's benefit in cancer therapy is minimal and inconclusive, but because of its immune-stimulating properties, it may prove to be a useful adjunct to conventional cancer therapies. An animal study demonstrated Echinacea's ability to enhance cellular immunity in leukemic mice, resulting in a suppressive effect on leukemia, via increased production of endogenous interferon-gamma.[18] In another animal study, peritoneal macrophages from immunosuppressed mice incubated with Echinacea polysaccharides showed increased production of TNF-α and enhanced macrophage activation. The mice in this study also exhibited restored resistance to *Listeria monocytogenes* and *Candida albicans*, lethal infections associated with their immunosuppressed state.[19]

Drug-Botanical Interactions

Because it is an immune stimulant, caution should be used in combining Echinacea with immunosuppressive drugs such as corticosteroids, cyclosporine, amiodarone, methotrexate, and ketoconazole.[20]

Side Effects and Toxicity

Historical use, modern research, and herbal reference publications show Echinacea to have an excellent safety profile. Echinacea use has been reported to occasionally cause reversible skin reactions, and for this reason, it should be used with caution in atopic individuals.[21]

Misinterpretation of the scientific literature regarding Echinacea's effect on the immune system has led to the development of several myths regarding Echinacea's therapeutic use including: (1) Echinacea is only appropriate for short-term use because it is not desirable to stimulate the immune system continuously,[8] and (2) Echinacea is an immune stimulator and as such, its use may be contraindicated in "progressive conditions" such as tuberculosis, leukemia, allergies, collagen disorders, multiple sclerosis, HIV/AIDS, and autoimmune disease.[22] However, the Native Americans' and Eclectics' high-quality, traditional-use data is a result of decades of extensive clinical experience, and does not support the suggested limitations. King[2] and Ellingwood[5] recommended long-term use of Echinacea for a variety of chronic conditions, including tuberculosis and autoimmune-related disorders. Similarly, neither modern research data nor authoritative herbal reference sources support the suggested limitations on Echinacea use. Numerous clinical studies of Echinacea have been conducted over the last 20-30 years that overwhelmingly demonstrate its therapeutic benefit and safety, even in patients with autoimmune disorders.[23,24] *The British Herbal Pharmacopoeia,*[25] *The British Herbal Compendium,*[26] and *The Encyclopedia of Common Natural Ingredients Used in Food, Drugs, and Cosmetics*[27] list no contraindications for Echinacea. Weiss also suggests Echinacea has an excellent safety profile and no side effects.[28]

Dosage

Echinacea is available in several forms, and dosages vary accordingly. Typical dosages for the various forms are:

- Dried root = 0.5 to 1.0 grams three times daily
- Tincture (1:5) = 1/2 to 1 teaspoon three times daily
- Dry, powdered extract (standardized to 3.5% echinacoside) = 300 mg three times daily
- Liquid Extract (1:1) = 1/4 to 1/2 teaspoon three times daily

References

1. Wagner H. Herbal immunostimulants. *Z Phytother* 1996;17:79-95.
2. King J. *The American Eclectic Dispensatory*. Cincinnati, OH: Moore, Wistach, and Keys;1854.
3. Bergner P. *The Healing Power of Echinacea and Goldenseal, and Other Immune System Herbs.* Rocklin, CA: Prima Publishing; 1997.
4. Schar D. *Echinacea, The Plant That Boosts Your Immune System.* London: Souvenir Press Ltd.; 1999.
5. Ellingwood F. *American Materia Medica, Therapeutics and Pharmacognosy.* Chicago, IL: Ellingwood's Therapeutist; 1919.
6. Melchart D, Linde K, Worku F, et al. Results of five randomized studies on the immunomodulatory activity of preparations of Echinacea. *J Altern Complement Med* 1995;1:145-160.
7. See DM, Broumand N, Sahl L, Tilles JG. *In vitro* effects of Echinacea and ginseng on natural killer and antibody-dependent cell cytotoxicity in healthy subjects and chronic fatigue syndrome or acquired immunodeficiency syndrome patients. *Immunopharmacology* 1997;35:229-235.
8. Bone K. Echinacea: When should it be used? *Altern Med Rev* 1997;2:451-458.
9. Melchart D, Linde K, Fischer P, Kaesmayr J. Echinacea for preventing and treating the common cold. *Cochrane Database Syst Rev* 2000;CD000530.
10. Henneicke-von Zepelin H, Hentschel C, Schnitker J, et al. Efficacy and safety of a fixed combination phytomedicine in the treatment of the common cold (acute viral respiratory tract infection): results of a randomised, double blind, placebo controlled, multicentre study. *Curr Med Res Opin* 1999;15:214-227.
11. Brinkeborn RM, Shah DV, Degenring FH. Echinaforce and other Echinacea fresh plant preparations in the treatment of the common cold. A randomized, placebo controlled, double-blind clinical trial. *Phytomedicine* 1999;6:1-6.

12. Lindenmuth GF, Lindenmuth EB. The efficacy of Echinacea compound herbal tea preparation on the severity and duration of upper respiratory and flu symptoms: a randomized, double-blind placebo-controlled study. *J Altern Complement Med* 2000;6:327-334.
13. Turner RB, Riker DK, Gangemi JD. Ineffectiveness of Echinacea for prevention of experimental rhinovirus colds. *Antimicrob Agents Chemother* 2000;44:1708-1709.
14. Grimm W, Muller HH. A randomized controlled trial of the effect of fluid extract of *Echinacea purpurea* on the incidence and severity of colds and respiratory infections. *Am J Med* 1999;106:138-143.
15. Tragni E, Galli CL, Tubaro A, et al. Anti-inflammatory activity of *Echinacea angustifolia* fractions separated on the basis of molecular weight. *Pharmacol Res Commun* 1988;20:S87-S90.
16. Tubaro A, Tragni E, Del Negro P, et al. Anti-inflammatory activity of a polysaccharide fraction of *Echinacea angustifolia*. *J Pharm Pharmacol* 1987;39:567-569.
17. Tragni E, Tubaro A, Melis S, Galli CL. Evidence from two classic irritation tests for an anti-inflammatory action of a natural extract, Echinacina B. *Food Chem Toxicol* 1985;23:317-319.
18. Hayashi I, Ohotsuki M, Suzuki I, Watanabe T. Effects of oral administration of *Echinacea purpurea* (American herb) on incidence of spontaneous leukemia caused by recombinant leukemia viruses in AKR/J mice. *Nihon Rinsho Meneki Gakkai Kaishi* 2001;24:10-20.
19. Steinmuller C, Roesler J, Grottrup E, et al. Polysaccharides isolated from plant cell cultures of *Echinacea purpurea* enhance the resistance of immunosuppressed mice against systemic infections with *Candida albicans* and *Listeria monocytogenes*. *Int J Immunopharmacol* 1993;15:605-614.
20. Miller LG. Herbal medicinals: selected clinical considerations focusing on known or potential drug-herb interactions. *Arch Intern Med* 1998;158:2200-2211.
21. Bauer R, Hoheisel O, Stuhlfauth I, Wolf H. Extract of the *Echinacea purpurea* herb: an allopathic phytoimmunostimulant. *Wien Med Wochenschr* 1999;149:185-189.
22. Bisset NG. *Herbal Drugs and Phytopharmaceuticals.* Wichtl M, ed., (German edition). Stuttgart/Boca Raton: Medpharm Scientific Publishers/CRC Press; 1994:182-184.
23. Jurcic K, Melchart D, Holzmann M, Martin P, et al. Zwei Probandenstudien zur stimulierung der granulozyten-phagozytose durch Echinacea-extrakt-haltige praparate. *Z Phytother* 1989;10:67-70.
24. Parnham MJ. Benefit-risk assessment of the squeezed sap of the purple coneflower (*Echinacea purpurea*) for long-term oral immunostimulation. *Phytomed* 1996;3:95-102.
25. British Herbal Medicine Association. *British Herbal Pharmacopoeia*. Cowling: BHMA; 1983:80-81.
26. British Herbal Medicine Association. *British Herbal Compendium. Vol 1*. Bournemouth: BHMA; 1992:81-83.
27. Leung AY, Forster S. *Encyclopedia of Common Natural Ingredients Used in Food, Drugs and Cosmetics.* 2nd ed. New York-Chichester: John Wiley; 1996:216-220.
28. Weiss RF. *Herbal Medicine*. (Translated by Meuss AR from the Sixth German Edition of *Lehrbuch der Phytotherapie*). Beaconsfield: Beaconsfield Publishers Ltd; 1988:229-230.

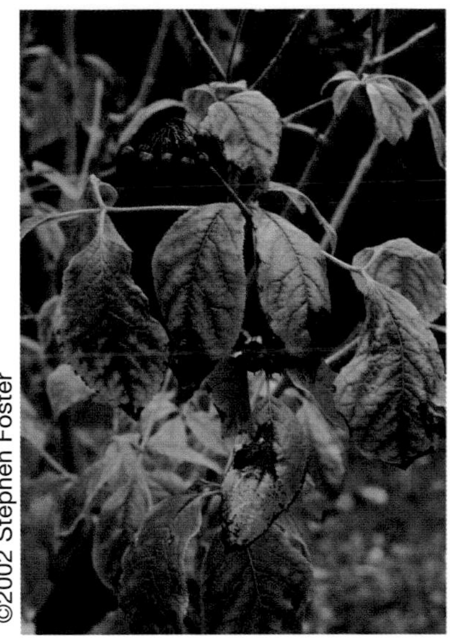
Eleutherococcus senticosus (Siberian ginseng)
©2002 Stephen Foster

Eleutherococcus senticosus

Description

Eleutherococcus senticosus (also known as Siberian ginseng, *Acanthopanax senticosus*, and *Ciwujia*) is an approximately two-meter high, hardy shrub native to the far eastern areas of the Russian taiga and the northern regions of Korea, Japan, and China.[1]

Active Constituents

The active ingredients of this plant are typically concentrated in the root and mainly consist of chemically distinct glycosides called Eleutherosides A-M.[2] Other phytochemicals found in the root structure include ciwujianosides (minor saponins), eleutherans (polysaccharides), beta sitosterol, isofraxidin (a coumarin derivative), sesamin (lignin), and friedelin (triterpene).[2] Eleutherosides I, K, L, and M have also been identified and isolated from the leaf of the plant.[2]

Mechanisms of Action

Eleutherococcus is primarily known as an adaptogen. This term, coined by researcher I.I. Brekhman, suggests such a plant has four general properties: (1) it is harmless to the host; (2) it has a general, rather specific, effect; (3) it increases the resistance of the recipient to a variety of physical, chemical, or biological stressors; and (4) for the user, it acts as a general stabilizer/normalizer.[3] Using animals to test his theory, Brekhman found Eleutherococcus decreases adrenal hypertrophy and the subsequent depletion of adrenal vitamin C levels in stressed rats.[4] Moreover, animals treated with an aqueous extract from the stem bark of this herb were able to increase their swimming time to exhaustion, confirming original research by Brekhman that mice exposed to Eleutherococcus have more stamina.[4,5]

In addition to its anti-fatigue and anti-stress effects, the plant also exhibits immunomodulatory effects. One study found intraperitoneal (i.p.) administration of an extract (primarily eleutherosides B and D) increased the cytostatic activity of natural killer cells by approximately 200 percent after one week.[6] A fluid extract of Eleutherococcus at doses of 1 to 0.1 mg/ml and 1 to 0.03 mg/ml, induced and enhanced the actions of IL-1 and IL-6, respectively, but not IL-2 *in vitro*.[7] Another *in vitro* study confirmed a liquid extract of the root inhibits replication of RNA viruses (human rhinovirus, respiratory syncytial virus, and influenza A virus), but not cells infected with DNA viruses such as adenovirus or herpes simplex type 1.[8]

Other pharmacological actions associated with Eleutherococcus root include radioprotection of the hematopoietic system in mice exposed to lethal radiation,[9] inhibition of histamine release from rat peritoneal cells, and inhibition of systemic anaphylaxis in rats.[10] Other research has noted the stem bark not only increases the concentration of biogenic amines (noradrenaline and dopamine) in the rat brain,[11] but also prevents stress-induced gastric ulcerations in rats[12] and induces apoptosis in human stomach cancer KATO III cells.[13]

Clinical Indications

Athletic Performance

Eleutherococcus has been touted as the herb that builds Russian athletes. In his review of the Russian scientific literature on this subject, Farnsworth notes a single 4 ml dose of the 33-percent ethanolic liquid extract given to five male skiers 1-1.5 hours before a 20-50 kilometer race increased skier resistance to hypoxemia and ability to adapt to increased exercise demands.[14] In another summary of the Russian studies, Halstead cites research on runners given either 2 ml ($n = 34$) or 4 ml ($n = 33$) of the extract 30 minutes before participating in a 10-kilometer race. The results were compared to 41 participants who did not take the herb (control). Those who took either 2 or 4 ml of the extract completed the race in an average time of 48.7 minutes and 45 minutes, respectively, compared to 52.6 minutes for the control group.[15] However, other research has not been able to reproduce the athletic-enhancing actions of Eleutherococcus. In a double-blind study involving nine endurance cyclists, 1,200 mg of a crude extract was taken daily for seven days prior to a simulated 10-kilometer time trial. Supplementation did not significantly alter the physiological responses of the athletes (e.g., oxygen consumption, respiratory exchange, heart rate, plasma lactate, plasma glucose, or perceived exertion) compared to placebo.[16]

After establishing baseline maximal work loads (control) using bicycle ergometry, six healthy male athletes (age 21-22) were consecutively given 2 ml (150 mg of the dried material) of a 33-percent ethanol extract of *Eleutherococcus senticosus* or a comparable placebo in the morning and evening 30 minutes before meals for eight days. Compared to control, individuals who took the herb had significant increases in overall work performance, including maximal oxygen uptake ($p < 0.01$), oxygen pulse ($p < 0.025$), total work ($p < 0.005$), and exhaustion time ($p < 0.005$). Moreover, there was a 23.3-percent increase in total work and a 16.3-percent increase in time to exhaustion in the Eleutherococcus group, compared to only a 7.5-percent and 5.4-percent increase in respective placebo values ($p < 0.05$).[17]

Immune Deficiency

In a controlled trial, 36 subjects were randomized to receive 10 ml of *Eleutherococcus senticosus* root extract or placebo three times per day after meals for one month. A flow cytometric evaluation of lymphocyte subpopulations was made before and after administration of Siberian ginseng or placebo. After four weeks of therapy, those in the active group had a significant increase in total lymphocyte ($p < 0.0001$), T-helper ($p < 0.00001$), T-suppressor ($p < 0.0001$), natural killer ($p < 0.1$) and B-lymphocyte ($p < 0.05$) cells compared to placebo.[18] Russian research on Eleutherococcus confirms the herb's immunomodulatory effects in healthy controls. Compared to placebo, 838 children utilizing the fluid extract on a daily basis for two months had a 25-percent increase in T-lymphocytes, a 20-percent increase in B-lymphocytes, a 10-percent reduction in overall infections, and a 60-percent decrease in the incidence of pneumonia.[19] However, this improvement in lymphocyte subsets was not confirmed in a recent placebo-controlled study in athletes using 8 ml of a 35-percent ethanolic extract of Siberian ginseng (equal to 4 grams crude herb) daily before breakfast for six weeks.[20]

Chronic Stress

In a double-blind study, 45 healthy volunteers (20 men, 25 women, ages 18-30) were randomized to receive two vials of *Eleutherococcus senticosus* or placebo for 30 days. Patients were subject to the Stroop Colour-Word (Stroop CW) test in order to assess their stress response, along with heart rate, and systolic and diastolic blood pressure before and after treatment. Unlike placebo, those employing the herb had a 40-percent reduction in heart rate response to the Stroop CW stressor. Moreover, in females but not males, the use of Siberian ginseng accounted for a 60-percent reduction in the systolic blood pressure response to the cognitive challenge test. These facts together suggest Siberian ginseng may be helpful for stress adaptation.[21]

Side Effects and Toxicity

Although Eleutherococcus is normally quite safe, individuals with hypertension are advised not to take this herb.[22] The literature has reported that oral use of the plant concomitantly with digoxin might result in dangerously high blood levels of digoxin.[23] However, it is likely the 74-year-old male presented in this latter case report consumed a product adulterated with a botanical similar in pronunciation to, and often confused with, Eleutherococcus (Ci-wuj-iia), called Wu jia (*Periploca sepium*).[24] This plant is known to contain digitalis glycosides and therefore would account for the adverse drug effects. Eleutherococcus increases the action of hexobarbitol given i.p. to rats and increases the efficacy of the antibiotic medications monomycin and kanamycin in humans treated for Shigella-positive dysentery and Proteus-induced enterocolitis.[25] Diabetics should monitor blood glucose levels due to the herb's reported hypoglycemic effects in animals.[26] The oral LD_{50} of the 33-percent ethanolic extract is estimated to be 14.5 g/kg.[25] Additionally, the extract is not considered to be teratogenic in mice at 10 mg/kg.[25] Safety in human pregnancy has not been established.

Dosage

In adults, dosage of the 33-percent ethanolic root extract is 10 ml three times per day.[17] Dosages of other extracts include the crude extract of the root at a dose of 2-3 grams daily and extracts standardized to eleutheroside B and E at a dose of 300-400 mg daily.[27] Any of these dosing regimens should be taken daily for 6-8 weeks, followed by a 2-week pause before continuing.[27]

References

1. Boon H, Smith M. *The Botanical Pharmacy*. Kingston, Ontario: Quarry Press; 1999:194.
2. Tang W, Eisenbrand G. *Chinese Drugs of Plant Origin*. Heidelberg: Springer Verlag; 1992:1.
3. Davydov M, Krikorian AD. *Eleutherococcus senticosus* (Rupr. & Maxim.) Maxim. (Araliaceae) as an adaptogen: a closer look. *J Ethnopharmacol* 2000;72:345-393.
4. Mills S, Bone K. *Principles and Practice of Phytotherapy*. New York: Churchill Livingston; 2000:536.
5. Nishibe S, Kinoshita H, Takeda H, et al. Phenolic compounds from stem bark of *Acanthopanax senticosus* and their pharmacological effect in chronic swimming stressed rats. *Chem Pharm Bull (Tokyo)* 1990;38:1763-1765.
6. Tang W, Eisenbrand G. *Chinese Drugs of Plant Origin*. Heidelberg: Springer Verlag; 1992:9.
7. Steinmann GG, Esperester A, Joller P. Immunopharmacological *in vitro* effects of *Eleutherococcus senticosus* extracts. *Arzneim Forsch/Drug Res* 2001;51:76-83.
8. Glattharr-Saalmuller B, Sacher F, Esperester A. Antiviral activity of an extract derived from roots of *Eleutherococcus senticosus*. *Antiviral Res* 2001;50:223-228.
9. Miyanomae T, Frindel E. Radioprotection of hemopoiesis conferred by *Acanthopanax senticosus* Harms (Shigoka) administered before or after irradiation. *Exp Hematol* 1988;16:801-806.
10. Yi JM, Kim MS, Seo SW, et al. *Acanthopanax senticosus* root inhibits mast-cell dependent anaphylaxis. *Clin Chim Acta* 2001;312:163-168.
11. Fujikawa T, Soya H, Hibasami H, et al. Effect of *Acanthopanax senticosus* Harms on biogenic monamine levels in the rat brain. *Phytother Res* 2002;16:474-478.
12. Fujikawa T, Yamaguchi A, Morita I, et al. Protective effects of *Acanthopanax senticosus* Harms from Hokkaido and its components on gastric ulcer in restrained cold water stressed rats. *Biol Pharm Bull* 1996;19:1227-1230.
13. Hibasami H, Fujikawa T, Takeda H, et al. Induction of apoptosis by *Acanthopanax senticosus* HARMS and its component sesamin in human stomach cancer KATO III cells. *Oncol Rep* 2000;7:1213-1216.
14. Farnsworth NR, Kinghorn AD, Soejarto DD, Waller DP. Siberian ginseng (*Eleutherococcus senticosus*): current status as an adaptogen. In: Wagner H, Hikino H, Farnsworth NR, eds. *Economic and Medicinal Plant Research Vol 1*. New York: Academic Press; 1985:155-215.
15. Halstead BW, Hood LL. *Eleutherococcus senticosus/Siberian ginseng: An Introduction to the Concept of Adaptogenic Medicine.* Long Beach, CA: Oriental Healing Arts Institute; 1984:28.
16. Eschbach LF, Webster MJ, Boyd JC, et al. The effects of Siberian ginseng (*Eleutherococcus senticosus*) on substrate utilization and performance. *Int J Sport Nutr Exerc Metab* 2000;10:444-451.
17. Asano K, Takahashi T, Miyashita M, et al. Effect of *Eleutherococcus senticosus* extract on human physical working capacity. *Planta Medica* 1986;3:175-177.
18. Bohn B, Nebe CT, Birr C. Flow-cytometric studies with *Eleutherococcus senticosus* extract as an immunomodulatory agent. *Arzneim-Forsch/Drug Res* 1987;37:1193-1196

19. Aicher B, Gund HJ, Schutz A. *Eleutherococcus senticosus*: therapie bei akuten grippalen infekten. *Pharm Ztg* 2001;41:11-18. [Article in German]
20. Gaffney BT, Hugel HM, Rich PA. The effects of *Eleutherococcus senticosus* and Panax ginseng on steroidal hormone indices of stress and lymphocyte subset numbers in endurance athletes. *Life Sciences* 2001;70:431-442.
21. Facchinetti F, Neri I, Tarabusi M. *Eleutherococcus senticosus* reduces cardiovascular response in healthy subjects: a randomized, placebo-controlled trial. *Stress Health* 2002;18:11-17.
22. Newall CA, Anderson LA, Phillipson JD. *Herbal Medicines*. London: The Pharmaceutical Press; 1996:143.
23. McRae S. Elevated serum digoxin levels in a patient taking digoxin and Siberian ginseng. *CMAJ* 1996;155:293-295.
24. Boon H, Smith M. *The Botanical Pharmacy*. Kingston, Ontario: Quarry Press; 1999:197-198.
25. Halstead BW, Hood LL. *Eleutherococcus senticosus/Siberian ginseng: An Introduction to the Concept of Adaptogenic Medicine*. Long Beach, CA: Oriental Healing Arts Institute; 1984:65.
26. Brinker F. *Herb Contraindications and Drug Interactions,* 2nd ed. Sandy, OR: Eclectic Medical Publications; 1998:123.
27. Brown DJ. *Herbal Prescriptions for Healing and Health*. Roseville, CA: Prima Publishing; 2000:94.

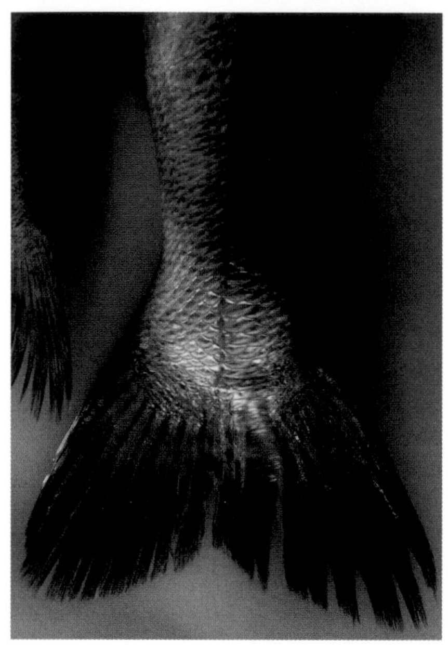

Fish Oil

Introduction

Many well-recognized problems are associated with excessive intake of dietary fat, including obesity, insulin resistance, coronary heart disease, and some forms of cancer. While intake of saturated fat, trans fatty acids, and arachidonic acid has been linked to the development of chronic disease, research shows omega-3 (n-3) fatty acids, specifically fish oils, are essential in the prevention and treatment of disease.

Biochemistry

Fish oils are mostly comprised of the essential fatty acids eicosapentaenoic acid (EPA, C20:5n-3) and docosahexaenoic acid (DHA, C22:6n-3), with lesser amounts of other fatty acids. EPA and DHA fall into a larger category of polyunsaturated fatty acids (PUFAs). Increasing the degree of unsaturation at a given carbon chain length increases the relative mobility and fluidity of the fatty acid, giving PUFAs physical properties not found in saturated fats, including increased bioavailablity.[1] EPA and DHA come from the PUFA alpha-linolenic acid (ALA) and are classified as omega-3 fatty acids. The nomenclature of an omega-3 fatty acid indicates the first carbon-carbon double bond occurs at the third carbon atom from the methyl end of the molecule.[2] Through a series of enzymatic reactions, ALA is converted first to EPA and then to DHA. Both EPA and DHA are deemed conditionally essential, as the body can synthesize them from ALA; however, while consumption of ALA can lead to significant increases in tissue EPA, it does not necessarily do so for DHA.[3] There are several circumstances where the requirement for DHA greatly exceeds the rate of synthesis, making supplementation necessary.

Mechanisms of Action

EPA and DHA compete with arachidonic acid (AA) for the enzyme cyclooxygenase. EPA is converted by platelet cyclooxygenase to thromboxane A3 (TXA3) – a very weak vasoconstrictor – unlike thromboxane A2 (TXA2), which is formed by the action of cyclooxygenase on AA and is a strong vasoconstrictor. However, prostacyclin I3 (PGI3), formed from EPA in the endothelium, is a potent vasodilator and inhibitor of platelet aggregation, as is prostacyclin I2 (PGI2) formed from AA. The net effect, therefore, of an

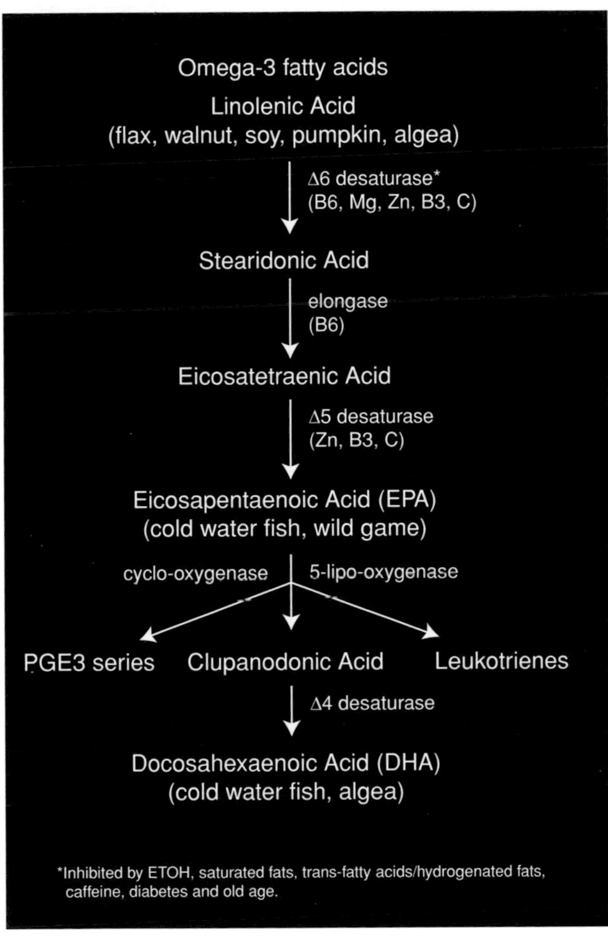

increased dietary EPA:AA ratio is relative vasodilation and platelet aggregation inhibition.[2] EPA yields 5-series leukotrienes, which are weakly chemotactic. A relative reduction in chemotaxis might be expected to be antiatherogenic. Fish oil decreases formation of very low density lipoproteins (VLDLs) and triglycerides due to inhibition of hepatic triglyceride synthesis. Because VLDL is a precursor to LDL, a reduction in LDL cholesterol is seen in some patients with hypertriglyceridemia; however, fish oil does not appear to lower plasma cholesterol in subjects with hypercholesterolemia.[4,5]

Clinical Indications

Arrhythmias

A series of animal studies by McLennan et al found diets supplemented with tuna oil (n-3 PUFA) significantly reduced the incidence and severity of arrhythmias, preventing ventricular fibrillation during coronary artery occlusion and reperfusion. These studies also found the severity of arrhythmias was significantly worsened by a diet supplemented with saturated fat.[6-8]

Coronary Heart Disease

The beneficial effects of fish oil on coronary heart disease (CHD) have been researched for more than two decades, particularly since the landmark study of Greenland Eskimos showed lower mortality rates from cardiovascular disease.[9] Fish oil has important metabolic effects, such as inhibiting platelet aggregation and lowering serum triglyceride levels, which could play a role in the prevention of CHD. A prospective study of European men found an inverse association between fatty fish consumption (but not lean or total fish consumption) and 20-year CHD mortality.[10] Fish oil has successfully been proven to reduce serum triglyceride levels in humans,[11] although the majority of studies have been conducted on men only. More recently, a study was conducted on the effects of n-3 fatty acid supplementation, specifically fish oil, on postmenopausal women. The fish oil supplement significantly reduced serum triglyceride concentrations by an average of 26 percent without affecting other lipid variables, regardless of hormone-replacement status. The effect was estimated to decrease CHD risk by 27 percent in postmenopausal women.[12] Thomas et al suggested fitness status, in addition to fish oil supplementation, may be an important factor in determining postprandial triglyceride levels. Sixty minutes of exercise, in addition to fish oil supplementation, decreased plasma triglyceride levels by 33 percent. It has been suggested that fish oil may inhibit lipoprotein lipase activity via its effect on insulin release.[13]

Cancer

Epidemiological, experimental, and mechanistic data implicate n-6 PUFAs as stimulators, and long chain n-3 PUFAs (specifically fish oil), as inhibitors of development and progression of a wide range of human cancers.[14,15] Studies have found the antitumor effect of EPA is mainly related to its suppression of cell proliferation. On the other hand, the effect of DHA appears to be related to its ability to induce apoptosis.[16,17] The dietary n-3/n-6 fatty acid ratio, rather than the quantity administered, appears to be the principal factor in the antitumor effect of n-3 PUFAs. An effective n-3/n-6 ratio appears to be in the range of 1.8-1.9.[16] EPA and DHA supplementation, in the form of fish oil, has also been found to suppress both breast and colon cancer tumor growth and metastasis.[18,19]

Cognitive Function

AA and DHA accrue rapidly in the prenatal human brain during the third trimester and the early postnatal period, when the rate of brain growth is maximal and most vulnerable to nutritional deficiencies. Postnatal deficiencies of DHA have specifically been found to relate negatively to visual acuity, neurodevelopment, and behavior. In general, breast milk contains sufficient amounts of long chain PUFAs, including DHA, to meet these needs, assuming the maternal diet is adequate. A study examining breast milk and DHA content in Pakistani mothers versus Dutch mothers found significantly lower amounts of DHA in Pakistanis, which was directly correlated to the decreased amount of fish eaten in North Pakistan.[20] It is also controversial at present whether infant formulas that contain only linoleic acid and alpha-linolenic acid are sufficient for brain development.[21]

Depression

In several observational studies, low concentrations of n-3 PUFAs were predictive of impulsive behaviors and greater severity of depression.[22,23] Dopaminergic and serotonergic functions in the frontal cortex seem to be affected by the fatty acid composition of the diet. An n-3 deficiency may be related to catecholaminergic disturbances in depression.[24] Recently it was demonstrated that EPA, DHA, and total n-3 fatty acid levels are significantly lower in red blood cell membranes of depressed subjects compared to controls.[25]

Diabetes

Rats that were fed diets high in fish oil, and with a low n-6/n-3 PUFA ratio, maintained normal insulin action. Diets high in saturated and mono-unsaturated fats led to profound insulin resistance in numerous tissues, as did diets high in omega-6 PUFAs.[1] Similar studies found that providing 5-10 percent of dietary energy from fish oil accelerated glucose uptake and maintenance of normal glucose metabolism, even at high levels of fat intake.[26] More importantly, the ability of fish oil to enhance the rate of glycogen storage allows skeletal muscle to increase its uptake of glucose, even under conditions where fatty acid oxidation is accelerated.[27] Fish oil enhances insulin secretion by incorporation of n-3 fatty acids into the plasma membrane to compete with AA production. This reduces the concentration of AA in the plasma membrane, decreasing the production of PGE2, which in turn suppresses the production of cAMP, a well-known enhancer of glucose-induced insulin secretion. Consequently, fish oil enhances insulin secretion from b-cells, regulating blood sugar.[28] The effect of fish oil on blood lipids should be evaluated in diabetics. A randomized trial conducted on 41 type 1 diabetics found 15 grams fish oil per day resulted in statistically significant elevations in LDL cholesterol.[29] It should be pointed out, however, that this study used a very high daily dose of fish oil – 15 grams versus an average daily therapeutic dose of 5 grams.

Rheumatoid Arthritis

Clinical and biochemical studies have shown fish oil, and to a lesser extent fish, can be used as a source of n-3 fatty acids in the treatment of rheumatoid arthritis. Studies found EPA and DHA reduced eicosanoid and proinflammatory cytokines. The synthesis of interleukin 1b decreased by 20 percent after a diet high in omega-3 fatty acids was consumed for two weeks, and decreased further at the end of four weeks. The synthesis of tumor necrosis factor-alpha decreased 40 percent after two weeks on the diet; at four weeks there was no further significant change.[3]

Other Therapeutic Considerations

Studies also show fish oil to be helpful in the treatment of asthma, acute respiratory distress syndrome, psoriasis, multiple sclerosis, and dysmenorrhea.[30-34]

Side Effects and Toxicity

Fish oil supplementation is generally safe and well tolerated. Few side effects have been reported. Studies to determine the maximum tolerated dose and dose-limiting toxicities of fish oil note occasional gastrointestinal complaints, mainly diarrhea.[35] Other areas of concern include heavy metal contamination of fish, specifically mercury. In the general population, diet is the major source of mercury exposure, primarily through fish consumption.[36] Quality control of products is an essential part of safety. To ensure quality, fish oil products should be purified by a process that removes environmental toxins such as dioxins, PCBs, and heavy metals.

Dosage

Clinical trials show dosages of 4g/day to be effective.[13] Other literature suggests dosage ranges from 1-10 g/day. The maximum tolerated dose was found to be 0.3g/kg per day of fish oil capsules; thus, a 70-kg patient can tolerate up to 21 grams per day.[35]

References

1. Storlien LH, Higgins JA, Thomas TC, et al. Diet composition and insulin action in animal models. *Br J Nutr* 2000;83:S85-S90.
2. Singleton CB, Walker BD, Cambell TJ. N-3 polyunsaturated fatty acids and cardiac mortality. *Aust N Z J Med* 2000;30;246-251.
3. Mantzioris E, Cleland LG, Gibson RA, et al. Biochemical effects of a diet containing foods enriched with n-3 fatty acids. *Am J Clin Nutr* 2000;72:42-48.
4. Schectman G, Kaul S, Kissebah AH. Heterogeneity of low-density lipoprotein responses to fish oil supplementation in hypertriglyceridemic subjects. *Arteriosclerosis* 1989;9:345.
5. Wilt TJ, Lofgren RP, Nichol KL et al. Fish oil supplementation does not lower plasma cholesterol in men with hypercholesterolaemia. *Ann Intern Med* 1989;109:465.
6. McLennan PL, Abeywardena MY, Charnock JS. Dietary fish oil prevents ventricular fibrillation following coronary artery occlusion and reperfusion. *Am Heart J* 1988;116:709.
7. McLennan PL, Abeywardena MY, Charnock JS. Dietary lipid modulation of ventricular fibrillation threshold in the marmoset monkey. *Am Heart J* 1992;123:1555.
8. McLennan PL. Relative effects of dietary saturated, monounsaturated and polyunsaturated fatty acids on cardiac arrhythmias in rats. *Am J Clin Nutr* 1993;57:207-212.
9. Kromann N, Green A. Epidemiological studies in the Upernavic district, Greenland. Incidence of some chronic diseases 1950-1974. *Acta Med Scand* 1980;208:401-406.
10. Oomen CM, Feskens JE, Rasanen L, et al. Fish consumption and coronary heart disease mortality in Finland, Italy, and the Netherlands. *Am J Epidemiol* 2000;151:999-1006.
11. Harris WS. n-3 fatty acids and serum lipoproteins: human studies. *Am J Clin Nutr* 1997;65:1645S-1654S.
12. Stark KD, Park EJ, Maines VA, et al. Effect of a fish-oil concentrate on serum lipids in postmenopausal women receiving and not receiving hormone replacement therapy in a placebo-controlled, double-blind trial. *Am J Clin Nutr* 2000;72:389-394.
13. Thomas TR, Fischer BA, Kist WB, et al. Effects of exercise and n-3 fatty acids on postprandial lipemia. *J Appl Physiol* 2000; 88:2199-2204.

14. Bougnoux P. n-3 polyunsaturated fatty acids and cancer. *Curr Opin Clin Nutr Metab Care* 1999;2:121-126.

15. deDecker EA. Possible beneficial effect of fish and fish n-3 polyunsaturated fatty acids in breast and colorectal cancer. *Eur J Cancer Prev* 1999;8:213-221.

16. Calviello G, Palozza P, Piccioni E, et al. Dietary supplementation with eicosapentaenoic and docosahexaenoic acid inhibits growth of morris hepatocarcinoma 3924a in rats: effects on proliferation and apoptosis. *Int J Cancer* 1998;75:699-705.

17. Lai PB, Ross JA, Fearon KC, et al. Cell cycle arrest and induction of apoptosis in pancreatic cancer cells exposed to eicosapentaenoic acid *in vitro*. *Br J Cancer* 1996;74:1375-1383.

18. Rose D, Connolly J, Rayburn J. Influence of diets containing eicosapentaenoic or docosahexaenoic acid on growth and metastasis of breast cancer cells in nude mice. *J Natl Cancer Inst* 1995;87:587-592.

19. Kontogiannea M, Gupta A, Ntanios F, et al. Omega-3 fatty acids decrease endothelial adhesions of human colorectal carcinoma cells. *J Surg Res* 2000;92:201-205.

20. Smit EN, Oelen EA, Frits AJ, et al. Breast milk docosahexaenoic acid (DHA) correlates with DHA status of malnourished infants. *Arch Dis Child* 2000;82:493-494.

21. Wainwright P. Nutrition and behaviour: the role of n-3 fatty acids in cognitive function. *Brit J Nutr* 2000;83:337-339.

22. Nettleton JA. Omega 3 fatty acids: comparison of plant and seafood sources in human nutrition. *J Am Diet Assoc* 1991;91:331-337.

23. Holman RT. The slow discovery of the importance of n-3 essential fatty acids in human health. *J Nutr* 1998;128:427S-433S.

24. Simon H, Scatton B, Le Moal M. Dopaminergic A10 neurons are involved in cognitive functions. *Nature* 1980;286:150-151.

25. Edwards R, Peet M, Shay J, et al. Depletion of docosahexaenoic acid in red blood cell membranes of depressive patients. *Biochem Soc Trans* 1998;26:S142.

26. Storlien LH, Kraegen WE, Chisholm DJ, et al. Fish oil prevents insulin resistance induced by high fat feeding in rats. *Science* 1987;237:885-888.

27. Storlien LH, Jenkins AB, Chisholm DJ, et al. Influence of dietary fat composition on development of insulin resistance in rats: relationship to muscle triglyceride and omega-3 fatty acids in muscle phospholipids. *Diabetes* 1991;40:280-289.

28. Ajiro K, Sawamura M, Ikeda K, et al. Beneficial effects of fish oil on glucose metabolism in spontaneously hypertensive rats. *Clin Exp Pharm Physiol* 2000;6:77-84.

29. Haines AP, Sanders TA, Imeson JD, et al. Effects of a fish oil supplement on platelet function, haemostatic variables and albuminuria in insulin-dependent diabetics. *Thromb Res* 1986;43:643-655.

30. Miller AL. The etiologies, pathophysiology, and alternative/complementary treatment of asthma. *Altern Med Rev* 2001;6:20-47.

31. Kumar KV, Manimala S, Gayani R, et al. Oxidant stress and essential fatty acids in patients with risk established ARDS. *Clin Chim Acta* 2000;298:111-112.

32. Dewsbury CE, et al. Topical eicosapentaenoic acid in the treatment of psoriasis. *Br J Dermatol* 1989;120:581.

33. Gallai V, Sarchielli P, Trequattrini A, et al. Cytokine secretion and eicosanoid production in the peripheral blood mononuclear cells of MS patients undergoing dietary supplementation with n-3 polyunsaturated fatty acids. *J Neuroimmunol* 1995;56:143-153.

34. Deutch B. Menstrual pain in Danish women correlated with low n-3 polyunsaturated fatty acid intake. *Eur J Clin Nutr* 1995;49:508-516.

35. Burns CP, Halabi S, Clamon GH, et al. Phase 1 clinical study of fish oil fatty acid capsules for patients with cancer cachexia: cancer and leukemia group B study 9473. *Clin Cancer Res* 1999;5:3942-3947.

36. Salonen JT, Seppanen K, Nyyssonen K, et al. Intake of mercury from fish, lipid peroxidation, and the risk of myocardial infarction and coronary, cardiovascular, and any death in eastern Finnish men. *Circulation* 1995;91:645-655.

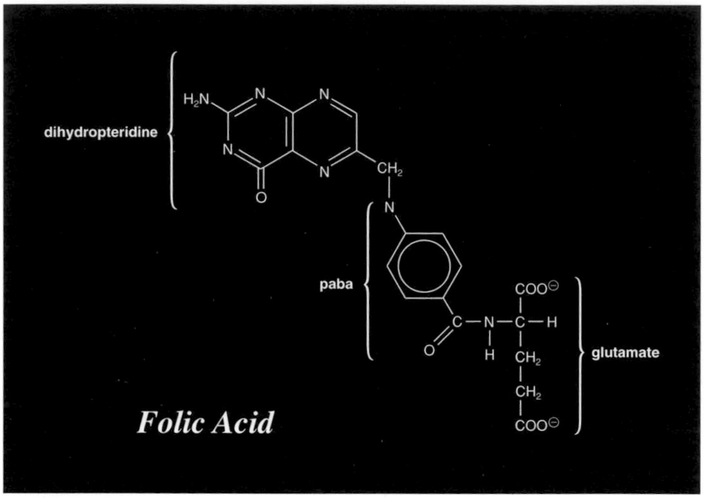

Folic Acid

Introduction

Folic acid, also known generically as folate or folacin, is a member of the B-complex family of vitamins, and works in concert with vitamin B12. Folic acid is necessary for DNA synthesis, in addition to being a methyl-group donor involved in many body processes. Therapeutically, folic acid can reduce homocysteine levels and the occurrence of neural tube defects, might play a role in preventing cervical dysplasia and protecting against neoplasia in ulcerative colitis, appears to be a rational aspect of a nutritional protocol to treat vitiligo, and can reduce inflammation of the gingiva. Neuropsychiatric conditions that may be secondary to folate deficiency include dementia, schizophrenia-like syndromes, insomnia, irritability, forgetfulness, endogenous depression, organic psychosis, peripheral neuropathy, myelopathy, and restless legs syndrome.

Biochemistry

Folic acid is a water-soluble member of the B-complex family of vitamins. In plants, folic acid is formed from a hetero-bicyclic pteridine ring, para-aminobenzoic acid (PABA), and glutamic acid. Humans cannot synthesize this compound; therefore, it is a dietary requirement.

Dietary folic acid is a complex and variable mixture of folate compounds, of which the majority occurs as polyglutamate (multiple glutamate molecules attached) conjugate compounds, reduced folates, and tetrahydrofolates. Despite the fact folic acid is the most common supplemental form of this vitamin, folic acid makes up 10 percent or less of the folates in the diet. Folates are abundant in the diet; however, cooking or processing readily destroys these compounds. The best folate source in food is green, leafy vegetables; sprouts, fruits, brewer's yeast, liver, and kidney also contain high amounts of folates.

Pharmacokinetics

Human pharmacokinetic studies indicate folic acid has very high bioavailability, with large oral doses of folic acid substantially raising plasma levels in healthy subjects in a time- and dose-dependent manner. Subsequent to high-dose oral administration of folic acid (ranging from 25 mg/day to 1,000 mg/day), red blood cell folate levels remain elevated for periods in excess of 40 days following discontinuation of the supplement. Folic acid is poorly transported to the brain and rapidly cleared from the central nervous system. The primary methods of elimination of absorbed folic acid are fecal (through bile) and urinary.[1-4]

After ingestion, the process of conversion of folic acid to the metabolically active coenzyme forms is relatively complex. Synthesis of the active forms of folic acid requires several enzymes, adequate liver and intestinal function, as well as adequate supplies of riboflavin (B2), niacin (B3), pyridoxine (B6), zinc, vitamin C, and serine. After the formation of the coenzyme forms of the vitamin in the liver, these metabolically active compounds are secreted into the small intestine with bile (the folate enterohepatic cycle), where they are reabsorbed and distributed to tissues throughout the body. Despite the biochemical complexity of this process, evidence suggests oral supplementation with folic acid is able to increase the body's pool of the active reduced folate metabolites (such as methyl-tetrahydrofolate) in healthy individuals.[5]

Enzyme defects, malabsorption or digestive system pathology, and liver disease result in impaired ability to activate folic acid into the required coenzyme forms in the body. Evidence indicates some individuals have a severe congenital deficiency of the enzyme methyl-tetrahydrofolate reductase, which is needed to activate folic acid into the 5-methyl-tetrahydrofolate coenzyme form of the vitamin. The existence of milder forms of this enzyme defect is strongly suspected and likely interacts with dietary folate status to determine risk for some disease conditions.[6-10] In individuals with a genetic defect of this enzyme (whether mild or severe), greater dietary exposure to foods rich in folates and supplemental folates in the form of folinic acid or 5-methyl-tetrahydrofolate might be preferable over folic acid supplementation.

Mechanisms of Action

Folic acid's primary mechanisms of action are through its role as a methyl donor in a range of metabolic and nervous system biochemical processes, as well as being necessary for DNA synthesis. Serine reacts with tetrahydrofolate, forming 5,10-methylene-tetrahydrofolate, the folate derivative involved in DNA synthesis. 5-methyl-tetrahydrofolate donates its methyl group to cobalamin (B12), forming methylcobalamin. With the help of the enzyme methionine synthase, methylcobalamin donates its methyl group to the amino acid metabolite homocysteine, converting it into the amino acid methionine. Methionine subsequently is converted into S-adenosylmethionine (SAMe), a methyl donor involved in numerous biochemical processes.

Deficiency States and Symptoms

Folic acid deficiency is considered to be one of the most common nutritional deficiencies. The following may contribute to a deficiency of folic acid: deficient food supply; defects in utilization, as in alcoholics or individuals with liver disease; malabsorption; increased needs in pregnant women, nursing mothers, and cancer patients; metabolic interference by drugs; folate losses in hemodialysis; and enzyme or cofactor deficiency needed for the generation of active folic acid.[11] Absorption of folic acid appears to be significantly impaired in HIV disease, irrespective of the stage of the disease.[12]

Signs and symptoms of folate deficiency include macrocytic anemia, fatigue, irritability, peripheral neuropathy, tendon hyper-reflexivity, restless legs syndrome, diarrhea, weight loss, insomnia, depression, dementia, cognitive disturbances, and psychiatric disorders.[13-18] Elevated plasma homocysteine can also indicate a dietary or functional deficiency of folic acid.

Clinical Indications

Anemia

Folic acid has a long history of use, in conjunction with vitamin B12, for the treatment of macrocytic anemia. Depending on the clinical status of the patient, the dose of folic acid required to reverse macrocytic anemia varies, but the therapeutic dose is usually about 1 mg per day. Duration of therapy to reverse macrocytic anemia can be as short as 15 days after initiation of supplementation, or it may require prolonged supplementation.[17,18]

Cervical Dysplasia

Research points to an association between folate status in adults and cervical dysplasia;[19-21] however, its role as an efficacious therapeutic intervention is unclear. A report suggests folic acid supplementation (10 mg folic acid for three months) was able to reverse cervical dysplasia in women taking oral contraceptives.[22] In another study, 154 individuals with grade 1 or 2 cervical intraepithelial neoplasia were randomly assigned either 10 mg of folic acid or a placebo daily for six months. No significant differences were observed between supplemented and unsupplemented subjects regarding dysplasia status, biopsy results, or prevalence of human papilloma virus type-16 infection.[23]

It is possible certain subsets of women (possibly those with an oral contraceptive-induced deficiency) might be more amenable to treatment; however, additional research is required to clarify the therapeutic role of folic acid in cervical dysplasia.

Gout

There is no evidence demonstrating efficacy of folic acid supplementation in gout. Although some *in vitro* evidence suggests folate compounds are potent inhibitors of xanthine oxidase activity,[24] it appears pterin aldehyde, a photolytic breakdown product of folic acid, and not folic acid itself, is responsible for the observed inactivation of xanthine oxidase.[25]

Available evidence has shown no ability of supplemental folic acid in doses up to 1,000 mg orally per day to significantly lower serum urate concentration, or to decrease urinary urate or total oxypurine excretion in hyperuricemic subjects.[26]

Homocysteinemia

Abnormally high plasma levels of homocysteine, the de-methylated derivative of the amino acid methionine, are an independent risk factor for cardiovascular disease. Elevated plasma homocysteine has been connected to increased risk of neural tube defects and other birth defects, as well as to schizophrenia, Alzheimer's disease, cognitive decline, osteoporosis, rheumatoid arthritis, kidney failure, and cancer.[27-31]

The activated coenzyme form of folic acid (5-methyltetrahydrofolate) is needed for optimal homocysteine metabolism, since it acts as a methyl-donor, providing a methyl-group to vitamin B12. The methylated form of vitamin B12 (methylcobalamin) subsequently transfers this methyl group to homocysteine. The result is a recycling of homocysteine to methionine and a subsequent reduction in elevated plasma homocysteine.

In healthy subjects, even low doses of folic acid can lower homocysteine levels. A dose of 250 mcg per day for four weeks reduced homocysteine an average of 11.4 percent in healthy 18-40-year-old women. A dose of 500 mcg per day over the same duration of time reduced levels by an average of almost 22 percent.[32] In a separate study, 650 mcg per day for six weeks resulted in an average plasma homocysteine reduction of 41.7 percent.[33]

In subjects with cardiovascular disease, 800 mcg per day of folic acid resulted in an average decrease of 23 percent in homocysteine levels,[27] while 2.5 mg per day resulted in an average decrease of 27 percent.[34] In subjects receiving the higher dose, 94 percent experienced some degree of reduction in homocysteine.[28] Evidence suggests individuals with higher initial homocysteine levels are likely to experience a greater reduction subsequent to folic acid supplementation.[34]

Despite the excellent results achieved with folic acid monotherapy, available evidence suggests an additive effect exists between folic acid and vitamins B6, B12, and betaine with respect to lowering homocysteine levels. Combinations of these nutrients typically produce greater reductions in homocysteine than does folic acid alone.[27-29,35]

Inflammatory Bowel Disease

Evidence suggests folic acid supplementation might lower the risk, in a dose-dependent fashion, of colonic neoplasia in patients with ulcerative colitis.[36,37]

Neuropsychiatric Applications

Neuropsychiatric diseases secondary to folate deficiency include dementia, schizophrenia-like syndromes, insomnia, irritability, forgetfulness, endogenous depression, organic psychosis, peripheral neuropathy, myelopathy, and restless legs syndrome.[14-18]

Lower serum and red blood cell folate concentrations have an association with depression, and deficiency might predict a poorer response to some antidepressant medications.[30,38-40] Several studies have documented improvement in depression in some patients subsequent to oral supplementation with the coenzyme form of folic acid (methyl-tetrahydrofolate) at doses between 15-50 mg per day.[41,42] Folic acid (500 mcg per day) significantly improved the antidepressant action of fluoxetine in subjects with major depression.[43]

Limited evidence implies supplemental folic acid might positively affect morbidity of some bi-polar patients placed on lithium therapy.[44]

A syndrome characterized by mild depression, permanent muscular and intellectual fatigue, mild symptoms of restless legs, depressed ankle jerk reflexes, diminution of vibration sensation in the legs, stocking-type hypoesthesia, and long-lasting constipation appears to respond to folic acid supplementation (5-10 mg per day for 6-12 months).[45]

Periodontal Disease

Folic acid can increase the resistance of the gingiva to local irritants and lead to a reduction in inflammation. A mouthwash containing 5 mg of folate per 5 ml of mouthwash used twice daily for four weeks, with a rinsing time of one minute, appears to be the most effective manner of application. The effect of folate on gingival health appears to be moderated largely, if not totally, through a local influence.[46-48]

Pregnancy

A low dietary intake of folic acid increases the risk for delivery of a child with a neural tube defect (NTD), and periconceptional folic acid supplementation significantly reduces the occurrence of NTD.[49-55]

Supplemental folic acid intake during pregnancy results in increased infant birth weight and improved Apgar scores, along with a concomitant decreased incidence of fetal growth retardation and maternal infections.[56-58]

Vitiligo

In some individuals, administration of folic acid appears to be a rational aspect of a nutritional protocol to treat vitiligo. Degrees of re-pigmentation ranging from complete re-pigmentation in six subjects and 80-percent re-pigmentation in two subjects was reported out of eight individuals who followed a three-year protocol with a dosage of 2 mg folic acid twice daily, 500 mg vitamin C twice daily, and intramuscular injections of vitamin B12 given every two weeks.[59]

A two-year study using a combination of folic acid, vitamin B12, and sun exposure for the treatment of vitiligo reported positive results. One hundred patients with vitiligo were treated, with re-pigmentation occurring in 52. Total re-pigmentation was seen in six patients and the spread of vitiligo was halted in 64 percent of the patients. Re-pigmentation was most evident on sun-exposed areas.[60]

Drug-Nutrient Interactions

- A number of drugs can interfere with the pharmacokinetics of folic acid. Cimetidine and antacids appear to reduce folate absorption.[61]
- Sulfasalazine interferes with folic acid absorption and conversion to the active form.[62] Supplementation with folic acid (15 mg/day for one month) prevents folate deficiency in patients with inflammatory bowel disease treated with salicylazosulfapyridine.[63]
- Continuous long-term use of aspirin, ibuprofen, acetaminophen, and other non-steroidal anti-inflammatory drugs appears to increase the body's need for folic acid.[62]
- Although the mechanism is unclear, anticonvulsants, antituberculosis drugs, alcohol, and oral contraceptives produce low serum and tissue concentrations of folate.[62,64]
- Folic acid reduces the elevated liver enzymes induced by methotrexate therapy in rheumatoid arthritis; however, it had no effect on the incidence, severity, and duration of other adverse events.[65]
- Folic acid supplementation prevents nitric oxide synthase dysfunction induced by continuous nitroglycerin use.[66]
- Anti-seizure medications, including carbamazepine and phenobarbitol, appear to utilize folic acid in their hepatic metabolism. Folic acid supplementation can increase metabolism of the drug, thus lowering blood levels of the drug and possibly resulting in breakthrough seizures. Initiating folic acid therapy after starting these drugs should be done with caution in these individuals.[67]
- The anticonvulsant drugs phenytoin and valproic acid appear to interfere with folate absorption.[68] Folic acid supplementation, at a time of day other than when taking an anticonvulsant, may be helpful to prevent deficiency.

There is conflicting information regarding the effects of folate supplementation in individuals treated with anti-folate medications such as methotrexate (MTX) and 5-fluorouracil (5-FU). There is evidence folic acid might inhibit the activity of these drugs, although in some cases it may increase their activity. In fact, the folic acid metabolite, folinic acid (also known as 5-formyltetrahydrofolate and leucovorin), is often used to "rescue" normal tissue after MTX or 5-FU therapy. Folic acid supplementation does not appear to interfere with methotrexate's anti-arthritic or anti-inflammatory activity. Since these medications are used to treat a wide range of malignant and nonmalignant disorders, indiscriminate use of folates should be avoided until further investigations are conducted.

Nutrient-Nutrient Interactions

Some concern exists that supplementation with high doses of folic acid could mask a vitamin B12 deficiency, resulting in neurological injury secondary to undiagnosed pernicious anemia. If there is any possibility of B12-induced anemia in an individual needing folate therapy, dual therapy with B12 and folate should be administered.

Some authors have suggested folic acid supplements might interfere with intestinal zinc absorption; however, at doses as high as 15 mg of folic acid daily, folic acid does not appear to have any significant effect on zinc status in healthy non-pregnant subjects.[67]

Side Effects and Toxicity

In doses typically administered for therapeutic purposes, folic acid is considered non-toxic. At doses of 15 mg per day and above, gastrointestinal complaints, insomnia, irritability, and fatigue have been mentioned as occasional side effects.

Folic acid is considered safe during pregnancy, with an established recommended intake of 800 mcg per day.

Dosage

The dose of folic acid required varies depending on the clinical condition. For lowering homocysteine, a minimum dose of 800 mcg per day is generally used. The most common therapeutic dose is in the range of 1-3 mg per day. Doses of greater than 10 mg per day have been used in conditions such as cervical dysplasia.

Dosages of over-the-counter folic acid supplements are restricted to no more than 800 mcg of folic acid per serving, although prescription forms of folic acid are available in higher doses.

References

1. Zettner A, Boss GR, Seegmiller JE. A long term study of the absorption of large oral doses of folic acid. *Ann Clin Lab Sci* 1981;11:516-524.
2. Schuster O, Weimann HJ, Muller J, et al. Pharmacokinctics and relative bioavailability of iron and folic acid in healthy volunteers. *Arzneimittelforschung* 1993;43:761-766. [article in German]
3. Gregory JF 3d, Bhandari SD, Bailey LB, et al. Relative bioavailability of deuterium-labeled monoglutamyl tetrahydrofolates and folic acid in human subjects. *Am J Clin Nutr* 1992;55:1147-1153.
4. Levitt M, Nixon F, Pincus JH, Bertino JR. Transport characteristics of folates in cerebrospinal fluid; a study utilizing doubly labeled 5-methyltetrahydrofolate and 5-formyltetrahydrofolate. *J Clin Invest* 1971;50:1301-1308.
5. Priest DG, Schmitz JC, Bunni MA. Accumulation of plasma reduced folates after folic acid administration. *Semin Oncol* 1999;26:S38-S41.
6. Yates JR, Ferguson-Smith MA, Shenkin A, et al. Is disordered folate metabolism the basis for the genetic predisposition to neural tube defects? *Clin Genet* 1987;31:279-287.
7. Lussier-Cacan S, Xhignesse M, Piolot A, et al. Plasma total homocysteine in healthy subjects: sex-specific relation with biological traits. *Am J Clin Nutr* 1996;64:587-593.
8. Kluijtmans LAJ, Van den Heuvel LPWJ,Boers GH, et al. Molecular genetic analysis in mild hyperhomocysteinemia: a common mutation in the methylenetetrahydrofolate reductase gene is a genetic risk factor in cardiovascular disease. *Am J Hum Genet* 1996;58:35-41.
9. Whitehead AS, Gallagher P, Mills JL. A genetic defect in 5,10 methylenetetrahydrofolate reductase in neural tube defects. *QJM* 1995;88:763-766.
10. Ulvik A, Evensen ET, Lien EA, et al. Smoking, folate and methylenetetrahydrofolate reductase status as interactive determinants of adenomatous and hyperplastic polyps of colorectum. *Am J Med Genet* 2001;101:246-254.
11. Halsted CH. The intestinal absorption of dietary folates in health and disease. *J Am Coll Nutr 1989*;8:650-658.
12. Revell P, O'Doherty MJ, Tang A, Savidge GF. Folic acid absorption in patients infected with the human immunodeficiency virus. *J Intern Med* 1991;230:227-231.
13. Botez MI. Folate deficiency and neurological disorders in adults. *Med Hypotheses* 1976;2:135-140.
14. Audebert M, Gendre JP, Le Quintrec Y. Folate and the nervous system. *Sem Hop* 1979;55:1383-1387. [article in French]
15. Young SN, Ghadirian AM. Folic acid and psychopathology. *Prog Neuropsychopharmacol Biol Psychiatry* 1989;13:841-863.
16. Metz J, Bell AH, Flicker L, et al. The significance of subnormal serum vitamin B12 concentration in older people: a case control study. *J Am Geriatr Soc* 1996;44:1355-1361.
17. Quinn K, Basu TK. Folate and vitamin B12 status of the elderly. *Eur J Clin Nutr* 1996;50:340-342.
18. Fine EJ, Soria ED. Myths about vitamin B12 deficiency. *South Med J* 1991;84:1475-1481.
19. Liu T, Soong SJ, Wilson NP, et al. A case control study of nutritional factors and cervical dysplasia. *Cancer Epidemiol Biomarkers Prev* 1993;2:525-530.
20. Grio R, Piacentino R, Marchino GL, Navone R. Antineoblastic activity of antioxidant vitamins: the role of folic acid in the prevention of cervical dysplasia. *Panminerva Med* 1993;35:193-196.
21. Kwasniewska A, Tukendorf A, Semczuk M. Folate deficiency and cervical intraepithelial neoplasia. *Eur J Gynaecol Oncol* 1997;18:526-530.
22. Butterworth CE Jr, Hatch KD, Gore H, et al. Improvement in cervical dysplasia associated with folic acid therapy in users of oral contraceptives. *Am J Clin Nutr* 1982;35:73-82.
23. Zarcone R, Bellini P, Carfora E, et al. Folic acid and cervix dysplasia. *Minerva Ginecol* 1996;48:397-400.

24. Lewis AS, Murphy L, McCalla C, et al. Inhibition of mammalian xanthine oxidase by folate compounds and amethopterin. *J Bio Chem* 1984;259:12-15.

25. Spector T, Ferone R. Folic acid does not inactivate xanthine oxidase. *J Biol Chem* 1984;259:10784-10786.

26. Boss GR, Ragsdale RA, Zettner A, Seegmiller JE. Failure of folic acid (pteroylglutamic acid) to affect hyperuricemia. *J Lab Clin Med* 1980;96:783-789.

27. Landgren F, Israelsson B, Lindgren A, et al. Plasma homocysteine in acute myocardial infarction: homocysteine-lowering effect of folic acid. *J Int Med* 1995;237:381-388.

28. Wilcken DE, Dudman NP, Tyrrell PA. Homocystinuria due to cystathionine beta-synthase deficiency – the effects of betaine treatment in pyridoxine-responsive patients. *Metabolism* 1985;12:1115-1121.

29. Dudman N, Wilcken D, Wang J, et al. Disordered methionine/homocysteine metabolism in premature vascular disease. Its occurence, cofactor therapy, and enzymology. *Arterioscler Thromb* 1993;13:1253-1260.

30. Fava M, Borus JS, Alpert JE, et al. Folate, vitamin B12, and homocysteine in major depressive disorder. *Am J Psychiatry* 1997;154:426-428.

31. Miller AL, Kelly GS. Homocysteine metabolism: nutritional modulation and impact on health and disease. *Altern Med Rev* 1997;2:234-254.

32. Brouwer IA, van Dusseldorp M, Thomas CMG, et al. Low-dose folic acid supplementation decreases plasma homocysteine concentrations: a randomized trial. *Indian Heart J* 2000;52:S53-S58.

33. Ubbink J, Vermaak W, van der Merwe A, et al. Vitamin requirements for the treatment of hyperhomocysteinemia in humans. *J Nutr* 1994;124:1927-1933.

34. Wald DS, Bishop L, Wald NJ, et al. Randomized trial of folic acid supplementation and serum homocysteine levels. *Arch Intern Med* 2001;161:695-700.

35. Wilcken DE, Wilcken B, Dudman NP, Tyrrell PA. Homocystinuria – the effects of betaine in the treatment of patients not responsive to pyridoxine. *N Engl J Med* 1983;309:448-453.

36. Lashner BA, Heidenreich PA, Su GL, et al. Effect of folate supplementation on the incidence of dysplasia and cancer in chronic ulcerative colitis. A case-control study. *Gastroenterology* 1989;97:255-259.

37. Lashner BA, Provencher KS, Seidner DL, et al. The effect of folic acid supplementation on the risk for cancer or dysplasia in ulcerative colitis. *Gastroenterology* 1997;112:29-32.

38. Abou-Saleh MT, Coppen A. Serum and red blood cell folate in depression. *Acta Psychiatr Scand* 1989;80:78-82.

39. Alpert JE, Fava M. Nutrition and depression: the role of folate. *Nutr Rev* 1997;55:145-149.

40. Wesson VA, Levitt AJ, Joffe RT. Change in folate status with antidepressant treatment. *Psychiatry Res* 1994;53:313-322.

41. Passeri M, Cucinotta D, Abate G, et al. Oral 5'-methyltetrahydrofolic acid in senile organic mental disorders with depression: results of a double-blind multicenter study. *Aging (Milano)* 1993;5:63-71.

42. Godfrey PS, Toone BK, Carney MW, et al. Enhancement of recovery from psychiatric illness by methylfolate. *Lancet* 1990;336:392-395.

43. Coppen A, Bailey J. Enhancement of the antidepressant action of fluoxetine by folic acid: a randomised, placebo controlled trial. *J Affect Disord* 2000;60:121-130.

44. Coppen A, Chaudhry S, Swade C. Folic acid enhances lithium prophylaxis. *J Affect Disord* 1986;10:9-13.

45. Botez MI, Peyronnard JM, Berube L, Labrecque R. Relapsing neuropathy, cerebral atrophy and folate deficiency. A close association. *Appl Neurophysiol* 1979;42:171-183.

46. Vogel RI, Fink RA, Schneider LC, et al. The effect of folic acid on gingival health. *J Periodontol* 1976;47:667-668.

47. Thomson ME, Pack AR. Effects of extended systemic and topical folate supplementation on gingivitis of pregnancy. *J Clin Periodontol* 1982;9:275-280.

48. Pack AR. Folate mouthwash: effects on established gingivitis in periodontal patients. *J Clin Periodontol* 1984;11:619-628.

49. MRC Vitamin Study Research Group. Prevention of neural tube defects: results of the Medical Research Council Vitamin Study. *Lancet* 1991;338:131-137.

50. Vergel RG, Sanchez LR, Heredero BL, et al. Primary prevention of neural tube defects with folic acid supplementation: Cuban experience. *Prenat Diag* 1990;10:149-152.

51. Milunsky A, Jick H, Jick SS, et al. Multivitamin/folic acid supplementation in early pregnancy reduces the prevalence of neural tube defects. *JAMA* 1989;262:2847-2852.

52. Czeizel AE, Dudas I. Prevention of the first occurrence of neural-tube defects by periconceptional vitamin supplementation. *N Engl J Med* 1992;327:1832-1835.

53. Bower C, Stanley FJ. Dietary folate as a risk factor for neural tube defects: evidence from a case-controlled study in Western Australia. *Med J Aust* 1989;150:613-619.

54. Werler MM, Shapiro S, Mitchell AA. Periconceptional folic acid exposure and risk of occurrent neural tube defects. *JAMA* 1993;269:1257-1261.

55. Shaw GM, Schaffer D, Velie EM, et al. Periconceptional vitamin use, dietary folate, and the occurrence of neural tube defects. *Epidemiology* 1995;6:219-226.

56. Tamura T, Goldenberg R, Freeberg L, et al. Maternal serum folate and zinc concentrations and their relationships to pregnancy outcome. *Am J Clin Nutr* 1992;56:365-370.

57. Scholl TO, Hediger ML, Schall JI, et al. Dietary and serum folate: their influence on the outcome of pregnancy. *Am J Clin Nutr* 1996;63:520-525.

58. Frelut ML, deCoucy GP, Christides JP, et al. Relationship between maternal folate status and foetal hypotrophy in a population with a good socio-economical level. *Int J Vitamin Nutr Res* 1995;65:267-271.

59. Montes LF, Diaz ML, Lajous J, Garcia NJ. Folic acid and vitamin B12 in vitiligo: a nutritional approach. *Cutis* 1992;50:39-42.

60. Juhlin L, Olsson MJ. Improvement of vitiligo after oral treatment with vitamin B12 and folic acid and the importance of sun exposure. *Acta Derm Venereol* 1997;77:460-462.

61. Russell RM, Golner BB, Krasinski SD, et al. Effect of antacid and H2 receptor antagonists on the intestinal absorption of folic acid. *J Lab Clin Med* 1988;112:458-463.

62. Lambie DG, Johnson RH. Drugs and folate metabolism. *Drugs* 1985;30:145-155.

63. Pironi L, Cornia GL, Ursitti MA, et al. Evaluation of oral administration of folic and folinic acid to prevent folate deficiency in patients with inflammatory bowel disease treated with salicylazosulfapyridine. *Int J Clin Pharm Res* 1988;8:143-148.

64. Backman N, Holm AK, Hanstrom L, et al. Folate treatment of diphenylhydantoin-induced gingival hyperplasia. *Scand J Dent Res* 1989;97:222-232.

65. van Ede AE, Laan RF, Rood MJ, et al. Effect of folic or folinic acid supplementation on the toxicity and efficacy of methotrexate in rheumatoid arthritis: a forty-eight week, multicenter, randomized, double-blind, placebo-controlled study. *Arthritis Rheum* 2001;44:1515-1524.

66. Gori T, Burstein JM, Ahmed S, et al. Folic acid prevents nitroglycerin-induced nitric oxide synthase dysfunction and nitrate tolerance: a human in vivo study. *Circulation* 2001;104:1119-1123.

67. Butterworth CE Jr, Tamura T. Folic acid safety and toxicity: a brief review. *Am J Clin Nutr* 1989;50:353-358.

68. Goggin T, Gough H, Bissessar A, et al. A comparative study of the relative effects of anticonvulsant drugs and dietary folate on the red cell folate status of patients with epilepsy. *Q J Med* 1987;65:911-919.

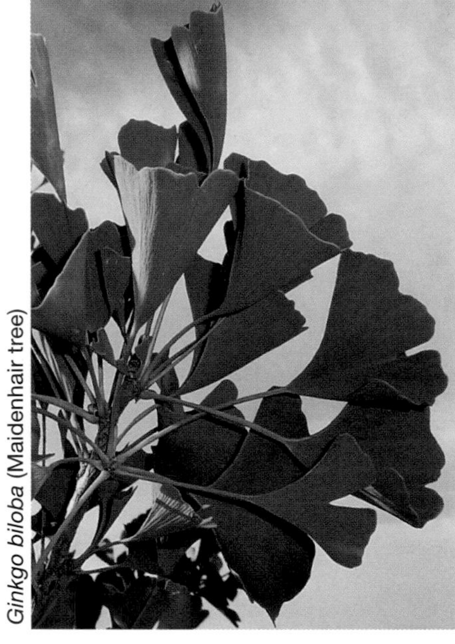
Ginkgo biloba (Maidenhair tree)

Ginkgo biloba

Description

Ginkgo biloba, also known as Maidenhair Tree, is the oldest living tree species, dating back approximately 200 million years. It is extremely resistant to pollution and disease, and is often planted as an ornamental tree. Because of its hardiness, Ginkgo trees can live as long as 1,000 years and grow to a height of 120 feet. Ginkgo seeds and leaves have been used in traditional Chinese medicine for over 5,000 years. In modern botanical medicine, extracts are made from the distinctive, fan-shaped leaves.

Active Constituents

Ginkgo biloba extracts utilized in clinical trials (EGb 761 and LI1370) are standardized in a multi-step procedure designed to concentrate the desired active principals from the plant. These extracts contain approximately 24-percent flavone glycosides (primarily composed of quercetin, kaempferol, and isorhamnetin) and 6-percent terpene lactones (2.8-3.4% ginkgolides A, B, and C, and 2.6-3.2% bilobalide). Other constituents include proanthocyanadins, glucose, rhamnose, organic acids (hydroxykinurenic, kynurenic, protocatechic, vanillic, shikimic), D-glucaric acid and ginkgolic acid, and related alkylphenols.

Mechanisms of Action

Ginkgo biloba extracts exhibit potent antioxidant activity,[1-4] and are capable, *in vitro*, of scavenging various reactive oxygen species,[5,6] and inhibiting or reducing the functional and morphological impairments observed after lipoperoxide release.[7,8] Animal and human studies note that Ginkgo extracts reduce clastogenic (chromosome-breaking) activity in the plasma after radiation exposure.[9] It is also possible that a large part of Ginkgo's anti-ischemic effect involves inhibition of free radical formation.[10]

One of the components of *Ginkgo biloba*, ginkgolide B, is a potent platelet-activating factor antagonist.[11] It is also likely that the flavonoid fraction, containing free radical scavengers, is important in this respect.[12] Extracts from the leaves of *Ginkgo biloba* are reported to be effective at increasing vascular relaxation via a nitric oxide pathway.[12] Ginkgo extracts (specifically the bilobalide component) can suppress hypoxia-induced membrane breakdown

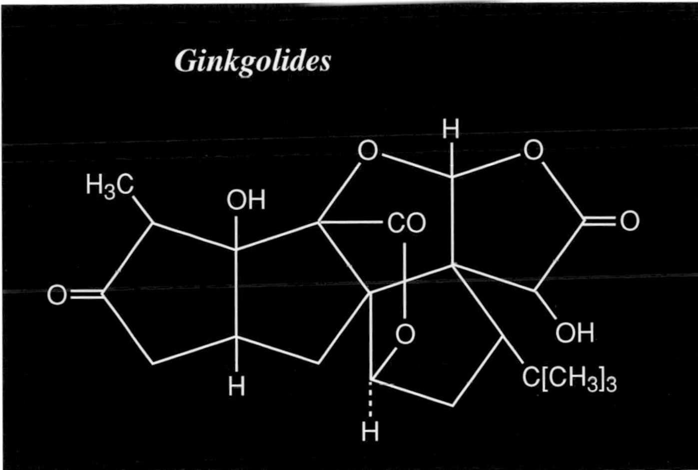

in the brain.[13] Oral administration can prevent the decline in muscarinic (cholinergic) receptor density in the hippocampus of rats,[14] and might inhibit degradation of acetylcholine by acetylcholinesterase.[15]

Experimental evidence indicates Ginkgo's effect on the central adrenergic system might also be involved in its therapeutic actions,[16] since the extract appears to reactivate noradrenergic activity,[17] particularly in aged animals.[18] Extracts of *Ginkgo biloba* leaves produce reversible inhibition of rat brain monoamine oxidase (MAO). Both MAO-A and -B types were inhibited to a similar extent.[19] The anti-stress and neuroprotective effects of *Ginkgo biloba* extract might also be related to its effect on glucocorticoid biosynthesis. Ginkgo extract – and specifically its components ginkgolide A and B – decreases corticosteroid synthesis.[20] *Ex vivo* treatment with Gingko extract has resulted in a 50-percent reduction of ACTH-stimulated corticosterone production by adrenocortical cells.[21]

Clinical Uses

Alzheimer's Disease/Senile Dementia

Research indicates Ginkgo extract may be efficacious in the treatment of a wide array of conditions associated with age-related physical and mental deterioration. Ginkgo extracts appear to be capable of stabilizing and, in some cases, improving cognitive performance and social functioning of patients with dementia.[22-25]

Cardiovascular Disease

Treatment with *Ginkgo biloba* extract lowers fibrinogen levels and decreases plasma viscosity.[26] Ginkgo administration might improve the clinical outcome following cardiopulmonary bypass by limiting oxidative stress.[27,28]

Cerebral Vascular Insufficiency and Impaired Cerebral Performance

Administration of *Ginkgo biloba* extracts has been shown to improve a variety of conditions associated with cerebral insufficiency,[29,30] including visual field disturbances associated with chronic lack of blood flow,[31] oculomotor and complex choice reaction,[32] vigilance and reaction times,[33] depressive mood,[34] memory and mental performance,[35,36] dizziness,[36] circulatory encephalopathy,[37] and decreased blood flow.[38]

Premenstrual Syndrome

Ginkgo extract is effective for the treatment of congestive (particularly breast symptoms) and neuropsychological symptoms of PMS,[39] and the alleviation of idiopathic cyclic edema.[40]

Antidepressant-Induced Sexual Dysfunction

Ginkgo extract has been used successfully to treat impotence and sexual dysfunction secondary to antidepressant medication use.[41] This includes selective serotonin reuptake inhibitors, serotonin and norepinephrine reuptake inhibitors, monoamine oxidase inhibitors, and tricyclics.[42]

Vascular Diseases

Research has shown positive findings in vascular complications such as intermittent claudication,[43-45] peripheral arterial occlusive disease,[46,47] chronic venous insufficiency,[48] and hemorrhoids.[49]

Liver Fibrosis

In a preliminary study, *Ginkgo biloba* was shown to be effective in arresting the development of liver fibrosis associated with chronic hepatitis B.[50]

Macular Degeneration

In spite of the small population sample, a statistically significant improvement in long distance visual acuity was observed in patients with macular degeneration after treatment with *Ginkgo biloba* extract.[51]

Tinnitus

Studies have shown contradictory results in the treatment of tinnitus, which might be due to the diverse etiology of this condition.[52-57]

Vertigo/Equilibrium Disorders

In a placebo-controlled, multi-center study, Ginkgo provided statistically and clinically significant relief of vertigo symptoms, with 47 percent of Ginkgo patients having total symptom relief, compared to 18 percent of those taking placebo.[58] Other studies have confirmed these results.[59-60]

Memory

Studies have shown improvements in attention, speed of memory, and quality of memory in healthy human subjects.[61-64]

Cancer

Phase two clinical trials have shown a good benefit-risk ratio of the combination of 5-fluorouracil and parenteral Ginkgo extract in the treatment of advanced colorectal and pancreatic cancer.[65,66]

Drug-Botanical Interactions

Ginkgo biloba should be avoided in patients with known hypersensitivity to the plant. The use of Ginkgo preparations during pregnancy and lactation has not been studied in humans.

The combined use of aspirin and *Ginkgo biloba* extracts has been reported to cause subdural hematoma in a few individuals.[67] Although the bleeding resolved after discontinuation of *Ginkgo biloba* extract, this combination, or the use of *Ginkgo biloba* extract with other blood thinners should be done with caution.[68,69] At least one case of retinal hemorrhage associated with Ginkgo and aspirin use has been reported.

Side Effects and Toxicity

Side effects are uncommon; however, gastrointestinal disturbances (nausea, vomiting, increased salivation, loss of appetite), headaches, dizziness, tinnitus, and hypersensitivity reactions, such as skin rash, have been reported to occur in some individuals.

The LD_{50} of *Ginkgo biloba* extract is 15.3 g/kg. No mutagenicity has been detected for the extract.

Dosage

The generally recommended daily dosage is 40-80 mg of a standardized extract two to three times daily. Recommended dosage for Alzheimer's disease is at the higher end of this range, or around 240 mg daily. In chronic conditions the extract should be administered for at least 6-8 weeks before evaluation of efficacy.

References

1. Rong Y, Geng Z, Lau BH. *Ginkgo biloba* attenuates oxidative stress in macrophages and endothelial cells. *Free Radic Biol Med* 1996;20:121-127.
2. Yan LJ, Droy-Lefaix MT, Packer L. *Ginkgo biloba* extract (EGb 761) protects human low density lipoproteins against oxidative modification mediated by copper. *Biochem Biophys Res Commun* 1995;212:360-366.
3. Shen JG, Zhou DY. Efficiency of *Ginkgo biloba* extract (EGb 761) in antioxidant protection against myocardial ischemia and reperfusion injury. *Biochem Mol Biol Int* 1995;35:125-134.

4. Marcocci L, Packer L, Droy-Lefaix MT, et al. Antioxidant action of *Ginkgo biloba* extract EGb 761. *Methods Enzymol* 1994;234:462-475.

5. Maitra I, Marcocci L, Droy-Lefaix MT, Packer L. Peroxyl radical scavenging activity of *Ginkgo biloba* extract EGb 761. *Biochem Pharmacol* 1995;49:1649-1655.

6. Hibatallah J, Carduner C, Poelman MC. *In-vivo* and *in-vitro* assessment of the free-radical-scavenger activity of Ginkgo flavone glycosides at high concentration. *J Pharm Pharmacol* 1999;51:1435-1440.

7. Dumont E, D'Arbigny P, Nouvelot A. Protection of polyunsaturated fatty acids against iron-dependent lipid peroxidation by a *Ginkgo biloba* extract (EGb 761). *Methods Find Exp Clin Pharmacol* 1995;17:83-88.

8. Droy-Lefaix MT, Cluzel J, Menerath JM, et al. Antioxidant effect of a *Ginkgo biloba* extract (EGb 761) on the retina. *Int J Tissue React* 1995;17:93-100.

9. Emerit I, Oganesian N, Sarkisian T, et al. Clastogenic factors in the plasma of Chernobyl accident recovery workers: anticlastogenic effect of *Ginkgo biloba* extract. *Radiat Res* 1995;144:198-205.

10. Pietri S, Maurelli E, Drieu K, Culcasi M. Cardioprotective and anti-oxidant effects of the terpenoid constituents of *Ginkgo biloba* extract (EGb 761). *J Mol Cell Cardiol* 1997;29:733-742.

11. Smith PF, Maclennan K, Darlington CL. The neuroprotective properties of the *Ginkgo biloba* leaf: a review of the possible relationship to platelet-activating factor (PAF). *J Ethnopharmacol* 1996;50:131-139.

12. Chen X, Salwinski S, Lee TJ. Extracts of *Ginkgo biloba* and ginsenosides exert cerebral vasorelaxation via a nitric oxide pathway. *Clin Exp Pharmacol Physiol* 1997;24:958-959.

13. Klein J, Chatterjee SS, Loffelholz K. Phospholipid breakdown and choline release under hypoxic conditions: inhibition by bilobalide, a constituent of *Ginkgo biloba*. *Brain Res* 1997;755:347-350.

14. Taylor JE. Neuromediator binding to receptors in the rat brain. The effect of chronic administration of *Ginkgo biloba* extract. *Presse Med* 1986;15:1491-1493. [Article in French]

15. Chopin P, Briley M. Effects of four non-cholinergic cognitive enhancers in comparison with tacrine and galanthamine on scopolamine-induced amnesia in rats. *Psychopharmacology* (Berl) 1992;106:26-30.

16. Brunello N, Racagni G, Clostre F, et al. Effects of an extract of *Ginkgo biloba* on noradrenergic systems of rat cerebral cortex. *Pharmacol Res Commun* 1985;17:1063-1072.

17. Racagni G, Brunello N, Paoletti R. Neuromediator changes during cerebral aging. The effect of *Ginkgo biloba* extract. *Presse Med* 1986;15:1488-1490. [Article in French]

18. Huguet F, Tarrade T. Alpha 2-adrenoceptor changes during cerebral aging. The effect of *Ginkgo biloba* extract. *J Pharm Pharmacol* 1992;44:24-27.

19. White HL, Scates PW, Cooper BR. Extracts of *Ginkgo biloba* leaves inhibit monoamine oxidase. *Life Sci* 1996;58:1315-1321.

20. Amri H, Ogwuegbu SO, Boujrad N, et al. *In vivo* regulation of peripheral-type benzodiazepine receptor and glucocorticoid synthesis by *Ginkgo biloba* extract EGb 761 and isolated ginkgolides. *Endocrinology* 1996;137:5707-5718.

21. Amri H, Drieu K, Papadopoulos V. *Ex vivo* regulation of adrenal cortical cell steroid and protein synthesis, in response to adrenocorticotropic hormone stimulation, by the *Ginkgo biloba* extract EGb 761 and isolated ginkgolide B. *Endocrinology* 1997;138:5415-5426.

22. Le Bars PL, Katz MM, Berman N, et al. A placebo-controlled, double-blind, randomized trial of an extract of *Ginkgo biloba* for dementia. North American EGb Study Group. *JAMA* 1997;278:1327-1332.

23. Kanowski S, Herrmann WM, Stephan K, et al. Proof of efficacy of the *Ginkgo biloba* special extract EGb 761 in outpatients suffering from mild to moderate primary degenerative dementia of the Alzheimer type or multi-infarct dementia. *Pharmacopsychiatry* 1996;29:47-56.

24. Le Bars PL, Kieser M, Itil KZ. A 26-week analysis of a double-blind, placebo-controlled trial of the *Ginkgo biloba* extract EGb 761 in dementia. *Dement Geriatr Cogn Disord* 2000;11:230-237.

25. Maurer K, Ihl R, Dierks T, et al. Clinical efficacy of *Ginkgo biloba* special extract EGb 761 in dementia of the Alzheimer type. *J Psychiatr Res* 1997;31:645-655.

26. Witte S, Anadere I, Walitza E. Improvement of hemorheology with *Ginkgo biloba* extract. Decreasing a cardiovascular risk factor. *Fortschr Med* 1992;110:247-250. [Article in German]

27. Pietri S, Seguin JR, d'Arbigny P, et al. *Ginkgo biloba* extract (EGb 761) pretreatment limits free radical-induced oxidative stress in patients undergoing coronary bypass surgery. *Cardiovasc Drugs Ther* 1997;11:121-131.

28. Liebgott T, Miollan M, Berchadsky Y, et al. Complementary cardioprotective effects of flavonoid metabolites and terpenoid constituents of *Ginkgo biloba* extract (EGb 761) during ischemia and reperfusion. *Basic Res Cardiol* 2000;95:368-377.

29. Kleijnen J, Knipschild P. *Ginkgo biloba* for cerebral insufficiency. *Br J Clin Pharmacol* 1992;34:352-358.

30. Gerhardt G, Rogalla K, Jaeger J. Drug therapy of disorders of cerebral performance. Randomized comparative study of dihydroergotoxine and *Ginkgo biloba* extract. *Fortschr Med* 1990;108:384-388. [Article in German]

31. Raabe A, Raabe M, Ihm P. Therapeutic follow-up using automatic perimetry in chronic cerebroretinal ischemia in elderly patients. Prospective double-blind study with graduated dose *Ginkgo biloba* treatment. *Klin Monatsbl Augenheilkd* 1991;199:432-438. [Article in German]

32. Schaffler K, Reeh PW. Double blind study of the hypoxia protective effect of a standardized *Ginkgo biloba* preparation after repeated administration in healthy subjects. *Arzneimittelforschung* 1985;35:1283-1286. [Article in German]

33. Gessner B, Voelp A, Klasser M. Study of the long-term action of a *Ginkgo biloba* extract on vigilance and mental performance as determined by means of quantitative pharmaco-EEG and psychometric measurements. *Arzneimittelforschung* 1985;35:1459-1465.

34. Eckmann F. Cerebral insufficiency – treatment with *Ginkgo-biloba* extract. Time of onset of effect in a double-blind study with 60 inpatients. *Fortschr Med* 1990;108:557-560. [Article in German]

35. Grassel E. Effect of *Ginkgo-biloba* extract on mental performance. Double-blind study using computerized measurement conditions in patients with cerebral insufficiency. *Fortschr Med* 1992;110:73-76. [Article in German]

36. Hofferberth B. The effect of *Ginkgo biloba* extract on neurophysiological and psychometric measurement results in patients with psychotic organic brain syndrome. A double-blind study against placebo. *Arzneimittelforschung* 1989;39:918-922. [Article in German]

37. Ivaniv OP. The results of using different forms of a *Ginkgo biloba* extract (EGb 761) in the combined treatment of patients with circulatory encephalopathy. *Lik Sprava* 1998:123-128.

38. Koltringer P, Eber O, Klima G, et al. Microcirculation in parenteral *Ginkgo biloba* extract therapy. *Wien Klin Wochenschr* 1989;101:198-200. [Article in German]

39. Tamborini A, Taurelle R. Value of standardized *Ginkgo biloba* extract (EGb 761) in the management of congestive symptoms of premenstrual syndrome. *Rev Fr Gynecol Obstet* 1993;88:447-457. [Article in French]

40. Lagrue G, Behar A, Kazandjian M, Rahbar K. Idiopathic cyclic edema. The role of capillary hyperpermeability and its correction by *Ginkgo biloba* extract. *Presse Med* 1986;15:1550-1553. [Article in French]

41. Sikora R, Sohn M, Deutz FJ, et al. *Ginkgo biloba* extract in the therapy of erectile dysfunction. *J Urol* 1989;141:188. [abstract]

42. Cohen AJ, Bartlik B. *Ginkgo biloba* for antidepressant-induced sexual dysfunction. *J Sex Marital Ther* 1998;24:139-143.

43. Ernst E. *Ginkgo biloba* in treatment of intermittent claudication. A systematic research based on controlled studies in the literature. *Fortschr Med* 1996;114:85-87. [Article in German]

44. Blume J, Kieser M, Holscher U. Placebo-controlled double-blind study of the effectiveness of *Ginkgo biloba* special extract EGb 761 in trained patients with intermittent claudication. *Vasa* 1996;25:265-274. [Article in German]

45. Peters H, Kieser M, Holscher U. Demonstration of the efficacy of *Ginkgo biloba* special extract EGb 761 on intermittent claudication – a placebo-controlled, double-blind multicenter trial. *Vasa* 1998;27:106-110.

46. Schweizer J, Hautmann C. Comparison of two dosages of *Ginkgo biloba* extract EGb 761 in patients with peripheral arterial occlusive disease Fontaine's stage IIb. A randomised, double-blind, multicentric clinical trial. *Arzneimittelforschung* 1999;49:900-904.

47. Li AL, Shi YD, Landsmann B, et al. Hemorheology and walking of peripheral arterial occlusive diseases patients during treatment with *Ginkgo biloba* extract. *Zhongguo Yao Li Xue Bao* 1998;19:417-421.

48. Janssens D, Michiels C, Guillaume G, et al. Increase in circulating endothelial cells in patients with primary chronic venous insufficiency: protective effect of Ginkor Fort in a randomized double-blind, placebo-controlled clinical trial. *J Cardiovasc Pharmacol* 1999;33:7-11.

49. Hep A, Robek O, Skricka T. Treatment of hemorrhoids from the viewpoint of the gastroenterologist. Personal experience with the Ginkor Fort preparation. *Vnitr Lek* 2000;46:282-285. [Article in Czech]

50. Li W, Dai QT, Liu ZE. Preliminary study on early fibrosis of chronic hepatitis B treated with *Ginkgo biloba* Composita. *Chung Kuo Chung Hsi I Chieh Ho Tsa Chih* 1995;15:593-595. [Article in Chinese]

51. Lebuisson DA, Leroy L, Rigal G. Treatment of senile macular degeneration with *Ginkgo biloba* extract. A preliminary double-blind drug vs. placebo study. *Presse Med* 1986;15:1556-1558. [Article in French]

52. Holgers KM, Axelsson A, Pringle I. *Ginkgo biloba* extract for the treatment of tinnitus. *Audiology* 1994;33:85-92.

53. Meyer B. Multicenter randomized double-blind drug vs. placebo study of the treatment of tinnitus with *Ginkgo biloba* extract. *Presse Med* 1986;15:1562-1564. [Article in French]

54. Meyer B. A multicenter study of tinnitus. Epidemiology and therapy. *Ann Otolaryngol Chir Cervicofac* 1986;103:185-188. [Article in French]

55. Jastreboff PJ, Zhou S, Jastreboff MM, et al. Attenuation of salicylate-induced tinnitus by *Ginkgo biloba* extract in rats. *Audiol Neurootol* 1997;2:197-212.

56. Drew S, Davies E. Effectiveness of *Ginkgo biloba* in treating tinnitus: double blind, placebo controlled trial. *Br Med J* 2001;322:72-78.

57. Ernst E, Stevinson C. *Ginkgo biloba* for tinnitus: a review. *Clin Otolaryngol* 1999;24:164-167.

58. Haguenauer JP, Cantenot F, Koskas H, Pierart H. Treatment of equilibrium disorders with *Ginkgo biloba* extract. A multicenter double-blind drug vs. placebo study. *Presse Med* 1986;15:1569-1572. [Article in French]

59. Claussen CF. Diagnostic and practical value of craniocorpography in vertiginous syndromes. *Presse Med* 1986;15:1565-1568. [Article in French]

60. Cesarani A, Meloni F, Alpini D, et al. *Ginkgo biloba* (EGb 761) in the treatment of equilibrium disorders. *Adv Ther* 1998;15:291-304.

61. Stough C, Clarke J, Lloyd J, et al. Neuropsychological changes after 30-day *Ginkgo biloba* administration in healthy participants. *Int J Neuropsychopharmacol* 2001;4:131-134.

62. Wesnes KA, Ward T, McGinty A, et al. The memory enhancing effects of a *Ginkgo biloba/Panax ginseng* combination in healthy middle-aged volunteers. *Psychopharmacology* (Berl) 2000;152:353-361.

63. Kennedy DO, Scholey AB, Wesnes KA. The dose-dependent cognitive effects of acute administration of *Ginkgo biloba* to healthy young volunteers. *Psychopharmacology* (Berl) 2000;151:416-423.

64. Mix JA, Crews WD Jr. An examination of the efficacy of *Ginkgo biloba* extract EGb 761 on the neuropsychologic functioning of cognitively intact older adults. *J Altern Complement Med* 2000;6:219-229.

65. Hauns B, Haring B, Kohler S, et al. Phase II study of combined 5-fluorouracil/ *Ginkgo biloba* extract (GBE 761 ONC) therapy in 5-fluorouracil pretreated patients with advanced colorectal cancer. *Phytother Res* 2001;15:34-38.

66. Hauns B, Haring B, Kohler S, Phase II study with 5-fluorouracil and *Ginkgo biloba extract* (GBE 761 ONC) in patients with pancreatic cancer. *Arzneimittelforschung* 1999;49:1030-1034.

67. Rowin J, Lewis SL. Spontaneous bilateral subdural hematomas associated with chronic *Ginkgo biloba* ingestion. *Neurology* 1996;46:1775-1776.

68. Miller LG. Herbal medicinals: selected clinical considerations focusing on known or potential drug-herb interactions. *Arch Intern Med* 1998;158:2200-2211.

69. Vaes LP, Chyka PA. Interactions of warfarin with garlic, ginger, ginkgo, or ginseng: nature of the evidence. *Ann Pharmacother* 2000;34:1478-1482.

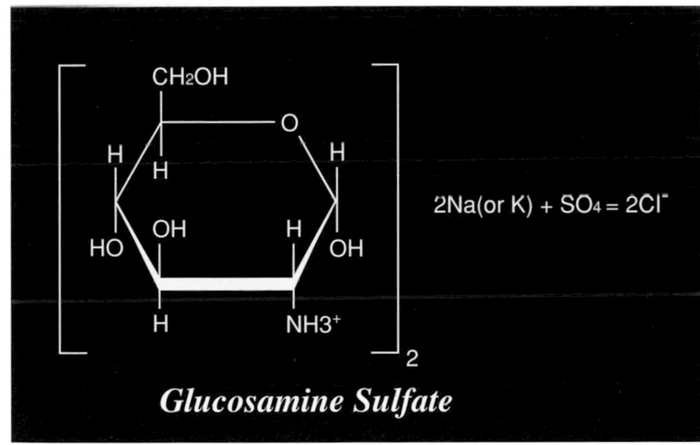

Glucosamine Sulfate

Glucosamine Sulfate

Introduction

Glucosamine sulfate's role in halting or reversing joint degeneration appears to be directly due to its ability to act as an essential substrate for, and to stimulate the biosynthesis of, glycosaminoglycans and the hyaluronic acid backbone needed for the formation of proteoglycans found in the structural matrix of joints. Successful treatment of osteoarthritis must effectively control pain and should slow down or reverse the progression of the degeneration. Biochemical and pharmacological data, combined with animal and human studies, demonstrate that glucosamine sulfate is capable of satisfying both of these criteria.

Glucosamine is the most fundamental building block required for biosynthesis of the classes of compounds including glycolipids, glycoproteins, glycosaminoglycans (formerly called mucopolysaccharides), hyaluronate, and proteoglycans. As a component of these macromolecules, glucosamine has a role in the synthesis of cell membrane lining, collagen, osteoid, and bone matrix. Glucosamine is also required for the formation of lubricants and protective agents such as mucin and mucous secretions.

Pharmacokinetics

In humans, about 90 percent of glucosamine, administered as an oral dose of glucosamine sulfate, is absorbed from the digestive tract.[1] After an oral dose, glucosamine concentrates in the liver, where it is incorporated into plasma proteins, degraded into smaller molecules, or utilized for other biosynthetic processes.[1] Elimination of glucosamine is primarily through the urine, with a small amount of glucosamine or its derivatives eliminated in the feces.[2,3]

Mechanisms of Action

Glucosamine sulfate is capable of stimulating proteoglycan synthesis, inhibiting the degradation of proteoglycans, and stimulating the regeneration of experimentally induced cartilage damage.[4,5] Some experts also believe glucosamine sulfate might promote the incorporation of sulfur into cartilage.[6] Researchers investigated the possibility that the symptomatic improvement seen with glucosamine sulfate use is at least partly mediated by the sulfate component of the molecule, and found serum and synovial fluid sulfate concentrations increased significantly after oral dosing of 1 gram of glucosamine sulfate;

however, oral sodium sulfate had no influence on these levels. The authors theorize, since sulfate is also necessary for glycosaminoglycan synthesis, the sulfate moiety might be responsible for the symptomatic improvement with glucosamine sulfate.[7]

Clinical Indications

Osteoarthritis

The primary therapeutic use of glucosamine sulfate has been in the treatment of degenerative diseases of the joints. Although many of the available studies have compared glucosamine sulfate to placebo, in the trials where glucosamine sulfate has been compared to NSAIDs, long-term reductions in pain are greater in patients receiving glucosamine sulfate.[8-13]

Symptoms such as articular pain, joint tenderness, and swelling often improve following a 6-8 week period of oral administration of glucosamine sulfate.[8-12,14,15] For most individuals, an expectation of a reduction in symptoms of from 50-70 percent is reasonable.[8] Improvements secondary to glucosamine sulfate therapy generally are sustained 6-12 weeks following cessation of the treatment regimen.[14]

For arthritis of the knee, evidence suggests that about 60 percent of patients will have a good to excellent response to this intervention, while an additional 35 percent will have a more moderate benefit. Preliminary evidence suggests patients with arthritis of the shoulder or elbow respond best to glucosamine sulfate (about 75 percent judged as good and only one percent judged as insufficient), while polyarticular arthritis and arthritis of the hip had the poorest response rate (only 43 percent and 49 percent, respectively).[14] Glucosamine sulfate is also used effectively in the treatment of temporomandibular joint osteoarthritis.[16]

Side Effects and Toxicity

No LD_{50} is established for glucosamine sulfate, since even at very high levels (5000 mg/kg oral, 3000 mg/kg IM and 1500 mg/kg IV) there is no mortality in mice or rats.[17] The incidence of mild side effects secondary to oral administration of glucosamine sulfate is reported to be 6-12 percent. The most commonly reported side effects include gastrointestinal disturbances (such as epigastric pain/tenderness, heartburn, diarrhea, nausea, dyspepsia, vomiting, and constipation), drowsiness, headaches, and skin reactions. These complaints are generally mild in character and are reversed when treatment with glucosamine sulfate is discontinued.[12,14]

Glucosamine sulfate has been administered safely to patients with a variety of disease conditions, including circulatory disease, liver disorders, diabetes, lung disorders, and depression, with no observed interference with either the course of the illness or pharmacological treatment for the conditions.[9] However, some concern exists regarding the use of glucosamine sulfate by individuals with type 2 diabetes, since evidence is suggestive of glucosamine sulfate contributing to insulin resistance.[18] Evidence also indicates that individuals with active peptic ulcers and individuals taking diuretics tend to have an increased incidence of side effects from glucosamine sulfate.[14]

Dosage

The advised oral dosage routine for glucosamine sulfate is 500 mg three times daily for a minimum of six weeks. Since obesity has been associated with a below average response to glucosamine sulfate,[14] a higher dose might be required by these individuals.

Warnings and Contraindications

The source of glucosamine sulfate in nutritional supplements is shellfish chitin. Therefore, individuals with a shellfish allergy should avoid glucosamine sulfate supplementation.

References

1. Setnikar I, Palumbo R, Canali S, Zanolo G. Pharmacokinetics of glucosamine in man. *Arzneim Forsch* 1993;43:1109-1113.
2. Setnikar I, Giachetti C, Zanolo G. Pharmacokinetics of glucosamine in the dog and in man. *Arzneim Forsch* 1986;36:729-733.
3. Setnikar I, Giachetti C, Zanolo G. Absorption, distribution, and excretion of radioactivity after a single intravenous or oral administration of [14C] glucosamine to the rat. *Pharmatherapeutica* 1984;3:538-550.
4. Karzel K, Lee KJ. Effect of hexosamine derivatives on mesenchymal metabolic processes of *in vitro* cultured fetal bone explants. *Z Rheumatol* 1982;41:212-218. [Article in German]
5. Setnikar I, Cereda R, Pacini MA, Revel L. Antireactive properties of glucosamine sulfate. *Arzneim Forsch* 1991;41:157-161.
6. Murray MT. Glucosamine sulfate: effective osteoarthritis treatment. *Amer J Nat Med* 1994; Sept:10-14.
7. Hoffer LJ, Kaplan LN, Hamadeh MJ, et al. Sulfate could mediate the therapeutic effect of glucosamine sulfate. *Metabolism* 2001;50:767-770.
8. D'Ambrosio ED, Casa B, Bompani R, et al. Glucosamine sulphate: a controlled clinical investigation in arthrosis. *Pharmatherapeutica* 1981;2:504-508.
9. Crolle G, D'Este E. Glucosamine sulphate for the management of arthrosis: a controlled clinical evaluation. *Curr Med Res Opin* 1980;7:104-109.
10. Vaz AL. Double-blind clinical evaluation of the relative efficacy of ibuprofen and glucosamine sulphate in the management of osteoarthrosis of the knee in out-patients. *Curr Med Res Opin* 1982;8:145-149.
11. Rovati LC. Clinical research in osteoarthritis: design and results of short-term and long-term trials with disease modifying drugs. *Int J Tissue React* 1992;14:243-251.
12. Qiu GX, Gao SN, Giacovelli G, et al. Efficacy and safety of glucosamine sulfate versus ibuprofen in patients with knee osteoarthritis. *Arzneim Forsch* 1998;48:469-474.
13. Reginster JY, Leroisy, Rovati LC, et al. Long-term effects of glucosamine sulphate on osteoarthritis progression: a randomised, placebo-controlled clinical trial. *Lancet* 2001;357:251-256.
14. Tapadinhas MJ, Rivera IC, Bignamini AA. Oral glucosamine sulfate in the management of arthrosis: report on a multi-centre open investigation in Portugal. *Pharmatherapeutica* 1982;3:157-168.
15. Pujalte JM, Llavore EP, Ylescupidez FR. Double-blind clinical evaluation of oral glucosamine sulphate in the basic treatment of osteoarthrosis. *Curr Med Res Opin* 1980;2:110-114.
16. Thie NM, Prasad NG, Major PW. Evaluation of glucosamine sulfate compared to ibuprofen for the treatment of temporomandibular joint osteoarthritis: a randomized double blind controlled 3 month clinical trial. *J Rheumatol* 2001;28:1347-1355.
17. Senin P, Makovec F, Rovati L. Stable compounds of glucosamine sulphate. *United States Patent* 4,642,340 1987.
18. Virkamaki A, Daniels MC, Hamalainen S, et al. Activation of the hexosamine pathway by glucosamine *in vivo* induces insulin resistance in multiple insulin sensitive tissues. *Endocrinology* 1997;138:2501-2507.

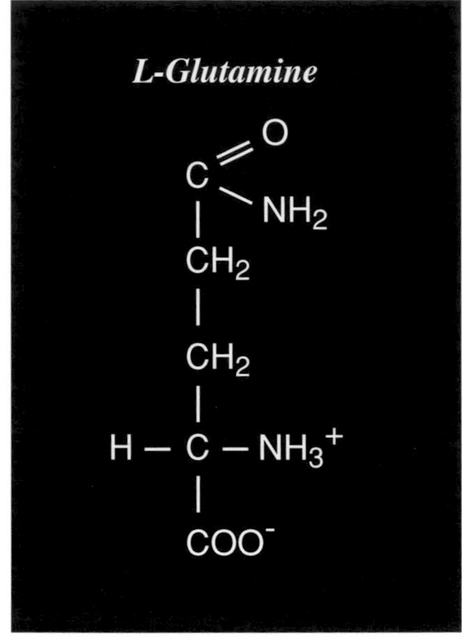

L-Glutamine

Introduction

L-glutamine is the most prevalent amino acid in the bloodstream and because human cells readily synthesize it, is usually considered a non-essential amino acid. It is found in high concentration in skeletal muscle, lung, liver, brain, and stomach tissue. Skeletal muscle contains the greatest intracellular concentration of glutamine, comprising up to 60 percent of total body glutamine stores, and is considered the primary storage depot and exporter of glutamine to other tissues. Under certain pathological circumstances the body's tissues need more glutamine than the amount supplied by diet and biosynthesis. During catabolic stress intracellular glutamine levels can drop more than 50 percent, and it is under these circumstances that supplemental glutamine becomes necessary.[1] In times of metabolic stress, glutamine is released into circulation, where it is transported to the tissue in need. Intracellular skeletal muscle glutamine concentration is affected by various insults, including injury, sepsis, prolonged stress, starvation, and the use of glucocorticoids. Therefore, glutamine has been re-classified as a conditionally essential amino acid. Research demonstrates glutamine supplementation may be beneficial when added to total parenteral nutrition (TPN) for surgery, trauma, and cancer patients. In addition, evidence suggests it may provide benefit for certain gastrointestinal conditions, wound healing, critically ill neonates, HIV/AIDS patients, immune enhancement in endurance athletes, and prevention of complications associated with chemotherapy, radiation, and bone marrow transplant.[1,2]

Biochemistry

L-glutamine accounts for 30-35 percent of the amino acid nitrogen in the plasma. It contains two ammonia groups, one from its precursor, glutamate, and the other from free ammonia in the bloodstream. One of glutamine's roles is to protect the body from high levels of ammonia by acting as a "nitrogen shuttle." Thus, glutamine can act as a buffer, accepting, then releasing excess ammonia when needed to form other amino acids, amino sugars, nucleotides, and urea. This capacity to accept and donate nitrogen makes glutamine the major vehicle for nitrogen transfer among tissues. Glutamine is one of the three amino acids involved in glutathione synthesis. Glutathione, an important intracellular antioxidant and hepatic detoxifier, is comprised of glutamic acid, cysteine, and glycine.[1,2]

Clinical Indications

Gastrointestinal Disease

The gastrointestinal tract is by far the greatest user of glutamine in the body, as enterocytes in the intestinal epithelium use glutamine as their principal metabolic fuel. Most of the research on glutamine and its connection to intestinal permeability has been conducted in conjunction with the use of TPN. Commercially available TPN solutions do not contain glutamine, which can result in atrophy of the mucosa and villi of the small intestine. Addition of glutamine to the TPN solution reverses mucosal atrophy associated with various gastrointestinal conditions.[3] Research has demonstrated glutamine-enriched TPN decreases villous atrophy, increases jejunal weight, and decreases intestinal permeability.[4,5] Trauma, infection, starvation, chemotherapy, and other stressors are all associated with a derangement of normal intestinal permeability. One potential consequence of increased intestinal permeability is microbial translocation. Bacteria, fungi, and their toxins may translocate across the mucosal barrier into the bloodstream and cause sepsis.[6] In numerous animal studies of experimentally induced intestinal hyperpermeability, the addition of glutamine or glutamine dipeptides (stable dipeptides of glutamine with alanine or glycine) to TPN improved gut barrier function, as well as immune activity in the gut.[7] Conditions characterized by increased intestinal permeability that might benefit from glutamine supplementation include food allergies and associated conditions, Crohn's disease, ulcerative colitis, and irritable bowel syndrome. A clinical study of ulcerative colitis patients demonstrated that feeding 30 g daily of glutamine-rich germinated barley foodstuff (GBF) for four weeks resulted in significant clinical and endoscopic improvement, independent of disease state. Disease exacerbation returned when GBF treatment was discontinued.[8] It has also been suggested that cabbage juice consumption may provide benefit to patients with gastric ulcers and gastritis, by virtue of its high glutamine content.

Wound Healing

The gastrointestinal tract has a large number of immune cells along its length - fibroblasts, lymphocytes, and macrophages. The ability of glutamine to nourish these immune cells may account for its positive impact on the gastrointestinal tract and immunity. Healing of surgical wounds, trauma injuries, and burns is accomplished in part by the actions of these immune cells. Their proper functioning is dependent on glutamine as a metabolic fuel for growth and proliferation. Therefore, depletion of intracellular glutamine can slow growth of these cells, and ultimately prolong healing.[1] A small clinical study conducted in Poland demonstrated glutamine-supplemented TPN rapidly improved a number of immune parameters in malnourished surgical patients with sepsis.[9] Additional clinical trials also suggest glutamine supplementation, as well as arginine and omega-3 fatty acids, may promote restoration of normal tissue function and intestinal permeability in post-operative patients.[10,11]

Infection and Immunity

Decreases in glutamine concentrations may result in an increased rate of infection in certain stressed patient populations. Critically ill newborn infants frequently display protein-calorie malnutrition due to the demands of sepsis and respiratory failure. A study of nine critically ill infants given a glutamine-supplemented enteral formula (0.3 g/kg glutamine daily for five days) demonstrated a significant decrease in infection and septic complications (20% in the glutamine group versus 75% in the control group).[12]

Endurance athletes also have decreased plasma glutamine concentrations after prolonged, strenuous exercise. This post-exercise glutamine depletion and associated immunosuppression may render the athlete more susceptible to infection. A group of 151 elite runners and rowers were given two drinks containing either glutamine or placebo immediately after, and two hours post-exercise, and were then asked to complete questionnaires regarding the incidence of infection during the seven days post-exercise. The percentage of patients infection-free during the seven days was significantly higher in the glutamine group (81%) than in the placebo group (49%).[13]

HIV/AIDS

HIV infection appears to induce glutamine deficiency, resulting in muscle protein wasting, particularly in the AIDS stage of the infection.[14] Approximately 20 percent of AIDS patients also have abnormal intestinal permeability.[15] Clinical studies have demonstrated glutamine supplementation has significant benefit in these patients. A double-blind, placebo-controlled study was conducted with 68 HIV-infected patients having documented weight loss who were given a nutrient mixture containing 14 g L-glutamine twice daily for eight weeks. Body weight, lean body mass, and fat mass were measured throughout the eight-week period. At eight weeks, patients taking the glutamine mixture had gained 3.0 ± 0.5 kg of body weight compared to 0.37 ± 0.84 kg in the placebo group. The body weight gain in the glutamine group was primarily lean body mass while the placebo group lost lean body mass. An additional benefit in the supplemented group was improved immune status as evidenced by increased CD3 and CD8 cell counts, and decreased HIV viral load.[16] In another double-blind, placebo controlled study of AIDS patients with abnormal intestinal permeability, glutamine supplementation (8 g daily for 28 days) resulted in stabilization of intestinal permeability and enhanced intestinal absorption.[15]

Cancer and Bone Marrow Transplantation

Like enterocytes, rapidly growing tumors have high glutaminase activity, using glutamine as their main fuel source.[17] Consequently, glutamine supplementation has been controversial in cancer patients. *In vitro* research has found glutamine added to tumor cell cultures increased cellular growth.[18,19] On the other hand, *in vivo* animal studies have not found glutamine increases tumor growth. In fact, one animal study demonstrated that glutamine supplementation actually reduced tumor growth by 40 percent and stimulated natural killer cell activity.[20]

Research has also suggested rapidly growing tumors can become "glutamine traps" and deplete muscle glutamine and glutathione,[17] although a clinical study of 32 colon cancer patients demonstrated colon tumors did not extract or "trap" more glutamine than intestinal tissue without tumor.[21]

Fluoruoracil/folinic acid chemotherapy for colorectal cancer often causes diarrhea. In a double-blind, placebo-controlled, randomized trial, glutamine (18 g daily) was given to 70 colorectal cancer patients five days prior to their first cycle of chemotherapy. Treatment continued for a total of 15 days and intestinal permeability and absorption were measured. When compared to baseline values, glutamine reduced changes in permeability and absorption induced by chemotherapy and may be of benefit in preventing chemotherapy-induced diarrhea.[22] A similar effect was seen in esophageal cancer patients undergoing radiation and chemotherapy, but the daily glutamine dose was higher, at 30 grams daily.[23]

Studies of glutamine's benefit in parenteral nutrition during and after bone marrow transplant (BMT) have yielded mixed results. Three earlier studies demonstrated glutamine supplementation during BMT was of some benefit in minimizing side effects of high-dose cytotoxic chemotherapy, namely oropharyngeal mucositis, decreased lymphocyte counts, and hepatic veno-occlusive disease.[24-26] More recent studies, however, demonstrated glutamine-enriched TPN solutions had only limited benefit in BMT patients, in regard to number of days on TPN, length of hospital stay, degree of mucositis, white blood cell counts, infection, and diarrhea.[27,28]

Side Effects and Toxicity

Numerous clinical trials in humans demonstrate that even at high doses, glutamine administration is without side effects and is well tolerated, even during times of physiologic stress.

Dosage

Glutamine is administered orally in bulk powder or in encapsulated form. Dosages vary greatly depending on the clinical situation, but are in the range of 2-4 grams daily in divided doses for general wound healing and intestinal support. For critically ill adults, cancer, and HIV patients, the dosage is much higher, ranging from 10-40 grams per day in divided doses. For these patients, the bulk powder form of glutamine eases administration of large doses.

References

1. Souba WW. *Glutamine Physiology, Biochemistry, and Nutrition in Critical Illness.* Austin, TX: R.G. Landes Co.; 1992.
2. Askanazi J, Carpenter YA, Michelsen CB, et al. Muscle and plasma amino acids following injury: Influence of intercurrent infection. *Ann Surg* 1980;192:78-85.
3. O'Dwyer ST, Smith RJ, Hwang TL, Wilmore DW. Maintenance of small bowel mucosa with glutamine-enriched parenteral nutrition. *J Parent Enteral Nutr* 1989;13:579-585.
4. Hwang TL, O'Dwyer ST, Smith RJ, et al. Preservation of small bowel mucosa using glutamine-enriched parenteral nutrition. *Surg Forum* 1987;38:56.
5. Li J, Langkamp-Henken B, Suzuki K, Stahlgren LH. Glutamine prevents parenteral nutrition-induced increases in intestinal permeability. *J Parent Enteral Nutr* 1994;18:303-307.
6. Barber AE, Jones WG, Minei JP, et al. Glutamine or fiber supplementation of a defined formula diet. Impact on bacterial translocation, tissue composition, and response to endotoxin. *J Parent Enteral Nutr* 1990;14:335-343.
7. Khan J, Iiboshi Y, Cui L, et al. Alanyl-glutamine-supplemented parenteral nutrition increased luminal mucus gel and decreased permeability in the rat small intestine. *J Parent Enteral Nutr* 1999;23:24-31.
8. Kanuchi O, Iwanaga T, Mitsuyama K. Germinated barley foodstuff feeding. A novel neutraceutical therapeutic strategy for ulcerative colitis. *Digestion* 2001;63:60-67.
9. Slotwinski R, Pertkiewicz M, Lech G, Szczygiel B. Cellular immunity changes after total parenteral nutrition enriched with glutamine in patients with sepsis and malnutrition. *Pol Merkuriusz Lek* 2000;8:405-408. [Article in Polish]
10. O'Flaherty L, Bouchier-Hayes DJ. Immunonutrition and surgical practice. *Proc Nutr Soc* 1999;58:831-837.
11. Jian ZM, Cao JD, Zhu XG, et al. The impact of alanyl-glutamine on clinical safety, nitrogen balance, intestinal permeability, and clinical outcome in postoperative patients; a randomized, double-blind, controlled study of 120 patients. *J Parenter Enteral Nutr* 1999;23:S62-S66.
12. Barbosa E, Moreira EA, Goes JE, Faintuch J. Pilot study with a glutamine-supplemented enteral formula in critically ill infants. *Rev Hosp Clin Fac Med Sao Paulo* 1999;54:21-24.
13. Castell LM, Poortmans JR, Newsholme EA. Does glutamine have a role in reducing infections in athletes? *Eur J Appl Physiol Occup Physiol* 1996;73:488-490.
14. Shabert JK, Wilmore DW. Glutamine deficiency as a cause of human immunodeficiency virus wasting. *Med Hypotheses* 1996;46:252-256.
15. Noyer CM, Simon D, Borczuk A, et al. A double-blind placebo-controlled pilot study of glutamine therapy for abnormal intestinal permeability in patients with AIDS. *Am J Gastroenterol* 1998;93:972-975.
16. Clark RH, Feleke G, Din M, et al. Nutritional treatment for acquired immunodeficiency virus-associated wasting using beta-hydroxy beta-methylbutyrate, glutamine, and arginine: a randomized, double-blind, placebo-controlled study. *J Parenter Enteral Nutr* 2000;24:133-139.
17. Klimberg VS, McClellan JL. Glutamine, cancer, and its therapy. *Am J Surg* 1996;172:418-424.
18. Ollenschlager G, Simmel A, Roth E. Availability of glutamine from peptides and acetylglutamine for human tumor-cell cultures. *Metabolism* 1989;38:S40-S42.
19. Moyer MP, Armstrong A, Aust JB, et al. Effects of gastrin, glutamine, and somatostatin on the *in vitro* growth of normal and malignant human gastric mucosal cells. *Arch Surg* 1986;121:285-288.
20. Fahr MJ, Kornbluth J, Blossom S, et al. Harry M. Vars Research Award. Glutamine enhances immunoregulation of tumor growth. *J Parenter Enteral Nutr* 1994;18:471-476.
21. van der Hulst RR, von Meyenfeldt MF, Deutz NE, Soeters PB. Glutamine extraction by the gut is reduced in patients with depleted gastrointestinal cancer. *Ann Surg* 1997;225:112-121.

22. Daniele B, Perrone F, Gallo C, et al. Oral glutamine in the prevention of fluorouracil induced intestinal toxicity: a double blind, placebo controlled, randomised trial. *Gut* 2001;48:28-33.
23. Yoshida S, Matsui M, Shirouzu Y, et al. Effects of glutamine supplements and radio-chemotherapy on systemic immune and gut barrier function in patients with advanced esophageal cancer. *Ann Surg* 1998;227:485-491.
24. Anderson PM, Ramsay NK, Shu XO, et al. Effect of low-dose oral glutamine on painful stomatitis during bone marrow transplantation. *Bone Marrow Transplant* 1998;22:339-344.
25. Brown SA, Goringe A, Fegan C, et al. Parenteral glutamine protects hepatic function during bone marrow transplantation. *Bone Marrow Transplant* 1998;22:281-284.
26. Ziegler TR, Bye RK, Persinger RL. Effects of glutamine supplementation on circulating lymphocytes after bone marrow transplantation: a pilot study. *Am J Med Sci* 1998;315:4-10.
27. Coghlin Dickson TM, Wong RM, Offrin RS, et al. Effect of oral glutamine supplementation during bone marrow transplantation. *J Parenter Enteral Nutr* 2000;24:61-66.
28. Schloerb PR, Skikne BS. Oral and parenteral glutamine in bone marrow transplantation: a randomized, double-blind study. *J Parenteral Enteral Nutr* 1999;23:117-122.

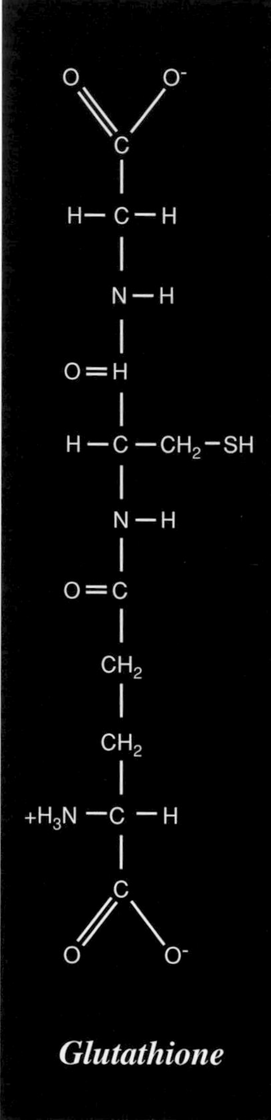

Glutathione

Glutathione

Introduction

Reduced glutathione, most commonly called glutathione or GSH, is a relatively small molecule ubiquitous in living systems.[1-3] Occurring naturally in all human cells, GSH is a water-phase orthomolecule. Its intracellular depletion ultimately results in cell death and its clinical relevance has been researched for decades.[4]

GSH is the smallest intracellular thiol (–SH) molecule. Its high electron-donating capacity (high negative redox potential) combined with high intracellular concentration (millimolar levels) generate great reducing power.[2] This characteristic underlies its potent antioxidant action and enzyme cofactor properties, and supports a complex thiol-exchange system, which hierarchically regulates cell activity.

GSH levels in human tissues normally range from 0.1 to 10 millimolar (mM), most concentrated in the liver (up to 10 mM) and in the spleen, kidney, lens, erythrocytes, and leukocytes.[5] Plasma concentration is in the micromolar range (approx. 4.5 µM).[6] Oxidative stressors that can deplete GSH include ultraviolet and other radiation;[7] viral infections;[2,8] environmental toxins, household chemicals, and heavy metals;[2] surgery, inflammation, burns, septic shock;[9,10] and dietary deficiencies of GSH precursors and enzyme cofactors.[11]

Biochemistry and Pharmacokinetics

Reduced glutathione (GSH) is a linear tripeptide of L-glutamine, L-cysteine, and glycine. Technically N-L-gamma-glutamyl-cysteinyl glycine or L-glutathione, the molecule has a sulfhydryl (–SH) group on the cysteinyl portion, which accounts for its strong electron-donating character. As electrons are lost the molecule becomes oxidized, and two such molecules become linked (dimerized) by a disulfide bridge to form glutathione disulfide or oxidized glutathione (GSSG). This linkage is reversible upon re-reduction. GSH is under tight homeostatic control both intracellularly and extracellularly.[2] A dynamic balance is maintained between GSH synthesis, its recycling from GSSG/oxidized glutathione, and its utilization.

GSH synthesis involves two closely linked, enzymatically-controlled reactions that utilize ATP.[12-14] First cysteine and glutamate are combined, by gamma-glutamyl cysteinyl synthetase. Second, GSH synthetase combines gamma-glutamylcysteine with glycine to generate GSH. As GSH levels rise, they self-limit further GSH synthesis; otherwise, cysteine availability is usually rate limiting. Fasting,[11] protein-energy malnutrition, or other dietary amino acid deficiencies[15] limit GSH synthesis.

GSH recycling is catalyzed by glutathione disulfide reductase, which uses reducing equivalents from NADPH to reconvert GSSG to 2GSH. The reducing power of ascorbate helps conserve systemic GSH.[16]

GSH is used as a cofactor by (1) multiple peroxidase enzymes, to detoxify peroxides generated from oxygen radical attack on biological molecules; (2) transhydrogenases, to reduce oxidized centers on DNA, proteins, and other biomolecules; and (3) glutathione S-transferases (GST) to conjugate GSH with endogenous substances (e.g., estrogens) and to exogenous electrophiles (e.g., arene oxides, unsaturated carbonyls, organic halides), and diverse xenobiotics. GST underactivity may increase risk for disease[17] but paradoxically, some GSH conjugates can also be toxic.[18,19]

Direct attack by free radical and other oxidative agents can also deplete GSH. The homeostatic glutathione redox cycle attempts to keep GSH repleted as it is being consumed.[20] Amounts available from foods are limited (less than 150 mg/day),[5] and oxidative depletion can outpace synthesis.

The liver is the largest GSH reservoir. The parenchymal cells synthesize GSH for P450 conjugation and numerous other metabolic requirements, then export GSH as a systemic source of –SH/reducing power.[12] GSH is carried in the bile to the intestinal luminal compartment. Epithelial tissues of the kidney tubules, intestinal lining, and lung, have substantial P450 activity and modest capacity to export GSH.[13]

GSH equivalents circulate in the blood predominantly as cystine, the oxidized and more stable form of cysteine. Cells import cystine from the blood, reconvert it to cysteine (likely using ascorbate as cofactor),[16] and from it synthesize GSH. Conversely, inside the cell GSH helps re-reduce oxidized forms of other antioxidants such as ascorbate and alpha-tocopherol.[16]

Mechanisms of Action

GSH is an extremely important cell protectant. It directly quenches reactive hydroxyl free radicals, other oxygen-centered free radicals, and radical centers on DNA and other biomolecules.[2] GSH is a primary protectant of skin, lens, cornea, and retina against radiation damage, and the biochemical foundation of P450 detoxication in the liver, kidneys, lungs, intestinal epithelia, and other organs.

GSH is the essential cofactor for many enzymes that require thiol-reducing equivalents, and helps keep redox-sensitive active sites on enzymes in the necessary reduced state.[21] Higher-order thiol cell systems – the metallothioneins, thioredoxins, and other redox regulator proteins – are ultimately regulated by GSH levels and the GSH/GSSG redox ratio. GSH/GSSG balance is crucial to homeostasis, stabilizing the cellular biomolecular spectrum, and facilitating cellular performance and survival.[2,21]

GSH and its metabolites also interface with energetics and neurotransmitter syntheses, through several prominent metabolic pathways.[20] GSH availability down-regulates the pro-inflammatory potential of leukotrienes and other eicosanoids. Recently discovered S-nitroso metabolites, generated *in vivo* from GSH and NO (nitric oxide) further diversify GSH's impact on metabolism.

Clinical Indications

Glutathione status is a highly sensitive indicator of cell functionality and viability. As intracellular GSH becomes reduced, the cell's functionality is progressively reduced until it dies. In humans, GSH depletion is linked to a number of disease states.[2,3,22]

Inherited Deficiencies

Individuals with inherited deficiencies of the GSH-synthesizing enzymes exhibit limited or generalized GSH deficiency,[3,14,22] with hemolytic anemia, spinocerebellar degeneration, peripheral neuropathy, myopathy, and aminoaciduria, and often develop severe neurological complications in the fourth decade of life. These conditions are not necessarily lethal because of their incomplete penetrance; in some tissues GSH can attain 50 percent of normal. In addition, some GSH is obtained from the diet. Low erythrocyte GSH also manifests in hereditary nonspherocytic lymphocytic leukemia, and glucose-6-phosphate dehydrogenase (G6PD) deficiency.

HIV Infection/Immunity

Immune cell functionality and proliferation rely on adequate intracellular GSH,[2,8] and healthy humans with low lymphocyte GSH can have low CD4 counts. HIV infection and sequelae feature systemic GSH depletion.[12] Oxidative stress is elevated at all stages of HIV disease; HIV infection lowers GSH in the plasma, erythrocytes, T-cells and other lymphocytes, and monocytes.[23] Children with HIV also demonstrate low plasma GSH.[8,22] The cachexia and wasting of AIDS may be amenable to GSH repletion.[12] HIV depletion of lung epithelial lining fluid (ELF) glutathione may predispose to opportunistic infections, and the ELF may be repleted using aerosolized GSH.[12]

Liver Cirrhosis, Hepatitis

Plasma and erythrocyte GSH can be low in patients with cirrhosis[6,24] or result from acute or chronic alcohol intake.[22] In nonalcoholic liver disease, liver GSH can be abnormally low and GSSG high.[25] Acetaminophen and other pharmaceutical or environmental xenobiotics can deplete liver GSH. Viral hepatitis can deplete GSH, and in hepatitis C patients monocyte GSH can be depleted.[26]

Pulmonary Disease

GSH deficiency has been linked to various pulmonary diseases,[3,12,22] including chronic obstructive pulmonary disease (COPD), acute respiratory distress syndrome (ARDS), neonatal lung damage, and asthma. The lung is particularly vulnerable to oxidative attack from inhalation of pure oxygen, airborne toxins, and oxygen radical release by lung phagocytes. GSH in lung ELF may be the first line of defense. The GSH content of ELF was found abnormally low in idiopathic pulmonary fibrosis, ARDS, and HIV-positive patients.[23] ARDS patients with sepsis had low GSH and high GSSG in their ELF.[12] GSH repletion can accelerate ARDS patient release from intensive care.[27]

GSH in the ELF can be lifesaving for premature infants. Pulmonary GSH levels have been found to be low in premature infants,[12] and in perinatal hypoxia cases umbilical blood GSH has also been found to be low.[3] Newborns with low GSH in the ELF may be at higher risk of chronic lung disease.[12]

Crohn's Disease, Gastrointestinal Inflammation

Gastric mucosa of aged subjects can have low GSH,[24] as can patients with gastritis and/or duodenal ulcer linked to *Helicobacter pylori* infection.[22] In Crohn's disease cases the affected ileal zones were found to have low GSH and high GSSG, and GSH enzymes were altered.[28]

Circulation

Acute myocardial infarction patients[29] and men with familial coronary artery disease[30] exhibit lowered GSH. Glutathione given i.v. prior to cardiopulmonary bypass surgery favorably influenced postoperative renal function while improving systemic arterial function.[31]

Infusion of GSH into patients with atherosclerosis enhanced microvascular vasodilation in response to acetylcholine, especially in subjects with baseline abnormal vessel wall reactivity.[30] Similar benefits were reported for the epicardial coronary artery system.[32] S-nitrosoglutathione also has platelet anti-aggregation activity in humans, as reviewed in Prasad et al.[30] The mechanism of vasodilation is suspected to be via glutathione's enhancement of nitric oxide.

Metal Storage/Wilson's Disease

In several copper-overloaded (Wilson's Disease) patients, hepatic GSH was markedly lowered.[2] This preliminary finding correlates with an impressive body of animal data.

Pancreatitis

Plasma GSH was significantly lowered in chronic pancreatitis linked to alcohol intake,[33] and patients with acute pancreatitis responded well to glutathione repletion.[2]

Diabetes

Subjects with impaired glucose tolerance, including early hyperglycemics, had reduced blood GSH.[34] In diabetics, the erythrocytes and platelets can be low in GSH.[22,35] Mild to moderate exercise can help normalize GSH status in diabetics,[22] although strenuous exercise can deplete GSH.[36,37]

Neurodegenerative Diseases

A variety of neurodegenerative diseases manifest abnormally low GSH.[2,3,22] In Alzheimer's a decrease in lymphoblast GSH has been reported. In Parkinson's disease the substantia nigra becomes greatly depleted of GSH.

The threshold of GSH depletion, below which the cell will usually die, is 70-80 percent.[2,22] The mitochondria, with their high oxygen radical flux, are particularly vulnerable.[38] Mitochondrial failure has been specifically implicated in retinal degeneration[7] and Parkinson's disease.[39]

Aging

The aging process is associated with deterioration of GSH homeostasis. Plasma GSH trends lower while GSSG becomes more elevated.[7] Limited data suggests higher GSH levels correlate with better health, regardless of age, and that subjects with chronic disease have poorer GSH status than those free of disease.[12] Exercise training can strengthen GSH homeostasis.[37] With progressively more disease states manifesting GSH deficiency, repletion is a viable preventive, therapeutic, and anti-aging strategy.

Glutathione Repletion Strategies

Oral/I.V. Glutathione

Tradition holds that GSH is not systemically bioavailable when given by mouth.[40] However, copious data confirm it is efficiently absorbed across the intestinal epithelium, by a specific uptake system.[41,42] Catabolism of newly-absorbed GSH after it reaches the portal blood intact but prior to reaching the liver accounts for the paradoxical findings.[43] Such breakdown of circulating GSH does not rule out its oral use for GI conditions such as Crohn's Disease.[28]

Results from two controlled trials suggest oral GSH had no significant benefit, but do not rule out benefit from high-dose GSH to depleted subjects.[4,40] In one trial, the plasma concentration was high-normal at baseline. In the second, the dose administered (to cirrhosis patients), at 300 mg/day for 28 days, may have been insufficient to replete liver GSH in the context of severe impairment of biosynthesis.[4]

Perlmutter reported case histories indicating success with GSH repletion in various neurodegenerative diseases.[44] He reported marked benefit from its intravenous administration in Parkinson's, and successful oral application of orthomolecular GSH precursors to cases of Alzheimer's, stroke, multiple sclerosis, amyotrophic lateral sclerosis, and post-polio syndrome.

N-acetylcysteine

Cysteine availability most often limits GSH biosynthesis *in vivo*. One orally bioavailable cysteine source is N-acetylcysteine (NAC). NAC is a potent antioxidant with antimutagenic and anticarcinogenic properties, and an established antidote for acetaminophen overdose known to deplete liver GSH. Oral dosing with NAC supplants oral L-cysteine, which is highly unstable and potentially toxic.[45]

Following its intestinal absorption, NAC is converted to circulating cysteine and can effectively replenish GSH in depleted patients.[46] In HIV/AIDS, plasma GSH and cysteine levels are often low. Two clinical trials, one of them double-blind, reported NAC had clinical benefit.[3] Administered intravenously or as an infusion over 15-30 minutes, it can replete glutathione in the ELF and improve lung function in patients with septic shock.[10] In one trial on pulmonary disease, oral NAC at 1800 mg/day failed to increase GSH.[47]

Alpha-Lipoic Acid

The antioxidant alpha-lipoic acid (ALA) is another effective GSH repleter. Orally, it raises GSH levels in HIV patients,[48] and is extremely safe and well tolerated.[49] ALA is a broad-spectrum, fat- and water-phase antioxidant with potent electron-donating capacity, and has added biochemical versatility as a Krebs cycle cofactor and transition metal chelator. It is superior to NAC in being recyclable *in vivo* from its oxidized form.

Methionine, Ascorbic Acid, Taurine

Oral L-methionine is a cysteine precursor but can cause nausea and vomiting, whereas its activated counterpart S-adenosylmethione (SAMe) is well tolerated. When given i.v. in high doses to cirrhotic patients, SAMe repleted erythrocyte GSH.[13] Ascorbate conserves intracellular glutathione and probably is a redox GSH cofactor.[16] Taurine is a sulfur amino acid which, given orally, can raise the platelet aggregation threshold and increase platelet GSH in healthy males.[2]

Other Methods of Glutathione Repletion

One synthetic cysteine delivery agent is L-2-oxothiazolidine-4-carboxylate (OTC, Procysteine), which can be enzymatically converted to cysteine within liver cells. Oral OTC is converted to GSH in humans.[12] Given intravenously to HIV patients, it increased blood GSH levels after six weeks of treatment.[50] In patients with coronary artery disease, oral OTC markedly improved arterial flow-mediated dilation.[51]

Glutathione esters have been heavily researched as potential oral delivery compounds but their long-term safety is in question. Their reported toxicity is perhaps attributable to metal impurities.[3]

Side Effects and Toxicity

GSH and other thiols tend to be sensitive to redox-active minerals, and care should be taken to omit these from therapeutic preparations.

Warnings and Contraindications

GSH use in cancer must be approached with caution, since some tumors may utilize it intracellularly to resist chemotherapy drugs.[19]

References

1. Kosower NS, Kosower EM. The glutathione status of cells. *Intl Rev Cytol* 1978;54:109-157.
2. Kidd PM. Glutathione: systemic protectant against oxidative and free radical damage. *Altern Med Rev* 1997;1:155-176.
3. Sen CK. Nutritional biochemistry of cellular glutathione. *Nutr Biochem* 1997;8:660-672.
4. Cook GC, Sherlock S. Results of a controlled clinical trial of glutathione in cases of hepatic cirrhosis. *Gut* 1965;6:472-476.
5. Bremer HJ, Duran M, Kamerling JP, et al. Glutathione. In: Bremer HJ, Duran M, Kamerling JP, et al, eds. *Disturbances of Amino Acid Metabolism:Clinical Chemistry and Diagnosis*. Baltimore-Munich: Urban and Schwarzenberg; 1981:80-82.
6. Chawla RK, Lewis FW, Kutner MH, et al. Plasma cysteine, cysteine, and glutathione in cirrhosis. *Gastroenterology* 1984;87:770-776.
7. Cai J, Nelson KC, Wu M, et al. Oxidative damage and protection of the RPE. *Progr Retinal Eye Res* 2000;19:205-221.
8. Look MP, Rockstroh JK, Rao GS, et al. Serum selenium, plasma glutathione (GSH) and erythrocyte glutathione peroxidase (GSH-Px)-levels in asymptomatic versus symptomatic human immunodeficiency virus-1 (HIV-1)-infection. *Eur J Clin Nutr* 1997;51:266-272.
9. Luo J-L, Hammarqvist F, Andersson K, et al. Surgical trauma decreases glutathione synthetic capacity in human skeletal muscle tissue. *Am J Physiol* 1998;275:E359-E365.
10. Spies CD, Reinhart K, Witt I, et al. Influence of N-acetylcysteine on direct indicators of tissue oxygenation in septic shock patients: results from a prospective, randomized, double-blind study. *Crit Care Med* 1994;22:1738-1746.
11. Whitcomb DC, Block GD. Association of acetaminophen hepatotoxicity with fasting and ethanol use. *JAMA* 1994;272:1845-1850.

12. Anderson ME. Glutathione and glutathione delivery compounds. *Adv Pharmacol* 1997;38:65-78.
13. Lomaestro BM, Malone M. Glutathione in health and disease: pharmacotherapeutic issues. *Ann Pharmacother* 1995;29:1263-1273.
14. Meister A, Larsson A. Glutathione synthetase deficiency and other disorders of the gamma-glutamyl cycle. In: Scriver CR, Kinzler KW, Valle D, et al, eds. *The Metabolic and Molecular Bases of Inherited Diseases*. New York: McGraw-Hill; 1995:1461-1477.
15. Verjee ZH, Behal R. Protein-calorie malnutrition: a study of red blood cell and serum enzymes during and after crisis. *Clin Chim Acta* 1976;70:139-147.
16. Meister A. Glutathione, ascorbate, and cellular protection. *Cancer Res* 1994;54:1969S-1975S.
17. Strange RC, Jones PW, Fryer AA. Glutathione S-transferase: genetics and role in toxicology. *Toxicol Letts* 2000;112-113:357-363.
18. Monks TJ, Lau SS. Glutathione conjugation as a mechanism for the transport of reactive metabolites. *Adv Pharmacol* 1994;27:183-205.
19. Mulder GJ, Ouwerkerk-Mahadevan S. Modulation of glutathione conjugation *in vivo*: how to decrease glutathione conjugation *in vivo* or in intact cellular systems *in vitro*. *Chem-Biol Interact* 1997;105:17-34.
20. Sen CK. Redox signaling and the emerging therapeutic potential of thiol antioxidants. *Biochem Pharmacol* 1998;55:1747-1758.
21. Weber GF. Final common pathways in neurodegenerative diseases: regulatory role of the glutathione cycle. *Neurosci Biobehav Rev* 1999;23:1079-1086.
22. Gul M, Kutay FZ, Temocin S, et al. Cellular and clinical implications of glutathione. *Indian J Exp Biol* 2000;38:625-634.
23. Pace GW, Leaf CD. The role of oxidative stress in HIV disease. *Free Rad Biol Med* 1995;19:523-528.
24. Loguercio C, Taranto D, Vitale LM, et al. Effect of liver cirrhosis and age on the glutathione concentration in the plasma, erythrocytes, and gastric mucosa of man. *Free Rad Biol Med* 1996;20:483-488.
25. Altomare E, Vendemiale G, Alano O. Hepatic glutathione content in patients with alcoholic and non alcoholic liver diseases. *Life Sci* 1998;43:991-998.
26. Suarez M, Beloqui O, Ferrer JV, et al. Glutathione depletion in chronic hepatitis C. *Intl Hepatol Commun* 1993;1:215-221.
27. Suter PM, Domenighetti G, Schaller MD, et al. N-acetylcysteine enhances recovery from acute lung injury in man. *Chest* 1994;105:190-194.
28. Iantomasi T, Marraccini P, Favilli F, et al. Glutathione metabolism in Crohn's disease. *Biochem Med Metab Biol* 1994;53:87-91.
29. Usal A, Acarturk E, Yuregir GT, et al. Decreased glutathione levels in acute myocardial infarction. *Jpn Heart J* 1996;37:177-182.
30. Prasad A, Andrews NP, Padder FA, et al. Glutathione reverses endothelial dysfunction and improves nitric oxide bioavailability. *J Am Coll Cardiol* 1999;34:507-514.
31. Amano J, Suzuki A, Sunamori M. Salutary effect of reduced glutathione on renal function in coronary artery bypass operation. *J Am Coll Surg* 1994;179:714-720.
32. Kugiyama K, Ohgushi M, Motoyama T, et al. Intracoronary infusion of reduced glutathione improves endothelial vasomotor response to acetylcholine in human coronary circulation. *Circulation* 1998;97:2299-2301.
33. Gut A, Chaloner C, Schofield D, et al. Evidence of toxic metabolite stress in black South Africans with chronic pancreatitis. *Clin Chim Acta* 1995;236:145-153.
34. Vijayalingam S, Parthiban A, Shanmugasundaram KR, et al. Abnormal antioxidant status in impaired glucose tolerance and non-insulin-dependent diabetes mellitus. *Diab Med* 1996;13:715-719.

35. Yoshida K, Hirokawa J, Tagami S, et al. Weakened cellular scavenging activity against oxidative stress in diabetes mellitus: regulation of glutathione synthesis and efflux. *Diabetol* 1995;38:201-210.

36. Grimble RF. Effect of antioxidative vitamins on immune function with clinical applications. *Intl J Vit Nutr Res* 1997;67:312-320.

37. Sen CK. Glutathione homeostasis in response to exercise training and nutritional supplements. *Mol Cell Biochem* 1999;196:31-42.

38. Meister A. Mitochondrial changes associated with glutathione deficiency. *Biochim Biophys Acta* 1995;1271:35-42.

39. Kidd PM. Parkinson's disease as multifactorial oxidative neurodegeneration: implications for integrative management. *Altern Med Rev* 2000;5:502-529.

40. Witschi A, Reddy S, Stofer B, et al. The systemic availability of oral glutathione. *Eur J Clin Pharmacol* 1992;43:667-669.

41. Hagen TM, Wierzbicka GT, Sillau AH, et al. Bioavailability of dietary glutathione: effect on plasma concentrations. *Am J Physiol* 1990;259:G524-529.

42. Vincenzini MT, Favilli F, Iantomasi T. Intestinal uptake and transmembrane transport systems of intact GSH; characteristics and possible biological role. *Biochim Biophys Acta* 1992;1113:13-23.

43. Aw TY, Wierzbicka G, Jones DP. Oral glutathione increases tissue glutathione *in vivo*. *Chem-Biol Interact* 1991;80:89-97.

44. Perlmutter D. BrainRecovery.com. Naples, FL: The Perlmutter Health Center; 2000.

45. Faintuch J, Aguilar PB, Nadalin W. Relevance of N-acetylcysteine in clinical practice: fact, myth or consequence? *Nutrition* 1999;15:177-179.

46. Traber J, Suter M, Walter P, et al. *In vivo* modulation of total and mitochondrial glutathione in rat liver. *Biochem Pharmacol* 1992;43:961-964.

47. Bridgeman MM, Marsden M, Selby C, et al. Effect of N-acetyl cysteine on the concentrations of thiols in plasma, bronchoalveolar lavage fluid and lung tissue. *Thorax* 1994;49:670-675.

48. Fuchs J, Schofer H, Milbradt R, et al. Studies on lipoate effects on blood redox state in human immunodeficiency virus infected patients. *Arzneimittelforschung* 1993;43:1359-1362.

49. Packer L, Witt EH, Tritschler HJ. Alpha-lipoic acid as a biological antioxidant. *Free Rad Biol Med* 1995;19:227-250.

50. Kalayjian RC, Skowron G, Emgushov R-T, et al. A phase I/II trial of intravenous L-2-oxothiazolidine-4-carboxylic acid (procysteine) in asymptomatic HIV-infected subjects. *J Acq Immune Def Syndr* 1994;7:369-374.

51. Vita JA, Frei B, Holbrook M. L-2-Oxothiazolidine-4-carboxylic acid reverses endothelial dysfunction in patients with coronary artery disease. *J Clin Invest* 1998;101:1408-1414.

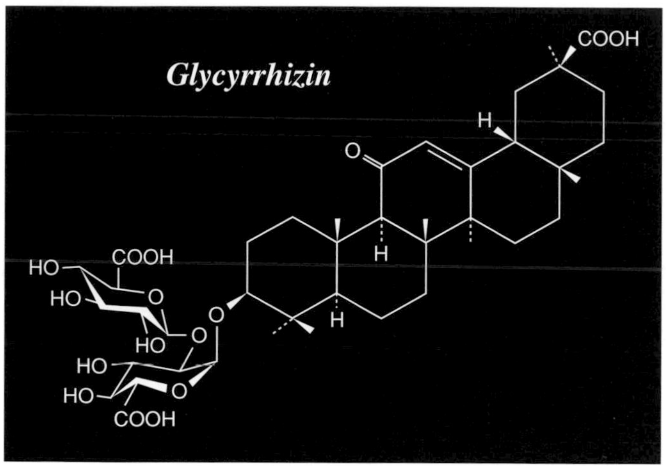

Glycyrrhiza glabra

Description

Glycyrrhiza glabra, also known as licorice and sweetwood, is native to the Mediterranean and certain areas of Asia. There are 20 different species of licorice in North and South America, Europe, South and Central Asia, and Australia. *Glycyrrhiza* is derived from the ancient Greek term *glykos,* meaning sweet, and *rhiza,* meaning root. Historically, the dried rhizome and root of this plant were employed medicinally by the Egyptian, Chinese, Greek, Indian, and Roman civilizations.

Active Constituents

A number of components have been isolated from licorice; among these is a water-soluble, biologically active complex that accounts for 40-50 percent of total dry material weight. This complex is composed of triterpene saponins, flavonoids, polysaccharides, pectins, simple sugars, amino acids, mineral salts, and various other substances.[1] The yellow color of licorice is due to the flavonoid content of the plant, which includes liquirtin, isoliquertin (a chalcone), and other compounds.[5]

Glycyrrhizen, a triterpenoid compound, accounts for the sweet taste of licorice root. This compound represents a mixture of potassium-calcium-magnesium salts of glycyrrhizic acid that varies within a 2-25 percent range. Among the natural saponins, glycyrrhizic acid is a molecule composed of a hydrophilic part, two molecules of glucuronic acid, and a hydrophobic fragment, glycyrrhetic acid. The similarity in structure of glycyrrhetic acid to the structure of hormones secreted by the adrenal cortex accounts for the mineral-corticoid and glucocorticoid activity of glycyrrhizic acid.[1]

Pharmacokinetics

After oral administration, licorice is metabolized to glycyrrhetinic acid by β-glucuronidase produced by intestinal bacteria.[3] After intravenous administration of licorice, both glycyrrhizin and glycyrrhetinic acid appear in the plasma. Intravenously administered glycyrrhizin is metabolized in the liver by lysosomal β-D-glucuronidase to 3-mono-glucuronide-glycyrrhitinic acid. The liver is not able to metabolize this molecule; therefore,

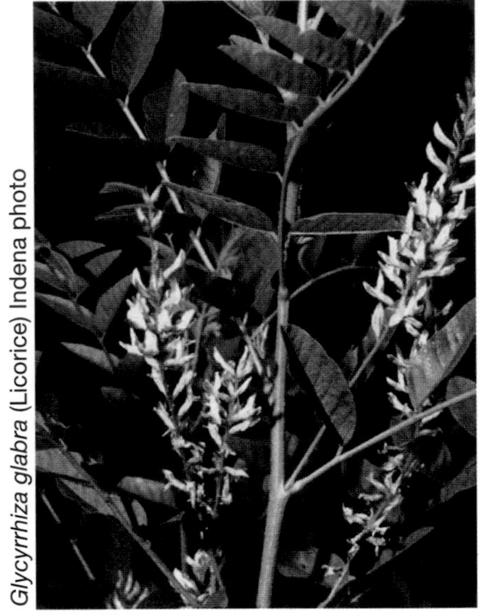

Glycyrrhiza glabra (Licorice) Indena photo

3-mono-glucoronide-glycyrrhetinic acid is excreted with bile into the intestine where it is further metabolized into glycyrrhetinic acid.[4]

After intravenous administration of glycyrrhizin in healthy volunteers, the terminal half-life and total body clearance were 2.7-4.8 h and 16-25 mL/h/kg, respectively.[5] After oral administration of 100 mg glycyrrhizin in the same healthy volunteers, no glycyrrhizin was found in the plasma and glycyrrhetinic acid was found at < 200 ng/mL. In the 24-hour period after oral administration, glycyrrhizin was found in the urine, suggesting it is partly absorbed as an intact molecule.

Mechanisms of Action

Licorice possesses anti-inflammatory and antiulcer activity, similar to the action of hydrocortisone. Glycyrrhizic acid and its derivatives exhibit properties of cortisone antagonists, in particular by blocking the antigranulomatous action of glucocorticoids. By doing so, the effects of endogenous glucocorticoids are potentiated, which suppresses oxidative phosphorylation and biosynthesis of sulfonated mucopolysaccharides, inhibits the activity of phospholipase A2, and increases the activity of glutamine transferase. Glycyrrhizic acid also affects the arachidonic acid cycle, thus inhibiting the biosynthesis of prostaglandins, specifically prostaglandin E2.[6]

Clinical Indications

Chronic Hepatitis

In Japan, glycyrrhizin has been used for more than 60 years as a treatment for chronic hepatitis. Stronger Neo-Minophagen C (SNMC), a glycyrrhizin preparation, has been extensively used with considerable success. SNMC has been shown to significantly lower aspartate transaminase (AST), alanine transaminase (ALT), and gamma-glutamyl transpeptide (GGT) concentrations, while simultaneously ameliorating histologic evidence of necrosis and inflammatory lesions in the liver.[7] In recent years, several studies have been performed exhibiting this action. Presently, interferon (IFN) therapy is the predominant treatment for chronic hepatitis; however, its efficacy is limited and an alternative treatment is highly desirable. SNMC has profound effects on the suppression of liver inflammation and is effective in improving chronic hepatitis and liver cirrhosis. It also appears to have considerably fewer side effects than IFN.[8]

In a double-blind, randomized, placebo-controlled trial investigating IV infusions of SNMC, short-term efficacy of licorice was confirmed with regard to ALT levels. The study showed the need for daily IV administration of SNMC, which is thought to be impractical for patients. The study also demonstrated that after cessation of therapy, the ALT-decreasing effect of licorice disappeared, suggesting the need for long-term administration.[9]

Oral Lichen Planus

In an open clinical trial, 17 hepatitis C-positive patients with oral lichen planus were given either routine dental care or 40 mL IV glycyrrhizin daily for one month. In comparison to the untreated group, 6/9 patients (66.7%) taking glycyrrhiza noted improved clinical symptoms, such as decreased redness, fewer white papules, and less erosion of the mucosa.[10]

Hepatocellular Carcinoma

In a retrospective study, long-term licorice administration for hepatitis C infection was effective in preventing hepatocellular carcinoma (HCC). Four hundred fifty-three patients diagnosed with hepatitis C were divided into three groups and given either licorice in the form of SNMC at a dose of 100 mL daily for two months or other natural treatments, such as vitamin K. The remaining group of patients was treated with a wider number of agents, including SNMC, corticosteroids, and immunosuppressive agents. As a result of this mixed medication regimen, this group was excluded from the study. After 10 years, analysis of the results showed 30/84 patients (35.7%) employing SNMC had normalized AST levels, compared with seven patients (6.4%) not treated with IV SNMC. Moreover, the 10- and 15-year appearance rate of HCC was 7 and 12 percent in the treated group, compared to 12 and 25 percent in the untreated group, respectively. A summary of the literature on HCC and the use of SNMC has confirmed that IV glycyrrhizin not only decreases ALT levels but also improves liver histology and decreases the incidence of hepatic cirrhosis.[11,12]

Aphthous Ulcers

In a double-blind, placebo-controlled trial, 24 patients with recurrent aphthous ulcers were randomly allocated to consume two grams of glycyrrhizin (carbenoxolone sodium) in 30 mL of warm water or a placebo three times per day, following meals, for four weeks. In contrast to the placebo group, the use of the oral licorice mouthwash significantly reduced the average number of ulcers per day, pain scores, and the development of new ulcers.[13]

Other Viral Illnesses

Studies show licorice, specifically glycyrrhizic acid, to have immune-modulating effects against *herpes simplex* virus (HSV), human immunodeficiency virus (HIV), *Varicella zoster*, and cytomegalovirus (CMV).[14-16] It has been reported that licorice inhibits growth and cytopathology of many unrelated DNA and RNA viruses, while not affecting cell activity or cellular replication.[17]In addition, glycyrrhizic acid has been shown to inactivate HSV irreversibly.[18]

A case report has shown that a 2-percent topical glycyrrhizic cream (carbenoxolone sodium) applied six times daily in 12 patients with acute oral herpetic infections resolved pain and dysphagia within 24-48 hours of beginning use. Moreover, the accompanying ulceration and lymphadenopathy gradually healed within 24-72 hours.[19]

CMV is the most common cause of congenital and perinatal viral infections throughout the world. It manifests with profound liver dysfunction and poor body weight gain. Both oral and IV preparations of licorice (SNMC) were administered to infants with CMV in a series of studies. Liver dysfunction and weight gain improved in nearly all cases compared to groups without treatment.[20-22]

Peptic Ulcer Disease

Licorice has been used as a demulcent and emollient for 2,000 years to promote the healing of ulcers by acting on the mucosal layer. In a double-blind, placebo-controlled study, 70 patients with endoscopically-confirmed gastric or duodenal ulcers were given glycyrrhizin (as carbenoxolone sodium) or placebo 300 mg per day during the first seven days, followed by 150 mg per day over the next several weeks. Carbenoxolone sodium speeds healing of gastric ulcers and protects against aspirin-induced damage to the gastric mucosa. The authors concluded those using carbenoxolone had an increase in pH at the stomach antrum from 1.1 to 6.0, and a reduction in basal and histamine-induced gastric acid secretion at pH 3 and 5. Overall, 70 percent of patients taking licorice extract healed their ulcers within three to five weeks of beginning therapy, compared to 36 percent employing placebo.[23]

Commonly, the side effects of licorice have limited its potential to be used on a long-term basis for treatment of peptic ulcer disease. A processed form of licorice, deglycyrrhizinated licorice (DGL), was produced to eliminate potential adverse effects, including licorice-induced hypertension.[24] In a double-blind trial, 100 patients were randomly chosen to chew Caved S (DGL plus antacid), two tablets three times per day, or take cimetidine 200 mg three times daily and 400 mg at night for 12 weeks. Endoscopy showed the healing rate between the two regimens was comparable at six (63 percent) and 12 weeks (91 percent). In addition, while both therapies reduced pain symptom scores in a comparable fashion during the day, cimetidine was more effective during the first two weeks at reducing nighttime pain.[25] A two-year follow-up trial comparing the two therapies in the prevention of gastric ulcer recurrence noted the outcomes were similar, with a reported relapse rate of 29 percent (9/31) in the Caved S group and 25 percent (8/32) in the cimetidine group.[26] Other studies have shown that 5,000-mg capsules per day for one month was not effective in the treatment of gastric ulcer when compared to placebo.[27]

A study was performed on the effects of licorice flavonoids on the growth of *Helicobacter pylori in vitro*. These flavonoid components showed promising anti-*H. pylori* activity against clarithromycin- and amoxicillin-resistant strains.[28]

Other Therapeutic Considerations

Studies also show licorice to have been effective in the treatment of melasma,[29] eosinophilic peritonitis,[30] postural hypotension,[31] erosive gastritis,[32] and as an anti-malarial[33] and anti-Leishmanial agent.[34]

Drug-Botanical Interactions

There is an increased likelihood of cardiac arrhythmias, particularly in those with ischemic heart disease, when licorice is used in conjunction with digoxin.[35]

Estrogen-based oral contraceptives may predispose some individuals to the mineralocorticoid side effects of licorice. This may be due in part to estrogens reacting with mineralocorticoid receptors, or inhibiting 11β-hydroxysteroid dehydrogenase.[36] Hypokalemia, commonly associated with metabolic acidosis, may co-present with essential benign hypertension in patients using diuretics and licorice simultaneously.[37]

Side Effects and Toxicity

One of the most commonly reported side effects with licorice supplementation is elevated blood pressure. This is due to licorice preparations suppressing the renin-angoitensin-aldosterone system. It is suggested licorice saponins are capable of potentiating aldosterone action while binding to mineralocorticoid receptors in the kidneys. The phenomenon is known as "pseudoaldosteronism." In addition to hypertension, patients may experience hypokalamia (potassium loss) and sodium retention in the form of edema. All symptoms usually disappear with discontinuation of therapy.[9] Many studies report no side effects during the course of treatment.[7,8] Generally, the onset and severity of symptoms depend on the size and duration of licorice intake, as well as individual susceptibility. The amount of licorice ingested daily by patients with mineralocorticoid excess syndromes appears to vary over a wide range, from as little as 1.5 grams per day to as much as 250 grams per day.[38]

Dosage

Because individual susceptibility to various licorice preparations is so vast, it is difficult to predict a dose that is appropriate for all individuals. Nevertheless, a daily oral intake of 1-10 mg of glycyrrhizin, which corresponds to 1-5 g licorice (2% glycyrrhizen), has been estimated to be a safe dose for most healthy adults.[39]

References:

1. Obolentseva GV, Litvinenko VI, Ammosov AS, et al. Pharmacological and therapeutic properties of licorice preparations (a review) *Pharm Chem J* 1999;33:24-31.
2. Evans WC. Licorice root. In: Evans WC, eds. *Pharacognosy.*14th ed. Philadelphia, PA:W.B. Saunders Company;1996:305.

3. Hattori M. Metabolism of glycyrrhizin by human intestinal flora II. Isolation and characterization of human intestinal bacteria capable of metabolizing glycyrrhizin and related compounds. *Chem Pharm Bull* 1985;33:210-217.
4. Akao T, Akao T, Hattori M, et al. Hydrolysis of glycerrhizin to 18 B-glycyrrhetyl monoglucuronide by lysosomal B-D-glucuronidase of animal livers. *Biochem Pharmacol* 1991;41:1025-1029.
5. Yamamura Y, Kawakami J, Snata T, et al. Pharmacokinetic profile of glycerrhizin in healthy volunteers by a new high-performance liquid chromatographic method. *J Pharm Sci* 1992;81:1042-1046.
6. Ohuchi K, Tsurufuji A. A study of the anti-inflammatory mechanism of glycyrrhizin. *Mino Med Rev* 1982;27:188-193.
7. Tsubota A, Kumada H, Arase Y, et al. Combined ursodeoxycholic acid and glycyrrhizin therapy for chronic hepatitis C virus infection: a randomized controlled trial in 170 patients. *Eur J Gastroenterol Hepatol* 1999;11:1071-1083.
8. Iino S, Tango T, Matsushima T, et al. Therapeutic effects of stronger neo-miniphagen C at different doses on chronic hepatitis and liver cirrhosis. *Hepatol Res* 2001;19:31-40.
9. Tekla GJ, Van Rossum MD, Vulto AG, et al. Glycyrrhizin-induced reduction of ALT in European patients with chronic hepatitis C. *Am J Gastroenterol* 2001;96:2432-2437.
10. Nagao Y, Sata M, Suzuki H, et al. Effectiveness of glycyrrhizin for oral lichen planus in patients with chronic HCV infection. *J Gastroenterol* 1996;31:691-695.
11. Arase Y, Ikeda K, Murashima N, et al. The long-term efficacy of glycyrrhizin in chronic hepatitis C patients. *Cancer* 1997;79:1494-1497.
12. Kumada H. Long-term treatment of chronic hepatitis C with glycyrrhizin [Stronger Neo-Minophagen C (SNMC)] for preventing liver cirrhosis and hepatocellular carcinoma. *Oncology* 2002;62:94-100.
13. Poswillo D, Partridge M. Management of recurrent aphthous ulcers. *Br Dent J* 1984;157:55-57.
14. Aikawa Y, Yoshiike T, Ogawa H. Effect of glycyrrhizin on pain and HLA-DR antigen expression on CD8-positive cells in peripheral blood of herpes zoster patients in comparison with other antiviral agents. *Skin Pharmacol* 1990;3:268-271.
15. Hattori T, Ikematsu S, Koito A, et al. Preliminary evidence for inhibitory effect of glycyrrhizin on HIV replication in patients with AIDS. *Antiviral Res* 1989;11:255-262.
16. Baba M, Shigeta S. Antiviral activity of glycyrrhizin against varicella-zoster virus in vitro. *Antiviral Res* 1987;7:99-107.
17. Ito M, Sato A, Hirabayashi K, et al. Mechanism of inhibitory effect of glycyrrhizin on replication of human immunodeficiency virus (HIV). *Antiviral Res* 1988;10:289-298.
18. Pompei R, Flore O, Marccialis MA, et al. Glycyrrhizic acid inhibits virus growth and inactivates virus particles. *Nature* 1979;281:689-690.
19. Partridge M, Poswillo DE. Topical carbenoxolone sodium in the management of herpes simplex infection. *Br J Oral Maxillofacial Surg* 1984;22:138-145.
20. Numazaki K, Umetsu M, Chiba S. Effect of glycyrrhizin in children with liver dysfunction associated with cytomegalovirus infection. *Tohuko J Exp Med* 1994;172:147-153.
21. Numazaki K, Chiba S. Natural course and trial of treatment for infantile liver dysfunction associated with cytomegalovirus infections. *In Vivo* 1993;7:477-480.
22. Numazaki K. Glycyrrhizin therapy for liver dysfunction associated with cytomegalovirus infection in immunocompetent children. *Antimicrobics Infect Dis Newsletter* 1998;17:70-71.
23. Loginov AS, Speransky MD, Speranskaya IE, et al. The effectiveness of carbenoxolone in the treatment of gastro-duodenal ulcer patients. *Scand J Gastroenterol Suppl* 1980;65:85-91.
24. Shibata S. A drug over the millennia: pharmacognosy, chemistry, and pharmacology of licorice. *Yakugaku Zasshi* 2000;120:849-862.

25. Morgan AG, McAdam WAF, Pacsoo C, et al. Comparison between cimetidine and Caved-S in the treatment of gastric ulceration, and subsequent maintenance therapy. *Gut* 1982;23:545-551.

26. Morgan AG, Pacsoo C McAdam WAF. Maintenance therapy: a two-year comparison between Caved-S and cimetidine treatment in the prevention of symptomatic gastric ulcer recurrence. *Gut* 1985;26:599-602.

27. Bardhan KD, Cumberland DC, Dixon RA, et al. Clinical trial of deglycyrrhizinised liquorice in gastric ulcer. *Gut* 1978;19:779-782.

28. Fukai T, Marumo A, Kaitou K, ct al. Anti-*Helicobacter pylori* flavonoids from licorice extract. *Life Sci* 2002;9:1449-1463.

29. Amer M, Metwalli M. Topical liquiritin improves melasma. *Int J Dermatol* 2000;39:299-301.

30. Takeda H, Ohta K, Niki H, et al. Eosinophilic peritonitis responding to treatment with glycyrrhizin. *Tokai J Exp Clin Med* 1991;16:183-186.

31. Basso A, Paola LD, Erle G, et al. Licorice ameliorates postural hypotension caused by diabetic autonomic neuropathy. *Diabetes Care* 1994;17:1356.

32. Kolarski V, Shopova-Petrova K, Vasileva E. Erosive gastritis and gastroduodenitis: clinical, diagnostic and therapeutic studies. *Vutr Boles* 1987;26:56-59. [article in Bulgarian]

33. Chen M, Theander TG, Christensen SB, et al. Licochalcone A, a new anti-malarial agent, inhibits in vitro growth of the human malaria parasite *Plasmodium falciparum* and protects mice from *P. yoelii* infection. *Antimicrob Agents Chemother* 1994;38:1470-1475.

34. Christensen SB, Ming C, Anderson L, et al. An anti-leishmanial chalcone from Chinese licorice roots. *Planta Medica* 1994;60:121-123.

35. Hoes AW, Grobbee DE, Peet TM. Do non-potassium sparing diuretics increase the risk of sudden cardiac death in hypertensive patients? Recent evidence. *Drugs* 1994;47:711-713.

36. Clyburn EB, Dipette DJ. Hypertension induced by drugs and other substances. *Semin Nephrol* 1995;15:72-86.

37. Olukoga A, Donaldson D. Liquorice and its health implications. *J R Soc Health* 2000;120:83-89.

38. Stormer F, Reistad R, Alexander J. Glycyrhhizic acid in liquorice – evaluation of health hazard. *Food Chem Toxicol* 1993;31:303-312.

39. Walker BR, Edwards CR. Licorice-induced hypertension and syndromes of apparent mineralcorticoid excess. *Endocrinol Metab Clin North Am* 1194;23:359-377.

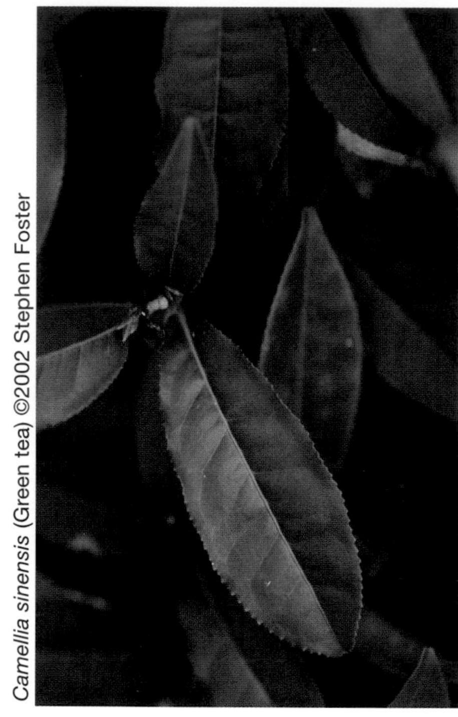
Camellia sinensis (Green tea) ©2002 Stephen Foster

Green Tea (*Camellia sinensis*)

Description

Tea is one of the most widely consumed beverages in the world, second only to water, and its medicinal properties have been widely explored. The tea plant, *Camellia sinensis*, is a member of the Theaceae family, and black, oolong, and green tea are produced from its leaves. It is an evergreen shrub or tree and can grow to heights of 30 feet, but is usually pruned to 2-5 feet for cultivation. The leaves are dark green, alternate and oval, with serrated edges, and the blossoms are white, fragrant, and appear in clusters or singly.

Active Constituents

Unlike black and oolong tea, green tea production does not involve oxidation of young tea leaves. Green tea is produced from steaming fresh leaves at high temperatures, thereby inactivating the oxidizing enzymes and leaving the polyphenol content intact. The polyphenols found in tea are more commonly known as flavanols or catechins, and comprise 30-40 percent of the extractable solids of dried green tea leaves. The main catechins in green tea are epicatechin, epicatechin-3-gallate, epigallocatechin, and epigallocatechin-3-gallate (EGCG), with the latter being the highest in concentration. Green tea polyphenols have demonstrated significant antioxidant, anticarcinogenic, anti-inflammatory, thermogenic, probiotic, and antimicrobial properties in numerous human, animal, and *in vitro* studies.[1,2]

Mechanisms of Action

The anticarcinogenic properties of green tea polyphenols, mainly EGCG, are likely a result of inhibition of tumor initiation and promotion, induction of apoptosis, and inhibition of cell replication rates, thus retarding the growth and development of neoplasms.[3,4] Green tea polyphenols' antioxidant potential is directly related to the combination of aromatic rings and hydroxyl groups that make up their structure, and is a result of binding and neutralization of free radicals by the hydroxyl groups. In addition, green tea polyphenols stimulate the activity of hepatic detoxification enzymes, thereby promoting detoxification of xenobiotic compounds, and are also capable of chelating metal ions, such as iron, that can generate radical oxygen species.[5,6]

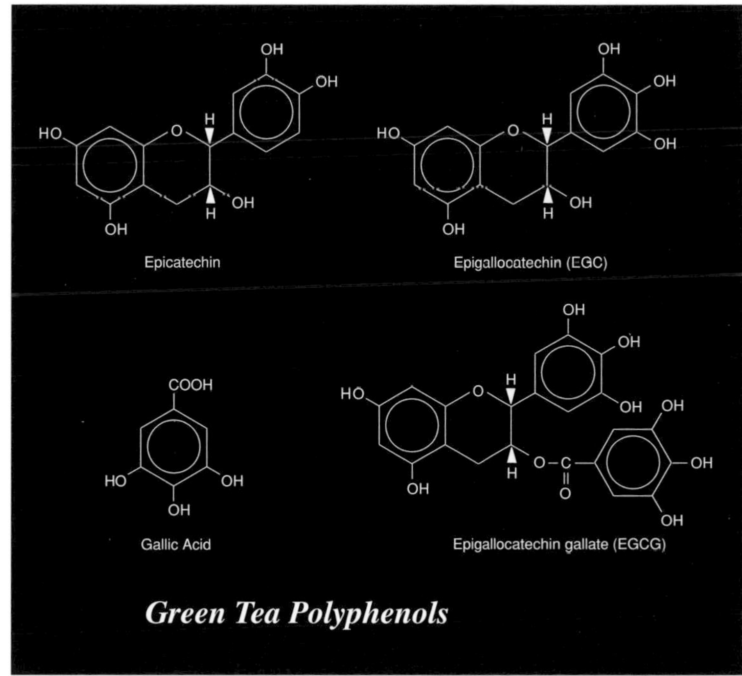

Green Tea Polyphenols

Green tea polyphenols inhibit the production of arachidonic acid metabolites such as pro-inflammatory prostaglandins and leukotrienes, resulting in a decreased inflammatory response. Human and animal studies have demonstrated EGCG's ability to block inflammatory responses to ultraviolet A and B radiation, as well as significantly inhibiting neutrophil migration that occurs during the inflammatory process.[7-9]

Research on green tea's thermogenic properties indicates a synergistic interaction between its caffeine content and catechin polyphenols that can result in prolonged stimulation of thermogenesis. Studies have also shown green tea extracts are capable of reducing fat digestion by inhibiting the activity of certain digestive enzymes.[10,11] Although the exact mechanism is unknown, green tea catechins have been shown to significantly raise levels of Lactobacilli and Bifidobacteria while decreasing levels of numerous potential pathogens.[12] Studies have also demonstrated green tea's antibacterial properties against a variety of gram-positive and gram-negative species.[13]

Clinical Indications

Cancer Prevention/Inhibition

Several studies have demonstrated green tea polyphenols' preventative and inhibitory effects against tumor formation and growth. While the studies are not conclusive, green tea polyphenols, particularly EGCG, may be effective in preventing cancer of the prostate, breast, esophagus, stomach, pancreas, and colon.[14] There is also some evidence that green tea polyphenols may be chemopreventive or inhibitory toward lung, skin, and liver cancer,[15-17] bladder and ovarian tumors,[18,19] leukemia,[20] and oral leukoplakia.[21]

Antioxidant Applications

Many chronic disease states and inflammatory conditions are a result of oxidative stress and subsequent generation of free radicals. Some of these include heart disease (resulting from LDL oxidation), renal disease and failure, several types of cancer, skin exposure damage caused by ultraviolet (A and B) rays, as well as diseases associated with aging. Green tea polyphenols are potent free radical scavengers due to the hydroxyl groups in their chemical structure. The hydroxyl groups form complexes with free radicals and neutralize them, preventing the progression of the disease process.[22]

Obesity/Weight Control

Recent studies on green tea's thermogenic properties have demonstrated a synergistic interaction between caffeine and catechin polyphenols that appears to prolong sympathetic stimulation of thermogenesis. A human study of green tea extract containing 90 mg EGCG taken three times daily concluded that men taking the extract burned 266 more calories per day than did those in the placebo group and that green tea extract's thermogenic effects may play a role in controlling obesity.[23] Green tea polyphenols have also beeen shown to markedly inhibit digestive lipases *in vitro*, resulting in decreased lipolysis of triglycerides, which may translate to reduced fat digestion in humans.[10,11]

Intestinal Dysbiosis and Infection

A small study in Japan demonstrated a special green tea catechin preparation (30.5% EGCG) was able to positively affect intestinal dysbiosis in nursing home patients by raising levels of Lactobacilli and Bifidobacteria while lowering levels of Enterobacteriaceae, Bacteroidaceae, and eubacteria. Levels of pathogenic bacterial metabolites were also decreased.[12] An *in vitro* study also demonstrated green tea possesses antimicrobial activity against a variety of gram-positive and gram-negative pathogenic bacteria that cause cystitis, pyelonephritis, diarrhea, dental caries,[24] pneumonia, and skin infections.[13]

Other Applications

Sickle cell anemia is characterized by a population of "dense cells" that may trigger vaso-occlusion and the painful sickle cell "crisis." One study demonstrated that 0.13 mg/mL green tea extract was capable of inhibiting dense-cell formation by 50 percent.[25]

Another potential therapeutic application of green tea is the treatment of psoriasis. The combination therapy of psoralens and ultraviolet A radiation is highly effective but has unfortunately been shown to substantially increase the risk for developing squamous cell carcinoma and melanoma. An *in vitro* study using human and mouse skin demonstrated that pre- and post-treatment with green tea extract inhibited DNA damage induced by the psoralen/ultraviolet A radiation exposure.[8]

Side Effects and Toxicity

Green tea is generally considered a safe, non-toxic beverage and consumption is usually without side effects. The average cup of green tea contains from 10-50 mg of caffeine, and over-consumption may cause irritability, insomnia, nervousness, and tachycardia. Because studies on its possible teratogenic effect are inconclusive, caffeine consumption is contraindicated during pregnancy. Lactating women should also limit caffeine intake to avoid sleep disorders in infants.[26]

Dosage

The dosage for green tea beverage varies, depending on the clinical situation and desired therapeutic effect. The phenolic content of green tea infusion is between 50-100 mg polyphenols per cup, depending on species, harvesting variables, and brewing methods,[27] with typical dosages range from 3 to 10 cups per day. Cancer preventative effects are usually associated with dosages in the higher end of the range.[28] Green tea extracts standardized to 80-percent total polyphenols are dosed at 500-1,500 mg per day.

References

1. Alschuler L. Green Tea: Healing tonic. *Am J Natur Med* 1998;5:28-31.
2. Graham HN. Green tea composition, consumption, and polyphenol chemistry. *Prev Med* 1992;21:334-350.
3. Nihal A, Hasan M. Green tea polyphenols and cancer: biological mechanisms and practical implications. *Nutr Rev* 1999;57:78-83.
4. Ahmad N, Feyes DK, Nieminen AL, et al. Green tea constituent epigallacatechin-3-gallate and induction of apoptosis and cell cycle arrest in human carcinoma cells. *J Natl Cancer Inst* 1997;89:1881-1886.
5. Serafini M, Ghiselli A, Ferro-Luzzi A. In vivo antioxidant effect of green and black tea in man. *Eur J Clin Nutr* 1996;50:28-32.
6. Erba D, Riso P, Colombo A, Testolin G. Supplementation of Jurkat T cells with green tea extract decreases oxidative damage due to iron treatment. *J Nutr* 1999;129:2130-2134.
7. Katiyar SK, Matsui MS, Elmets CA, Mukhtar H. Polyphenolic antioxidant (-)-epigallocatechin-3-gallate from green tea reduces UVB-induced inflammatory responses and infiltration of leukocytes in human skin. *Photochem Photobiol* 1999;69:148-153.
8. Zhao JF, Zhang YJ, Jin XH, et al. Green tea protects against psoralen plus ultraviolet A-induced photochemical damage to skin. *J Invest Dermatol* 1999;113:1070-1075.
9. Hofbauer R, Frass M, Gmeiner B, et al. The green tea extract epigallocatechin gallate is able to reduce neutrophil transmigration through monolayers of endothelial cells. *Wien Klin Wochenschr* 1999;111:276-282.
10. Dulloo AG, Seydoux J, Girardier L, et al. Green tea and thermogenesis: interactions between catechin-polyphenols, caffeine, and sympathetic activity. *Int J Obes Relat Metab Disord* 2000;24:252-258.
11. Juhel C, Armand M, Pafumi Y, et al. Green tea extract (AR25) inhibits lipolysis of triglycerides in gastric and duodenal medium in vitro. *J Nutr Biochem* 2000;11:45-51.
12. Goto K, Kanaya S, Nishikawa T, et al. Green tea catechins improve gut flora. *Ann Long-Term Care* 1998;6:1-7.

13. Chou CC, Lin LL, Chung KT. Antimicrobial activity of tea as affected by the degree of fermentation and manufacturing season. *Int J Food Microbiol* 1999;48:125-130.
14. Katiyar SK, Mukhtar H. Tea antioxidants in cancer chemoprevention. *J Cell Biochem* 1997;27:S59-S67.
15. Lee IP, Kim YH, Kang MH, et al. Chemopreventative effect of green tea (*Camellia sinensis*) against cigarette smoke-induced mutations (SCE) in humans. *J Cell Biochem* 1997;27:S68-S75.
16. Picard D. The biochemistry of green tea polyphenols and their potential application in human skin cancer. *Altern Med Rev* 1996;1:31-42.
17. Hirose M, Hoshiya T, Akagi K, et al. Effects of green tea catechins in a rat multi-organ carcinogenesis model. *Carcinogenesis* 1993;14:1549-1553.
18. Sato D. Inhibition of urinary bladder tumors induced by N-butyl-N-(4-hydroxybutyl)-nitrosamine in rats by green tea. *Int J Urol* 1999;6:93-99.
19. Sugiyama T, Sadzuka Y. Enhancing effects of green tea components on the antitumor activity of adriamycin against M5076 ovarian sarcoma. *Cancer Lett* 1998;133:19-26.
20. Otsuka T, Ogo T, Eto T, et al. Growth inhibition of leukemic cells by (-)-epigallocatechin gallate, the main constituent of green tea. *Life Sci* 1998;63:1387-1403.
21. Khafif A, Schantz SP, al-Rawi M, et al. Green tea regulates cell cycle progression in oral leukoplakia. *Head Neck* 1998;20:528-534.
22. Ichihashi M, Ahmed NU, Budiyanto A, et al. Preventive effect of antioxidant on ultraviolet-induced skin cancer in mice. *J Dermatol Sci* 2000;23:S45-S50.
23. Dulloo AG, Duret C, Rohrer D, et al. Efficacy of a green tea extract rich in catechin polyphenols and caffeine in increasing 24-h energy expenditure and fat oxidation in humans. *Am J Clin Nutrition* 1999;70:1040-1045.
24. You S. Study on feasibility of Chinese green tea polyphenols (CTP) for preventing dental caries. *Chung Hua Kou Hsueh Tsa Chih* 1993;28:197-199.
25. Ohnishi ST, Ohnishi T, Ogunmola GB. Sickle cell anemia: a potential nutritional approach for a molecular disease. *Nutrition* 2000;16:330-338.
26. DerMarderosian A. *The Review of Natural Products.* St. Louis, MO: Facts and Comparisons, Wolters Kluwer Co. 1999.
27. Yamimoto T, Juneja LR, Djoing-Chu C, Kim M. *Chemistry and Applications of Green Tea.* Boca Raton, FL: CRC Press, 1997:51-52,
28. Imai K, Suga K, Nakachi K. Cancer-preventative effects of drinking tea among a Japanese population. *Prev Med* 1997;26:769-775.

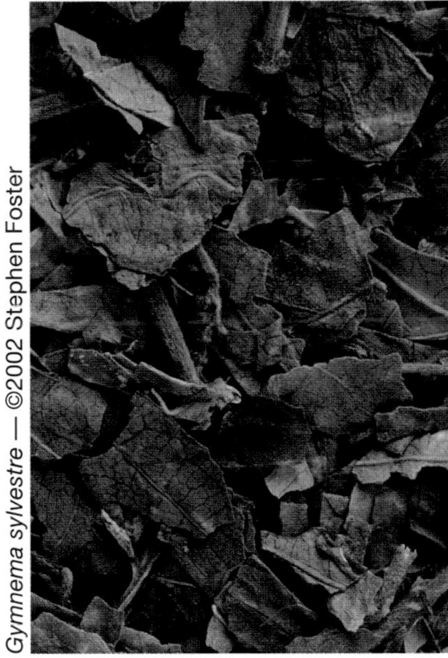
Gymnema sylvestre — ©2002 Stephen Foster

Gymnema sylvestre

Description

Gymnema sylvestre is a woody, climbing plant, native to India. The leaves of this plant have been used in India for 2,000 years to treat madhu meha, or "honey urine," an early term for glucosuria detected by pouring the patients urine onto the ground and observing whether or not insects were attracted to it. Chewing the leaves also destroys the ability to discriminate "sweet" taste, giving it its common name, gurmar or "sugar destroyer."

Active Constituents

Plant constituents include two resins (one soluble in alcohol), six-percent gymnemic acids, saponins, stigmasterol, quercitol, and the amino acid derivatives betaine, choline, and trimethylamine.[1]

Mechanisms of Action

Gymnema sylvestre is a stomachic, diuretic, refrigerant, astringent, and tonic.[1] The herb has been found to increase urine output and reduce hyperglycemia in both animal and human studies.

The antidiabetic activity of Gymnema appears to be due to a combination of mechanisms. Two animal studies on beryllium nitrate- and streptozotocin-diabetic rats found Gymnema extracts to double the number of insulin-secreting beta cells in the pancreas, and to return blood sugars to almost normal.[2,3] Gymnema increases the enzymes responsible for glucose uptake and utilization,[4] and inhibits peripheral utilization of glucose by somatotropin and corticotrophin.[5] Plant extracts have also been found to inhibit epinephrine-induced hyperglycemia.[6]

Clinical Indications

The primary clinical application for this botanical is as an antidiabetic agent. Gymnema has been the object of considerable research since the 1930s, with promising results for both type 1 and 2 diabetes. Numerous animal studies have confirmed the hypoglycemic effect of *Gymnema sylvestre*.[7-9]

Type 1 Diabetes

In a controlled study, a standardized extract of the plant was given to 27 type 1 diabetics at a dose of 400 mg daily for 6-30 months. Thirty-seven other diabetics continued on insulin therapy alone and were tracked for 10-12 months. In the Gymnema group, insulin requirements were decreased by one-half and the average blood glucose decreased from 232 mg/dL to 152 mg/dL. The control group showed no significant decreases in blood sugar or insulin requirement. In addition, there was a statistically significant decrease in glycosylated hemoglobin (HbA1c) after 6-8 months on Gymnema when compared to pretreatment levels or the control group.[10]

Type 2 Diabetes

Twenty-two type 2 diabetics were administered 400 mg Gymnema extract daily for 18-20 months along with their oral hypoglycemic medications. This group experienced significant decreases in average blood sugar and HbA1c, and an increase in pancreatic release of insulin. Medication dosages were decreased and five participants were able to discontinue their medications entirely.[11]

Lipid-lowering

Preliminary animal studies indicate Gymnema may be beneficial for lowering blood lipids. When fed to rats on either a high- or normal-fat diet for 10 weeks, *Gymnema sylvestre* suppressed body weight gain and liver lipid accumulation to the same extent as chitosan in those on a high-fat diet.[12] In a three-week study in rats, Gymnema feeding decreased total cholesterol and triglycerides and increased fecal fat elimination.[13] Further research is warranted to determine whether Gymnema has this same lipid-lowering effect in clinical practice.

Side Effects and Toxicity

No significant adverse effects have been reported, aside from the expected hypoglycemia.[14] Safety in pregnancy has not been established.

Dosage

The typical therapeutic dose of an extract standardized to contain 24-percent gymnemic acids is 400-600 mg daily. It is not clear from examining the studies whether divided doses is ideal but, because it is being used to regulate blood sugar, three divided doses with meals seems preferable.

References

1. Kapoor LD. *Handbook of Ayurvedic Medicinal Plants.* Boca Raton, FL: CRC Press, Inc; 1990:200-201.
2. Prakash AO, Mather S, Mather R. Effect of feeding *Gymnema sylvestre* leaves on blood glucose in beryllium nitrate treated rats. *J Ethnopharmacol* 1986;18:143-146.
3. Shanmugasundaram ER, Gopinath KL, Shanmugasundaram KR, Rojendran VM. Possible regeneration of the islets of Langerhans in streptozotocin-diabetic rats given *Gymnema sylvestre* leaf extracts. *J Ethnopharmacol* 1990;30:265-279.
4. Shanmugasundaram KR, Panneerselvam C, Samudram P, Shanmugasundaram ER. Enzyme changes and glucose utilisation in diabetic rabbits: the effect of *Gymnema sylvestre*, R.Br. *J Ethnopharmacol* 1983;7:205-234.
5. Gupta SS, Variyar MC. Experimental studies on pituitary diabetes IV. Effect of *Gymnema sylvestre* and *Coccinia indica* against the hyperglycemia response of somatotropin and corticotrophin hormones. *Indian J Med Res* 1964;52:200-207.
6. Gupta SS. Inhibitory effect of *Gymnema sylvestre* (Gurmar) on adrenaline induced hyperglycemia in rats. *Indian J Med Sci* 1961;15:883-887.
7. Srivasta Y, Bhatt HV, Prem AS, et al. Hypoglycemic and life-prolonging properties of *Gymnema sylvestre* leaf extract in diabetic rats. *Isr J Med Sci* 1985;21:540-542.
8. Okabayashi Y, Tani S, Fujisawa T, et al. Effect of *Gymnema sylvestre*, R.Br. on glucose homeostasis in rats. *Diabetes Res Clin Pract* 1990;9:143-148.
9. Venkatakrishna-Bhatt H, Srivastava Y, Jhala CI, et al. Effect of *Gymnema sylvestre,* R.Br. leaves on blood sugar and longevity of alloxan diabetic rats. *Indian J Pharmacol* 1981;13:99.
10. Shanmugasundaram ER, Rajeswari G, Baskaran K, et al. Use of *Gymnema sylvestre* leaf in the control of blood glucose in insulin-dependent diabetes mellitus. *J Ethnopharmacol* 1990;30:281-294.
11. Baskaran K, Ahamath BK, Shanmugasundaram KR, Shanmugasundaram ER. Antidiabetic effect of a leaf extract from *Gymnema sylvestre* in non-insulin-dependent diabetes mellitus patients. *J Ethnopharmacol* 1990;30:295-305.
12. Sigematsu N, Asano R, Shimosaka M, Okazaki M. Effect of long term-administration with *Gymnema sylvestre* R.Br. on plasma and liver lipid in rats. *Biol Pharm Bull* 2001;24:643-649.
13. Shigematsu N, Asano R, Shimosaka M, Okazaki M. Effect of administration with the extract of *Gymnema sylvestre* R.Br. leaves on lipid metabolism in rats. *Biol Pharm Bull* 2001;24:713-717.
14. Facts and Comparisons Publishing Group. *The Review of Natural Products.* St. Louis, MO: Facts and Comparisons, a Wolters Kluwer Co; 1996.

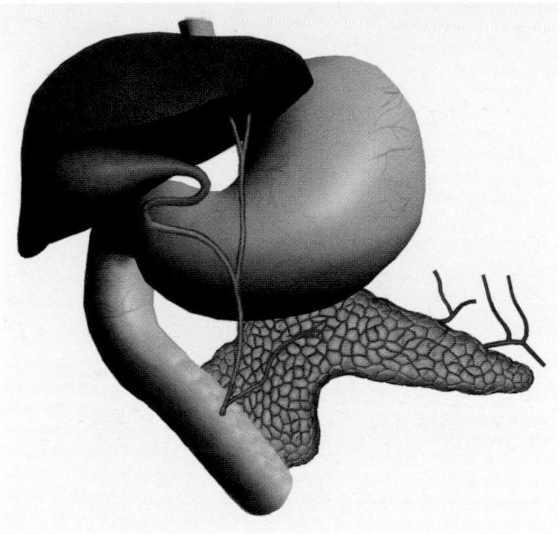

Hydrochloric acid

Introduction

Hydrochloric acid (HCl) assists protein digestion, renders the stomach sterile against orally ingested pathogens, prevents bacterial and fungal overgrowth of the small intestine, encourages the flow of bile and pancreatic enzymes, and facilitates the absorption of a variety of nutrients, including folic acid, ascorbic acid, beta-carotene, non-heme iron, and some forms of calcium, magnesium, and zinc. Case reports suggest therapeutic potential as replacement therapy under circumstances of impaired HCl secretion in skin disorders, childhood asthma, B-vitamin deficiencies, anemia, and gastrointestinal disorders.

Historically, hydrochloric acid was prescribed for many symptoms and clinical conditions and was listed as a therapeutic intervention in various pharmacopoeias. However, beginning in the late 1920s and early 1930s, its common use by the medical establishment began to decline. The therapeutic efficacy of oral administration of HCl is still equivocal, largely due to a scarcity of outcome-focused clinical intervention studies; however, proponents suggest a therapeutic value of exogenous HCl supplementation in conditions associated with impaired HCl secretion.

Biochemistry and Mechanism of Action

HCl secretion is required for protein digestion by activating pepsinogen to pepsin. Food enters the stomach as chyme, stimulating the release of the hormone gastrin. The presence of gastrin in the blood stimulates the parietal cells of the stomach to release HCL, concentrated to a pH of 0.8. This high concentration of hydrogen ions requires a tremendous amount of energy to be formed (1,500 calories of energy per liter of gastric juice).

Deficiency States

Numerous signs and symptoms have been attributed to decreased HCl secretion, as well as several clinical conditions. While these symptoms, signs, and conditions may help identify patients with hypo- or achlorhydria, analysis with the Heidelberg pH capsule or other diagnostic testing should be used to confirm low stomach acid. Common symptoms of low gastric acidity include bloating after eating, diarrhea, constipation, flatulence, heartburn, food allergies, and indigestion. Clinical conditions associated with low gastric acidity include, but are not limited to, anemia, arthritis, asthma, celiac disease, osteoporosis, various skin diseases, and flatulent dyspepsia. Numerous studies have also shown HCl secretion declines with age[1]

Clinical Indications

Nutrient Absorption

In patients with histamine-fast achlorhydria, both ferric chloride and ferrous ascorbate were better absorbed when given with an acid solution. The acid solution did not alter absorption of hemoglobin iron.[2]

HCl appears to play an important role in the absorption of B-complex vitamins. Supplementation of HCl in conjunction with B-complex vitamins in functionally achlorhydric individuals improved patients' therapeutic response to B-vitamin therapy.[3] A case report of an individual with a 17-year history of depression along with clinical signs and symptoms of B-vitamin deficiency that was refractory to B-vitamin therapy reported that adding HCl before meals to B-vitamin therapy resulted in rapid recovery.[4] Evidence indicates folic acid absorption is enhanced in individuals with gastric atrophy when HCl is supplemented.[5]

Absorption of other nutrients such as zinc,[6-8] calcium,[9] ascorbic acid,[10] and beta-carotene[11] is decreased under circumstances of impaired HCl secretion; however, studies have not been conducted on the impact of HCl replacement therapy on the absorption of these nutrients in subjects with inadequate HCl secretion.

Skin Diseases

In a series of 400 patients with skin disorders including acne rosacea, eczema, psoriasis, seborrheic dermatitis, urticaria, and vitiligo that were resistant to local treatment, a high prevalence were found to have impaired HCl secretion. An improvement in general health and skin condition was observed following replacement therapy with oral HCl and B complex (as brewer's yeast) in virtually all patients. Cases with moderate HCl deficiency showed the most rapid improvement.[3]

Other clinical case reports have suggested improvements in eczema and vitiligo subsequent to HCl administration in subjects with functional hypoacidity or achlorhydria.[12,13]

Diabetic Neuritis

Case reports indicate diabetic patients with impaired HCl secretion and severe neuritis refractive to thiamine supplementation may experience marked improvement after receiving HCl supplementation.[14]

Asthma

One-hundred-and-sixty asthmatic children with low HCl levels avoided known food allergens and were supplemented with HCl before or during meals. An immediate improvement in appetite, weight, and sleep was observed. Asthma attacks were shorter in duration and of lesser intensity.[15]

Wright has commented on hypochlorhydria and low pepsin production resulting in incomplete digestion of food and macromolecule absorption, increasing both the number and severity of food allergies, while simultaneously impairing micronutrient nutrition. He also comments on the benefit of HCl administration as part of an integrated treatment protocol for childhood asthma.[16]

Anemia

Glutamic acid HCl was dosed at 5 grains three times daily before meals to 25 diabetic patients with blood cell counts of 4.2 million or less. Following treatment with glutamic acid HCl, the average red blood cell (RBC) count increased from 4.06 to 4.56 million. A subsequent combination of glutamic acid HCl with inorganic iron (ferrous carbonate 6 3/4 grains three times daily) increased RBC count to 4.85 million.[14]

Other Indications

Twenty-seven achlorhydric patients were supplemented with betaine HCl and pepsin for six months. General improvement in physical condition and strength was noted in all subjects. Indigestion and excessive gas were relieved in all patients with this complaint. Signs of oral mucosal inflammation improved in 78 percent of the patients, and of 22 patients with a complaint of a chronic sore mouth, five had complete relief and 11 others noted improvement.[17]

Administration of HCl between meals (but not with meals) to subjects with achlorhydria results in indican metabolism improving markedly; however, no change in urinary indican levels occurs in patients with normal gastric secretion following HCl supplementation, irrespective of when administered.[18]

Side Effects and Toxicity

It is recommended that HCl supplementation be avoided during periods of active peptic ulcer. Subjective sensations of heaviness in the chest, warmth, and occasionally pain or burning have been reported at high doses.

Dosage

Hydrochloric acid is available primarily as betaine HCl, although glutamic acid HCl is found in some formulas.

The potency of a capsule or tablet preparation may vary from 5-10 grains, with 1 grain equal to approximately 64.75 mg HCl. Clinically, practitioners have reported administering dosages of HCl from as little as 5 grains three times daily with meals to levels as high as 60-80 grains three times daily with meals in some patients. Other clinicians utilize a protocol where one capsule is given before, during, and after each meal.

If HCl is being administered for an individual with intestinal bacterial or fungal overgrowth due to lack of basal HCl production, it is recommended that one capsule of betaine HCl be supplemented three times daily between meals.

References

1. Kelly G. Hydrochloric acid: physiologic functions and clinical implications. *Altern Med Rev* 1997;2:116-127.
2. Jacobs A, Bothwell TH, Charleton RW. Role of hydrochloric acid in iron absorption. *J Appl Physiol* 1964;19:187-188.
3. Allison JR. The relation of hydrochloric acid and vitamin B complex deficiency in certain skin diseases. *South Med J* 1945;38:235-241.
4. Keuter EJW. Deficiency of vitamin B complex, presenting itself psychiatrically as an atypical endogenous depression. *Nutr Abstr Rev* 1959;29:273. [Abstract]
5. Russell RM, Krasinski SD, Samloff IM. Correction of impaired folic acid (PteGlu) absorption by orally administered HCl in subjects with gastric atrophy. *Am J Clin Nutr* 1984;39:656.
6. Sturniolo GC, Montino MC, Rossetto L, et al. Inhibition of gastric acid secretion reduces zinc absorption in man. *J Amer Col Nutr* 1991;10:372-375.
7. Henderson LM, Brewer GJ, Dressman JB, et al. Effect of intragastric pH on the absorption of oral zinc acetate and zinc oxide in young healthy volunteers. *JPEN* 1995;19:393-397.
8. Sandstrom B, Abrahamsson H. Zinc absorption and achlorhydria. *Eur J Clin Nutr* 1989;43:877-879.
9. Hunt JN, Johnson C. Relation between gastric secretion of acid and urinary excretion of calcium after oral supplements of calcium. *Dig Dis Sci* 1983;28:417-421.
10. O'Connor HJ, Schorah CJ, Habibzedah N, et al. Vitamin C in the human stomach: relation to gastric pH, gastroduodenal disease, and possible sources. *Gut* 1989;30:436-442.
11. Tang G, Serfaty-Lacrosniere C, Camilo ME, et al. Gastric acidity influences the blood response to a B-carotene dose in humans. *Am J Clin Nutr* 1996;64:622-626.
12. Ayers S. Gastric secretion in psoriasis, eczema, and dermatitis herpetiformis. *Arch Dermatol Syph* 1929;20:854-857.
13. Francis HW. Achlorhydia as an etiological factor in vitiligo, with report of four cases. *Nebraska Med J* 1931;16:25-26.
14. Rabinowitch IM. Achlorhydria and its clinical significance in diabetes mellitus. *Am J Dig Dis* 1949;16:322-332.
15. Bray GW. The hypochlorhydria of asthma of childhood. *Quart J Med* 1931;24:181-197.
16. Wright JV. Treatment of childhood asthma with parenteral vitamin B12, gastric re-acidification, and attention to food allergy, magnesium and pyridoxine. Three case reports with background and an integrated hypothesis. *J Nutr Med* 1990;1:277-282.
17. Sharp GS, Fister HW. The diagnosis and treatment of achlorhydria: ten-year study. *J Amer Ger Soc* 1967;15:786-791.
18. Brummer P, Kasanen A. The effect of hydrochloric acid on the indican metabolism in achlorhydria. *Acta Medica Scan* 1956;155:11-14.

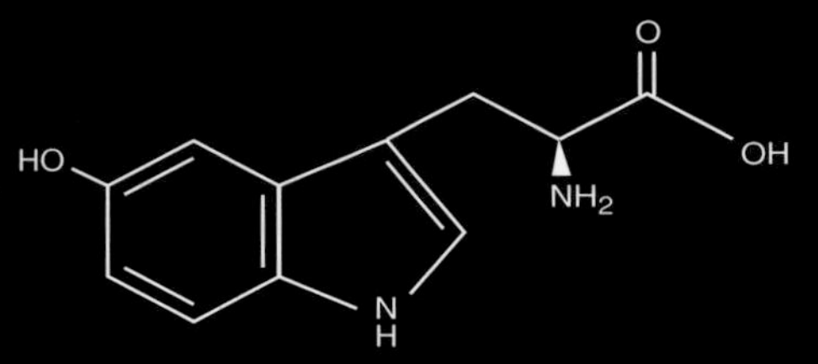

5-Hydroxytryptophan

5-Hydroxytryptophan

Introduction

5-Hydroxytryptophan (5-HTP) is the intermediate metabolite of the amino acid L-tryptophan (LT) in the serotonin pathway. It is dedicated to this pathway; i.e., it cannot be converted back into tryptophan, but can only go on to serotonin and its metabolites. This conversion is dependent on the presence of the active form of vitamin B6, pyridoxal-5' phosphate. Therapeutic use of 5-HTP bypasses the conversion of LT into 5-HTP by the enzyme tryptophan hydrolase, which is the rate-limiting step in the synthesis of serotonin. Tryptophan hydrolase can be inhibited by numerous factors, including stress, insulin resistance, vitamin B6 deficiency, insufficient magnesium, and increasing age.[1] In addition, these same factors can increase the conversion of LT to kynurenine via tryptophan oxygenase, making LT unavailable for serotonin production.

5-HTP is used therapeutically to treat depression, obesity, chronic headaches, insomnia, and fibromyalgia, and is commercially produced by extraction from the seeds of the African plant,*Griffonia simplicifolia*.

Pharmacokinetics

5-HTP is well absorbed from an oral dose, with about 70 percent reaching the bloodstream.[2,3] Absorption of 5-HTP is not affected by the presence of other amino acids; therefore it may be taken with meals without reducing its effectiveness. Unlike LT, 5-HTP cannot be shunted into niacin or protein production.

Serotonin levels in the brain are highly dependent on levels of 5-HTP and LT in the central nervous system (CNS). 5-HTP easily crosses the blood-brain barrier, not requiring the presence of a transport molecule. LT, on the other hand, requires use of a transport molecule to gain access to the CNS. Since it shares this transport molecule with several other amino acids, the presence of these competing amino acids can inhibit LT transport into the brain.

Mechanisms of Action

5-HTP acts primarily by increasing levels of serotonin within the central nervous system. Other neurotransmitters and CNS chemicals, such as melatonin, dopamine, norepinephrine, and beta-endorphin have also been shown to increase following oral administration of 5-HTP.[4-7]

Clinical Indications

Depression

Numerous open and double-blind studies of patients with either unipolar or bipolar depression have demonstrated significant clinical response in 2 to 4 weeks at doses of 50-300 mg 5-HTP three times per day.[8-14] In a study comparing 5-HTP and the serotonin reuptake inhibitor fluvoxamine, 5-HTP was as effective as fluvoxamine in relieving depressive symptoms.[15]

Fibromyalgia

Fibromyalgia patients have been found to have low serotonin levels, which can contribute to a low pain threshold. Three clinical trials of 5-HTP administration, totaling 300 patients, demonstrated significant improvement in fibromyalgia symptoms, including pain, morning stiffness, anxiety, and fatigue.[16-19]

Obesity

Decreased caloric intake during dieting can lower serum tryptophan and CNS serotonin levels. Low serotonin levels in obese patients have been associated with carbohydrate cravings and resultant binge eating. Three studies with 5-HTP in obese patients resulted in decreased food intake and subsequent weight loss.[20-22] In a double-blind, placebo-controlled study, patients took either 300 mg 5-HTP three times per day or placebo, and followed no specific dietary regimen for six weeks. During the following six weeks, both groups were instructed to continue supplementation and follow a 1,200-calorie per day diet. The 5-HTP group spontaneously reduced carbohydrate intake and total caloric intake in the first six-week period, and was able to follow the decreased caloric intake in the second six-week period, resulting in significant weight loss compared to placebo.[20]

Insomnia

5-HTP has been shown to be beneficial in treating insomnia, especially in improving sleep quality by increasing REM sleep.[23-26]

Chronic Headache

5-HTP has been used successfully in the prevention of chronic headaches of various types, including migraine, tension headaches, and juvenile headaches.[16,27-34]

Drug-Nutrient Interactions

Although no reports have been published, it is possible that 5-HTP, when taken in combination with a selective serotonin reuptake inhibitor (SSRI) antidepressant such as Prozac®, Paxil®, or Zoloft®, may cause a condition known as serotonin syndrome. This syndrome is characterized by agitation, confusion, delirium, tachycardia, diaphoresis, and blood pressure fluctuations.

Side Effects and Toxicity

Because some patients may experience mild nausea when initiating treatment with 5-HTP, it is advisable to begin with a 50 mg dose and titrate upward.

Dosage

Initial dosage for 5-HTP is usually 50 mg three times per day with meals. If clinical response is inadequate after two weeks, dosage may be increased to 100 mg three times per day. For depression, doses of 50-300 mg 5-HTP three times per day have been used. In fibromyalgia, 100 mg twice or three times per day has been successful. Obesity studies used a higher dose, 300 mg three times per day. For insomnia, the dosage is usually 100-300 mg before bedtime. For chronic headaches, 200 mg three times per day has been used.

Warnings and Contraindications

5-HTP should not be used in patients currently being treated or who have recently been treated with an SSRI antidepressant.

References

1. Hussain AM, Mitra AK. Effect of aging on tryptophan hydroxylase in rat brain: implications on serotonin level. *Drug Metab Dispos* 2000;28:1038-1042.
2. Magnussen IE, Nielsen-Kudsk F. Bioavailability and related pharmacokinetics in man of orally administered L-5-hydroxytryptophan in a steady state. *Acta Pharmacol Toxicol* 1980;46:257-262.
3. Magnussen I, Jensen TS, Rand JH, Van Woert MH. Plasma accumulation of metabolism of orally administered single dose L-5-hydroxytryptophan in man. *Acta Pharmacol Toxicol* 1981;49:184-189.
4. van Praag HM, Lemus C. Monoamine precursors in the treatment of psychiatric disorders. In: Wurtman RJ, Wurtman JJ, eds. *Nutrition and the Brain.* New York: Raven Press; 1986:89-139.
5. den Boer JA, Westenberg HG. Behavioral, neuroendocrine, and biochemical effects of 5-hydroxytryptophan administration in panic disorder. *Psychiatry Res* 1990;31:267-278.
6. Chadwick D, Jenner P, Harris R, et al. Manipulation of brain serotonin in the treatment of myoclonus. *Lancet* 1975;2:434-435.
7. Guilleminault C, Tharp BR, Cousin D. HVA and 5HIAA CSF measurements and 5HTP trials in some patients with involuntary movements. *J Neurol Sci* 1973;18:435-441.
8. van Praag H, de Hann S. Depression vulnerability and 5-hydroxytryptophan prophylaxis. *Psychiatry Res* 1980;3:75-83.
9. Loo H, Zarifian E, Wirth JF, Deniker P. Open study of L-5-H.T.P. in melancholic depressed patients over 50 years of age. *Encephale* 1980;6:241-246.

10. van Hiele LJ. L-5-Hydroxytryptophan in depression: the first substitution therapy in psychiatry? The treatment of 99 out-patients with "therapy-resistant" depressions. *Neuropsychobiology* 1980;6:230-240.

11. Angst J, Woggon B, Schoepf J. The treatment of depression with L-5-hydroxytryptophan versus imipramine. Results of two open and one double-blind study. *Arch Psychiatr Nervenkr* 1977;224:175-186.

12. Alino JJ, Gutierrez JL, Iglesias ML. 5-Hydroxytryptophan (5-HTP) and a MAOI (nialamide) in the treatment of depressions. A double-blind controlled study. *Int Pharmacopsychiatry* 1976;11:8-15.

13. Takahashi S, Kondo H, Kato N. Effect of L-5-hydroxytryptophan on brain monoamine metabolism and evaluation of its clinical effect in depressed patients. *J Psychiatr Res* 1975;12:177-187.

14. Persson T, Roos BE. 5-hydroxytryptophan for depression. *Lancet* 1967;2:987-988.

15. Poldinger W, Calanchini B, Schwartz W. A functional-dimensional approach to depression: serotonin deficiency as a target syndrome in a comparison of 5-hydroxytryptophan and fluvoxamine. *Psychopathology* 1991;24:53-81.

16. Nicolodi M, Sicuteri F. Fibromyalgia and migraine, two faces of the same mechanism. Serotonin as the common clue for pathogenesis and therapy. *Adv Exp Med Biol* 1996;398:373-379.

17. Puttini PS, Caruso I. Primary fibromyalgia syndrome and 5-hydroxy-L-tryptophan: a 90-day open study. *J Int Med Res* 1992;20:182-189.

18. Caruso I, Sarzi Puttini P, Cazzola M, Azzolini V. Double-blind study of 5-hydroxytryptophan versus placebo in the treatment of primary fibromyalgia syndrome. *J Int Med Res* 1990;18:201-209.

19. Neeck G. Neuroendocrine and hormonal perturbations and relations to the serotonergic system in fibromyalgia patients. *Scand J Rheumatol* 2000;113;8-12.

20. Cangiano C, Ceci F, Cascino A, et al. Eating behavior and adherence to dietary prescriptions in obese adult subjects treated with 5-hydroxytryptophan. *Am J Clin Nutr* 1992;56:863-867.

21. Cangiano C, Ceci F, Cairella M, et al. Effects of 5-hydroxytryptophan on eating behavior and adherence to dietary prescriptions in obese adult subjects. *Adv Exp Med Biol* 1991;294:591-593.

22. Ceci F, Cangiano C, Cairella M, et al. The effects of oral 5-hydroxytryptophan administration on feeding behavior in obese adult female subjects. *J Neural Transm* 1989;76:109-117.

23. Soulairac A, Lambinet H. Effect of 5-hydroxytryptophan, a serotonin precursor, on sleep disorders. *Ann Med Psychol* 1977;1:792-798.

24. Guilleminault C, Cathala JP, Castaigne P. Effects of 5-hydroxytryptophan on sleep of a patient with a brain-stem lesion. *Electroencephalogr Clin Neurophysiol* 1973;34:177-184.

25. Wyatt RJ, Zarcone V, Engelman K, et al. Effects of 5-hydroxytryptophan on the sleep of normal human subjects. *Electroencephalogr Clin Neurophysiol* 1971;30:505-509.

26. Python A, Steimer T, de Saint Hilaire Z, et al. Extracellular serotonin variations during vigilance states in the preoptic area of rats: a microdialysis study. *Brain Res* 2001;910:49-54.

27. Nicolodi M, Sicuteri F. L-5-hydroxytryptophan can prevent nociceptive disorders in man. *Adv Exp Med Biol* 1999;467:177-182.

28. Riberio CA. L-5-Hydroxytryptophan in the prophylaxis of chronic tension-type headache: a double-blind, randomized, placebo-controlled study. For the Portuguese Head Society. *Headache* 2000;40:451-456.

29. Maissen CP, Ludin HP. Comparison of the effect of 5-hydroxytryptophan and propranolol in the interval treatment of migraine. *Schweiz Med Wochenschr* 1991;121:1585-1590.

30. De Giorgis G, Miletto R, Iannuccelli M, et al. Headache in association with sleep disorders in children: a psychodiagnostic evaluation and controlled clinical study-L-5-HTP versus placebo. *Drugs Exp Clin Res* 1987;13:425-433.

31. Titus F, Davalos A, Alom J, Codina A. 5-Hydroxytryptophan versus methysergide in the prophylaxis of migraine. Randomized clinical trial. *Eur Neurol* 1986;25:327-329.

32. De Benedittis G, Massei R. Serotonin precursors in chronic primary headache. A double-blind cross-over study with L-5-hydroxytryptophan vs. placebo. *J Neurosurg Sci* 1985;29:239-248.

33. Longo G, Rudoi I, Iannuccelli M, et al. Treatment of essential headache in developmental age with L-5-HTP (cross over double-blind study versus placebo). *Pediatr Med Chir* 1984;6:241-245.

34. Bono G, Criscuoli M, Martignoni E, et al. Serotonin precursors in migraine prophylaxis. *Adv Neurol* 1982;33:357-363.

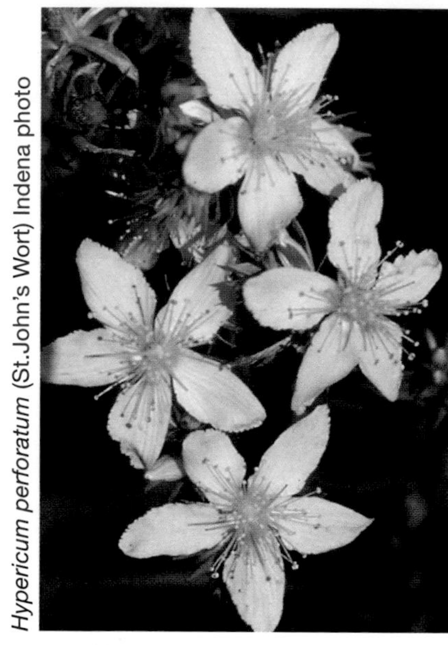

Hypericum perforatum (St.John's Wort) Indena photo

Hypericum perforatum

Description

Hypericum perforatum L. (St. John's wort) is a five-petalled, yellow-flowered perennial weed common to the western United States, Europe, and Asia.[1] Close examination of the flowers reveals small black dots that, when rubbed between the fingers, produce a red stain. This red pigment contains the constituent hypericin. Held up to light, the leaves of the plant display a number of bright, translucent dots. This perforated look led to the botanical name perforatum. The plant is currently cultivated in Europe, North and South America, Australia, and China.[2] The aerial parts of the plant are harvested during the flowering season and used in modern, standardized extracts.

Dioscorides, the foremost physician of ancient Greece, as well as Pliny and Hippocrates, recommended the herb for a host of ailments including sciatica and poisonous bites. The name St. John's wort has its origin in Christian folk tradition. The golden flowers of the plant are thought to be particularly abundant on June 24, the day traditionally celebrated as the birthday of John the Baptist.[3] St. John's wort has a long history of use in traditional European herbal medicine. It was, and continues to be, used as a topical treatment for wounds and burns. It has also been used as a folk remedy for kidney and lung ailments, as well as mood disorders.

Active Constituents

St. John's wort has a complex and diverse chemical makeup. Constituents include volatile oils (0.05 to 0.3%, including α-pinene, and cineole), anthraquinones, carotenoids, cumarine, flavonoids (0.5 to 1.0%, including hyperoside and rutin), naphthodianthrones (0.1 to 0.3% of which 80-90% are hypericin and psuedohypericin), carbolic acids, phloroglucins (up to 3% hyperforin), xanthones, and proanthocyanidins.[1] The naphthodianthrones hypericin and pseudohypericin previously received most of the attention in pharmacological studies. This is based on their contributions to the antiviral properties of the plant as well as speculation (based on early in vitro data) that they may also contribute to the plant's antidepressant actions.[4] This may partially explain why many extracts continue to be standardized to contain measured amounts of hypericin. Recent research, however, indicates that other constituents such as hyperforin[5,6] and possibly flavonoid compounds may also contribute to the antidepressant actions of the plant.

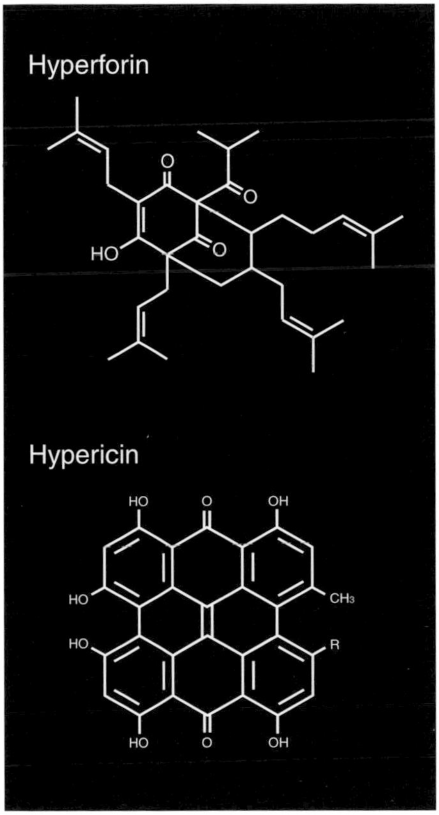

Hyperforin

Hypericin

Mechanisms of Action

A number of proposed mechanisms exist for St. John's wort's antidepressant effect, involving several neurotransmitters and hormones. Initially, inhibition of monoamine oxidase (MAO) was believed to be the primary mode of action,[7] and was thought to be due primarily to hypericin.[8] More recent research indicates constituents of St. John's wort exert MAO inhibition only at concentrations higher than those typically found in commercially available extracts.[9,10]

Attention over the past few years has shifted to the ability of St. John's wort and the constituent hyperforin to inhibit synaptosomal re-uptake of serotonin, norepinephrine, and dopamine.[11,12] Two human pharmacological studies demonstrating an increase in cortisol levels following administration of two different St. John's wort extracts have recently been reported to support this proposed mechanism of action.[13,14] Although this has been the topic of much debate among European researchers, it has led to some commercial extracts providing standardized amounts (3-5%) of hyperforin.

Clinical Indications

Depression

A meta-analysis published in1996 of 23 studies involving over 1,500 individuals found significantly positive responses to St. John's wort based on analysis of the Hamilton Depression Scale (HAMD) before and after treatment.[15] This was supported by a more recent meta-analysis covering clinical trials published through 2000.[16] In 2000, the Annals of Internal Medicine featured a two-part overview and critique of newer drug therapies for depression and dysthymia (a chronic but milder form of depression) and included St. John's wort as a potential treatment for both conditions.[17,18] Both reviews conclude St. John's wort is more effective than placebo for the treatment of mild to moderate depression and less likely to cause side effects than commonly prescribed antidepressants. However, the authors suggest that problems with publication bias leading to overzealous reporting of results as well as lack of standardized dosing should be addressed in future clinical studies. Additionally, they suggest future studies be longer in duration and include more head-to-head comparisons with newer antidepressants such as the SSRIs.

The 2000 meta-analysis of St. John's wort clinical trials lists 16 placebo-controlled trials on persons with mild to moderate depression.[16] These studies lasted from 4 to 12 weeks, with doses varying between 500-900 mg per day. Many of these trials were completed using 300 mg of the LI 160 extract (standardized to 0.3% hypericin) three times per day.[19-21] A significant decrease in HAMD scores compared to placebo was found in all trials. Similar results have been noted for an extract designated ZE 117,[22] as well as an extract standardized to 0.3% hyperforin with the designator WS 5572.[23,24]

A well-publicized 8-week, placebo-controlled trial published in the Journal of the American Medical Association found 900-1200 mg of St. John's wort per day was ineffective in treating severe depression.[25] The study results have been challenged due to the low placebo response reported (18.6%), the dose used, and the inclusion of patients with more severe depression than in previous trials with St. John's wort.

At least 12 clinical trials have compared St. John's wort directly to prescription antidepressants, including imipramine, amitriptyline, and fluoxetine in persons with mild to moderate depression.[16] Earlier clinical trials comparing 900 mg of St. John's wort per day with imipramine (75 mg/day) or amitriptyline (75 mg/day) in patients with mild to moderate depression found St. John's wort extract (LI 160) to be equally effective in lowering HAMD scores, with fewer side effects.[26,27] However, these trials have been criticized due to the low dose of the standard antidepressant and lack of a placebo group. One trial comparing 1,050 mg of St. John's wort per day with 100 mg/day of imipramine or placebo did find St. John's wort was safe and effective in treating mild to moderate depression.[28] More recently, 500 mg of the ZE 117 extract was as effective as 150 mg of imipramine in a six-week clinical trial that also lacked a placebo arm.[29]

Two double-blind, randomized trials (with no placebo arm) have suggested that 500 mg[30] or 800 mg[31] per day of St. John's wort is as effective as 20 mg/day of fluoxetine (Prozac®). Both trials lasted six weeks and noted that patients taking St. John's wort reported fewer side effects. A small, seven-week pilot study found St. John's wort (900 mg/day) was as effective as 75 mg/day of sertraline (Zoloft®).[32] A larger (340 participants) eight-week trial of St. John's wort compared to sertraline and placebo in major depression noted a high placebo response that resulted in neither St. John's wort extract nor sertraline being significantly different from placebo. However, it did show that St. John's wort was as effective as the prescription drug.[33]

Seasonal Affective Disorder

A small pilot study and a larger open-label study suggested patients suffering from seasonal affective disorder (SAD) may benefit from taking 300 mg St. John's wort extract three times per day for eight weeks.[34,35] Placebo-controlled trials are needed to confirm the efficacy of St. John's wort for SAD.

Drug-Botanical Interactions

Concomitant use of St. John's wort extract with selective serotonin reuptake inhibitors (SSRIs) has resulted in serotonin syndrome in two previous case reports[36,37] and was reported in two individuals in a recent report on the safety and efficacy of St. John's wort based on a local survey completed by the University of Missouri.[38]

Case reports and/or pharmacological studies have indicated that St. John's wort may reduce serum levels of the following drugs: indinavir, cyclosporine, theophylline, digoxin, warfarin, and oral birth control pills.[39-47] The most direct effect on serum levels in patients taking St. John's wort has been found with cyclosporine[40-43] and indinavir.[39] Patients taking these medications should avoid concomitant use of St. John's wort. The popular opinion for these interactions is based on in vitro studies suggesting St. John's wort causes induction of the cytochrome P450 isoenzyme CYP3A4.[48,49] However, both *in vitro* and *in vivo* studies have not supported this finding.[50,51] Further studies will hopefully clarify the extent St. John's wort interacts with the cytochrome P450 system and provide more focus to potential drug interactions for the herb.

Safety and Toxicity

In a drug monitoring study of 3,250 patients taking 900 mg/day of St. John's wort, adverse events were reported in 2.4 percent of subjects, the most common being gastrointestinal irritation, restlessness, fatigue, and allergic skin reactions.[52]

St. John's wort may cause the skin and eyes to become photosensitive.[53] There is a case report of a woman experiencing neuropathy (nerve injury and pain) in sun-exposed skin areas after taking 500 mg of whole St. John's wort for four weeks.[54] However, one pharmacological study found doses as high as 3,600 mg (11.25 mg of hypericin) did not increase photosensitivity.[55] Fair-skinned individuals should take precautions when exposed to the sun while taking St. John's wort. It is advisable that elderly people taking St. John's wort also use protective eyewear when exposed to the sun. Although the German Commission E lists no contraindications to use of St. John's wort during pregnancy or lactation,[56] the basis for this statement appears to be based more on historical use than actual safety studies.

Patients taking St. John's wort as an antidepressant should be closely questioned about any history of bipolar disorder. There have been several case reports of St. John's wort causing mania in patients with this history.[57-60]

Dosage

Typical daily dosages of standardized St. John's wort extracts range from 500 to 1,050 mg for the treatment of mild to moderate depression. The dose is typically divided over two to three doses throughout the day. It may take two to four weeks to notice clinical results.

References

1. Wichtl M. *Herbal Drugs and Phytopharmaceuticals*. Boca Raton, FL: CRC Press; 1994:273-275.
2. Blumenthal M, Goldberg A, Brinckmann J, eds. *Herbal Medicine: Expanded Commission E Monographs.* Newton, MA: Integrative Medicine Communications; 2000:359-366.
3. Foster S, Tyler VE. *Tyler's Honest Herbal*. New York: Haworth Press; 1999:331-333.
4. Schulz V, Hansel R, Tyler VE. *Rational Phytotherapy: A Physicians' Guide to Herbal Medicine*. Berlin: Springer-Verlag; 2001:57-77.
5. Chatterjee SS, Bhattacharya SK, Wonnemann M, et al. Hyperforin as a possible antidepressant component of Hypericum extracts. *Life Sciences* 1998;63:499-510.
6. Muller WE, Singer A, Wonnemann M. Hyperforin–antidepressant activity by a novel mechanism of action. *Pharmacopsychiatry* 2001;34:S98-S102.
7. Suzuki O, Katsumata Y, Oya M. Inhibition of monoamine oxidase by hypericin. *Planta Med* 1984;50:272-274.
8. Holzl J, Demisch L, Gollnik B. Investigations about antidepressive and mood changing effects of *Hypericum perforatum. Planta Med* 1989;55:643.
9. Bladt S, Wagner H. Inhibition of MAO by fractions and constituents of Hypericum extract. *J Geriatr Psychiatry Neurol* 1994;7:S57-S59.
10. Thiede HM, Walper A. Inhibition of MAO and COMT by Hypericum extracts and Hypericin. *J Geriatr Psychiatry Neurol* 1994;7:S54-S56.
11. Muller WE, Rolli M, Schafer C, Hafner U. Effects of hypericum extract (LI 160) in biochemical models of antidepressant activity. *Pharmacopsychiatry* 1997;30:S102-S107.
12. Muller WE, Singer A, Wonnemann M, et al. Hyperforin represents the neurotransmitter reuptake inhibiting constituent of hypericum extract. *Pharmacopsychiatry* 1998;31:S16-S21.
13. Schule C, Baghai T, Ferrera A, Laakmann G. Neuroendocrine effects of Hypericum extract WS 5570 in 12 healthy male volunteers. *Pharmacopsychiatry* 2001;34: S127-S133.
14. Franklin M, Cowen PJ. Researching the antidepressant actions of *Hypericum perforatum* (St. John's wort) in animals and man. *Pharmacopsychiatry* 2001;34: S29-S37.
15. Linde K, Ramirez G, Mulrow C, et al. St. John's wort for depression – an overview and meta-analysis of randomized clinical trials. *BMJ* 1996;313:253-261.
16. Kasper S. *Hypericum perforatum*–a review of clinical studies. *Pharmacopsychiatry* 2001;34:S51-S55.
17. Snow V, Lascher S, Mottur-Pilson C. Pharmacologic treatment of acute major depression and dysthymia: Clinical guideline, Part 1. *Ann Intern Med* 2000;132:738-742.
18. Williams JW, Mulrow CD, Chiquette E, et al. A systematic review of newer pharmacotherapies for depression in adults–evidence report summary: Clinical guideline, Part 2. *Ann Intern Med* 2000;132:743-756.
19. Sommer H, Harrer G. Placebo-controlled double blind study examining the effectiveness of an Hypericum preparation in 105 mildly depressed patients. *J Geriatr Psychiatry Neurol* 1994;7:S9-S11.
20. Hansgen KD, Vesper J, Ploch M. Multicenter double-blind study examining the antidepressant effectiveness of the Hypericum extract LI 160. *J Geriatr Psychiatry Neurol* 1994;7:S15-S18.

21. Montgomery SA, Hubner WD, Grigoleit HG. Efficacy and tolerability of St. John's wort extract compared with placebo in patients with mild to moderate depressive disorder. *Phytomedicine* 2000;7:S107.
22. Schrader E, Meier B, Brattsrom A. Hypercium treatment of mild-moderate depression in a placebo-controlled study. A prospective, double-blind, randomized, placebo-controlled, multicenter study. *Human Psychopharmacol* 1998;13:163-169.
23. Laakman G, Schule C, Baghai T, Kieser M. St. John's wort in mild to moderate depression: the relevance of hyperforin for the clinical efficacy. *Pharmacopsychiatry* 1998;31:S54-S59.
24. Kalb R, Trautmann-Sponsel RD, Kieser M. Efficacy and tolerability of Hypericum extract WS 5572 versus placebo in mildly to moderately depressed patients. *Pharmacopsychiatry* 2001;34:96-103.
25. Shelton RC, Keller MB, Gelenberg A, et al. Effectiveness of St. John's wort in major depression: A randomized trial. *JAMA* 2001;285:1978-1986.
26. Vorbach EU, H¸bner WD, Arnoldt KH. Effectiveness and tolerance of the Hypericum extract LI 160 in comparison with imipramine: Randomized double-blind study with 135 outpatients. *J Geriatr Psychiatry Neurol* 1994;7:S19-S23.
27. Wheatley D. LI 160, an extract of St. John's wort versus amitriptyline in mildly to moderately depressed outpatients–controlled six week clinical trial. *Pharmacopsychiatry* 1997;30:S77-S80.
28. Philipp M, Kohnen R, Hiller KO. Hypericum extract versus imipramine or placebo in patients with moderate depression: randomized multicenter study of treatment for eight weeks. *BMJ* 1999;319:1534-1539.
29. Woelk H. Comparison of St. John's wort and imipramine for treating depression: Randomized controlled trial. *BMJ* 2000;321:536-539.
30. Schrader D. Equivalence of St. John's wort extract (ZE 117) and fluoxetine: a randomized, controlled study in mild-moderate depression. *Intl Clin Psychopharmacol* 2000;15:61-68.
31. Harrer G, Schmidt U, Kuhn U, Biller A. Comparison of equivalence between the St. John's wort extract LoHyp-57 and fluoxetine. *Arzneimittelforschung* 1999;49:289-296.
32. Brenner R, Azbel V, Madhusoodanan S, Pawlowska M. Comparison of an extract of Hypericum (LI 160) and sertraline in the treatment of depression: A double-blind, randomized pilot study. *Clin Ther* 2000;22:411-419.
33. Hypericum Depression Trial Study Group. Effect of *Hypericum perforatum* (St. John's wort) in major depressive disorder: a randomized controlled trial. *JAMA* 2002;287:1807-1814.
34. Kasper S. Treatment of seasonal affective disorder (SAD) with Hypericum extract. *Pharmacopsychiatry* 1997;30:S89-S93.
35. Wheatley D. Hypericum in seasonal affective disorder (SAD). *Curr Med Res Opin* 1999;15:33-37.
36. Demott K. St. John's wort tied to serotonin syndrome. *Clin Psychiatry News* 1998;26:28.
37. Gordon JB. SSRIs and St. John's wort: possible toxicity? *Am Family Physician* 1998;57:950.
38. Bekman SE, Sommi RW, Switzer J. Consumer use of St. John's wort: A survey on effectiveness, safety, and tolerability. *Pharmacotherapy* 2000;20:568-5674.
39. Piscitelli SC, Burstein AH, Chaitt D, et al. Indinavir concentrations and St. John's wort. *Lancet* 2000;355:547-548. [letter]
40. Ruschitzka F, Meier P, Turina M, et al. Acute transplant rejection due to Saint John's wort. *Lancet* 2000;355:548-549. [letter]
41. Breidenbach T, Hoffmann MW, Becker T, et al. Drug interaction of St. John's wort with cyclosporin. *Lancet* 2000;355:1912. [letter]
42. Karilova M, Treichel U, Malago M, et al. Interaction of *Hypericum perforatum* (St. John's wort) with cyclosporine A metabolism in a patient after liver transplantation. *J Hepatology* 2000;33:853-855.
43. Barone GW, Gurley BJ, Ketel BL, et al. Drug interaction between St. John's wort and cyclosporine. *Ann Pharmacother* 2000;34:1013-1016.

44. Nebel A, Schneider BJ, Baker RK, Kroll DJ. Potential metabolic interaction between St. John's wort and theophylline. *Ann Pharmacother* 1999;33:502. [letter]

45. Maurer A, Johne A, Bauer S, et al. Interaction of St. John's wort extract with phenprocoumon. *Eur J Clin Pharmacol* 1999;55:A22.

46. Johne A, Brockmuller J, Bauer S, et al. Pharmacokinetic interaction of digoxin with an herbal extract from St. John's wort (*Hypericum perforatum*). *Clin Pharmacol Ther* 1999;66:338-345.

47. Ernst E. Second thoughts about safety of St. John's wort. *Lancet* 1999;354:2014-2016. [letter]

48. Roby CA, Anderson GD, Kantor E, et al. St. John's wort: Effect on CYP3A4 activity. *Clin Pharmacol Ther* 2000;67:451-457.

49. Moore LB, Goodwin B, Jones SA, et al. St. John's wort induces hepatic drug metabolism through activation of the pregnane X receptor. *Proc Natl Acad Sci USA* 2000;97:7500-7502.

50. Noldner M, Chatterjee S. Effects of two different extracts of St. John's wort and some of their constituents on cytochrome P450 activities in rat liver microsomes. *Pharmacopsychiatry* 2001;34:S108-S110.

51. Markowitz JS, DeVane CL, Boulton DW, et al. Effect of St. John's wort (*Hypericum perforatum*) on cytochrome P-450 2D6 and 3A4 activity in healthy volunteers. *Pharmacol Letters* 2000;66:133-139.

52. Woelk H, Burkhard G, Grunwald J. Benefits and risks of the Hypericum extract LI 160: Drug monitoring study with 3250 patients. *J Geriat Psychiatry Neurol* 1994;7:S34-S38.

53. Lane-Brown MM. Photosensitivity associated with herbal preparations of St. John's wort *(Hypericum perforatum). Med J Aust* 2000;172:302. [letter]

54. Bove GM. Acute neuropathy after exposure to sun in a patient treated with St John's Wort. *Lancet* 1998;352:1121-1122. [letter]

55. Brockmoller J, Reum T, Bauer S, et al. Hypericin and pseudohypericin: Pharmacokinetics and effects on photosensitivity in humans. *Pharmacopsychiatry* 1997;30:S94-S101.

56. Blumenthal M, Busse WR, Goldberg A, et al, eds. *The Complete Commission E Monographs*. Boston, MA: Integrative Medicine Communications; 1998:214-215.

57. Nierenberg AA, Burt T, Matthews J, Weiss AP. Mania associated with St. John's wort. *Biol Psychiatry* 1999;46:1707-1708.

58. Moses EL, Mallinger AG. St. John's wort: Three cases of possible mania induction. *J Clin Psychopharmacol* 2000;20:115-117.

59. O'Breasail AM, Argouarch S. Hypomania and St John's wort. *Can J Psychiatry* 1998;43:746-747. [letter]

60. Schneck C. St. John's wort and hypomania. *J Clin Psychiatry* 1998;59:689. [letter]

Idebenone

Introduction

Idebenone [2,3-dimethoxy-5-methyl-6-(10-hydroxydecyl)-1,4-benzoquinone] is a synthetic analogue of coenzyme Q10 (CoQ10), the vital cell membrane antioxidant and essential constituent of the ATP-producing mitochondrial electron transport chain (ETC). Idebenone is a potent antioxidant, with the ability to operate under low oxygen tension situations. Because of its ability to inhibit lipid peroxidation, idebenone protects cell membranes and mitochondria from oxidative damage. Its antioxidant properties protect against cerebral ischemia and nerve damage in the central nervous system. Idebenone also interacts with the ETC, preserving ATP formation in ischemic states. This compound has also been shown to stimulate nerve growth factor, a characteristic that could be important in the treatment of Alzheimer's and other neurodegenerative diseases.

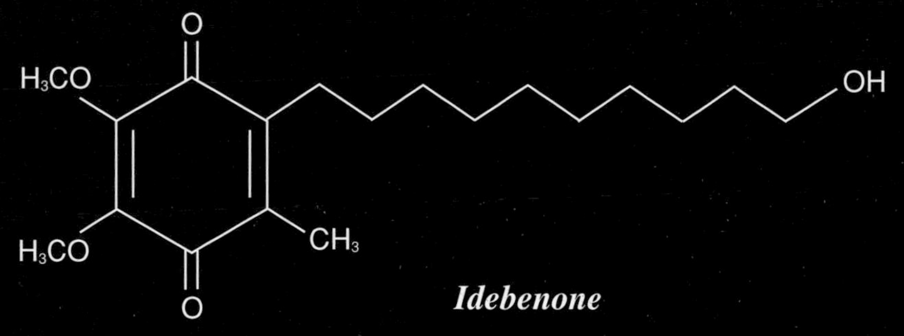

Idebenone

Pharmacokinetics

Idebenone is rapidly absorbed and reaches peak concentrations in the brain comparable to those in plasma.[1] Animal studies showed a peak plasma level 15 minutes after oral administration, with a half-life of 2.2-15.4 hours. Idebenone was well distributed in tissues, with higher concentrations in the gut, liver, and kidney. Excretion was via both urine and feces, mostly as metabolites.[2] A human pharmacokinetic and safety study found a half-life of 18 hours, with biphasic elimination.[3] Researchers found no long-term tissue accumulation in humans or rats.[2,3]

Mechanisms of Action

As with other antioxidants, idebenone exists in a reduced and an oxidized state. In a study of idebenone's effect on astroglial cells, idebenone, in either redox state, significantly inhibited the enzymatic metabolism of arachidonic acid by cyclooxygenase and lipoxygenase. This effect was stronger with the reduced form, and showed potential central nervous system anti-inflammatory activity.[4]

Introduction of iron and ascorbate to a cell mixture or a group of isolated cells can establish experimental cellular oxidant injury. Synaptosomes isolated from rat brain cortex were treated with iron and ascorbate. Idebenone prevented both the formation of reactive oxygen species in the cytosol and mitochondria, as well as a decrease in protein-sulfhydryl content (an indicator of protein oxidation), compared to controls.[5]

It appears that, in addition to functioning as an antioxidant, idebenone functions as an electron carrier in the ETC, similar to CoQ10. To illustrate, researchers in Japan introduced idebenone into a canine CoQ10-depleted brain mitochondrial preparation, which prevented the loss of ETC activity normally seen with CoQ10 depletion. Idebenone also inhibited mitochondrial lipid peroxidation,[6] which can be interpreted as protecting against mitochondrial membrane damage. Other animal studies confirm the mitochondrial membrane protective effects of idebenone.[7,8]

Idebenone treatment of rats with experimental cerebral ischemia inhibited the loss of acetylcholine in forebrain regions, prevented increases in lactate and free fatty acids, and preserved ATP content in the cerebral cortex. These results indicate idebenone protects against ischemic damage and promotes ATP production in the brain.[9,10]

Clinical Indications

Alzheimer's Disease

Nerve growth factor plays an important role in the growth, survival, and preservation of cholinergic neurons in the central nervous system. In Alzheimer's disease, cholinergic neurons can become damaged and die. In a rat study, oral administration of idebenone stimulated increases in nerve growth factor protein, mRNA, and choline acetyltransferase activity in basal forebrain lesioned rats. Idebenone also improved behavioral deficits in habituation, water maze, and passive avoidance tasks, which suggests idebenone might stimulate nerve growth factor synthesis *in vivo*. Similar results were found in aged rats.[11-13]

Amyloid beta-peptide (ABP), the major constituent of senile plaques in Alzheimer's disease, is neurotoxic, possibly via an oxidative stress mechanism. Rats given an intracerebroventricular infusion of ABP demonstrated significant impairment of memory and behavior, which was prevented when idebenone and alpha tocopherol were given orally before and during ABP infusion.[14] In a double-blind, placebo-controlled multi-center human study, 450 patients were given either placebo for 12 months, followed by idebenone 90 mg three times per day for another 12 months; 90 mg three times per day for 24 months; or 120 mg three times per day for 24 months. Significant dose-dependent improvements were seen in measurements of clinical status and in neuropsychiatric tests compared to placebo. These improvements continued over the two-year study.[15]

Three hundred patients with mild-to-moderate Alzheimer's disease were randomized to receive either placebo, idebenone 30 mg three times per day, or 90 mg three times per day for six months. Statistically significant improvement was noted in the total score of the Alzheimer's Disease Assessment Scale (ADAS-total), and in one cognitive parameter (ADAS-cog). An analysis of therapy responders revealed significant improvement in three outcome measures (clinical global response, ADAS-Cog, and non-cognitive scores) in the idebenone 90 mg three times per day group, compared to placebo.[16] Other studies have confirmed these findings.[17]

Liver Disease

Oxidative stress has been implicated in a number of hepatic diseases, including bile acid-induced liver injury in hepatic cholestasis, which was evaluated in an *in vitro* study. Treatment with idebenone protected against bile acid-induced rat hepatocellular injury and lipid peroxidation, and prevented hydroperoxide production in hepatic mitochondria.[18]

Cerebrovascular Disease

In a small human study of nine patients with cerebrovascular disease, 90 mg idebenone was given daily, and electroencephalograms and clinical symptoms were monitored. The results suggested that idebenone supplementation produced improvements in EEG and clinical symptoms in these patients.[19]

Friedreich's Ataxia

Friedreich's ataxia (FA), an autosomal recessive spinal ataxia, is characterized by unsteady gait, weakness, sensory loss, upper extremity ataxia, mental decline, and progressive cardiomyopathy. The pathophysiology of FA is due to a deficiency of frataxin, a protein involved in regulation of mitochondrial iron content, which causes oxidative damage from mitochondrial iron overload. This leads to a deficiency in mitochondrial enzymes, reduced energy output, and mitochondrial damage. Idebenone dosing (5 mg/kg daily for 8 weeks) in FA patients significantly decreased a marker of oxidative DNA damage.[20] Idebenone prevented iron-induced lipoperoxidation and cardiac muscle injury in three patients given 5 mg/kg daily for 4-9 months, resulting in a reduction of left ventricular enlargement in these patients.[21]

Side Effects and Toxicity

Two hundred Alzheimer's disease patients received either 90 mg or 270 mg idebenone per day for six months. No significant adverse events or changes in vital signs, ECG or clinical laboratory parameters were noted.[16] Barkworth et al gave 10 healthy male volunteers 300 mg per day for 35 days. No changes were seen in blood and urine lab values, and the dose was well tolerated.[3] Safety and tolerability of idebenone were good and similar to placebo during a two-year study utilizing doses up to 360 mg per day.[15] A 900 mg per day dose was given to 17 men for four weeks, with no adverse effects seen on electroretinography, auditory evoked potentials, or visual analogue scales.[22]

Dosage

Typical clinical dosages are 100-300 mg per day.

Warnings and Contraindications

Idebenone has been found to inhibit platelet aggregation *in vitro*, by inhibition of phospholipase B2 production,[23] which might contraindicate its use in patients already on anti-clotting therapy or in those with a history of – or at risk for – hemorrhagic stroke.

References

1. Parnetti L. Clinical pharmacokinetics of drugs for Alzheimer's disease. *Clin Pharmacokinet* 1995;29:110-129.
2. Torii H, Yoshida K, Kobayashi T, et al. Disposition of idebenone (CV-2619), a new cerebral metabolism improving agent, in rats and dogs. *J Pharmacobiodyn* 1985;8:457-467.
3. Barkworth MF, Dyde CJ, Johnson KI, Schnelle K. An early phase I study to determine the tolerance, safety and pharmacokinetics of idebenone following multiple oral doses. *Arzneimittelforschung* 1985;35:1704-1707.
4. Civenni G, Bezzi P, Trotti D, et al. Inhibitory effect of the neuroprotective agent idebenone and arachidonic acid metabolism in astrocytes. *Eur J Pharmacol* 1999;370:161-167.
5. Cardoso SM, Pereira C, Oliveira CR. The protective effect of vitamin E, idebenone and reduced glutathione on free radical mediated injury in rat brain synaptosomes. *Biochem Biophys Res Commun* 1998;246:703-710.
6. Imada I, Fujita T, Sugiyama Y, et al. Effects of idebenone and related compounds on respiratory activities of brain mitochondria, and on lipid peroxidation of their membranes. *Arch Gerontol Geriatr* 1989;8:323-341.
7. Suno M, Nagaoka A Inhibition of lipid peroxidation by idebenone in brain mitochondria in the presence of succinate. *Arch Gerontol Geriatr* 1989;8:291-297.
8. Suno M, Nagaoka A. Inhibition of brain mitochondrial swelling by idebenone. *Arch Gerontol Geriatr* 1989;8:299-305.
9. Kakihana M, Yamazaki N, Nagaoka A. Effects of idebenone on the levels of acetylcholine, choline, free fatty acids, and energy metabolites in the brains of rats with cerebral ischemia. *Arch Gerontol Geriatr* 1989;8:247-256.

10. Kakihana M, Yamazaki N, Nagaoka A. Effects of idebenone (CV-2619) on the concentrations of acetylcholine and choline in various brain regions of rats with cerebral ischemia. *Jpn J Pharmacol* 1984;36:357-363.

11. Nitta A, Murakami Y, Furukawa Y, et al. Oral administration of idebenone induces nerve growth factor in the brain and improves learning and memory in basal forebrain-lesioned rats. *Naunyn Schmiedebergs Arch Pharmacol* 1994;349:401-407.

12. Nabeshima T, Nitta A, Fuji K, et al. Oral administration of NGF synthesis stimulators recovers reduced brain NGF content in aged rats and cognitive dysfunction in basal-forebrain-lesioned rats. *Gerontology* 1994;40:S46-S56.

13. Nitta A, Hasegawa T, Nabeshima T. Oral administration of idebenone, a stimulator of NGF synthesis, recovers reduced NGF content in aged rat brain. *Neurosci Lett* 1993;163:219-222.

14. Yamada K, Tanaka T, Han D, et al. Protective effects of idebenone and alpha-tocopherol on beta-amyloid-(1-42)-induced learning and memory deficits in rats: implication of oxidative stress in beta-amyloid-induced neurotoxicity *in vivo*. *Eur J Neurosci* 1999;11:83-90.

15. Gutzmann H, Hadler D. Sustained efficacy and safety of idebenone in the treatment of Alzheimer's disease: update on a 2-year double-blind multicentre study. *J Neural Transm* 1998;54:S301-S310.

16. Weyer G, Babej-Dolle RM, Hadler D, et al. A controlled study of two doses of idebenone in the treatment of Alzheimer's disease. *Neuropsychobiology* 1997;36:73-82.

17. Bergamasco B, Scarzella L, La Commare P. Idebenone, a new drug in the treatment of cognitive impairment in patients with dementia of the Alzheimer type. *Funct Neurol* 1994;9:161-168.

18. Shivaram KN, Winklhofer-Roob BM, Straka MS, et al. The effect of idebenone, a coenzyme Q analogue, on hydrophobic bile acid toxicity to isolated rat hepatocytes and hepatic mitochondria. *Free Radic Biol Med* 1998;25:480-492.

19. Nakano T, Miyasaka M, Mori K, et al. Effects of idebenone on electroencephalograms of patients with cerebrovascular disorders. *Arch Gerontol Geriatr* 1989;8:355-366.

20. Schulz JB, Dehmer T, Schols L, et al. Oxidative stress in patients with Friedreich's ataxia. *Neurology* 2000;55:1719-1721.

21. Rustin P, von Kleist-Retzow JC, Chantrel-Groussard K, et al. Effect of idebenone on cardiomyopathy in Friedreich's ataxia: a preliminary study. *Lancet* 1999;354:477-479.

22. Schaffler K, Hadler D, Stark M. Dose-effect relationship of idebenone in an experimental cerebral deficit model. Pilot study in healthy young volunteers with piracetam as reference drug. *Arzneimittelforschung* 1998;48:720-726.

23. Suno M, Terashita Z, Nagaoka A. Inhibition of platelet aggregation by idebenone and the mechanism of the inhibition. *Arch Gerontol Geriatr* 1989;8:313-321.

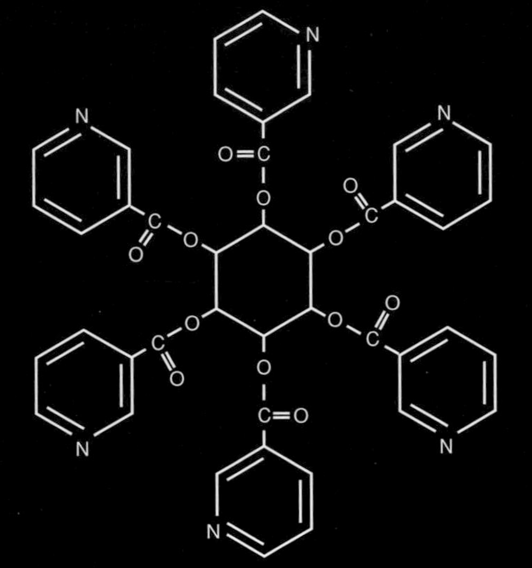

Inositol Hexaniacinate

Inositol Hexaniacinate

Introduction

Inositol hexaniacinate (IHN), also known as inositol hexanicotinate and inositol nicotinate, is the hexanicotinic acid ester of meso-inositol. This compound consists of six molecules of nicotinic acid (niacin) with an inositol molecule in the center (see figure). Pharmacokinetic studies indicate the molecule is, at least in part, absorbed intact, and hydrolyzed in the body with release of free niacin and inositol.[1] It appears to be metabolized slowly, not reaching maximum serum levels until approximately 10 hours after ingestion.[2]

Mechanisms of Action

Inositol hexaniacinate's actions in the body are believed to be the same as those for niacin. These include initiating a decrease in free fatty acid mobilization; a decrease in very-low-density lipoprotein (VLDL) synthesis in the liver resulting in a decrease in LDL cholesterol, total cholesterol, and triglycerides; inhibition of cholesterol synthesis in the liver; an increase in high-density lipoprotein (HDL) levels by decreasing its catabolism;[3] and fibrinolysis.[4,5]

Clinical Indications

Hyperlipidemia

Studies report significant lipid-lowering effects of IHN at doses of 400 mg 3-4 times daily.[6] Welsh and Eade found IHN more effective than niacin in its hypocholesterolemic, antihypertensive and lipotropic effects.[2]

Raynaud's Disease

A review of the literature reveals numerous positive studies on the use of IHN in Raynaud's Disease.[2,4,5,7-9] The mechanism of action appears to be more than just a transient vasodilation, involving lipid-lowering and fibrinolysis.[4,5] This explains the need for long-term administration.

Intermittent Claudication

The use of niacin esters for the treatment of intermittent claudication secondary to atherosclerosis has been examined extensively. Significant improvement has been reported by several investigators at dosages of 2 grams twice daily, typically for at least three months.[10-13] While arterial dilation may be a factor, it has been postulated that reduction in fibrinogen, improvement in blood viscosity, and resultant improvement in oxygen transport are involved in the therapeutic effects.[11]

Other Peripheral Vascular Diseases

IHN appears to have application in the treatment of other conditions resulting from peripheral vascular insufficiency, including threatened amputation from gangrene, restless leg syndrome, stasis dermatitis, atherosclerosis-related migraines, and hypertension.[2]

Dermatological Conditions

IHN has been used for the treatment of various dermatological conditions, including scleroderma, acne, dermatitis herpetiformis, exfoliative glossitis, and psoriasis. IHN appeared to help four out of five patients with dermatitis herpetiformis.[2] One patient with sclerodermal skin lesions was reported to have improved significantly on 1200 mg IHN daily.[2] Results with other skin conditions have been less promising. It appears the dermatological problems most benefited by IHN are those related to vascular insufficiency.[2]

Drug-Nutrient Interactions

Although no adverse reactions between inositol hexaniacinate and other nutrients or drugs have been reported, due to its fibrinolytic effect it should be used with caution in conjunction with anticoagulant medications.

Side Effects and Toxicity

No adverse effects have been reported from the use of inositol hexaniacinate in dosages as high as 4 grams daily.[4,6,8,9] Conversely, numerous toxic reactions, both acute and chronic, have been reported from the use of other forms of high-dose niacin. Reactions to niacin range from acute symptoms of flushing, pruritis, and GI complaints to chronic symptoms of hepatotoxicity, hyperuricemia, and impaired glucose tolerance. Despite the lack of reported adverse reactions, use of IHN in patients with known liver disease should be avoided. In addition, if high doses (2 grams or greater daily) are being administered, liver enzymes should be monitored every 2-3 months for at least the first six months.

Dosage

The typical dosage for Raynaud's disease is 1 gram four times per day for several months.

Recommended dosage for lipid-lowering and improving conditions related to peripheral vascular insufficiency ranges from 1500 mg to 4 grams daily, in divided dosages of two to three times daily.

References

1. Harthon L, Brattsand R. Enzymatic hydrolysis of pentaerythritoltetranicotinate and meso-inositolhexanicotinate in blood and tissues. *Arzneim-Forsch* 1979;29:1859-1862.
2. Welsh AL, Eade M. Inositol hexanicotinate for improved nicotinic acid therapy. *Int Record Med* 1961;174:9-15.
3. El-Enein AMA, Hafez YS, Salem H, Abdel M. The role of nicotinic acid and inositol hexaniacinate as anticholesterolemic and antilipemic agents. *Nutr Reports Int* 1983;28:899-911.
4. Holti G. An experimentally controlled evaluation of the effect of inositol nicotinate upon the digital blood flow in patients with Raynaud's phenomenon. *J Int Med Res* 1979;7:473-483.
5. Aylward M. Hexopal in Raynaud's disease. *J Int Med Res* 1979;7:484-491.
6. Dorner V, Fischer FW. The influence of m-inositol hexanicotinate ester on the serum lipids and lipoproteins. *Arzneim-Forsch* 1961;11:110-113.
7. Ring EF, Bacon PA. Quantitative thermographic assessment of inositol nicotinate therapy in Raynaud's phenomena. *J Int Med Res* 1977;5:217-222.
8. Ring EFJ, Porto LO, Bacon PA. Quantitative thermal imaging to assess inositol nicotinate treatment for Raynaud's syndrome. *J Int Med Res* 1981;9:393-400.
9. Sunderland GT, Belch JJF, Sturrock RD, et al. A double blind randomized placebo controlled trial of Hexopal in primary Raynaud's disease. *Clin Rheum* 1988;7:46-49.
10. O'Hara J. A double-blind placebo-controlled study of Hexopal in the treatment of intermittent claudication. *J Int Med Res* 1985;13:322-327.
11. O'Hara J, Jolly PN, Nicol CG. The therapeutic efficacy of inositol nicotinate (Hexopal) in intermittent claudication: a controlled trial. *Br J Clin Practice* 1988;42:377-383.
12. Tyson VCH. Treatment of intermittent claudication. *Practitioner* 1979;223:121-126.
13. Seckfort H. Treating circulatory problems with inositol nicotinic acid ester. *Med Klin* 1959;10:416-418.

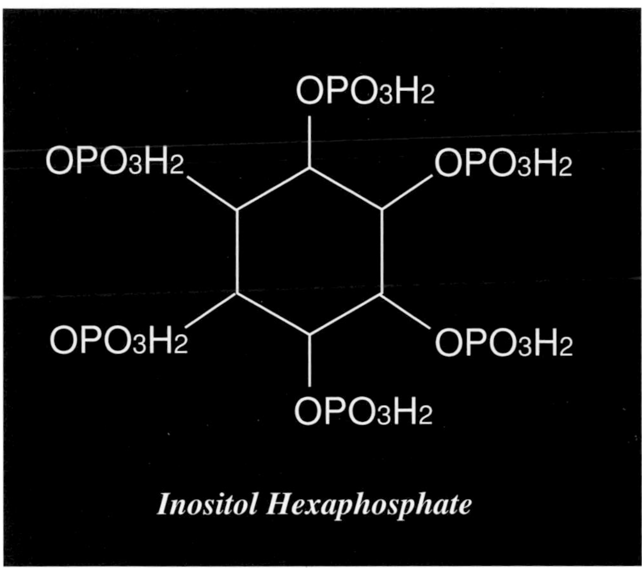

Inositol Hexaphosphate

Inositol Hexaphosphate

Introduction

Inositol hexaphosphate (IP6), also known as myo-inositol hexaphosphate and phytic acid, is a naturally occurring compound first identified in 1855. IP6 is found in substantial amounts in whole grains, cereals, legumes, nuts, and seeds, and is the primary energy source for the germinating plant.[1,2] IP6 and its lower phosphorylated forms are also found in most mammalian cells, where they assist in regulating a variety of important cellular functions.[2] IP6 functions as an antioxidant by chelating divalent cations such as copper and iron, preventing the generation of reactive oxygen species responsible for cell injury and carcinogenesis.[3] Recently, both *in vivo* and *in vitro* studies utilizing IP6 have revealed a significant anticancer activity with a variety of tumor types, possibly via inhibition of tumor cell growth and differentiation.[4] *In vitro* studies with colon, liver, and rhabdomyosarcoma cell lines, and animal models of mammary, colon, intestinal, and liver cancer, as well as rhabdomyosarcoma, have all demonstrated IP6's anticancer properties. Currently, human clinical trials in cancer are lacking. Other properties of IP6 include an anti-platelet aggregating and lipid-lowering effect, suggesting a potential role in cardiovascular disease; inhibition of HIV-1 virus replication; modulation of insulin secretion in pancreatic beta cells; and inhibition of urinary calcium oxalate crystallization, thereby preventing renal stone development.

Biochemistry and Pharmacokinetics

Independent of the route of administration, IP6 has been found to be absorbed almost instantaneously, transported intracellularly and dephosphorylated into lower inositol phosphates. IP6 reached targeted tumor tissue as early as one hour post-administration in rats.[7] When incubated with a human mammary cancer cell line, low intracellular levels of IP6 were detected as early as one minute post-incubation.[6] Pharmacokinetic studies of IP6 in humans are lacking.

Mechanisms of Action

The mechanisms of action for IP6 are not completely understood. A recent study supported earlier research that IP6 functions as an antioxidant by chelating divalent cations such as copper and iron, preventing the formation of reactive oxygen species responsible for cell injury and carcinogenesis.[7] The chelation hypothesis, however, does not completely explain IP6's antineoplastic activity. It is reasonable to conclude that, in addition to its antioxidant role, IP6 probably exerts its action via control of cell division. In a recent study it was shown that IP6 decreased S phase and arrested cells in the G0/G1 phase of the cell cycle. A significant decrease in the expression of proliferation markers indicated IP6 disengaged cells from actively cycling.[8] In addition, IP6 has been shown to enhance NK-cell activity, thereby boosting NK-cell cytotoxicity.[9] Although mechanisms of action pertaining to IP6's anti-platelet aggregating and lipid-lowering effect, its inhibition of HIV-1 replication, and its ability to modulate insulin secretion remain somewhat unclear, it is likely they are a function of IP6's antioxidant properties or its ability to influence a variety of cellular functions. Studies of IP6 and urolithiasis have indicated it inhibits crystallization of calcium oxalate salts in the urine, preventing renal stone development.[10]

Deficiency States

Deficiencies of IP6 have been associated with an increase in calcium oxalate crystals in the urine and resulting increased risk for kidney stone formation.[10] Due to its antioxidant and antineoplastic properties, IP6 deficiency may also pose an increased risk for disease states mediated by reactive oxygen species, such as cardiovascular disease and cancer.

Clinical Indications

Colon Cancer

Epidemiological studies and animal research have suggested an inverse relationship between colon cancer and consumption of high-fiber foods. Among the many components of fiber, inositol hexaphosphate has been studied extensively for its inhibitory effects against colon carcinogenesis. Rat studies have demonstrated IP6 reduces tumor prevalence, frequency, and size in a dose-dependent manner during the initiation and post-initiation stages.[11,12] Another study examining the preventive effects of wheat bran fractions in rat colon cancer showed that removal of both IP6 and lipids from wheat bran significantly increased colon tumor multiplicity and volume. Removal of IP6 or lipids independent of each other had no significant effect on colon tumor incidence,[13] possibly suggesting the two fractions operate together to inhibit carcinogenesis.

Breast Cancer

Based on studies of IP6's antineoplastic properties in colon cancer models, animal studies have been conducted to assess its effect on mammary carcinoma. A consistent, reproducible, and significant inhibition of mammary cancer by IP6 has been shown in 7,12-dimethylbenz[a]anthracene (DMBA)-induced mammary cancer in rats. A significant reduction was observed in tumor number, multiplicity (number of tumors per tumor-bearing animal), and tumor burden. It was also noted that IP6 protected rats from spontaneous mammary tumors. This study demonstrated IP6 was more effective than a high fiber diet in preventing experimental mammary tumors.[14] Thompson and Zhang also reported a reduction of carly markers of experimental mammary carcinogenesis.[15] In another study by Vucenik et al, IP6 and inositol were examined for their effect on DMBA-induced rat mammary tumors. Tumor-bearing animals were given IP6 alone, inositol alone, or IP6 plus inositol, with controls receiving neither substance. Rats treated with IP6 plus inositol showed a 48-percent reduction in tumor multiplicity as well as slight decreases in tumor size and incidence, when compared with control animals. Data from this study suggests IP6 plus inositol may be protective against mammary carcinoma in animals. Additional studies in humans are warranted.[16]

Hepatocellular Carcinoma

IP6 has demonstrated both *in vivo* and *in vitro* inhibition of the human liver cancer cell line, HepG2. Research conducted by Vucenik et al assessed whether IP6 could inhibit tumorigenicity and suppress or regress growth of HepG2 cells in a transplanted nude mouse model. In mice receiving HepG2 cells pretreated with IP6, no tumor was found, compared to a 71-percent tumor incidence in mice receiving untreated HepG2 control cells. In the tumor suppression/regression arm of the study, tumors were allowed to reach a diameter of 8-10 mm at which point intra-tumoral injection of IP6 was performed for 12 consecutive days. At autopsy, tumor weight in IP6-treated animals was 86-1180 percent (340-percent average) less than in control mice. This data indicates IP6 inhibits formation of liver cancer and regresses pre-existing human hepatic cancer xenografts.[17]

Rhabdomyosarcoma

Rhabdomyosarcoma (RMS) is a tumor of mesenchymal origin and is the most common soft tissue sarcoma in children. Patients with advanced metastatic RMS frequently do not respond to therapies currently available.

In vitro and *in vivo* research of IP6's effect on human rhabdomyosarcoma cell line demonstrated IP6 suppressed the growth *in vitro* in a time and dose-dependent manner and also induced cell differentiation. A 50-percent inhibition of cell growth was seen with < 1.0 mM IP6. However, the removal of IP6 from the media after 72 hours of treatment allowed the cancerous cells to recover their growth. In xenografted nude mice IP6 suppressed RMS cell growth *in vivo*. IP6-treated mice produced 25-fold smaller tumors after two weeks of treatment when compared to controls. When the treatment period was extended to five weeks, a 49-fold reduction in tumor size was noted.[18] The results of this research suggest a potential therapeutic role for IP6 in RMS and possibly other mesenchymal neoplasms.

Cardiovascular Disease

Dyslipidemia

IP6's antioxidant function allows it to form complexes with cations linked to the etiology of hypercholesterolemia. The effect of IP6 was examined in rats fed both standard rodent chow (low in saturated fat) plus monopotassium phytate, and chow plus cholesterol and monopotassium phytate. In the treated groups, IP6 resulted in a 19-percent decrease in total cholesterol in the chow group and a 32-percent decrease in total cholesterol in the cholesterol-enriched chow group. The mean triglyceride level decreased also by an average of 65 percent in both groups.[19]

Platelet Aggregation

Platelet adhesion to endothelial cells and subsequent aggregation are key steps in the development of atherosclerosis. A study of IP6's effect on platelet aggregation was conducted using whole blood obtained from 10 healthy volunteers. Aggregation of activated platelets, incubated with IP6, was significantly inhibited in a dose-dependent manner, suggesting a potential role in reducing cardiovascular disease risk.[20]

HIV

In vitro studies have indicated that IP6 incubated with HIV-1 infected T cells inhibited the replication of HIV-1.[21],[22] Although the mechanisms of IP6 action have not yet been determined, the researchers speculate that it acts on HIV-1 early replicative stage since the IP6 was only in actual contact with the cells during the period of viral infection. IP6 was subsequently removed and cells were cultured for five days.[22]

Excess Insulin Secretion

Research has shown an influx of extracellular calcium is one of the events that drives insulin release.[23] IP6 may be a key element in modulating insulin secretion via its effect on calcium channel activity and the fact that it is the dominant inositol phosphate in insulin-secreting pancreatic beta cells.[24] The mechanism of action is not fully understood but it appears IP6 specifically inhibits serine threonine protein phosphatase activity, which in turn opens intracellular calcium channels, driving insulin release.[23]

Urolithiasis

Research has shown IP6 significantly inhibits the precipitation of urinary calcium oxalate crystals. Inadequate intake of IP6 in the diet results in a deficiency of urinary IP6 and may pose an increased risk for the development of calcium oxalate kidney stones.[12,25,26]

Drug-Nutrient Interactions

IP6 strongly binds divalent minerals such as magnesium, iron, calcium, and zinc, and may cause mineral deficiencies if not taken away from meals and mineral supplements. One study demonstrated that phytate-enriched infant formula given to infants younger than four months resulted in a decrease in bioavailability of zinc.[27] The U.S. Department of Agriculture is currently developing first-generation low-phytate hybrid lines of maize, barley, rice, and soybean in an attempt to circumvent mineral depletion by IP6.[28]

Side Effects and Toxicity

Animal studies have shown IP6 is very safe and without toxic effects, even when administered long term and/or at high doses.[14,29] Regarding toxicity in humans, sodium-IP6 administered to 35 patients at a dose of 8.8 grams per day (in divided doses) for several months resulted in no apparent toxicity.[30]

Dosage

Dosage information for humans is limited and the optimal IP6 dosage for cancer treatment is yet to be determined. It is typically dosed at two grams and above daily in divided doses. A study in which IP6 was given to patients at risk for kidney stones utilized doses of 8.8 grams daily.[30]

Warnings and Contraindications

Due to its strong binding affinity for minerals, inositol hexaphosphate should be taken separately from meals, mineral supplements, and multivitamins containing minerals to prevent the potential deficiency that may result.

References

1. Graf E. Applications of phytic acid. *J Am Oil Chem Soc* 1983;60:1861-1867.
2. Szwergold BS, Graham RA, Brown TR. Observation of inositol pentakis- and hexakis-phosphates in mammalian tissues by 31P NMR. *Biochem Biophys Res Commun* 1987;149:874-881.
3. Harland BF, Oberleas D. Phytate in foods. *Wld Rev Nutr Diet* 1987;52:235-259.
4. Shamsuddin AM, Vucenik I, Cole KE. IP6: a novel anti-cancer agent. *Life Sci* 1997;61:343-354.
5. Sakamoto K, Vucenik I, Shamsuddin AM. [3H]phytic acid (inositol hexaphosphate) is absorbed and distributed to various tissues in rats. *J Nutr* 1993;123:713-720.

6. Vucenik I, Shamsuddin AM. [3H]inositol hexaphosphate (phytic acid) is rapidly absorbed and metabolized by murine and human malignant cells *in vitro*. *J Nutr* 1994;124:861-868.
7. Midorikawa K, Murata M, Oikawa S, et al. Protective effect of phytic acid on oxidative DNA damage with reference to cancer chemoprevention. *Biochem Biophys Res Commun* 2001;288:552-557.
8. El-Sherbiny YM, Cox MC, Ismail ZA, et al. G0/G1 arrest and S phase inhibition of human cancer cell lines by inositol hexaphosphate (IP6). *Anticancer Res* 2001;21:2393-2403.
9. Shamsuddin AM. Reduction of cell proliferation and enhancement of NK-cell activity. 1992. U.S. Patent #5,082,833.
10. Grases F, Costa-Bauza A. Phytate (IP6) is a powerful agent for preventing calcifications in biological fluids: usefulness in renal lithiasis treatment. *Anticancer Res* 1999;19:3717-3722.
11. Reddy BS. Prevention of colon carcinogenesis by components of dietary fiber. *Anticancer Res* 1999;19:3681-3683.
12. Ullah A, Shamsuddin AM. Dose-dependent inhibition of large intestinal cancer by inositol hexaphosphate in F344 rats. *Carcinogenesis* 1990;11:2219-2222.
13. Reddy BS, Hirose Y, Cohen LA, et al. Preventive potential of wheat bran fractions against experimental colon carcinogenesis: implications for human colon cancer prevention. *Cancer Res* 2000;60:4792-4797.
14. Shamsuddin AM, Vucenik I. Mammary tumor inhibition by IP6: a review. *Anticancer Res* 1999;19:3671-3674.
15. Thompson LU, Zhang L. Phytic acid and minerals: effect on early markers of risk for mammary and colon carcinogenesis. *Carcinogenesis* 1991;12:2041-2045.
16. Vucenik I, Sakamoto K, Bansal M, Shamsuddin AM. Inhibition of rat mammary carcinogenesis by inositol hexaphosphate (phytic acid). A pilot study. *Cancer Lett* 1993;75:95-102.
17. Vucenik I, Zhang ZS, Shamsuddin AM. IP6 in treatment of liver cancer II. Intra-tumoral injection of IP6 regresses pre-existing human liver cancer xenotransplanted in nude mice. *Anticancer Res* 1998;18:4091-4096.
18. Vucenik I, Kalebic T, Tantivejkul K, Shamsuddin AM. Novel anticancer function of inositol hexaphosphate: Inhibition of human rhabdomyosarcoma *in vitro* and *in vivo*. *Anticancer Res* 1998;18:1377-1384.
19. Jariwalla RJ. Inositol hexaphosphate (IP6) as an anti-neoplastic and lipid-lowering agent. *Anticancer Res* 1999;19:3699-3702.
20. Vucenik I, Podczasy JJ, Shamsuddin AM. Antiplatelet activity of inositol hexaphosphate (IP6). *Anticancer Res* 1999;19:3689-3693.
21. Otake T, Shimonaka H, Kanai M, et al. Inhibitory effect of inositol hexasulfate and inositol hexaphosphoric acid (phytic acid) on the proliferation of the human immunodeficiency virus (HIV) *in vitro*. *Kansenshogaku Zasshi* 1989;63:676-683.
22. Otake T, Mori H, Morimoto M, et al. Anti-HIV-1 activity of myo-inositol hexaphosphoric acid (IP6) and myo-inositol hexasulfate (IS6). *Anticancer Res* 1999;19:3723-3726.
23. Larsson O, Barker CJ, Sjoholm A, et al. Inhibition of phosphatases and increased Ca^{2+} channel activity by inositol hexaphosphate. *Science* 1997;278:471-474.
24. Barker CJ, Berggren P. Inositol hexakisphosphate and beta-cell stimulus secretion coupling. *Anticancer Res* 1999;19:3737-3742.
25. Grases F, Simonet BM, March JG, Prieto RM. Inositol hexakisphosphate in urine: the relationship between oral intake and urinary excretion. *BJU Int* 2000;85:138-142.
26. Grases F, March JG, Prieto RM, et al. Urinary phytate in calcium oxalate stone formers and healthy people – dietary effects on phytate excretion. *Scand J Urol Nephrol* 2000;34:162-164.
27. Bosscher D, Lu Z, Janssens G, et al. *In vitro* availability of zinc from infant foods with increasing phytic acid contents. *Br J Nutr* 2001;86:241-247.
28. Raboy V. Progress in breeding low phytate crops. *J Nutr* 2002;132:503S-505S.
29. Dong Z, Huang C, Ma WY. PI-3 in signal transduction, cell transformation, and as a target for chemoprevention of cancer. *Anticancer Res* 1999;19:3743-3747.
30. Henneman PH, Benedict PH, Forbes AP, Dudley HR. Idiopathic hypercalciuria. *N Engl J Med* 1958;17:802-807.

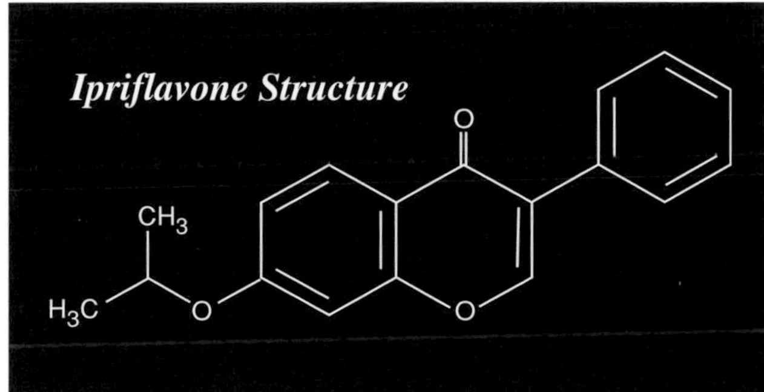

Ipriflavone

Introduction

Ipriflavone (IP), chemical structure 7-isopropoxy-isoflavone, is an isoflavone, synthesized from the soy isoflavone, daidzein. Ipriflavone was discovered in the 1930s but has only recently begun to be embraced by the medical community in this country. Over 150 studies on safety and effectiveness, both animal and human, have been conducted in Italy, Hungary, and Japan. As of 1997, 2,769 patients had been treated and studied, for a total of 3,132 patient years.[1] From the weight of the evidence, ipriflavone holds great promise in the prevention and treatment of osteoporosis and other metabolic bone diseases.

Pharmacokinetics

Ipriflavone is metabolized mainly in the liver and excreted in the urine. Food appears to enhance its absorption. When given to healthy male volunteers, 80 percent of a 200-mg dose of ipriflavone was absorbed when taken after breakfast.[2] Ipriflavone metabolism was not found to be significantly different in elderly osteoporotic or mild kidney failure patients than in younger, healthy subjects.[3] Studies using labeled IP in rats found it concentrated primarily in the gastrointestinal tract, liver, kidneys, bones, and adrenal glands.[3]

Mechanisms of Action

Anti-resorptive Mechanisms

An animal study found ipriflavone inhibited parathyroid hormone-, vitamin D-, PGE2-, and interleukin 1β-stimulated bone resorption.[4] Bonnuci et al found parathyroid-stimulated osteoclastic activity and resulting hypercalcemia were inhibited in a dose-dependent manner by ipriflavone supplementation in rats.[5]

Bone-forming Mechanisms

An *in vitro* examination of the osteoblastic effect of ipriflavone and its metabolites resulted in interesting findings. Ipriflavone and one of its metabolites stimulated cell proliferation of an osteoblast-like cell line (UMR-106a – a cell line often used to determine the effect of various hormones and drugs on bone metabolism). IP and another metabolite increased alkaline phosphatase activity, while another metabolite enhanced collagen formation; IP alone inhibited parathyroid hormone activity.[6]

Lack of Direct Estrogen Effect

One of the benefits of ipriflavone in the treatment of osteoporosis is its lack of direct estrogenic effect. Melis et al administered ipriflavone or placebo to a group of 15 postmenopausal women. LH, FSH, prolactin, and estradiol were measured after a single oral dose of 600 or 1,000 mg, and after 7, 14, and 21 days of treatment with 600 or 1,000 mg doses. No differences in endocrine effect were noted between the ipriflavone and placebo groups. Vaginal cytology was unchanged after 21 days of IP or placebo compared to a significant increase in superficial vaginal cells in the estrogen group.[7]

In vitro investigation of the interaction between ipriflavone and preosteoclastic cell lines found it was not mediated by direct interaction with estrogen receptors.[8] Instead, unique binding cites for ipriflavone were identified in the nucleus of preosteoclastic cells. The presence of IP binding sites was confirmed by Miyauchi et al. They identified two classes of binding sites in chicken osteoclasts and their precursors.[9] Similar ipriflavone binding sites have been identified in human leukemic cells, a line with similar characteristics to osteoclast precursors.

Calcitonin secretion is modulated by estrogen and, while ipriflavone alone did not enhance calcitonin levels, it acted synergistically with estrogen, necessitating lower doses of estrogen to achieve normal calcitonin secretion. It appears IP increases the sensitivity of the thyroid gland to estrogen-stimulated calcitonin secretion.[10]

Clinical Indications

In the last decade there have been over 60 human studies – many double blind and placebo controlled – on the use of ipriflavone for the prevention and reversal of bone loss. An overview of these studies follows.

Postmenopausal Osteoporosis

Ipriflavone has been studied in numerous double-blind, placebo-controlled trials conducted in Italy, Hungary, and Japan. The same protocol was used throughout most of the studies – 200 mg ipriflavone or placebo three times daily. In most of the studies, calcium (500-1000 mg) was given to both ipriflavone and placebo groups. Several two-year studies looked at women immediately postmenopause (age 50-65) and found bone mass was maintained or improved slightly in the ipriflavone groups while those in the placebo groups experienced significant bone loss.[11-14]

It appears ipriflavone may be particularly effective for the treatment of so-called "senile osteoporosis" (osteoporosis in women or men over the age of 65) as evidenced by the results of two studies in seven Italian centers.[1,15] In these studies a total of 112 subjects aged 65-79 were followed for two years. Subjects took either 600 mg ipriflavone plus 1 g calcium daily or placebo plus 1 g calcium. A four- to six-percent increase in bone density was observed in the ipriflavone groups, whereas the placebo groups experienced as much as a three-percent decrease in bone density. The most clinically relevant finding in the larger of the two studies was a decrease in fracture rates in the IP group (2 of 41 patients experienced fractures in the IP group, whereas 11 of 43 experienced fractures in the placebo group).[1]

A recent four-year study published in *JAMA* found no significant change in bone mineral density in a group of postmenopausal osteoporotic women taking ipriflavone (n=234) at a dose of 200 mg three times daily when compared to placebo (n=240). While bone density did not increase significantly, neither was significant loss reported in either group. Unlike previous studies, this study did not divide the treatment groups according to age but combined all ages (45-75 years).[16]

Ipriflavone for Osteoporosis in Combination with Other Nutrients or Medications

Ipriflavone has been found to enhance the effect of other bone-preserving agents, including 1α vitamin D (a form commonly used in Japan for osteoporosis).[17]

A number of studies have examined the effect of ipriflavone and estrogen for the treatment of osteoporosis. While low doses of conjugated estrogen (0.15-0.30 mg/day) typically are high enough to prevent hot flashes and other neurovegetative symptoms of menopause, a somewhat higher dose (0.625 mg/day or higher) is generally necessary for bone protection. Some studies, however, have found that when combining ipriflavone and estrogen, lower doses of estrogen afford protection.[18-20]

Ipriflavone versus Salmon Calcitonin

An open, controlled 12-month trial compared ipriflavone with salmon calcitonin in 40 postmenopausal women. Significant increases in bone density were observed in both groups after 12 months: a 4.3 percent increase in BMD in the ipriflavone group and a 1.9-percent increase in the calcitonin group.[21]

Ipriflavone in the Prevention of Surgical or Drug-induced Osteoporosis

Researchers examined the effect of ipriflavone in restraining bone loss induced by gonadotropin hormone-releasing hormone agonists (GnRH-A) such as Lupron®, used to induce ovarian atrophy for the treatment of endometriosis, uterine fibroids, etc. In a double-blind, placebo-controlled trial 78 women treated with GnRH-A (3.75 mg leuproreline every 30 days for six months) were randomly assigned to receive either ipriflavone (600 mg/day) or placebo; both groups received 500 mg calcium daily. In placebo subjects, markers of bone turnover (urinary hydroxyproline and plasma bone Gla) were significantly elevated while BMD decreased significantly after six months. Conversely, there were no changes in BMD or bone markers in the ipriflavone-treated group.[22]

Animal studies have found ipriflavone inhibited bone loss associated with long-term steroid use[23] and immobilization.[24,25]

Other Conditions

Several other pathological conditions involving bone may be helped by ipriflavone, including Paget's disease of the bone,[26] hyperparathyroidism,[27] otosclerosis,[28] and renal osteodystrophy.[29]

Drug-Nutrient Interactions

A reduction in theophylline metabolism and increased serum theophylline was observed in a patient being treated with ipriflavone.[30] Animal studies have indicated this may be due to inhibition of certain cytochrome p450 enzymes, resulting in diminished elimination of the drug via the liver.[31,32] While ipriflavone does not have a directly estrogenic effect, it appears to act synergistically with estrogen to normalize calcitonin levels.[10]

Side Effects and Toxicity

In general, ipriflavone appears to be quite safe and well tolerated. As of 1997, long-term safety of ipriflavone (for periods ranging from 6-96 months) had been assessed in 2,769 patients for a total of 3,132 patient years in 60 human studies.[1] The incidence of adverse reactions in the ipriflavone-treated patients was 14.5 percent, while the incidence in the placebo groups was 16.1 percent. Side effects were mainly gastrointestinal (GI). Since the placebo groups in most studies received calcium, it is not unreasonable to assume calcium may have as much to do with GI effects as ipriflavone. Other symptoms observed to a lesser extent include skin rashes, headaches, depression, drowsiness, and tachycardia. Minor transient abnormalities in liver, kidney, and hematological parameters were documented in a small percent of subjects. One study found subclinical lymphocytopenia as a side effect of treatment in 29 of 474 postmenopausal participants.[16] Why this effect on white blood cell count had not been found in previous studies is unclear; however, it might be prudent to conduct periodic CBCs on patients using long-term ipriflavone therapy.

Dosage

Dosage for treatment of osteoporosis has been consistent – 200 mg three times daily. The most successful dosage for Paget's disease was 1,200 mg daily for 30 days, followed by 600 mg daily.[26] Hyperparathyroidism was treated with 1,200 mg daily,[27] otosclerosis with doses of 200 mg four times daily,[28] and renal osteodystrophy with doses of 400-600 mg daily.[29]

References

1. Agnusdei D, Bufalino L. Efficacy of ipriflavone in established osteoporosis and long-term safety. *Calcif Tissue Int* 1997;61:S23-S27.
2. Saito AM. Pharmacokinetic study of ipriflavone (TC80) by oral administration in healthy male volunteers. *Jpn Pharm Ther J* 1985;13:7223-7233.
3. Reginster JYL. Ipriflavone pharmacological properties and usefulness in postmenopausal osteoporosis. *Bone Miner* 1993;23:223-232.
4. Tsutsumi N, Kawashima K, Nagata H, et al. Effects of KCA-098 on bone metabolism: comparison with those of ipriflavone. *Jpn J Pharmacol* 1994;65:343-349.
5. Bonucci E, Ballanti P, Martelli A, et al. Ipriflavone inhibits osteoclast differentiation in parathyroid transplanted parietal bone of rats. *Calcif Tissue Int* 1992;50:314-319.
6. Benvenuti S, Tanini A, Frediani U, et al. Effects of ipriflavone and its metabolites on a clonal osteoblastic cell line. *J Bone Miner Res* 1991;6:987-996.
7. Melis GB, Paoletti AM, Cagnacci L, et al. Lack of any estrogenic effect of ipriflavone in postmenopausal women. *J Endocrin Invest* 1992;15:755-761.
8. Petilli M, Fiorelli G, Benvenuti U, et al. Interactions between ipriflavone and the estrogen receptor. *Calcif Tissue Int* 1995;56:160-165.
9. Miyauchi A, Notoya K, Taketomi S, et al. Novel ipriflavone receptors coupled to calcium influx regulate osteoclast differentiation and function. *Endocrinology* 1996;137:3544-3550.
10. Yamazaki I, Kinoshita M. Calcitonin secreting property of ipriflavone in the presence of estrogen. *Life Sci* 1986;38:1535-1541.
11. Adami S, Bufalino L, Cervetti R, et al. Ipriflavone prevents radial bone loss in postmenopausal women with low bone mass over 2 years. *Osteoporos Int* 1997;7:119-125.
12. Gennari C, Adami S, Agnusdei D, et al. Effect of chronic treatment with ipriflavone in postmenopausal women with low bone mass. *Calcif Tissue Int* 1997;61:S19-S22.
13. Agnusdei D, Crepaldi G, Isaia G, et al. A double blind, placebo-controlled trial of ipriflavone for prevention of postmenopausal spinal bone loss. *Calcif Tissue Int* 1997;61:142-147.
14. Valente M, Bufalino L, Castiglione GN, et al. Effects of 1-year treatment with ipriflavone on bone in postmenopausal women with low bone mass. *Calcif Tissue Int* 1994;54:377-380.
15. Passeri M, Biondi M, Costi D, et al. Effect of ipriflavone on bone mass in elderly osteoporotic women. *Bone Miner* 1992;19:S57-S62.
16. Alexandersen P, Toussaint A, Christiansen C, et al. Ipriflavone in the treatment of osteoporosis: a randomized controlled trial. *JAMA* 2001;285:1482-1488.
17. Ushiroyama T, Okamura S, Ikeda A, Ueki M. Efficacy of ipriflavone and 1α vitamin D therapy for the cessation of vertebral bone loss. *Int J Gynaecol Obstet* 1995;48:283-288.
18. Melis GB, Paoletti AM, Bartolini R, et al. Ipriflavone and low doses of estrogen in the prevention of one mineral loss in climacterium. *Bone Miner* 1992;19:S49-S56.
19. Gambacciani M, Ciaponi M, Cappagli B, et al. Effects of combined low dose of the isoflavone derivative ipriflavone and estrogen replacement on bone mineral density and metabolism in postmenopausal women. *Maturitas* 1997;28:75-81.
20. Agnusdei D, Gennari C, Bufalino L. Prevention of early postmenopausal bone loss using low doses of conjugated estrogens and the non-hormonal, bone-active drug ipriflavone. *Osteoporos Int* 1995;5:462-466.
21. Cecchettin M, Bellometti S, Cremonesi G, et al. Metabolic and bone effects after administration of ipriflavone and salmon calcitonin in postmenopausal osteoporosis. *Biomed Pharmacother* 1995;49:465-468.
22. Gambacciani M, Cappagli B, Piagessi L, et al. Ipriflavone prevents the loss of bone mass in pharmacological menopause induced by GnRH-agonists. *Calcif Tissue Int* 1997;61:15-18.

23. Yamazaki I, Shino A, Shimizu Y, et al. Effect of ipriflavone on glucocorticoid-induced osteoporosis in rats. *Life Sci* 1986;38:951-958.

24. Notoya K, Yoshia K, Tsukuda R, et al. Increase in femoral bone mass by ipriflavone alone and in combination with 1α-hydroxyvitamin D_3 in growing rats with skeletal unloading. *Calcif Tissue Int* 1996;58:88-94.

25. Foldes I, Rapcsak M, Szoor A, et al. The effect of ipriflavone treatment on osteoporosis induced by immobilization. *Acta Morphologica Hungarica* 1988;36:79-93.

26. Agnusdei D, Camporeale A, Gonnelli S, et al. Short-term treatment of Paget's disease of bone with ipriflavone. *Bone Miner* 1992;19:S35-S42.

27. Mazzuoli G, Romagnoli E, Carnevale V, et al. Effects of ipriflavone on bone remodeling in primary hyperparathyroidism. *Bone Miner* 1992;19:S27-S33.

28. Sziklai I, Komora V, Ribari O. Double-blind study of the effectiveness of a bioflavonoid in the control of tinnitus in otosclerosis. *Acta Chirurgica Hungarica* 1992-93;33:101-107.

29. Hyodo T, Ono K, Koumi T, et al. A study of the effects of ipriflavone administration in hemodialysis patients with renal osteodystrophy: preliminary report. *Nephron* 1991;58:114-115.

30. Takahashi J, Kawakatsu K, Wakayama T, Sawaoka H. Elevation of serum theophylline levels by ipriflavone in a patient with chronic obstructive pulmonary disease. *Eur J Clin Pharmacol* 1992;43:207-208.

31. Monostory K, Vereczky L, Levai F, Szatmari I. Ipriflavone as an inhibitor of human cytochrome p450 enzymes. *Br J Pharmacol* 1998;123:605-610.

32. Monostory K, Vereczky L. Interaction of theophylline and ipriflavone at the cytochrome p450 level. *Eur J Drug Metab Pharmacokinet* 1995;20:40-47.

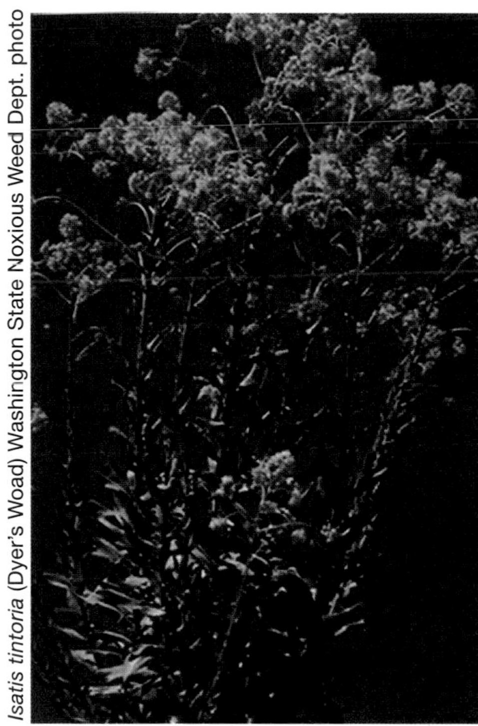
Isatis tintoria (Dyer's Woad) Washington State Noxious Weed Dept. photo

Isatis tinctoria

Description

Isatis tinctoria (also known as dyer's woad), a member of the Brassica family, is a plant native to the grasslands of southeastern Russia that cultivation spread widely across Asia and Europe. In addition to its medicinal use, Isatis has a long history of use as an indigo dye. Isatis is a commonly used herb in traditional Chinese medicine. Root extracts of the herb are known as Ban Lang Gen and leaf extracts are known as Da Qing Ye. An indigo dye extract containing other herbs in addition to Isatis is referred to as Qing Dai. Documented medicinal use of Isatis in the western tradition extends back to at least the first century A.D. Both the leaves and roots have been used medicinally.

Active Constituents

Isatis leaves contain an alkaloid known as tryptanthrin,[1] which is strongly inhibitory to the cyclooxygenase-2 (COX-2) enzyme, and is theorized to be largely responsible for the anti-inflammatory action of Isatis. The leaves also contain several derivatives of hydroxycinnamic acid, including ferulic acid and sinapic acid.[2] These agents are thought to be important in the anti-inflammatory and anti-allergic activity of Isatis leaf preparations.[3]

Indirubin, a compound found in Isatis root, has undergone screening for anti-cancer activity. Indirubin is thought to inhibit DNA replication in neoplastic cells without causing significant marrow suppression.[4]

Like many Brassica plants, Isatis contains a number of indole compounds.[2] Dietary indoles are thought to have a number of anti-cancer effects,[5] and may help explain the traditional use of Isatis in the treatment of cancer.

Complete analysis of the constituents of Isatis root has not been published to date. Some of the major known ingredients of the root not listed above include indoxyl-beta-glucoside, beta-sitosterol, and isatin.[6] While both leaf and root extracts of Isatis clearly have a strong antimicrobial action, the constituents responsible for this action remain elusive.

Clinical Indications

Infection

Isatis leaves have been used in traditional medicine mainly for treatment of infections; specifically, encephalitis, upper respiratory infection, and gastroenteritis are considered major indications for Isatis.[6]

Isatis root extracts have also been used to treat infection. The anti-microbial action of the root is likely more broad spectrum than that of the leaves. *In vitro* and human studies from China have shown Isatis root extract to be anti-bacterial, anti-viral, and anti-parasitic.[6]

Cancer

Root extracts have also been used to treat patients with solid tumors and leukemia, a traditional usage that led to purification of the component compound indirubin. Review of several published trials from China found oral administration of 150-200 mg of purified indirubin per day led to remission in 60 percent of patients with chronic myelocytic leukemia.[4]

Inflammation

Inflammatory conditions are also considered a major indication for Isatis leaf.[1] In traditional Chinese medicine, leaf extracts are used to clear heat and toxins from the blood.[7]

Isatis root was a constituent of the botanical formula PC-SPES, which demonstrated a therapeutic effect against prostate cancer in preliminary trials.[8] However, PC-SPES was subsequently pulled off the market after it was discovered it contained the synthetic drugs diethylstilbestrol, indomethacin, and warfarin.[9] The relative importance of Isatis in this formula remains to be elucidated.

Side Effects and Toxicity

Clinical trials have not assessed the safety of Isatis leaf or root preparations. Traditional Chinese herbal texts do not list adverse effects, but do caution against the use of Isatis in cases of weak constitution.[7]

Animal studies using pure indirubin in doses up to 1,000 mg/kg showed no gross pathological effect.[4] Adverse effects of indirubin in humans include abdominal pain, diarrhea, nausea, vomiting, thrombocytopenia, and rare marked bone marrow suppression.[4]

Dosage

A typical adult dosage of Isatis dried root is 1-2 grams per day, in divided doses.

References

1. Danz H, Stoyanova S, Wippich P, et al. Identification and isolation of the cyclooxygenase-2 inhibitory principle in *Isatis tinctoria*. *Planta Med* 2001;67:411-416.
2. Hartleb I, Seifert K. Acid constituents from *Isatis tinctoria*. *Planta Med* 1995;61:95-96.
3. Diel F, Well S, Ficht F, Paetzold M. Tea of *Isatis tinctoria* (woad) responses by allergic patients *in vivo* and *in vitro*. *Aktuel Ernahrungsmed* 1992;17:34-36. [Article in German]
4. Mingzhu M, Bangyuan Y. Progress in indirubin treatment of myelocytic leukemia. *J Tradit Chin Med* 1983;3:245-248.
5. Brignall M. Prevention and treatment of cancer with indole-3-carbinol. *Altern Med Rev* 2002;6:580-589.
6. Benske D, Gamble A. *Chinese Herbal Medicine Materia Medica*. Seattle, WA: Eastland Press; 1986.
7. Yeung HC. *Handbook of Chinese Herbs and Formulas*. Los Angeles, CA: No publisher listed; 1985.
8. Oh WK, George DJ, Hackmann K, et al. Activity of the herbal combination, PC-SPES, in the treatment of patients with androgen-independent prostate cancer. *Urology* 2001;57:122-126.
9. Sovak M, Seligson AL, Konas M, et al. Herbal composition PC-SPES for management of prostate cancer: identification of active principles. *J Natl Cancer Inst* 2002;94:1275-1280.

Lactobacillus sporogenes

Description

Lactobacillus sporogenes is a gram-positive, spore-forming, lactic-acid producing bacillus. It was originally isolated and described in 1933. The organism requires a complex mixture of organic substrates for growth, including fermentable carbohydrates and peptides.

Pharmacokinetics

Subsequent to oral administration, *L. sporogenes* passes through the stomach in its spore form and, upon arrival in the duodenum, germinates and multiplies rapidly.[1]

Estimates suggest the average duration of time between oral dosing and germination is four hours.[1] After germination, *L. sporogenes* is metabolically active in the intestines, producing lactic acid.

L. sporogenes is considered a semi-resident, as it takes up only a temporary residence in the human intestines. Spores of *L. sporogenes* are excreted slowly via the feces for approximately seven days after discontinuation of administration.[1]

Mechanisms of Action

Despite the transient nature of this organism in the digestive tract, the changes this lactic acid bacillus produces shift the environment in support of a complex gastrointestinal flora.[1,2]

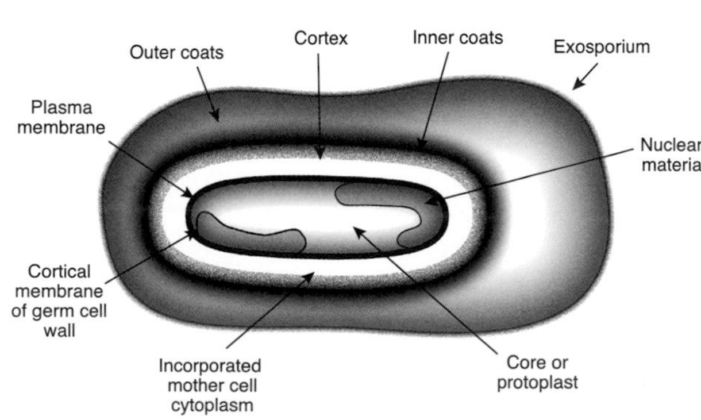

The mechanism of action is presumed to be a result of improving gastrointestinal ecology by replenishing the quantity of desirable obligate microorganisms and antagonizing pathogenic microbes.[2,3]

Two isomeric forms of lactic acid can be produced by lactic acid-producing bacteria – levorotatory (L (+)) lactic acid and dextrorotatory (D(-)) lactic acid. L(+) lactic acid is completely metabolized in the body; however, D(-) lactic acid is not completely metabolized, resulting in a degree of metabolic acidosis. *L. sporogenes* produces only L(+) lactic acid.[1]

L. sporogenes is assumed to produce bacteriocins[2] and short chain fatty acids. As the organism grows, it assimilates and incorporates cholesterol into its cellular structure.[1]

L. sporogenes possesses significant β-galactosidase (lactase) activity *in vitro*.[4]

Clinical Indications

Lipid Disorders

Administration of *L. sporogenes* to rabbits resulted in a 90-percent inhibition in the rise of serum cholesterol secondary to feeding of high cholesterol diets.[5]

Oral *L. sporogenes* supplementation (360 million spores/day) decreased total serum cholesterol from an average of 330 mg/dL to 226 mg/dL in 17 subjects with type II hyperlipidemia over a three-month time interval. HDL-cholesterol increased slightly. No changes in serum triglyceride levels were observed.[6]

Digestive Disorders

In laboratory animals with bacterial dysbiosis, *L. sporogenes* supplementation inhibits growth of pathogenic microorganisms and results in renewal of desirable obligate gastrointestinal organisms to normal levels.[3] Reports suggest that supplementation produces a rapid resolution of acute gastrointestinal infection induced by pathogenic bacteria in calves.[3]

It has been reported that the efficacy of treatment in patients with bacterial dysbiosis receiving *L. sporogenes* was 20-30 percent higher than traditional probiotics such as *Lactobacillus acidophilus* or Bifidobacteria.[2]

Seventy percent of individuals suffering from chronic constipation treated with 300-750 million spores per day of *L. sporogenes* for two to 10 days experienced an amelioration of abdominal distention and a normalization of stools.[7]

Reports suggest a benefit in neonatal diarrhea.[7]

Aphthous Stomatitis

Reports suggest efficacy in the treatment of aphthous stomatitis with resolution occurring within two to three days.[8,9]

Vaginitis

Vaginal administration of *L. sporogenes* was investigated in non-specific vaginitis. Subjects with Trichomonas or Candida vaginitis were excluded from the study. Complete relief of pruritis and discharge was reported by 93 percent of subjects. Postmenopausal subjects had a slower response to therapy.[10]

Side Effects and Toxicity

Acute toxicity studies in animals have been conducted with doses as high as 50 g/kg for seven days. No abnormalities, either during supplementation or in the period after withdrawal of the supplement, were observed. Chronic supplementation of doses as high as 5 g/kg for 15 months in animals results in no observed toxicity. In humans, adverse reactions following supplementation have not been reported.

Dosage

A reasonable dose is 100 mg two to three times daily, with each 100 mg containing approximately 1.5 billion colony-forming units.

References

1. Majeed M, Prakash L. *Lactospore®: The Effective Probiotic*. Piscataway, NJ: NutriScience Publishers, Inc.; 1998.
2. Voichishina LG, Chaplinskii VI, V'iunitskaia VA. The use of sporulating bacteria in treating patients with dysbacteriosis. *Vrach Delo* 1991;12:73-75. [Article in Russian]
3. Smirnov VV, Reznik SR, V'iunitskaia VA, et al. The effect of the complex probiotic sporolact on the intestinal microbiocenosis of warm-blooded animals. *Mikrobiol Z* 1995;57:42-49. [Article in Russian]
4. Kim YM, et al. Studies on the production of b-galactosidase by *Lactobacillus sporogenes*. Properties and applications of b-galactosidase. *Korean J Applied Microbiol Bioeng* 1985;13;355-360.
5. Kumar ORM, Christopher KJ. Feeding of *L. sporogenes* to rabbits. *Ind Vet J* 1989;66:896-898.
6. Mohan JC, Arora R, Khalilullah M. Preliminary observations on effect of *Lactobacillus sporogenes* on serum lipid levels in hypercholesterolemic patients. *Indian J Med Res* 1990;92:431-432.
7. Dhongade RK, Anjaneyulu R. *Maharashtra Medical J* 1977;23:473-474. [abstract]
8. Mathur SN, et al. Sporlac therapy in treatment of apthous stomatitis. *Uttar Pradesh State Dent J* 1970;11:7-12.
9. Sharma JK, Kapoor KK, Mukhija RD. Clinical trial of Sporlac in the treatment of recurrent aphthous ulceration. *Uttar Pradesh State Dent J* 1980;11:7-12.
10. Shirodkar NV, Sankholkar PC, Ghosh S, Nulkar SM. Multi-centre clinical assessment of myconip vaginal tablets in non-specific vaginitis. *Indian Pract* 1980;33:207-210.

Ligusticum wallichii

Description

A member of the Umbelliferae family, *Ligusticum wallichii* is used in Chinese medicine for a variety of hematological disorders, including ischemia and thrombosis. When combined with Astragalus, Ligusticum has demonstrated a notable immunopotentiating effect. Included in many classic Chinese formulations, it is also part of the Japanese and Korean herbal formularies. Classically, it is prescribed for headaches, abdominal pain, arthralgias, and menstrual disorders due to blood stasis.[1] Ligusticum's active ingredients include tetramethylpyrazine, ferulic acid, chrysophanol, sedanoic acid, and 1-2 percent essential oils.

Clinical Indications

Ischemia

One-hundred-and-fifty-eight subjects with transient ischemic attacks were randomly divided into a Ligusticum group (111 cases) and an aspirin group (47 cases). The total effective rate in the Ligusticum group was 89.2 percent, compared to 61.7 percent in the aspirin group ($P<0.01$). Ligusticum increased cerebral blood flow, accelerated the velocity of blood flow, dilated the spastic artery, and decreased peripheral arterial resistance.[2] In another study, Ligusticum was evaluated in the treatment of ischemic stroke. Injectable preparations were shown to improve brain microcirculation through inhibiting thrombus formation, decreasing platelet aggregation, and improving blood viscosity. The effect of Ligusticum was the same or better than controls using papaverine, dextran, and aspirin-persantin.[3]

Antibacterial/Antifungal

Ligusticum has demonstrated *in vitro* antibacterial activity against several strains of pathogenic bacteria including *Pseudomonas aeruginosa, Shigella sonnei, Salmonella typhi* and *Vibrio cholera*, as well as many dermatomycoses.[4]

Inflammation

When given to guinea pigs with histamine/acetylcholine-induced bronchospasm, Ligusticum decreased plasma levels of thromboxane B2, relaxed tracheal muscle, increased the forced expiratory volume, and inhibited synthesis and release of thromboxane A2, with no adverse side effects. The total effective rate was 92 percent, compared with 62 percent in the control group ($p <0.01$).[5] In a Japanese study, the active ingredients in Ligusticum, tetramethylpyrazine and ferulic acid, were found to have both significant anti-inflammatory and analgesic effects.[6]

Dosage and Toxicity

Ligusticum is prescribed in traditional Chinese decoctions at dosages up to 9 grams, administered over several days. Overdose symptoms may include vomiting and dizziness.[1]

References

1. Hong YH. *Oriental Materia Medica: A Concise Guide.* Long Beach, CA: Oriental Healing Arts Institute; 1986.
2. Chen DR. Clinical and experimental study of *Ligusticum wallichii* and aspirin in the treatment of transient ischemic attack. *Zhongguo Zhong Xi Yi Jie He Za Zhi* 1992;12:672-674. [article in Chinese]
3. Chen KJ, Chen K. Ischemic stroke treated with *Ligusticum chuanxiong*. *Chin Med J* (Engl) 1992;105:870-873.
4. Bensky D, Gamble A. *Chinese Herbal Medicine: Materia Medica, Revised Edition.* Seattle, WA: Eastland Press; 1993.
5. Shao CR, Chen FM, Tang YX. Clinical and experimental study on *Ligusticum wallichi* mixture in preventing and treating bronchial asthma. *Zhongguo Zhong Xi Yi Jie He Za Zhi* 1994;14:465-468. [article in Chinese]
6. Ozaki Y. Anti-inflammatory effect of tetramethylpyrazine and ferulic acid. *Chem Pharm Bull (Tokyo)* 1992;40:954-956.

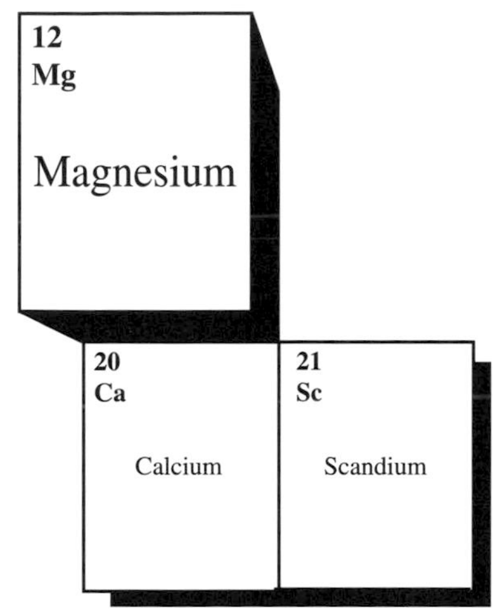

Magnesium

Introduction

Although American diets generally do not contain adequate amounts of magnesium,[1] physiological magnesium deficiencies are more likely to occur in those on diuretics or high sodium diets,[2] with malabsorption syndromes,[3] or with diabetes.[4] Because magnesium plays such a diverse and essential role in human physiology, subclinical magnesium deficiency can manifest in symptoms such as fatigue and muscle weakness.[3] Magnesium deficits can also exacerbate an already existing disease state or increase the risk of complications in specific conditions, including diabetes, cardiovascular conditions, renal stones, osteoporosis, hypertension, preeclampsia, and asthma.

Magnesium exists mostly as an intracellular cation with 99 percent of body stores in intracellular spaces. Approximately 66 percent is found in bone, and 33 percent in cardiac muscle, skeletal muscle, and liver.[3]

Pharmacokinetics

Absorption of magnesium is proportional to the amount ingested, with fractional absorption decreasing the larger the dosage. It is absorbed in both the small intestine and colon, with the distal jejunum and ileum the sites of most efficient absorption, via both active and passive transport. It is taken up in the cells by a carrier-mediated transport system and excreted via the kidneys.

Enteric-coated magnesium salts are less well absorbed than non-enteric-coated supplements.[5] Salts with high solubility such as magnesium citrate appear to be better absorbed than less soluble forms such as magnesium oxide.[6]

Mechanisms of Action

Magnesium is involved in over 300 enzymatic reactions in the body, including ATP synthesis, protein synthesis, glycogen breakdown, fatty acid oxidation, and maintenance of membrane stability of the cardiovascular, neuromuscular, neuroendocrine, and immune systems.[7] Magnesium plays a regulatory role in the sodium-potassium ATPase pump, with a magnesium deficiency impairing movement of potassium into the cell.[4] This may explain the clinical phenomenon of hypokalemia that is remedied only when magnesium supplementation is used.[8] Magnesium also acts as a calcium channel blocker, with magnesium deficiency resulting in increased intracellular calcium. Conversely, higher levels of magnesium inhibit intra- and extracellular calcium flux.[9] Magnesium affects parathormone (PTH) secretion; hypomagnesemia induces hypocalcemia as a chronic magnesium deficiency impairs PTH production.[10] Magnesium deficiency also impairs the synthesis of 1,25(OH)2 vitamin D and can lead to peripheral resistance to the effects of vitamin D as well as resistance to PTH.[11]

Deficiency States and Symptoms

Magnesium deficiency may be precipitated by a multitude of factors, including acute renal tubular damage, diabetes,[3] caffeine use,[12] cocaine use, alcohol abuse, malabsorption syndromes, short bowel syndrome, pancreatitis, diarrhea, laxative use, phosphorus depletion (found in eating disorders), parenteral feeding, hyperthyroidism, acute myocardial infarction, cardiac bypass surgery, major trauma, burns,[3] and AIDS.[13]

The symptoms of magnesium deficiency are diverse and include cardiac arrhythmias,[14] hypertension, vasospasm, electrocardiogram changes, and muscle fasciculations.[15] Bronchospasm, muscle weakness, headache, hypokalemia, and insulin resistance also occur in non-critical patients with low magnesium.[16]

Clinical Indications

Asthma

Epidemiological evidence indicates a relationship between declining magnesium intake and increased prevalence of asthma.[17] Children with asthma have lower leukocyte magnesium levels during bronchial obstruction and acute attacks compared to children without asthma.[18] There is good evidence, in acute episodes, that intravenous magnesium acts as a large airway bronchodilator.[19-22] Not only does magnesium have a relaxing effect on bronchial airways, it has a positive effect on reducing mast cell degranulation, pulmonary muscle contractility, and neuro-hormonal mediator release.[23] The majority of research has involved either intravenous or nebulized magnesium sulfate in acute asthma attacks and in chronic asthma.[24]

A single-blind, placebo-controlled, cross-over study found significant reduction in airway resistance in stable asthmatics in response to 2.5 g intravenous magnesium sulfate.[19] The effect lasted for 20 minutes post-infusion, which was the extent of the monitoring period. This work has been replicated by several researchers,[25,26] and although no studies have looked at oral magnesium supplementation in asthma, there is a significant correlation between increased bronchial reactivity and lowered intracellular magnesium levels in asthmatics.[27]

Several authors have suggested oral magnesium salts are beneficial in the treatment of asthma and other reactive airway diseases.[17,23,24,28] Harari[24] studied 38 asthmatic patients who were treated at a clinic on the Dead Sea, an environment where both the water and the ambient air are high in magnesium and bromides. At the end of 28 days, all patients had experienced a significant decrease in their peak flow index, 36.8 percent had suspended their medications, and 43 percent had reduced the frequency of medication use.

Cardiovascular and Cerebrovascular Disease

Using a variety of assays for tissue magnesium stores, studies of patients with vasospastic angina, coronary artery disease, and cardiovascular mortality revealed low magnesium stores in the majority of those tested.[29]

Ischemia-Reperfusion Injury

Magnesium has been shown to reduce ischemia-reperfusion injury in the myocardium.[29] When blood flow is re-established in ischemic tissue, free radicals and an influx of leukocytes can cause further damage to this tissue. Ischemia-reperfusion injury occurs in 23-27 percent of all patients receiving thrombolytic therapy during an acute myocardial infarction.[30] Magnesium can prevent and reverse free radical-mediated damage to the endothelium.[30,31]

Stroke

Epidemiological evidence indicates risk for stroke and stroke-related mortality is reduced in populations that have magnesium-rich diets.[32] A 1997 study found 98 of 105 stroke patients (many below age 55) had deficient levels of serum ionized magnesium.[33] The levels of magnesium in the study were found to cause rapid, prolonged, and often irreversible contraction and spasm of cultured, cerebral-vascular smooth muscle cells. Both animal and human studies have shown low magnesium levels correlate with greater cerebral infarct size.[34,35]

Mitral Valve Prolapse

Mitral valve prolapse (MVP) is particularly prevalent among women of childbearing age. A randomized study of 141 patients with echocardiogram-confirmed MVP found 60 percent had an abnormally low serum magnesium level (<0.7 mMol/L).[36] Seventy patients with low RBC magnesium levels received either oral magnesium supplementation or a placebo for a five-week period. The magnesium group received 1,800 mg/day of magnesium carbonate (510 mg of elemental magnesium) for the first week, then 1,200 mg/day of magnesium carbonate (340 mg of elemental magnesium) for the remaining four weeks. The average number of MVP symptoms in the patients treated with magnesium decreased from 10.4 to 5.6 after treatment. At the beginning of the study, anxiety was present in 54 percent of the supplemented patients and five weeks later was present in only 15 percent. The level of norepinephrine excreted in the urine also declined markedly after magnesium supplementation, and increased in the placebo group. The researchers concluded MVP symptoms were linked to magnesium deficiency in the study population and hypothesized the deficiency may be caused by an increased release of epinephrine and norepinephrine in MVP patients. The beneficial effect of magnesium was speculated to be a result of magnesium's ability to inhibit the toxic effects of an excessive release of catecholamines.

Hyperlipidemia

One uncontrolled, pilot study in 16 hyperlipidemic adults with abnormally low HDL (35.2 ± 8.7) found supplementation with magnesium chloride reduced total cholesterol an average of 40 points (from 297.6 ± 56.9 to 257.1 ± 39.1).[37]

The author's proposed mechanism for magnesium's hypocholesterolemic effect is the ability of magnesium to partially inactivate the catecholaminergic response of the adrenal gland and sympathetic nervous system, diminishing lipolysis. Magnesium also increases lipoprotein lipase through a similar mechanism.

Hypertension

Magnesium has been effective in lowering elevated blood pressure in long-term diuretic users, those on high-sodium diets, in hypertension associated with diabetes, and those with high renin levels.[38,39] Approximately 50 percent of magnesium-depleted subjects have hypertension that responds to restoration of normal serum magnesium levels.[40]

Pregnancy

Magnesium is essential for the release of parathyroid hormone in pregnancy. Epidemiological studies show an inverse relationship between magnesium levels in drinking water and risk of stillbirth.[41] Randomized studies are conflicting in their assessment of magnesium supplementation in pregnancy and its effects on preeclampsia, reduced risk of preterm labor, maternal hospitalization, and increasing birth weight.[42,43] However, when given during pregnancy, magnesium sulfate reduces risk of eclampsia in women with pregnancy-induced hypertension.[44]

Osteoporosis

Women with osteoporosis have demonstrated significantly low serum magnesium, evidence of magnesium depletion in magnesium loading test, and low levels of magnesium in bone tissue.[45-47] Magnesium intake has been positively correlated with forearm bone mineral content in women aged 23-75.[48] Prospective studies of osteoporotic women given tolerance-dosed (up to 750 mg per day) magnesium hydroxide for two years resulted in significant increases in trabecular bone density in the wrist during the first year of the study. In the second year, the bone density measurements simply leveled off.[45]

A trial in ovariectomized rats, shown to be a useful model for research relating to postmenopausal women, utilized a high-magnesium, high-calcium diet to evaluate the effect of magnesium on bone strength and bone resorption.[49] Magnesium supplementation at 0.15 percent of the total diet (the equivalent of 1,300 mg magnesium/day in an adult female) increased osteocalcin (a marker for osteoblastic activity), reduced parathyroid hormone and deoxypyridinoline (a bone resorption marker), and increased bone strength and fracture resistance of the femur. Bone formation, prevention of bone resorption, and increase in dynamic strength of bone occurred even though intestinal calcium absorption was reduced in rats on the high-magnesium diet.

Magnesium supplementation also appears to have benefit in osteoporosis secondary to malabsorption in gluten-sensitive enteropathy (GSE).[50] In five patients with GSE and osteoporosis of the hip and spine, 500-575 mg magnesium hydroxide daily resulted in statistically significant increases in femoral neck and total proximal femoral bone density. This increase, which took place after two years, occurred along with an increase in erythrocyte magnesium levels.

Diabetes and Insulin Resistance

Diabetics, especially those with type 1 diabetes, are at risk for magnesium deficiency because glycosuria and insulin insensitivity increase renal loss of magnesium and decrease magnesium absorption from the intestine.[51-53] There is a positive correlation between elevations in glycosylated hemoglobin and the severity of magnesium deficiency in diabetes.[4] Conversely, studies indicate magnesium supplementation improves glucose handling in nondiabetics and improves insulin sensitivity in type 1 and 2 diabetes.[54-56]

Magnesium deficiency appears to play a role in the development of diabetic retinopathy, as magnesium levels are lower in diabetics with retinopathy and magnesium deficiency states may contribute to circulatory damage that leads to microangiopathy.[57,58]

Kidney Stones

Several studies have addressed the efficacy of both magnesium and citrate separately in the prevention of recurrent calcium oxalate stones.[59,60] Citrate forms insoluble complexes with calcium, inhibiting the formation of calcium phosphate and oxalate stones.[61] When citrate is given as a salt (in combination with sodium or potassium), it increases urinary pH, inhibiting uric acid stone formation.[62] In idiopathic calcium-stone formers, low erythrocyte magnesium levels indicate possible magnesium deficiency as a factor in stone formation.[63]

Magnesium supplementation alone has been shown to reduce oxalate levels in the urine and prevent recurrent stone formation. In a controlled study, 55 patients who had an average of 0.8 stones per year, were given 500 mg elemental magnesium daily.[64] After a period of 2-4 years, the rate of stone formation was reduced to 0.08 stones/person/year, a 90-percent reduction. Eighty-five percent of patients remained stone free during the trial. A control group of 43 patients experienced an increase in incidence of stone formation with 59 percent developing new stones in the four-year follow-up period. In another controlled trial, 45 out of 56 patients (80%) were stone free after 200 mg magnesium hydroxide twice daily for two years. In the control group, 44 percent experienced recurrences.[65]

Magnesium and potassium, supplemented in combination as magnesium-potassium citrate, were able to produce a higher level of urinary citrate than either alone.[61] An uncontrolled study in patients with calcium renal stones found magnesium-potassium citrate supplementation resulted in a significant decrease in the ability to form calcium oxalate stones in those with idiopathic calcium urolithiasis.[66] Patients were given magnesium-potassium citrate in doses that supplied 185 mg elemental magnesium with 22 mMol potassium daily. Uric acid levels in those patients decreased by 60 percent, urinary pH rose by 80 percent, and calcium oxalate formation declined significantly.

Headache

Migraine and cluster headaches have been associated with low free magnesium levels in the brain, with the lowest levels in those with the most severe migraine symptomology.[67] Multiple studies have also found low serum and erythrocyte magnesium levels in the majority of those with either migraine or cluster headaches.[68,69] Magnesium has been used effectively intravenously for symptom relief, and oral supplementation of 360 mg elemental magnesium has shown relief in premenstrual migraine.[70,71]

Physical Exertion/Altitude Sickness

Athletes are at risk for magnesium deficiency.[72] An uncontrolled study of four mountain climbers reported significant improvement in altitude sickness symptom scores at 3,700-4,600 meter elevations after taking magnesium citrate at daily doses of 900-1,200 mg.[73] The climbers reported feeling less fatigue and muscular discomfort; no adverse effects were reported.

Chemical Toxicity

Magnesium is one of the most common nutrient deficiencies in those with environmentally-induced illness.[74] Patients found to retain chemical residues and heavy metals were also found to excrete high amounts of magnesium in their urine.[75] This deficiency leads to decreased cytochrome p450 and NADPH cytochrome reductase activity, both of which are essential for proper drug and chemical biotransformation. Magnesium deficiency, particularly in chemically toxic individuals, also limits metabolism of aniline and aminopyrene, both carcinogens. Supplementation with magnesium can reverse the effects of these deficits.[75]

Premenstrual Syndrome

Some subpopulations of women with premenstrual syndrome (PMS) demonstrate low magnesium levels. In a double-blind, placebo-controlled study, women with PMS were given 360 mg magnesium three times daily or placebo from day 15 of their menstrual cycle until menses. Magnesium significantly improved some measurements of mood changes.[76]

Fibromyalgia

Abnormalities in magnesium status have been noted in patients with fibromyalgia, including elevated hair magnesium,[77] high leukocyte magnesium, and low erythrocyte magnesium.[78] Supplementation of magnesium combined with malic acid has reduced severity of pain and tenderness associated with fibromyalgia.[79]

Drug-Nutrient Interactions

Medications that cause magnesium deficiency include diuretics (especially loop diuretics), amphotericin-B, platinum-based chemotherapy, aminoglycosides, cyclosporine, and albuterol and other beta agonists.[3]

Digoxin causes increased urinary magnesium loss; this can be dangerous, as magnesium deficiency increases the toxicity of digoxin, which develops at significantly lower blood levels when the patient is magnesium deficient.[81]

Magnesium can interfere with the absorption of tetracyclines. It is advised to supplement with magnesium at a time of day other than when taking tetracyclines.

Side Effects and Toxicity

Dosages over 500 mg magnesium hydroxide or oxide have resulted in gastrointestinal disturbances and diarrhea (probably due to poor absorption), and may induce net phosphate loss.[80] Elevated blood levels of magnesium occur infrequently in renal insufficiency and in chronic use of magnesium-containing laxatives and antacids. Magnesium supplementation is contraindicated in renal insufficiency.[3]

Dosage

Therapeutic effects appear in oral dosages as low as 250 mg elemental magnesium in magnesium-deficient individuals but may need to be increased to 12 mg per kg body weight for therapeutic interventions.[82] Both magnesium citrate and magnesium citrate-malate are significantly more soluble and absorbable than the oxide or hydroxide forms.[6,83]

References

1. Pennington JA. Current dietary intakes of trace elements and minerals. In: Bogden J, Klevay LM, eds. *Clinical Nutrition of the Essential Trace Elements and Minerals*. Totowa: Humana Press; 2000:49-67.
2. Massry SG, Coburn JW, Chapman LW, Kleeman CR. Effect of NaCl infusion on urinary Ca^{++} and Mg^{++} during reduction in their filtered loads. *Am J Physiol* 1967;213:1218-1224.
3. Dacey MJ. Hypomagnesemic disorders. *Crit Care Clin* 2001;17:155-173.
4. Sjogren A, Floren CH, Nilsson A. Magnesium deficiency in IDDM related to level of glycosylated hemoglobin. *Diabetes* 1986;35:459-463.
5. Hendler SS, Rorvik D. *PDR for Nutritional Supplements*, 1st ed. Des Moines, IA: Medical Economics – Thompson Healthcare; 2001.

6. Fine KD, Santa Ana CA, Porter JL, Fordtran JS. Intestinal absorption of magnesium from food and supplements. *J Clin Invest* 1991;88:396-402.

7. Ebel H, Gunther T. Magnesium metabolism: a review. *J Clin Chem Biochem* 1980;18:T257-270.

8. Whang R, Oei O, Aikawa JK, et al. Predictors of clinical hypomagnesemia. Hypokalemia, hypophosphatemia, hyponatremia, and hypocalcemia. *Arch Intern Med* 1984;144:1794-1796.

9. White RE, Hartzell HC. Effects of intracellular free magnesium on calcium current in isolated cardiac myocytes. *Science* 1988;239:778-780.

10. Martini L. Magnesium supplementation and bone turnover. *Nutr Rev* 1999;57:227-229.

11. Freitag JJ, Martin KJ, Conrades MB, et al. Evidence for skeletal resistance to parathyroid hormone in magnesium deficiency. *J Clin Invest* 1979;64:1238-1244.

12. Yeh JK, Aloia JF, Semla HM, Chen SY. Influence of injected caffeine on the metabolism of calcium and the retention and excretion of sodium, potassium, phosphorus, magnesium, zinc and copper in rats. *J Nutr* 1986;116:273-280.

13. Skirnik JH, Bogden JD, Baker H, et al. Micronutrient profiles in HIV-1-infected heterosexual adults. *J Acquir Immune Defic Syndr Hum Retrovirol* 1996;12:75-83.

14. Arsenian MA. Magnesium and cardiovascular disease. *Prog Cardiovasc Dis* 1993;35:271-310.

15. Foley C, Zaritsky A. Should we measure ionized magnesium? *Crit Care Med* 1998;26:1949-1950.

16. Ferrari R, Albertini A, Curello S, et al. Myocardial recovery during post-ischaemic reperfusion: effects of nifedepine, calcium and magnesium *J Mol Cell Cardiol* 1986;18:487-498.

17. Soutar A, Seaton A, Brown K. Bronchial reactivity and dietary antioxidants. *Thorax* 1997;52:166-170.

18. Mircetic RN, Dodig S, Raos M, et al. Magnesium concentration in plasma, leukocytes and urine in children with intermittent asthma. *Clin Chim Acta* 2001;312:197-203.

19. Sharma SK, Bhargava A, Pande JN. Effect of parenteral magnesium sulfate on pulmonary functions in bronchial asthma. *J Asthma* 1994;31:109-115.

20. Noppen M, Vanmaele L, Impens N, et al. Effect of inhaled magnesium sulfate on sodium metabisulfate induced bronchoconstriction in asthma. *Chest* 1997;111:858-861.

21. Skobeloff EM, Spivey WH, McNamara RM, Greenspon L. Intravenous magnesium sulfate for the treatment of acute asthma in the emergency department. *JAMA* 1989;262;1210-1213.

22. Skorodin MS, Tenholder MF, Yetter B, et al. Magnesium sulfate in exacerbations of chronic obstructive pulmonary disease. *Arch Intern Med* 1995;155:496-500.

23. Mathew R, Altura BM. Magnesium and the lungs. *Magnesium* 1988;7:173-187.

24. Harari M, Barzillai R, Shani J. Magnesium in the management of asthma: critical review of acute and chronic treatments, and Deutsches Medizinisches Zentrum's (DMZ's) clinical experience at the Dead Sea. *J Asthma* 1998;35:525-536.

25. Okayama H, Aikawa T, Okayama M, et al. Bronchodilating effect of intravenous magnesium sulfate in bronchial asthma. *JAMA* 1987;257:1076-1078.

26. Rolla G, Bucca C, Bugiana M, et al. Reduction of histamine-induced bronchoconstriction by magnesium in asthmatic patients. *Allergy* 1987;42:186-188.

27. Dominguez LJ Barbagallo M, DiLorenzo G, et al. Bronchial reactivity and intracellular magnesium: a possible mechanism for the bronchodilating effects of magnesium in asthma. *Clin Sci* 1998;95:137-142.

28. Durlach J, Durlach V, Bac P, et al. Magnesium and therapeutics. *Magnes Res* 1994;7:313-328.

29. Gomez MN. Magnesium and cardiovascular disease. *Anesthesiology* 1998;89:222-240.

30. Shechter M, Sharir M, Labrador MJ, et al. Oral magnesium therapy improves endothelial function in patients with coronary artery disease. *Circulation* 2000;102:2353-2358.

31. Tofukuji M, Stamler A, Li J, et al. Effects of magnesium cardioplegia on regulation of the porcine coronary circulation. *J Surg Res* 1997;233-239.

32. Iso H, Stampfer MJ, Manson JE, et al. Prospective study of calcium, potassium, and magnesium intake and risk of stroke in women. *Stroke* 1999;30:1772-1779.

33. Altura BT, Memon ZI, Zhang A, et al. Low levels of serum ionized magnesium are found in patients early after stroke which results in rapid elevation in cytosolic free calcium and spasm in cerebral vascular muscle cells. *Neurosci Lett* 1997;230:37-40.

34. Lee EJ, Ayoub IA, Harris FB, et al. Mexiletine and magnesium independently, but not combined, protect against permanent focal cerebral ischemia in Wistar rats. *J Neurosci Res* 1999;58:442-448.

35. Lampl Y, Geva D, Gilad R, et al. Cerebrospinal fluid magnesium level as a prognostic factor in ischaemic stroke. *J Neurol* 1998;245:584-588.

36. Lichodziejewska B, Klos J, Rezler J, et al. Clinical symptoms of mitral valve prolapse are related to hypomagnesemia and attenuated by magnesium supplementation. *Am J Cardiol* 1997;79:768-772.

37. Davis WH, Leary WP, Reyes AJ, et al. Monotherapy with magnesium increases abnormally low high density lipoprotein cholesterol: a clinical assay. *Curr Ther Res* 1984;36:341-346.

38. Dyckner T, Wester PO. Effect of magnesium on blood pressure. *Br Med J* 1983;286:1847-1849.

39. Saito K, Hattori K, Omatsu T, et al. Effects of oral magnesium on blood pressure and red cell sodium transport in patients receiving long-term thiazide diuretics for hypertension. *Am J Hypertens* 1988;1:71S-74S.

40. Altura BM, Altura BT. Magnesium ions and contraction of vascular smooth muscles: relationship to some vascular diseases. *Fed Proc* 1981;40:2672-2679.

41. Klebanoff MA, Shiono PH, Berendes HW, Rhoads GG. Facts and artifacts about anemia and preterm delivery. *JAMA* 1989;262:511-515.

42. Spatling L, Spatling G. Magnesium supplementation in pregnancy. A double-blind study. *Brit J Obstet Gynaecol* 1988;95:120-125.

43. Sibai BM, Villar MA, Bray E. Magnesium supplementation during pregnancy: A double-blind randomized controlled clinical trial. *Am J Obstet Gynecol* 1989;161:115-119.

44. Lindheimer MD. Pre-eclampsia-eclampsia 1996: preventable? Have disputes on its treatment been resolved? *Curr Opin Nephrol Hyperten* 1996;5:452-458.

45. Stendig-Lindberg G, Tepper R, Leichter I. Trabecular bone density in a two year controlled trial of peroral magnesium in osteoporosis. *Magnes Res* 1993;6:155-163.

46. Cohen L, Laor L. Correlation between bone magnesium concentration and magnesium retention in the intravenous magnesium load test. *Magnes Res* 1990;3:271-274.

47. Cohen L. Laor L, Kitzes R. Magnesium malabsorption in postmenopausal osteoporosis. *Magnesium* 1983;2:139-143.

48. Angus RM, Sambrook PN, Pocock NA, Eisman JA. Dietary intake and bone mineral density. *Bone Miner* 1988;4:265-277.

49. Toba Y, Kajita Y, Masuyama R, et al. Dietary magnesium supplementation affects bone metabolism and dynamic strength of bone in ovariectomized rats. *J Nutr* 2000;130:216-220.

50. Rude RK. Olerich M. Magnesium deficiency: possible role in osteoporosis associated with gluten-sensitive enteropathy. *Osteoporos Int* 1996;6:453-461.

51. Elamin A, Tuvemo T. Magnesium and insulin-dependent diabetes mellitus. *Diabetes Res Clin Pract* 1990;10:203-209.

52. Paolisso G, Sgambato S, Passariello N, et al. Insulin induces opposite changes in plasma and erythrocyte magnesium concentrations in normal man. *Diabetologia* 1986;29:644-647.

53. de Valk HW. Magnesium and diabetes mellitus. *Neth J Med* 1999;54:139-146.

54. Paolisso G, Sgambato S, Pizza G, et al. Improved insulin response and action by chronic magnesium administration in aged NIDDM subjects. *Diabetes Care* 1989;12:265-269.

55. Paolisso G, Sgambato S, Gambardella A, et al. Daily magnesium supplements improve glucose handling in elderly subjects. *Am J Clin Nutr* 1992;55:1161-1167.

56. Sjogren A, Floren CH, Nilsson A. Oral administration of magnesium hydroxide to subjects with insulin-dependent diabetes mellitus: effects on magnesium and potassium levels and on insulin requirements. *Magnesium* 1988;7:117-122.

57. Williams B, Schrier RW. Characterization of glucose-induced in situ protein kinase C activity in cultured vascular smooth muscle cells. *Diabetes* 1992;41:1464-1472.

58. Ceriello A, Guigliano D, Dello Russo P, Passariello N. Hypomagnesemia in relation to diabetic retinopathy. *Diabetes Care* 1982;5:558-559.

59. Pak CY, Fuller C. Idiopathic hypocitraturic calcium-oxalate nephrolithiasis successfully treated with potassium citrate. *Ann Intern Med* 1986:104:33-37.

60. Hallson PC, Rose GA, Sulaiman S. Magnesium reduces calcium oxalate crystal formation in human whole urine. *Clin Sci* 1982;62:17-19.

61. Koenig K, Padalino P, Alexandrides G, Pak CY. Bioavailability of potassium and magnesium, and citraturic response from potassium-magnesium citrate. *J Urol* 1991;145:330-334.

62. Pak CY, Sakhaee K, Fuller C. Successful management of uric acid nephrolithiasis with potassium citrate. *Kidney Int* 1986;30:422-428.

63. Schmiedl A, Schwille PO. Magnesium status in idiopathic calcium urolithiasis – an orientational study in younger males. *Eur J Clin Chem Clin Biochem* 1996;34:393-400.

64. Johansson G, Backman U, Danielson BG, et al. Effects of magnesium hydroxide in renal stone disease. *J Am Coll Nutr* 1982;1:179-185.

65. Johansson G, Backman U, Danielson BG, et al. Magnesium metabolism in renal stone formers. Effects of therapy with magnesium hydroxide. *Scand J Urol Nephrol Suppl* 1980;53:125-134.

66. Pak CY, Koenig K, Khan R, et al. Physiochemical action of potassium-magnesium citrate in nephrolithiasis. *J Bone Miner Res* 1992;7:281-285.

67. Lodi R, Iotti S, Cortelli P, et al. Deficient energy metabolism is associated with low free magnesium in the brains of patients with migraine and cluster headache. *Brain Res Bull* 2001;54:437-441.

68. Sarchielli P, Costa G, Firenze C, et al. Serum and salivary magnesium levels in migraine and tension-type headaches. Results in a group of adult patients. *Cephalalgia* 1992;12:21-27.

69. Soriani S, Arnaldi C, De Carlo L, et al. Serum and red blood cell magnesium levels in juvenile migraine patients. *Headache* 1995;35:14-16.

70. Mauskop A, Altura BT, Cracco RQ, Altura BM. Intravenous magnesium sulfate relieves migraine attacks in patients with low serum ionized magnesium levels: a pilot study. *Clin Sci* 1995;89:633-636.

71. Facchinetti F, Sances G, Borella P, et al. Magnesium prophylaxis of menstrual migraine: effects on intracellular magnesium. *Headache* 1991;31:298-301.

72. Lukaski HC. Magnesium, zinc, and chromium nutriture and physical activity. *Am J Clin Nutr* 2000;72:585S-593S.

73. Dumont L, Mardirosoff C, Soto-Debeuf G, Tassonyi E. Magnesium and acute mountain sickness. *Aviat Space Environ Med* 1999;70:625.

74. Rea W. *Chemical Sensitivity.* Boca Raton, Fl: CRC Press; 1992:vol 1:307.

75. Crinnion W. Environmental Medicine. In Pizzorno J, Murray M, eds. *The Textbook of Natural Medicine.* 2nd ed. New York: Churchill Livingstone; 1999:297.

76. Facchinetti F, Borella P, Sances G, et al. Oral magnesium successfully relieves premenstrual mood changes. *Obstet Gynecol* 1991;78:177-181.

77. Ng SY. Hair calcium and magnesium levels in patients with fibromyalgia: a case center study. *J Manipulative Physiol Ther* 1999;22:586-593.

78. Eisinger J, Plantamura A, Marie PA, Ayavou T. Selenium and magnesium status in fibromyalgia. *Magnes Res* 1994;7:285-288.

79. Russell IJ, Michalek JE, Flechas JD, Abraham GE. Treatment of fibromyalgia syndrome with Super Malic: a randomized, double blind, placebo controlled, crossover pilot study. *J Rheumatol* 1995;22:953-958.

80. Murray M, Pizzorno J. Hypertension. In Pizzorno J, Murray M, eds. *The Textbook of Natural Medicine.* 2nd ed. New York: Churchill Livingstone; 1999:1306.

81. Young IS, Goh EM, McKillop UH, et al. Magnesium status and digoxin toxicity. *Br J Clin Pharmacol* 1991;32:717-721.

82. Spencer H. Minerals and mineral interactions in human beings. *J Am Diet Assoc* 1986:86:864-867.

83. Basso LE, Ubbink JB, Delport R, et al. Effect of magnesium supplementation on the fractional absorption of 45CaCl2 in women with a low erythrocyte magnesium concentration. *Metabolism* 2000;49:1092-1096.

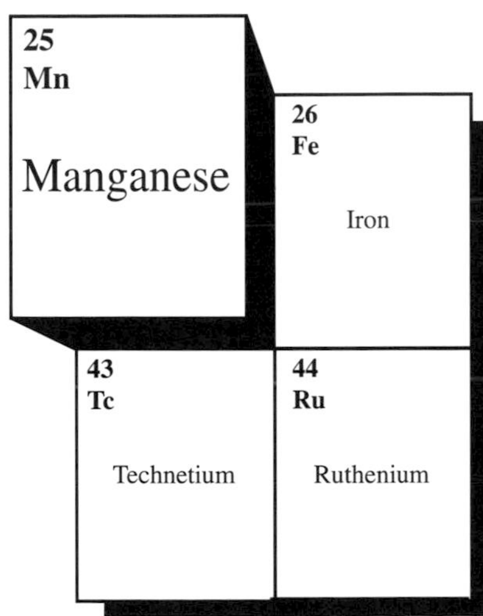

Manganese

Introduction

Manganese is considered to be a trace mineral, of which the average adult needs 2-5 mg per day to meet the Estimated Safe and Adequate Daily Dietary Intake (ESADDI).[1] Americans, however, especially women, consume less than these levels.[2] Even at 2-5 mg per day, women can be in negative manganese balance, with the daily excretion of manganese exceeding intake.[3]

Manganese is necessary for the production of manganese superoxide dismutase, an antioxidant enzyme that quenches the superoxide radical. Many environmental and dietary factors, including ozone,[4] alcohol,[5] high polyunsaturated fat diet, and oxidative stress[6] increase the need for superoxide dismutase and may increase the biological need for manganese.

Biochemistry and Mechanisms of Action

Manganese concentrates in mitochondrial tissue and in the bone, liver, pancreas, and kidney.[7] Manganese is an essential component of carbohydrate metabolism, reproductive function, and skeletal and cartilage development.[8] Manganese is the critical element in the metalloenzymes pyruvate decarboxylase and superoxide dismutase that are involved in energy production and immune function. Manganese also activates phosphatases, kinases, decarboxylases, and glycosyltransferases, facilitating the synthesis of protein and DNA in the production of mucopolysaccharides found in cartilage.[3] Superoxide dismutase – an enzyme that protects cell membranes from lipid peroxidation,[9] radiation- or chemical-induced carcinogenesis,[10] reperfusion injury,[11] and inflammation[12] – has been found at low levels in manganese deficiency.[13] In animal studies, manganese supplementation has significantly elevated levels of superoxide dismutase.[13]

Pharmacokinetics

Manganese is absorbed in the small intestine, but absorptive efficiency is poor. Absorbed manganese is very quickly secreted (within minutes) into the gut in bile. It is estimated that six percent of ingested manganese is absorbed.[14] This low absorption and rapid elimination serves as a protective mechanism against manganese toxicity.[15] Absorbed manganese is transported in the blood bound to plasma carrier proteins and is eliminated primarily through the feces.

Deficiency States

Human manganese deficiency is uncommon. Severely manganese-deficient animals exhibit symptoms of growth retardation, dermatitis, and reproductive failure, as well as metabolic changes including reduced HDL cholesterol and diabetic-like glucose intolerance.[16,17] Decreased serum manganese has been found in epileptics,[18-20] diabetics,[21,22] and persons with osteoporosis.[23]

The case of a well-known basketball player who had a history of recurrent non-healing fracture, bone pain, and no measurable blood manganese was brought to the attention of researchers at the University of California at San Diego.[24] The reversal of this condition with supplemental manganese, calcium, zinc, and copper initiated more research in the area of manganese metabolism and bone physiology. Other patients with slow fracture-healing rates were also shown to have low blood manganese, copper, and zinc levels.[24]

Clinical Indications

Osteopenia/Osteoporosis

Multiple studies in animals have shown manganese-deficient diets in rats prevent cartilage formation and produce osteopenia, the result of an imbalance between osteoblastic and osteoclastic activity.[25] In controlled studies of postmenopausal women with and without bone density changes, the serum manganese levels in the osteoporotic women were significantly lower.[23] In a randomized, controlled, two-year trial, the same researchers used a trace mineral combination of 15 mg zinc, 2.5 mg copper, and 5 mg manganese with calcium citrate-malate (1,000 mg elemental calcium) against placebo and calcium citrate-malate alone in postmenopausal women.[23] The increase in bone gain was greatest in those given trace minerals plus calcium, although the change did not reach statistical significance. Although this trial was unable to look at the effect of single element supplementation, evidence for a synergistic effect exists. Supplementation with manganese appears to be warranted in those at risk for osteoporosis, particularly if manganese levels are low.

Epilepsy

Several studies have found low levels of manganese in blood or hair of epileptic adults and children.[18-20] In one study of 52 epileptics, the difference between manganese levels was significant; blood manganese levels in epileptics were 24-percent lower than control levels ($p<0.002$).[18] In those with significantly lower manganese, the frequency of seizure activity and cases of non-trauma-related epilepsy were positively correlated with depressed manganese levels. One case study of pediatric seizure disorder involved a boy with blood manganese levels of 50 percent of normal values.[26] After supplementation of 20 mg per day, seizure frequency decreased and speech, gait, and cognitive function improved.

Diabetes

Levels of both erythrocyte and lymphocyte manganese levels have been shown to be significantly depressed in type 1 diabetics.[21,22] Manganese has been shown to have hypoglycemic effects in type 1. A case report of a 21-year-old male with type 1 diabetes revealed consistent depressions in blood glucose levels, even with hypoglycemic events, after 3-5 mg oral manganese chloride supplementation.[27] Manganese deficiency, in addition to a role in inhibiting gluconeogenesis and altering carbohydrate metabolism,[28] appears to play a role in the pathology of diabetes through decreased levels of the antioxidant enzyme manganese superoxide dismutase.[29] In animal studies, manganese-deficient diets in diabetic rats decreased the production of manganese superoxide dismutase in the kidney and liver, and increased lipid peroxidation. Increased oxidative damage is linked to nephropathy in animal models of diabetes and possibly vascular and neural complications in human diabetes.[30] In young, female non-diabetics 15 mg manganese had a significant elevating effect on lymphocyte manganese superoxide dismutase.[31]

Side Effects and Toxicity

Manganese balance studies reveal some people can be in positive balance with intakes of 2.5-15 mg per day, while others may be in negative manganese balance at the same level of dietary intake. This wide variance in need for manganese may be related to factors that inhibit manganese absorption: dietary calcium, iron, phosphorus, and phytate.[15] Another difficulty in understanding manganese nutrition is that in rats, at least 37 percent of absorbed manganese is excreted in bile.[32] Studies showing greater levels of biliary manganese excreted with concomitant heavy metal administration may indicate a relationship between manganese loss and heavy metal accumulation and elimination.[33,34]

There is only one published case of "supplemental manganese" toxicity in the literature in an elderly man who had been taking unknown amounts of manganese for several years.[35] He had significantly elevated serum manganese levels, symptoms of dementia, and a Parkinson-like syndrome.

Elevated plasma manganese levels have been documented in parenteral manganese supplementation and in patients with impaired liver function or biliary secretion. Manganese toxicity has been documented in chronic inhalation in manganese miners and arc welders. Toxicity symptoms include anorexia, growth depression, aggressive behavior, reproductive failure, anemia, severe psychiatric disorders, and neurological disorders resembling schizophrenia and Parkinson's disease.[36]

Manganese is considered non-toxic when administered orally. Research on oral manganese has shown the body is protected from oral toxicity by low absorption levels and a high rate of elimination by the liver.[15] In several small studies, elevated hair manganese levels have been suspected to contribute to aggressive behavior,[37] attention deficit disorder,[38] dementia,[39] and learning disorders.[40,41] It is unclear whether these correlations hold merit, but some practitioners have opted to use caution with supplemental manganese.

Dosage

Case studies cited above used 5-20 mg doses for treatment of manganese deficiency. The Tolerable Upper Intake Level (the highest level of daily nutrient intake likely to pose no risk of adverse health effect in almost all individuals) is 11 mg daily.[42]

References

1. Pennington JA. Current dietary intakes of trace elements and minerals. In: Bogden JD, Klevay LM, eds. *Clinical Nutrition of the Essential Trace Elements and Minerals*. Totowa, NJ: Humana Press; 2000:49-68.
2. National Research Council. *Recommended Dietary Allowances*. 10th ed. Washington, DC: National Academic Press; 1989.
3. Manganese bioavailability overview. In: Kies C, ed. *Nutritional Bioavailability of Manganese*. Washington, DC: American Chemical Society; 1987:1-8.
4. Heng H, Rucker RB, Crotty J, Dubick MA. The effects of ozone on lung, heart, and liver superoxide dismutase and glutathione peroxidase activities in the protein-deficient rat. *Toxicol Lett* 1987;38:225-237.
5. Keen CL, Tamura T, Lonnerdal B, et al. Changes in hepatic superoxide dismutase activity in alcoholic monkeys. *Am J Clin Nutr* 1985;41:929-932.
6. Davis CD, Ney DM, Greger JL. Manganese, iron and lipid interactions in rats. *J Nutr* 1990;120:507-513.
7. Nickolova PI. Effect of manganese on essential trace element metabolism. Tissue concentrations and excretion of manganese, iron, copper, cobalt and zinc. *Trace Elem Med* 1993;10:141-147.
8. Matkovic V, Badenhop N, Ilich JK. Trace element and mineral nutrition in adolescents. In: Bogden JD, Klevay LM, eds. *Clinical Nutrition of the Essential Trace Elements and Minerals.* Totowa, NJ: Humana Press; 2000:49-68.
9. Pucheu S, Coudray C, Tresallet N, et al. Effect of iron overload in the isolated ischemic and reperfused rat heart. *Cardiovasc Drugs Ther* 1993;7:701-711.
10. Borek C, Troll W. Modifiers of free radicals inhibit *in vitro* the oncogenic action of x-rays, bleomycin, and the tumor promotor 12-O-tetradecanoylphorbol 13-acetate. *Proc Natl Acad Sci USA* 1983;801:1304-1307.
11. Lutz J, Augustin A, Friedrich E. Severity of oxygen free radical effects after ischemia and reperfusion in intestinal tissue and the influence of different drugs. *Adv Exp Med Biol* 1990;277:683-690.
12. Nimrod A, Beck Y, Hartman JR, et al. Recombinant human manganese superoxide dismutase (r-hMnSOD) is a potent anti-inflammatory agent. In: Hayaishi O, Niki E, Kondo M, eds. *Medical, Biochemical, and Chemical Aspects of Free Radicals.* Amsterdam: Elsevier/North Holland; 1988:743-746.
13. Paynter DI. Changes in activity of the manganese superoxide dismutase enzyme in tissues of the rat with changes in dietary manganese. *J Nutr* 1980;110:437-447.
14. Davidsson L, Cederblad A, Lonnerdal B, Sandstrom B. Manganese retention in man: a method for estimating manganese absorption in man. *Am J Clin Nutr* 1989;49:170-179.
15. Greger JL. Dietary standards for manganese: overlap between nutritional and toxicological studies. *J Nutr* 1998;128:368S-371S.
16. Baly DL, Schneiderman JS, Garcia-Welsh AL. Effect of manganese deficiency on insulin binding, glucose transport and metabolism in rat adipocytes. *J Nutr* 1990;120:1075-1079.
17. Keen CL, Zidenberg-Cherr S. Manganese. In: Ziegler EE, Filer L, eds. *Present Knowledge in Nutrition.* 7th ed. Washington, DC: ILSI press; 1996:334-343.

18. Carl GF, Keen CL, Gallagher BB, et al. Association of low blood manganese concentrations with epilepsy. *Neurology* 1986;36:1584-1587.

19. Dupont CL, Tanaka Y. Blood manganese levels in children with convulsive disorder. *Biochem Med* 1985;33:246-255.

20. Papavasiliou PS, Kutt H, Miller ST, et al. Seizure disorders and trace metals: manganese tissue levels in treated epileptics. *Neurology* 1979;29:1466-1473.

21. Shvets NV, Kramarenko LD, Vydyborets SV, Gaidukova SN. Disordered trace element content of the erythrocytes in diabetes mellitus. *Lik Sprava* 1994;1:52-55. [Article in Russian]

22. Ekmekcioglu C, Prohaska C, Pomazal K, et al. Concentrations of seven trace elements in different hematological matrices in patients with type 2 diabetes as compared to healthy controls. *Biol Trace Elem Res* 2001;79:205-219.

23. Reginster JY, Strause LG, Saltman PD, et al. Trace elements and postmenopausal osteoporosis: a preliminary study of decreased serum manganese. *Med Sci Res* 1988;16:337-338.

24. Saltman PD, Strause LG. Role of manganese in bone metabolism. In: Kies C, ed. *Nutritional Bioavailability of Manganese*. Washington, DC: American Chemical Society; 1987:46-55.

25. Strause LG, Saltman PD, Glowacki J. The effect of deficiencies of manganese and copper on osteoinduction and on resorption of bone particles in rats. *Calcif Tissue Int* 1987;41:145-150.

26. Tanaka Y. Low manganese level may trigger epilepsy. *JAMA* 1977;238:1805.

27. Rubenstein AH. Hypoglycemia induced by manganese. *Nature* 1962;194:188-189.

28. Rognstad R. Possible sites of Mn(II) action on carbohydrate metabolism in the liver. In: Schramm VL, Wedler FC, eds. *Manganese in Metabolism and Enzyme Function*. New York, NY: Academic Press; 1986:133-146.

29. Thompson KH, Godin DV, Lee M. Tissue antioxidant status in streptozotocin-induced diabetes in rats. Effects of dietary manganese deficiency. *Biol Trace Elem Res* 1992;35:213-224.

30. Asayama K, Hayashibe H, Dobashi K, et al. Antioxidant enzyme status and lipid peroxidation in various tissues of diabetic and starved rats. *Diabetes Res* 1989;12:85-91.

31. Davis CD, Greger JL. Longitudinal changes of manganese-dependent superoxide dismutase and other indexes of manganese and iron status in women. *Am J Clin Nutr* 1992;55:747-752.

32. Davis CD, Zech L, Greger JL. Manganese metabolism in rats: an improved methodology for assessing gut endogenous losses. *Proc Soc Exp Biol Med* 1993;202:103-108.

33. Malecki EA, Radzanowski GM, Radzanowski TJ, et al. Biliary manganese excretion in conscious rats is affected by acute and chronic manganese intake but not by dietary fat. *J Nutr* 1996;126:489-498.

34. Thompson TN, Klaassen CD. Presystemic elimination of manganese in rats. *Toxicol Appl Pharmacol* 1982;64:236-243.

35. Banta RG, Markesbery WR. Elevated manganese levels associated with dementia and extrapyramidal signs. *Neurology* 1977;27:213-216.

36. Hurley LS, Keen CL. Manganese. In: Mertz W, ed. *Trace Elements in Human and Animal Nutrition,* 5th ed. San Diego, CA: Academic Press; 1989:185-221.

37. Marlow M. Hair trace element content of violence prone male children. *J Advancement Med* 1994;7:15-18.

38. Barlow PJ. A pilot study on the metal levels in the hair of hyperactive children. *Med Hypotheses* 1983;11:309-318.

39. Mena I. Manganese. In: Bronner F, Coburn JW, eds. *Disorders of Mineral Metabolism. Trace Minerals.* New York, NY: Academic Press; 1981:233-270.

40. Pihl RO, Parkes M. Hair element content in learning disabled children. *Science* 1977;198:204-206.

41. Collipp PJ, Chen SY, Maitinsky S. Manganese in infant formula and learning disability. *Ann Nutr Metab* 1983;27:488-494.

42. Food and Nutrition Board: Institute of Medicine. Manganese. In: *Dietary Reference Intakes*. Washington, DC: National Academy Press

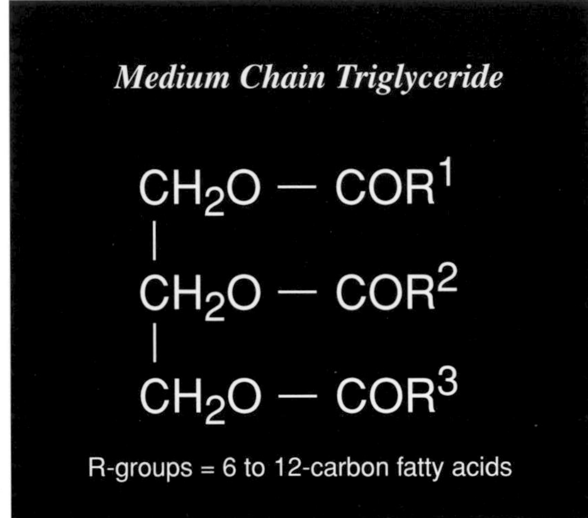

Medium Chain Triglycerides

Introduction

Medium chain triglycerides (MCTs) are a class of lipids in which three saturated fats are bound to a glycerol backbone. What distinguishes MCTs from other triglycerides is the fact that each fat molecule is between six and twelve carbons in length. MCTs are a component of many foods, with coconut and palm oils being the dietary sources with the highest concentration of MCTs. MCTs are also available as a dietary supplement.

Pharmacokinetics

MCTs have a different pattern of absorption and utilization than long-chain triglycerides (LCT) that make up 97 percent of dietary fats. For absorption of LCT to occur, the fatty acid chains must be separated from the glycerol backbone by the lipase enzyme. These fatty acids form into micelles, are then absorbed, reattached to glycerol, and the resultant triglycerides travel through the lymphatics en route to the bloodstream. Up to 30 percent of MCTs are absorbed intact across the intestinal barrier and directly enters the portal vein. This allows for much quicker absorption and utilization of MCTs compared to LCT. MCTs are transported into the mitochondria independent of the carnitine shuttle, which is necessary for LCT mitochondrial absorption. Oxidation of MCTs provides 8.3 calories per gram. For more information on the absorption and utilization of MCTs, consult Ruppin and Middleton.[1]

Clinical Indications

Malabsorption

The use of MCTs is clearly indicated in malabsorption states. Children with cystic fibrosis supplemented with up to 75 ml of MCTs per day experienced greater weight gain and reduced fecal fat compared to a trial period on a control diet.[2] When MCTs are given concurrently with a pancreatic enzyme preparation, absorption is improved.[3] MCTs have been used in other malabsorption syndromes, including short-bowel syndrome, celiac disease, and hepatic disease.[4]

HIV/AIDS

MCTs may help with weight maintenance in AIDS patients. An enteral formula containing 85 percent of fat calories from MCTs (35% of total calories from fat) led to decreases in stool fat, number of bowel movements, and abdominal symptoms, as well as increased fat absorption compared to baseline.[5] No improvement was seen in subjects taking a control LCT-containing formula. Another controlled trial confirmed these results.[6] MCT-containing caloric supplements do not appear to cause weight gain in AIDS patients compared to a control diet.[7]

Cachexia

In chronically ill patients receiving total parenteral nutrition, preparations containing 50 percent of fat calories from MCTs led to a significantly lower production of tumor necrosis factor-alpha (TNFα) compared to a solution with 100 percent LCT.[8] TNFα is a cytokine thought to be responsible for at least some symptoms of cachexia.

MCTs have been used as part of a ketogenic diet to treat children with intractable seizures and cancer. The ketogenic diet varies, but generally contains 60 percent of calories from MCT oil, 20 percent from protein, 10 percent from carbohydrate, and 10 percent from other dietary fats. Although some preliminary data are available showing reduced sugar metabolism at tumor sites,[9] use of ketogenic diets to treat active cancers remains unproven. A small study showed an enteral formula containing MCTs and hydrolyzed casein protein led to better weight maintenance during radiation therapy than an ad libitum diet.[10]

Weight Loss Programs

In a randomized, crossover trial, 12 non-obese women fed a diet providing 80 percent of fat calories as MCTs (40% of total calories from fat) exhibited a greater rate of oxidation of long-chain saturated fats for energy.[11] Another study demonstrated an increased metabolic rate in response to substitution of just 20 percent of fat calories with MCTs.[12] Obese women fed an 800 kcal/day diet with 24 percent of calories from MCTs had no more weight loss than women eating a similar diet without MCTs.[13] While some authors have theorized a role for MCTs in weight control,[14] this role has yet to be fully defined.

Exercise Nutrition

It has been theorized that MCTs improve energy utilization during exercise, but this has not been conclusively demonstrated in clinical trials. One study found similar exercise performance among subjects fed 400 kcal as MCTs, LCT, or carbohydrate.[15] Subjects used MCTs as an energy source more efficiently than LCT, but less efficiently than carbohydrate. Another clinical trial found cyclists ingesting a 5-percent MCT solution actually had decreased exercise performance compared to those taking a carbohydrate solution or placebo.[16] This decrease in exercise performance was thought to be due to gastrointestinal upset. When MCTs were given concurrently with carbohydrate, no negative effect on performance was noted.

Diabetes

In the inpatient setting, an experimental diet containing 78 percent of fat calories as MCTs (31% of total energy intake) increased glucose metabolism in patients with type 2 diabetes mellitus.[17] In five outpatients with type 2 diabetes, an experimental diet containing 18 percent of calories from MCTs led to a slight reduction in post-prandial blood sugar and no effect on fasting blood sugar.[18] The role of MCTs in the management of diabetes remains to be decided.

Side Effects and Toxicity

Due to its unique absorption characteristics, MCTs tend to be well tolerated, even in individuals with severe malabsorption. While fat malabsorption symptoms are generally fewer with MCTs than with LCT, some steatorrhea can occur.[3] Mild gastrointestinal upset has been reported in trials using high doses of MCTs.[16]

MCTs significantly raised serum cholesterol in subjects with prior mild hypercholesterolemia.[19] In another study, MCT administration led to an increase in serum lipids compared to corn oil, but a decrease in serum lipids when compared to butter.[20] MCTs significantly increased serum triglycerides and decreased HDL cholesterol compared to LCT in one study,[21] and significantly lowered plasma triglycerides versus LCT in another study.[22] In addition, MCT administration has been associated with a slight increase in serum insulin.[23]

Dosage

Appropriate doses of MCTs vary with condition. Studies involving MCTs have typically used 15-30 ml of MCTs per day in children, and 50-100 mL per day in adults. Higher doses may be required in patients with severe cachexia.

References

1. Ruppin DC, Middleton WRJ. Clinical use of medium chain triglycerides. *Drugs* 1980;20:216-224.
2. Kuo PT, Huang NN. The effect of medium chain triglyceride upon fat absorption and plasma lipid and depot fat of children with cystic fibrosis of the pancreas. *J Clin Invest* 1965;44:1924-1933.
3. Durie PR, Newth CJ, Forstner GG, Gall DG. Malabsorption of medium-chain triglycerides in infants with cystic fibrosis: correction with pancreatic enzyme supplements. *J Pediatr* 1980;96:862-865.
4. Gracey M, Burke V, Anderson CM. Medium chain triglycerides in paediatric practice. *Arch Dis Child* 1970;45:445-452.
5. Craig CB, Darnell BE, Weinsier RL, et al. Decreased fat and nitrogen losses in patients with AIDS receiving medium-chain-triglyceride-enriched formula vs those receiving long-chain-triglyceride-containing formula. *J Am Diet Assoc* 1997;97:605-611.

6. Wanke CA, Pleskow D, Degirolami PC, et al. A medium chain triglyceride-based diet in patients with HIV and chronic diarrhea reduces diarrhea and malabsorption: a prospective, controlled trial. *Nutrition* 1996;12:766-771.

7. Gibert CL, Wheeler DA, Collins G, et al. Randomized, controlled trial of caloric supplements in HIV infection. *J Acquir Immune Defic Syndr* 1999;22:253-259.

8. Gogos CA, Zoumbos N, Makri M, Kalfarentzos F. Medium- and long-chain triglycerides have different effects on the synthesis of tumor necrosis factor by human mononuclear cells in patients under total parenteral nutrition. *J Am Coll Nutr* 1994;13:40-44.

9. Nebeling LC, Lerner E. Implementing a ketogenic diet based on medium-chain triglyceride oil in pediatric patients with cancer. *J Am Diet Assoc* 1995;95:693-697.

10. Bounous G, Le Bei E, Shuster J, et al. Dietary protection during radiation therapy. *Strahlentherapie* 1975;149:476-483.

11. Papamandjaris AA, White MD, Raeini-Sarjaz M, Jones PJH. Endogenous fat oxidation during medium chain versus long chain triglyceride feeding in healthy women. *Int J Obesity* 2000;24:1158-1166.

12. Matsuo T, Matsuo M, Taguchi N, Takeuchi H. The thermic effect is greater for structured medium- and long-chain triacylglycerols versus long-chain triacylglycerols in healthy young women. *Metabolism* 2001;50:125-130.

13. Yost TJ, Eckel RH. Hypocaloric feeding in obese women: metabolic effects of medium chain triglyceride substitution. *Am J Clin Nutr* 1989;49:326-330.

14. Papamandjaris AA, MacDougall DE, Jones PJH. Medium chain fatty acid metabolism and energy expenditure: obesity treatment implications. *Life Sci* 1998;62:1203-1213.

15. Satabin P, Portero P, Defer G, et al. Metabolic and hormonal responses to lipid and carbohydrate diets during exercise in man. *Med Sci Sports Exerc* 1987;19:218-223.

16. Jeukendrup AE, Thielen JJHC, Wagenmakers AJM, et al. Effect of medium-chain triacylglycerol and carbohydrate ingestion during exercise on substrate utilization and subsequent cycling performance. *Am J Clin Nutr* 1998;67:397-404.

17. Eckel RH, Hanson AS, Chen AY, et al. Dietary substitution of medium chain triglycerides improves insulin-mediated glucose metabolism in non-insulin dependent diabetics. *Diabetes* 1992;41:641-647.

18. Yost TJ, Erskine JM, Gregg TS, et al. Dietary substitution of medium chain triglycerides in subjects with non-insulin-dependent diabetes mellitus in an ambulatory setting: impact on glycemic control and insulin-mediated glucose metabolism. *J Am Coll Nutr* 1994;13:615-622.

19. Cater NB, Heller HJ, Denke MA. Comparison of the effects of medium-chain triacylglycerols, palm oil, and high oleic acid sunflower oil on plasma triacylglycerol fatty acids and lipid and lipoprotein concentrations in humans. *Am J Clin Nutr* 1997;65:41-45.

20. Hashim SA, Arteaga A, Van Itallie TB. Effect of a saturated medium-chain triglyceride on serum-lipids in man. *Lancet* 1960;i:1105-1108.

21. Swift LL, Hill JO, Peters JC, Greene HL. Plasma lipids and lipoproteins during 6 d of maintenance feeding with long-chain, medium-chain, and mixed-chain triglycerides. *Am J Clin Nutr* 1992;56:881-886.

22. Calabrese C, Myer S, Munson S, et al. A cross-over study of the effect of a single oral feeding of medium chain triglyceride oil vs. canola oil on post-ingestion plasma triglyceride levels in healthy men. *Altern Med Rev* 1999;4:23-28.

23. Tamir I, Grant DB, Fosbrooke AS, et al. Effects of a single oral load of medium-chain triglyceride on serum lipid and insulin levels in man. *J Lipid Res* 1968;9:661-666.

Methylcobalamin

Introduction

Methylcobalamin is one of the two coenzyme forms of vitamin B12 (the other being adenosylcobalamin). It is a cofactor in the enzyme methionine synthase, which functions to transfer methyl groups for the regeneration of methionine from homocysteine.

Pharmacokinetics

Evidence indicates methylcobalamin is utilized more efficiently than cyanocobalamin to increase levels of one of the coenzyme forms of vitamin B12. Experiments have demonstrated similar absorption of methylcobalamin following oral administration. The quantity of cobalamin detected following a small oral dose of methylcobalamin is similar to the amount following administration of cyanocobalamin; but significantly more cobalamin

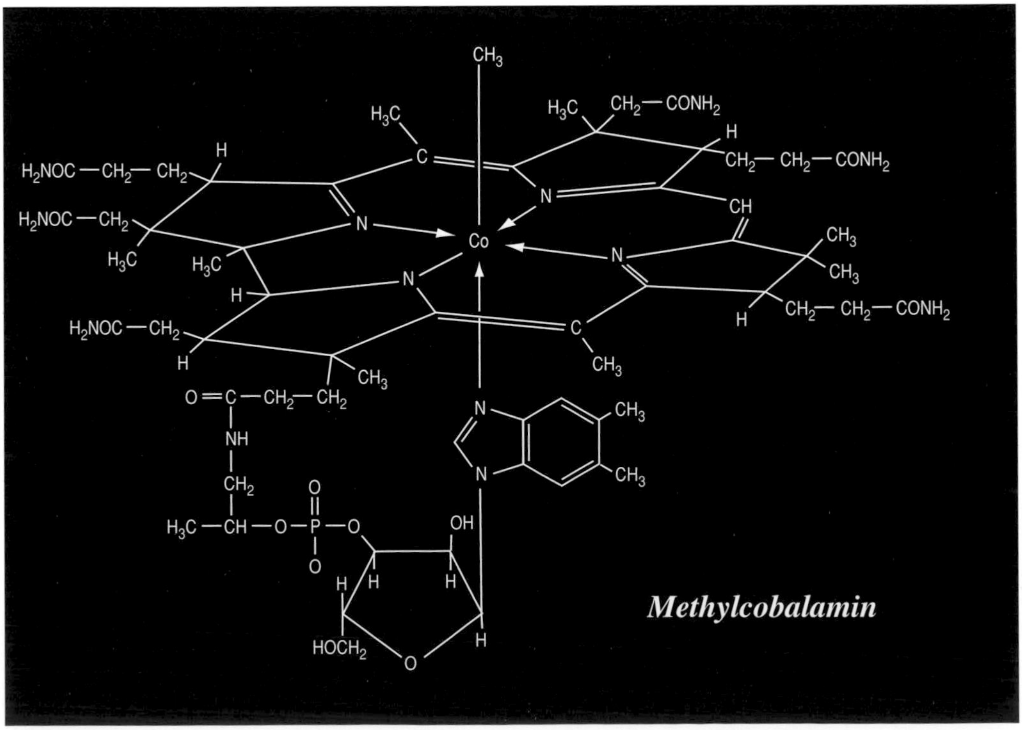

Methylcobalamin

accumulates in liver tissue following administration of methylcobalamin. Human urinary excretion of methylcobalamin is about one-third that of a similar dose of cyanocobalamin, indicating substantially greater tissue retention.[1]

Clinical Indications

Bell's Palsy

Evidence suggests methylcobalamin dramatically shortened the recovery time for facial nerve function in Bell's palsy.[2]

Cancer

Cell culture and *in vivo* experimental results indicated methylcobalamin can inhibit the proliferation of malignant cells.[3] Methylcobalamin enhanced survival time and reduced tumor growth following inoculation of mice with Ehrlich ascites tumor cells.[4] Methylcobalamin has been shown to increase survival time of leukemic mice. Under the same experimental conditions, cyanocobalamin was inactive.[5] Although more research is required to verify findings, experimental evidence suggested methylcobalamin might enhance the efficacy of methotrexate.[6]

Diabetic Neuropathy

Oral administration of methylcobalamin (500 mcg three times daily for four months) resulted in subjective improvement in burning sensations, numbness, loss of sensation, and muscle cramps. An improvement in reflexes, vibration sense, lower motor neuron weakness, and sensitivity to pain was also observed.[7]

Eye Function

Experiments indicated chronic administration of methylcobalamin protected cultured retinal neurons against N-methyl-D-aspartate-receptor-mediated glutamate neurotoxicity.[8] Deterioration of accommodation following visual work has also been shown to improve in individuals receiving methylcobalamin.[9]

Heart Rate Variability

Heart rate variability is a means of detecting the relative activity and balance of the sympathetic/parasympathetic nervous systems. Methylcobalamin produces improvements in several components of heart rate variability, suggesting a balancing effect on the nervous system.[10]

HIV

Under experimental conditions, methylcobalamin inhibited HIV-1 infection of normal human blood monocytes and lymphocytes.[11]

Homocysteinemia

Elevated levels of homocysteine can be a metabolic indication of decreased levels of the methylcobalamin form of vitamin B12. Therefore, it is not surprising that elevated homocysteine levels were reduced from a mean value of 14.7 to 10.2 nmol/ml following parenteral treatment with methylcobalamin.[12]

Male Infertility

In one study, methylcobalamin, at a dose of 6 mg per day for 16 weeks, improved sperm count by 37.5 percent.[13] In a separate investigation, methylcobalamin, given at a dose of 1,500 micrograms per day for 4-24 weeks, resulted in sperm concentration increases in 38 percent of cases, total sperm count increases in 54 percent of cases, and sperm motility increases in 50 percent of cases.[14]

Sleep Disturbances

The use of methylcobalamin in the treatment of a variety of sleep-wake disorders is very promising. Although the exact mechanism of action is not yet elucidated, it is possible that methylcobalamin is needed for the synthesis of melatonin, since the biosynthetic formation of melatonin requires the donation of a methyl group. Supplementation appears to have a great deal of ability to modulate melatonin secretion, enhance light-sensitivity, normalize circadian rhythms, and normalize sleep-wake rhythm.[15-20]

Side Effects and Toxicity

Methylcobalamin has excellent tolerability and no known toxicity.

Dosage

The dosage for clinical effect is 1,500-6,000 mcg per day. No significant therapeutic advantage appears to occur from dosages exceeding this maximum dose. Methylcobalamin has been administered orally, intramuscularly, and intravenously; however, positive clinical results have been reported irrespective of the method of administration. It is not clear whether any therapeutic advantage is gained from the non-oral methods of administration.

References

1. Okuda K, Yashima K, Kitazaki T, Takara I. Intestinal absorption and concurrent chemical changes of methylcobalamin. *J Lab Clin Med* 1973;81:557-567.
2. Jalaludin MA. Methylcobalamin treatment of Bell's palsy. *Methods Find Exp Clin Pharmacol* 1995;17:539-544.
3. Nishizawa Y, Yamamoto T, Terada N, et al. Effects of methylcobalamin on the proliferation of androgen-sensitive or estrogen-sensitive malignant cells in culture and *in vivo*. *Int J Vitam Nutr Res* 1997;67:164-170.
4. Shimizu N, Hamazoe R, Kanayama H, et al. Experimental study of antitumor effect of methyl-B12. *Oncology* 1987;44:169-173.
5. Tsao CS, Myashita K. Influence of cobalamin on the survival of mice bearing ascites tumor. *Pathology* 1993;61:104-108.
6. Miasishcheva NV, Gerasimova GK, Il'ina NS, Sof'ina ZP. Effect of methylcobalamin on methotrexate transport in normal and tumorous tissues. *Biull Eksp Biol Med* 1985;99:736-738. [Article in Russian]
7. Yaqub BA, Siddique A, Sulimani R. Effects of methylcobalamin on diabetic neuropathy. *Clin Neurol Neurosurg* 1992;94:105-111.
8. Kikuchi M, Kashii S, Honda Y, et al. Protective effects of methylcobalamin, a vitamin B12 analog, against glutamate-induced neurotoxicity in retinal cell culture. *Invest Ophthalmol Vis Sci* 1997;38:848-854.
9. Iwasaki T, Kurimoto S. Effect of methylcobalamin in accommodative dysfunction of eye by visual load. *Sangyo Ika Daigaku Zasshi* 1987;9:127-132.
10. Yoshioka K, Tanaka K. Effect of methylcobalamin on diabetic autonomic neuropathy as assessed by power spectral analysis of heart rate variations. *Horm Metab Res* 1995;27:43-44.
11. Weinberg JB, Sauls DL, Misukonis MA, Shugars DC. Inhibition of productive human immunodeficiency virus-1 infection by cobalamins. *Blood* 1995;86:1281-1287.
12. Araki A, Sako Y, Ito H. Plasma homocysteine concentrations in Japanese patients with non-insulin-dependent diabetes mellitus: effect of parenteral methylcobalamin treatment. *Atherosclerosis* 1993;103:149-157.
13. Moriyama H, Nakamura K, Sanda N, et al. Studies on the usefulness of a long-term, high-dose treatment of methylcobalamin in patients with oligozoospermia. *Hinyokika Kiyo* 1987;33:151-156.
14. Isoyama R, Kawai S, Shimizu Y, et al. Clinical experience with methylcobalamin (CH3-B12) for male infertility. *Hinyokika Kiyo* 1984;30:581-586.
15. Uchiyama M, Mayer G, Okawa M, Meier-Ewert K. Effects of vitamin B12 on human circadian body temperature rhythm. *Neurosci Lett* 1995;192:1-4.
16. Tomoda A, Miike T, Matsukura M. Circadian rhythm abnormalities in adrenoleukodystrophy and methyl B12 treatment. *Brain Dev* 1995;17:428-431.
17. Yamada N. Treatment of recurrent hypersomnia with methylcobalamin (vitamin B12): a case report. *Psychiatry Clin Neurosci* 1995;49:305-307.
18. Ohta T, Ando K, Iwata T, et al. Treatment of persistent sleep-wake schedule disorders in adolescents with methylcobalamin (vitamin B12). *Sleep* 1991;14:414-418.
19. Mayer G, Kroger M, Meier-Ewert K. Effects of vitamin B12 on performance and circadian rhythm in normal subjects. *Neuropsychopharmacology* 1996;15:456-464.
20. Hashimoto S, Kohsaka M, Morita N, et al. Vitamin B12 enhances the phase-response of circadian melatonin rhythm to a single bright light exposure in humans. *Neurosci Lett* 1996;220:129-132.

Modified Citrus Pectin

Introduction

Modified citrus pectin (MCP), also known as fractionated pectin, is a complex polysaccharide obtained from the peel and pulp of citrus fruits. Modified citrus pectin is rich in galactoside residues, giving it an affinity for certain types of cancer cells. Metastasis is one of the most life-threatening aspects of cancer and the lack of effective anti-metastatic therapies has prompted research on MCP's effectiveness in blocking metastasis of certain types of cancers, including melanomas, prostate, and breast cancers.

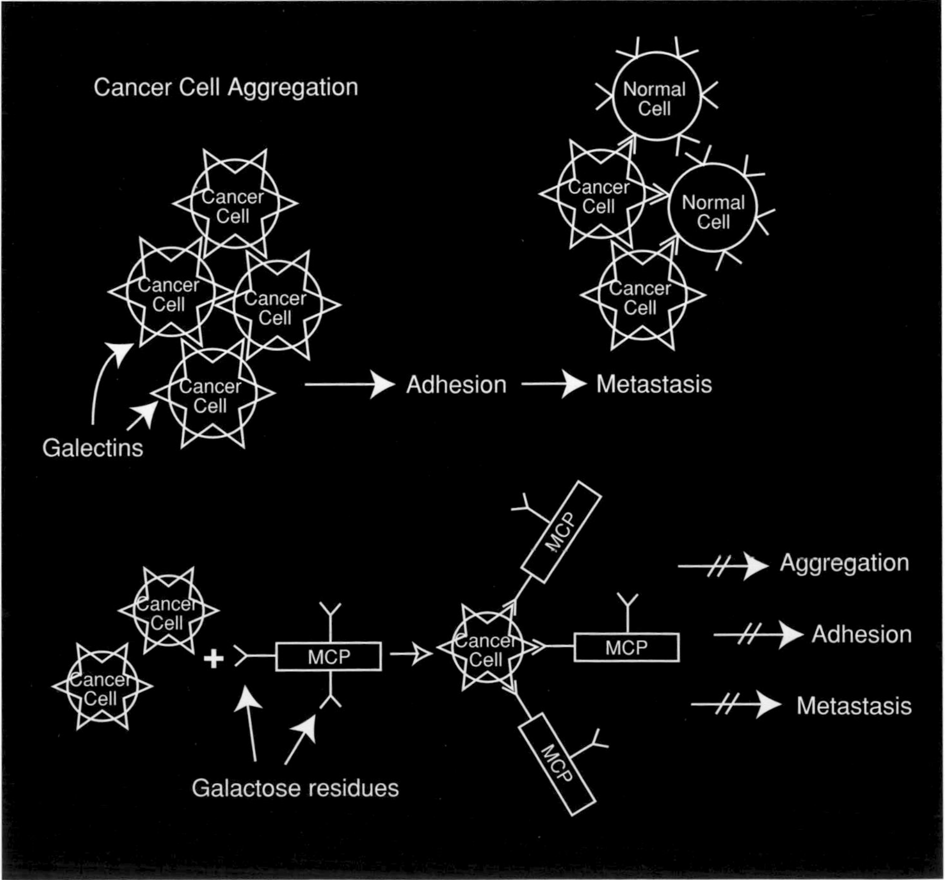

Biochemistry

Modified citrus pectin is produced from citrus pectin via pH and temperature modification that breaks it into shorter, non-branched, galactose-rich carbohydrate chains. These shorter chains dissolve more readily in water and are better absorbed and utilized by the body than ordinary, long-chain pectins. It is believed the shorter polysaccharide units afford MCP its ability to access and bind tightly to galactose-binding lectins (galectins) on the surface of certain types of cancer cells.[1]

Mechanism of Action

Research indicates that in order for metastasis to occur, cancerous cells must first aggregate; galectins on their surface are thought to be responsible for much of this metastatic potential. Galactose-rich, modified citrus pectin has a binding affinity for galectins on the surface of cancer cells, resulting in an inhibition, or blocking, of cancer cell aggregation, adhesion, and metastasis.[1,2] Due to the life-threatening nature of metastatic cancer, most research on anti-metastatic therapies has either been in *in vitro* cell cultures or in animal studies. Although it is still unclear exactly how these study results translate to humans, MCP studies are promising.[3]

Clinical Indications

Prostate Cancer

Pienta et al examined modified citrus pectin's effectiveness against prostate cancer metastasis in the Dunning rat model. Rats were injected with prostate adenocarcinoma cell lines and given drinking water containing various MCP concentrations. Oral MCP did not affect primary tumor growth, but significantly reduced metastases when compared to control animals.[4] In one human study, Strum et al examined the effect of MCP on prostate specific antigen (PSA) doubling time in seven prostate cancer patients. PSA is an enzymatic tumor marker, and its doubling time reflects the speed at which the cancer is growing. Modified citrus pectin was administered orally at a dosage of 15 grams per day in three divided doses. Four of seven patients exhibited more than 30-percent lengthening of PSA doubling time. Lengthening of the doubling time represents a decrease in the cancer growth rate.[1]

Breast Cancer

As with prostate adenocarcinoma, research demonstrates metastasis of breast cancer cell lines requires aggregation and adhesion of cancerous cells to tissue endothelium for invasion into neighboring tissue.[5] The anti-adhesive properties of modified citrus pectin were studied in an *in vitro* model utilizing breast carcinoma cell lines MCF-7 and T-47D. MCP blocked the adhesion of malignant cells to blood vessel endothelia, thus inhibiting metastasis.[6]

A more recent human study examined galectin expression in 27 patients with invasive breast cancer. The study revealed that increasing histologic grades of breast cancer exhibited a decrease in galectin-3 expression, possibly resulting in increased cancer cell motility and metastasis.[7]

Melanoma

One of the better animal models for studying metastasis is the highly metastatic mouse B16-F1 melanoma. Using this system Platt and Raz determined that MCP significantly decreased tumor metastases to the lung by more than 90 percent. In comparison, regular citrus pectin administration resulted in a significant increase (up to three-fold) in tumor metastases. The researchers concluded MCP's interference in the metastatic process might lead to a reduced ability to form tumor cell aggregates and metastases.[8]

Colon Cancer

Mice implanted with human colon-25 tumor cells were given 1 ml daily of a solution containing 0.8 mg/ml or 1.6 mg/ml modified citrus pectin. A significant decrease in primary tumor growth was observed in these mice, compared to controls receiving distilled water.[9] This is the first study showing modified citrus pectin administration causing a reduction in growth of a primary solid tumor.

Side Effects and Toxicity

Because it is a soluble fiber, administration of modified citrus pectin is unlikely to result in gastric intolerance, even at high doses. No pattern of adverse reaction has been recorded in the scientific literature. As with any dietary fiber, MCP at high doses may result in mild cases of loose stool, but this is usually self-limiting and does not warrant discontinuing treatment.

Dosage

A typical adult dose of modified citrus pectin is 6-30 grams daily, in divided doses. This may be modified by the practitioner depending on the patient's clinical status, type of cancer, and degree of (or potential for) metastasis. MCP powder can be blended in a small amount of water, then diluted with a juice of choice.

References

1. Strum S, Scholz M, McDermed J, et al. Modified citrus pectin slows PSA doubling time: a pilot clinical trial. Presentation: International Conference on Diet and Prevention of Cancer, Tampere, Finland. May 28, 1999 – June 2, 1999.
2. Raz A, Loton R. Endogenous galactoside-binding lectins: a new class of functional cell surface molecules related to metastasis. *Cancer Metastasis Rev* 1987;6:433-452.
3. Nicolson GL. Cancer metastasis: tumor cell and host organ properties important in metastasis to specific secondary sites. *Biochim Biophys Acta* 1988;948:175-224.
4. Pienta KJ, Naik H, Akhtah A, et al. Inhibition of spontaneous metastasis in a rat prostate cancer model by oral administration of modified citrus pectin. *J Natl Cancer Inst* 1995;87:348-353.
5. Glinsky VV, Huflejt ME, Glinsky GV, et al. Effects of Thomsen-Friedenreich antigen-specific peptide P-30 on beta-galactoside-mediated homotypic aggregation and adhesion to the endothelium of MDA-MB-435 human breast carcinoma cells. *Cancer Res* 2000;60:2584-2588.
6. Naik H, Pilat MJ, Donat T, et al. Inhibition of *in vitro* tumor cell-endothelial adhesion by modified citrus pectin: a pH modified natural complex carbohydrate. *Proc Am Assoc Cancer Res* 1995;36:Abstract 377.
7. Idikio H. Galectin-3 expression in human breast carcinoma: correlation with cancer histologic grade. *Int J Oncol* 1998;12:1287-1290.
8. Platt D, Raz A. Modulation of the lung cell colonization of B16-F1 melanoma cells by citrus pectin. *J Natl Cancer Inst* 1992;18:438-442.
9. Hayashi A, Gillen A, Lott J. Effects of daily oral administration of quercetin chalcone and modified citrus pectin on implanted colon-25 tumor growth in Balb-c mice. *Altern Med Rev* 2000;5:546-552.

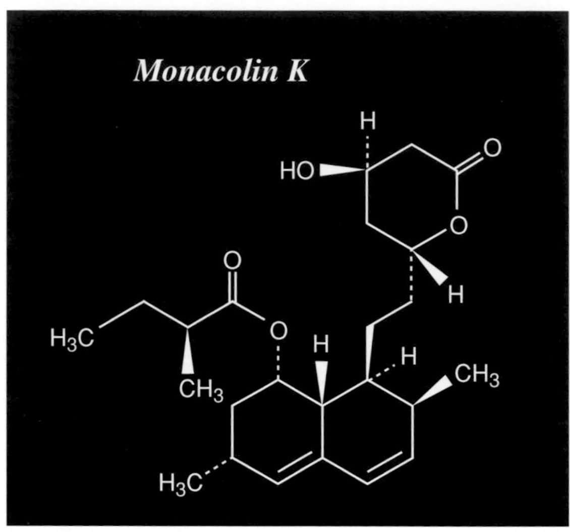

Monascus purpureus (Red Yeast Rice)

Description

Red yeast rice, a fermented product of rice on which red yeast (*Monascus purpureus*) has been grown, has been used in Chinese cuisine and as a medicinal food to promote "blood circulation" for centuries. In Asian countries, red yeast rice is a dietary staple and is used to make rice wine, as a flavoring agent, and to preserve the flavor and color of fish and meat.[1] Red yeast rice forms naturally occurring HMG-CoA reductase inhibitors known as monacolins. The medicinal properties of red yeast rice favorably impact lipid profiles of hypercholesterolemic patients.

Active Constituents

The HMG-CoA reductase activity of red yeast rice comes from a family of naturally occurring substances called monacolins. Monacolin K, also known as mevinolin or lovastatin, is the ingredient in red yeast rice that Merck & Co., pharmaceutical manufacturer of Mevacor (lovastatin), asserts is a patented pharmaceutical. However, red yeast rice contains a family of nine different monacolins, all of which have the ability to inhibit HMG-CoA reductase. Other active ingredients in red yeast rice include sterols (beta-sitosterol, campesterol, stigmasterol, sapogenin), isoflavones, and monounsaturated fatty acids.[2]

Mechanisms of Action

The first documentation of the biomolecular action of red yeast rice was published in 2002. The results indicate one of the anti-hyperlipidemic actions of red yeast rice is a consequence of an inhibitory effect on cholesterol biosynthesis in hepatic cells.[3] It is unclear whether the lipid-lowering effect of red yeast rice is due solely to the monacolin K content, or if other monacolins, sterols, and isoflavones contribute to its cholesterol-lowering effect.

The monacolin K content of one proprietary preparation of red yeast rice used in a clinical trial was calculated to be 0.2 percent of the total product.[2] This trial used a daily dosage of 2.4 grams of red yeast rice (the corresponding monacolin K dosage would be 4.8 mg). The dosages used in clinical trials of lovastatin are 20-40 mg per day.[4] It is unlikely the lipid-lowering effects found in this study was a result of the monacolin K content alone.

Clinical Indications

Hypercholesterolemia

The first human trial, an eight-week study conducted in China, evaluated the effect of 1.2 g/day red yeast rice on 324 hypercholesterolemic adults (total cholesterol above 230 mg/dL) who also had elevated LDL (over 130 mg/dL) and low HDL (under 40 mg/dL) versus controls.[5] Total cholesterol, LDL cholesterol, and triglycerides dropped by 23, 31, and 34 percent, respectively. Serum HDL levels increased by 20 percent. The second study included 83 hypercholesterolemic adults on 2.4 g red yeast rice daily or placebo.[2] Participants were asked to maintain a diet of 30-percent fat, 10-percent saturated fat, and a maximum of 300 mg cholesterol daily. After eight weeks the treatment group had an 18-percent lower mean total cholesterol level compared to placebo and a 17-percent drop in total cholesterol from baseline. There was also a 23-percent difference in LDL between the treatment group and the placebo group and a 23-percent drop in the treatment group, evident at eight weeks. Triglycerides also dropped 16 percent in the treatment population. The drops in total cholesterol and LDL were consistent at eight and 12 weeks. There were no changes in HDL levels.

A multi-center, self-controlled, open-labeled study used the American Heart Association's Step I diet for four weeks followed by red yeast rice 2.4 grams daily for eight weeks in 187 hypercholestrolemic patients. There were no significant differences with the diet alone, but after eight weeks of red yeast rice, total cholesterol decreased 16.4 percent, LDL by 21 percent, triglycerides by 24.5 percent, and HDL increased 14.6 percent.[6]

Clinical trials using red yeast rice with hyperlipidemic elderly patients[7] as well as HIV-related dyslipidemic patients[8] have also demonstrated ability of red yeast rice to improve lipid profiles.

Drug-Nutrient Interactions

Because HMG-CoA reductase inhibitors reduce the production of coenzyme Q10 (CoQ10),[9] supplementation of CoQ10 with long-term use of red yeast rice extract may be prudent. Theoretically, the drug-related contraindications for lovastatin are probably prudent to adhere to with red yeast rice preparations as well, including avoidance of co-administration with niacin, gemfibrozil, cyclosporin, azole anti-fungals, erythromycin, clarithromycin, nefazodone, and protease inhibitors.[10]

Side Effects and Toxicity

Toxicity evaluations of red yeast rice in animals for as long as four months have shown no toxicity.[1] Human trials have not shown elevations of liver enzymes or renal impairment.[2,5] Side effects have been limited to headaches, gastrointestinal discomfort, and temporary and harmless red coloring of the stool.

Although larger, long-term trials will be helpful in understanding the efficacy and potential long-term effects of red yeast rice, the apparent lack of statin-like side effects in these short-term studies warrants further investigation of this hypolipidemic agent.

Dosage

No dosage standards have been established for red yeast rice. Adult dosages used in clinical studies range from 1.2-2.4 g per day[2,5] to 0.8 g/kg/day.[1] In Asian countries the average daily intake of red yeast rice is 14-55 grams.[11]

It should be noted the monacolin content of red yeast rice varies significantly according to the strain. Total monacolin content of nine different commercially available preparations evaluated by high performance liquid chromatography (HPLC) varied from zero to 0.58 percent.[12] Findings of clinical trials using red yeast rice with a standardized level and profile of monocolins may not be applicable to all commercially available red yeast rice preparations.

Warnings and Contraindications

Theoretically, the contraindications for lovastatin use are probably prudent to adhere to with monacolin K-containing red yeast rice preparations, including pregnancy, breast feeding, and hepatic or renal impairment.[10]

References

1. Li C, Zhu Y, Wang Y, et al. *Monascus purpureus* fermented rice (red yeast rice): A natural food product that lowers blood cholesterol in animal models of hypercholesterolemia. *Nutr Res* 1998;18:71-81.
2. Heber D, Yip I, Ashley JM, et al. Cholesterol-lowering effects of a proprietary Chinese red-yeast-rice dietary supplement. *Am J Clin Nutr* 1999;69:231-236.
3. Man RY, Lynn EG, Cheung F, et al. Cholestin inhibits cholesterol synthesis and secretion in hepatic cells (HepG2). *Mol Cell Biochem* 2002;233:153-158.
4. Bradford RH, Shear CL, Chremos AN, et al. Expanded Clinical Evaluation of Lovastatin (EXCEL) study results: two-year efficacy and safety follow-up. *Am J Cardiol* 1994;74:667-673.
5. Wang J, Lu Z, Chi J, et al. Multicenter clinical trial of the serum lipid-lowering effects of a *Monascus purpureus* (red yeast) rice preparation from traditional Chinese medicine. *Cur Ther Res* 1997;58:964-978.
6. Rippe J, Bonovich K, Colfer H. A multi-center, self-controlled study of Cholestin™ in subjects with elevated cholesterol. 39th Annual Conference on Cardiovascular Disease Epidemiology and Prevention. Orlando, FL: 1999; March 24-27:1123.
7. Qin S, Zhang W, Qi P, et al. Elderly patients with primary hyperlipidemia benefited from treatment with a *Monascus purpureus* rice preparation: a placebo-controlled, double-blind clinical trial. 39th Annual Conference on Cardiovascular Disease Epidemiology and Prevention. Orlando, FL: 1999; March 24-27:1123.
8. Keithley JK, Swanson B, Sha BE, et al. A pilot study of the safety and efficacy of cholestin in treating HIV-related dyslipidemia. *Nutrition* 2002;18:201-204.
9. Farmer JA, Torre-Amione G. Comparative tolerability of HMG-CoA-reductase inhibitors. *Drug Safety* 2000;23:197-213.
10. Mortom I, Hall J. *The Avery Complete Guide to Medicines*. New York, NY: Penguin Putnam; 2001:513-514.
11. Havel R. Dietary supplement or drug? The case of cholestin. *Am J Clin Nutr* 1999;69:175-176.
12. Heber D, Lembertas A, Lu QY, et al. An analysis of nine proprietary Chinese red yeast rice dietary supplements: implications of variability in chemical profile and contents. *J Altern Complement Med* 2001;7:133-139.

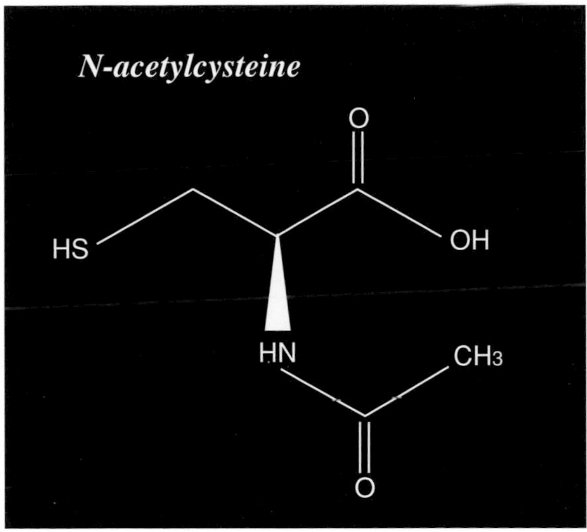

N-acetylcysteine

Introduction

N-acetylcysteine (NAC) is the acetylated derivative of the amino acid L-cysteine. Historically NAC has been used as a mucolytic agent in chronic respiratory illnesses, as well as an antidote for hepatotoxicity due to acetaminophen overdose. More recently, animal and human studies have shown NAC to be a powerful antioxidant and potential therapeutic agent in the treatment of cancer, heart disease, HIV infection, heavy metal toxicity, and other diseases characterized by oxidative damage. NAC has also been shown to be of value in Sjogren's syndrome, influenza, hepatitis C, and myoclonus epilepsy.

Biochemistry and Pharmacokinetics

NAC is a sulfhydryl-containing compound rapidly absorbed into various tissues following an oral dose, deacetylated and metabolized in the intestines and liver, and its metabolites incorporated into proteins and peptides. Peak plasma levels of NAC occur approximately one hour after an oral dose; at 12 hours post-dose it is undetectable in plasma. Despite a relatively low bioavailability of only 4-10 percent, oral administration of NAC appears to be clinically effective.[1] The biological activity of NAC is attributed to its sulfhydryl group, while its acetyl-substituted amino group affords it protection against oxidative and metabolic processes.[2,3] NAC administration is an effective method of increasing plasma glutathione (GSH) levels, as incorporation of cysteine into GSH appears to be the rate-limiting step in GSH synthesis.

Mechanisms of Action

NAC's effectiveness is primarily attributed to its ability to reduce extracellular cystine to cysteine, and as a source of sulfhydryl groups. NAC stimulates glutathione synthesis, enhances glutathione-S-transferase activity, promotes liver detoxification by inhibiting xenobiotic biotransformation, and is a powerful nucleophile capable of scavenging free radicals.[4,5] NAC's effectiveness as a mucolytic agent results from its sulfhydryl group interacting with disulfide bonds in mucoproteins, with mucus subsequently being broken into smaller, less viscous units. NAC may also act as an expectorant by stimulating ciliary action and the gastro-pulmonary vagal reflex, thereby clearing mucus from the airways.[6] Studies have also shown NAC to be of benefit in heart disease by lowering homocysteine and lipoprotein(a) levels via dissociation of disulfide bonds,[7,8] protecting against ischemia and reperfusion damage via replenishment of the glutathione redox system,[9] as well as potentiating the activity of nitroglycerin.[10]

Clinical Indications

Respiratory Illness

Several animal and human studies have explored NAC's effectiveness as a therapeutic agent for various types of respiratory illness. While results vary, NAC administration has resulted in improved expectoration, with decreased cough severity[11] and diaphragm fatigue.[12] In a small study of 18 patients with fibrosing alveolitis – a condition characterized by severe oxidative stress and decreased glutathione levels – NAC 600 mg three times daily for 12 weeks resulted in improvement in pulmonary function and glutathione levels.[13] Studies of patients with chronic bronchitis, severe airway obstruction, and cystic fibrosis showed a slight, although not statistically significant, decrease in exacerbations.[14,15]

HIV Infection

Human immunodeficiency virus (HIV)-positive individuals usually exhibit low GSH and cysteine levels, which has prompted studies on NAC's effectiveness as a therapeutic tool for these patients. Research suggests NAC is capable of enhancing T cell immunity by stimulating T cell colony formation[16] and blocking NF kappa B expression.[17,18] In a double-blind, placebo-controlled trial, NAC positively impacted plasma cysteine levels and CD4+ lymphocyte cell counts.[19] More studies are needed, but it appears NAC may help prevent progression to AIDS when given to HIV-positive patients early in the course of disease.

Cancer/Chemoprevention

Research has shown NAC to have potential as a chemopreventive agent and as a treatment in certain types of cancer, including lung, skin, head and neck, breast, and liver cancer.[20] *In vitro* studies have demonstrated NAC to be directly anti-mutagenic and anti-carcinogenic. NAC also inhibits the mutagenicity of certain compounds *in vivo*.[21] NAC.administration in cell cultures and animal studies selectively protects normal cells, but not malignant ones, from chemotherapy and radiation toxicity.[22] Other *in vitro* studies note NAC's inhibition of cell growth and proliferation in human melanoma, prostate, and astrocytoma cell lines.[23-25]

Acetaminophen and Other Poisonings

Historically the most prevalent and well-accepted use of NAC has been as an antidote for acetaminophen (Tylenol®, paracetamol) poisoning. The resultant liver toxicity is due to an acetaminophen metabolite that depletes hepatocytes of glutathione, and causes hepatocellular damage and possibly even death. NAC administered intravenously or orally within 24 hours of overdose is effective at preventing liver toxicity; however, improvement is most notable if treatment is initiated within 8-10 hours of acetaminophen overdose. NAC's effectiveness declines when treatment is delayed beyond 10 hours, at which time the risk of mortality significantly increases.[26-28] NAC has also been effective for heavy metal poisoning by gold, silver, copper, mercury, lead, and arsenic, as well as in cases of poisoning by carbon tetrachloride, acrylonitriles, halothane, paraquat, acetaldehyde, coumarin, and interferon.[6] Information involving these substances is primarily from animal studies or single case reports; therefore, additional studies are needed to establish NAC's effectiveness in this area.

Viral Hepatitis

The standard therapy for chronic hepatitis C (CHC) involves the usage of interferon-alpha (IFN); however, many patients are either resistant to IFN therapy or they become resistant after a period of time. A pilot study found six-month NAC supplementation (600 mg three times daily) enhanced the response to IFN therapy in chronic hepatitis C patients resistant to IFN, with normalization of serum alanine aminotransferase (ALT) in 41 percent of patients.[29] In a subsequent study of 147 CHC patients, 1,800 mg per day NAC plus IFN for six months resulted in a small increase in sustained virological response – 5.5 percent versus 4.1 percent on IFN alone.[30] Significant improvements were seen in ALT, viral load, and redox balance in 77 patients on NAC plus IFN, compared to IFN alone, in a more recent study.[31]

Heart Disease

Several small clinical studies have demonstrated NAC may be an effective therapeutic agent in the management of heart disease. Wiklund et al found NAC reduced plasma homocysteine levels by 45 percent,[8] while Gavish and Breslow demonstrated NAC's (2-4 grams daily for eight weeks) ability to decrease lipoprotein(a) by 70 percent.[7] Due to its ability to significantly increase tissue GSH, NAC may also be useful in treating ischemia and reperfusion seen in acute myocardial infarction and the resultant depletion in cellular sulfhydryl groups.[9] In addition, NAC appears to potentiate nitroglycerin's coronary dilating and anti-platelet properties, and therefore may be a useful combination therapy in patients with unstable angina pectoris and myocardial infarction.[32,33]

Other Clinical Indications

Clinical studies have also demonstrated NAC's therapeutic benefit in the treatment of Sjogren's syndrome,[34] myoclonus epilepsy,[35] influenza,[36] and illness associated with cigarette smoking.[37]

Side Effects and Toxicity

NAC is generally safe and well tolerated even at high doses. The most common side-effects associated with high oral doses are nausea, vomiting, and other gastrointestinal disturbances; therefore, oral administration is contraindicated in persons with active peptic ulcer. Infrequently, anaphylactic reactions due to histamine release occur and can consist of rash, pruritis, angioedema, bronchospasm, tachycardia, and changes in blood pressure.[6] Intravenous administration has, in rare instances, caused allergic reactions generally in the form of rash or angioedema.[38] NAC is "Ames test" negative, but animal studies on embryotoxicity are equivocal. In addition, studies in pregnant women are inadequate; therefore, NAC should be used with caution during pregnancy, and only if clearly indicated.[39] Oral administration of NAC and charcoal at the same time is not recommended, as charcoal may cause a reduction in the absorption of NAC.[40] In addition, as with any single antioxidant nutrient, NAC at therapeutic doses (even as low as 1.2 grams daily) has the potential to have pro-oxidant activity and is not recommended at these doses in the absence of significant oxidative stress.[41]

Dosage

The typical oral dose for NAC as a mucolytic agent and for most other clinical indications is 600-1,500 mg daily in three divided doses. In patients with cancer or heart disease the therapeutic dosage is higher, usually in the range of 2-4 grams daily. For acetaminophen poisoning, NAC is administered orally with a loading dose of 140 mg/kg and 17 subsequent doses of 70 mg/kg every four hours. In acetaminophen poisoning it is important to begin administering NAC within 8-10 hours of overdose to ensure effectiveness.[6]

Warnings and Contraindications

NAC may have a protective effect on normal tissue in individuals utilizing many cancer chemotherapeutic agents;[42-47] however, two studies noted that NAC inhibits cytotoxicity of the cancer chemotherapy drug cisplatin,[48,49] and an animal study suggests NAC might reduce the anti-neoplastic action of doxorubicin. These combinations should be avoided unless further information recommends otherwise.[50]

References

1. Borgstrom L, Kagedal B, Paulsen O. Pharmacokinetics of N-acetylcysteine in man. *Eur J Clin Pharmacol* 1986;31:217-222.
2. Bonanomi L, Gazzaniga A. Toxicological, pharmacokinetic and metabolic studies on acetylcysteine. *Eur J Respir Dis* 1980;61:45-51.
3. Sjodin K, Nilsson E, Hallberg A, Tunek A. Metabolism of N-acetyl-l-cysteine. *Biochem Pharm* 1989;38:3981-3985.
4. De Vries N, De Flora S. N-Acetyl-l-cysteine. *J Cell Biochem* 1993;17F:S270-S277.
5. De Flora S, Bennicelli C, Camoirano A, et al. In vivo effects of N-acetylcysteine on glutathione metabolism and on the biotransformation of carcinogenic and/or mutagenic compounds. *Carcinogenesis* 1985;6:1735-1745.
6. Zimet I. Acetylcysteine: A drug that is much more than a mucokinetic. *Biomed Pharmacother* 1988;42:513-520.
7. Gavish D, Breslow JL. Lipoprotein(a) reduction by N-acetylcysteine. *Lancet* 1991;337:203-204.
8. Wiklund O, Fager G, Andersson A, et al. N-acetylcysteine treatment lowers plasma homocysteine but not serum lipoprotein(a) levels. *Atherosclerosis* 1996;119:99-106.
9. Ceconi C, Curello S, Cargnoni A, et al. The role of glutathione status in the protection against ischaemic and reperfusion damage: effects of N-acetyl cysteine. *J Mol Cell Cardiol* 1988;20:5-13.
10. Horowitz JD, Henry CA, Syrjanen ML, et al. Nitroglycerine/N-acetylcysteine in the management of unstable angina pectoris. *Eur Heart J* 1988;9:95-100.
11. Jackson IM, Barnes J, Cooksey P. Efficacy and tolerability of oral acetylcysteine (Fabrol) in chronic bronchitis: a double-blind placebo controlled study. *J Int Med Res* 1984;12:198-206.
12. Hida W, Shindo C, Satoh J, et al. N-acetylcysteine inhibits loss of diaphragm function in streptozotocin-treated rats. *Am J Respir Crit Care Med* 1996;153:1875-1879.
13. Behr J, Maier K, Degenkolb B, et al. Antioxidative and clinical effects of high-dose N-acetylcysteine in fibrosing alveolitis. Adjunctive therapy to maintenance immunosuppression. *Am J Respir Crit Care Med* 1997;156:1897-1901.
14. British Thoracic Society Research Committee. Oral N-acetylcysteine and exacerbation rates in patients with chronic bronchitis and severe airways obstructions. *Thorax* 1985;40:832-835.
15. Gotz M, Kraemer R, Kerrebijn KF, Popow C. Oral acetylcysteine in cystic fibrosis. A co-operative study. *Eur J Respir Dis* 1980;61:S122-S126.
16. Wu J, Levy M, Black PH. 2-Mercaptoethanol and n-acetylcysteine enhance T cell colony formation in AIDS and ARC. *Clin Exp Immunol* 1989;77:7-10.
17. Breithaupt TB, Vazquez A, Baez I, Eylar EH. The suppression of T cell function and NF(kappa)B expression by serine protease inhibitors is blocked by N-acetylcysteine. *Cell Immunol* 1996;173:1323-1329.
18. Droge W, Eck H-P, Mihm S. HIV-induced cysteine deficiency and T-cell dysfunction – a rationale for treatment with N-acetylcysteine. *Immun Today* 1992;13:211-214.
19. Akerlund B, Jarstrand C, Lindeke B, et al. Effect of N-acetylcysteine(NAC) treatment on HIV-1 infection: a double-blind placebo-controlled trial. *Eur J Clin Pharmacol* 1996;50:457-461.
20. De Flora S, Cesarone CF, Izzotti A, et al. N-acetylcysteine as antimutagen and anticarcinogen. *Toxicol Lett* 1992;53:Abstract W4/L2.
21. De Flora S, Rossi GA, De Flora A. Metabolic, desmutagenic and anticarcinogenic effects of N-acetylcysteine. *Respiration* 1986;50:S43-S49.
22. De Flora S, D'Agostini F, Masiello L, et al. Synergism between N-acetylcysteine and doxorubicin in the prevention of tumorigenicity and metastasis in murine models. *Int J Cancer* 1996;67:842-848.
23. Chiao JW, Chung F, Krzeminski J, et al. Modulation of growth of human prostate cancer cells by the N-acetylcysteine conjugate of phenethyl isothiocyanate. *Int J Oncol* 2000;16:1215-1219.
24. Redondo P, Badres E, Solano T, et al. Vascular endothelial growth factor (VEGF) and melanoma. N-acetylcysteine downregulates VEGF production in vitro. *Cytokine* 2000;12:374-378.
25. Arora-Kuruganti P, Lucchesi PA, Wurster RD. Proliferation of cultured human astrocytoma cells in response to an oxidant and antioxidant. *J Neurooncol* 1999;44:213-221.

26. Smilkstein MJ, Knapp GL, Kulig KW, Rumack BH. Efficacy of oral N-acetylcysteine in the treatment of acetaminophen overdose. Analysis of the national multicenter study (1976 to 1985). *N Engl J Med* 1988;319:2557-2562.

27. Wang PH, Yang MJ, Lee WL, et al. Acetaminophen poisoning in late pregnancy. A case report. *J Reprod Med* 1997;42:367-371.

28. Perry HE, Shannon MW. Efficacy of oral versus intravenous N-acetylcysteine in acetaminophen overdose: results of an open-label, clinical trial. *J Pediatr* 1998;132:149-152.

29. Beloqui O, Prieto J, Suarez M, et al. N-acetylcysteine enhances the response to interferon-alpha in chronic hepatitis C: a pilot study. *J Interferon Res* 1993;13:279-282.

30. Grant PR, Black A, Garcia N, et al. Combination therapy with interferon-alpha plus N-acetylcysteine for chronic hepatitis C: a placebo controlled double-blind multicentre study. *J Med Virol* 2000;61:439-442.

31. Neri S, Ierna D, Antoci S, et al. Association of alpha-interferon and acetyl cysteine in patients with chronic C hepatitis. *Panminerva Med* 2000;42:187-192.

32. Winniford MD, Kennedy PL, Wells PJ, Hillis LD. Potentiation of nitroglycerin-induced coronary dilatation by N-acetylcysteine. *Circulation* 1986;73:138-142.

33. Chirkov YY, Horowitz JD. N-Acetylcysteine potentiates nitroglycerin-induced reversal of platelet aggregation. *J Cardiovasc Pharmacol* 1996;28:375-380.

34. Walters MT, Rubin CE, Keightley SJ, Ward CD. A double-blind, cross-over, study of oral N-acetylcysteine in Sjogren's syndrome. *Scand J Rheumatol Suppl* 1986;61:253-258.

35. Hurd RW, Wilder BJ, Helveston WR, Uthman BM. Treatment of four siblings with progressive myoclonus epilepsy of the Unverricht-Lundborg type with N-acetylcysteine. *Neurology* 1996;47:1264-1268.

36. De Flora S, Grassi C, Carati L. Attenuation of influenza-like symptomatology and improvement of cell-mediated immunity with long-term N-acetylcysteine treatment. *Eur Respir J* 1997;10:1535-1541.

37. Rogers DF, Jeffery PK. Inhibition by oral N-acetylcysteine of cigarette smoke-induced "bronchitis" in the rat. *Exp Lung Res* 1986;10:267-283.

38. Tenenbein M. Hypersensitivity-like reactions to N-acetylcysteine. *Vet Hum Toxicol* 1984;26:S3-S5.

39. Threlkeld DS, ed. *Drug Facts and Comparisons*. St Louis, Missouri: Facts and Comparisons;1997:1090-1094.

40. Klein-Schwartz W, Oderda GM. Adsorption of oral antidotes for acetaminophen poisoning (methionine and N-acetylcysteine) by activated charcoal. *Clin Toxicol* 1981;18:283-290.

41. Kleinveld HA, Demacker PNM, Stalenhoef APH. Failure of N-acetylcysteine to reduce low-density lipoprotein oxidizability in healthy subjects. *Eur J Clin Pharmacol* 1992;43:639-642.

42. Levy L, Vredevoe DL. The effect of N-acetylcysteine on cyclophosphamide immunoregulation and antitumor activity. *Semin Oncol* 1983;10:S7-S16.

43. Harrison EF, Fuquay ME, Hunter HL. Effect of N-acetylcysteine on the antitumor activity of cyclophosphamide against Walker-256 carcinosarcoma in rats. *Semin Oncol* 1983;10:S25-S27.

44. Palermo MS, Olabuenaga SE, Giordano M, Isturiz MA. Immunomodulation exerted by cyclophosphamide is not interfered with by N acetylcysteine. *Int J Immunopharmac* 1986;8:651-655.

45. Slavik M, Saiers JH. Phase I clinical study of acetylcysteine's preventing ifosfamide-induced hematuria. *Semin Oncol* 1983;10:S62-S65.

46. Holoye PY, Duelge J, Hansen RM, et al. Prophylaxis of ifosfamide toxicity with oral acetylcysteine. *Semin Oncol* 1983;10:S66-S71.

47. Sheikh-Hamad D, Timmins K, Jalali Z. Cisplatin-induced renal toxicity: possible reversal by N-acetylcysteine treatment. *J Am Soc Nephrol* 1997;8:1640-1644.

48. Roller A, Weller M. Antioxidants specifically inhibit cisplatin cytotoxicity of human malignant glioma cells. *Anticancer Res* 1998;18:4493-4497.

49. Miyajima A, Nakashima J, Tachibana M, et al. N-acetylcysteine modifies cis-dichlorodiammineplatinum induced effects in bladder cancer cells. *Jpn J Cancer Res* 1999;90:565-570.

50. Schmitt-Graff A, Scheulen ME. Prevention of adriamycin cardiotoxicity by niacin, isocitrate, or N-acetylcysteine in mice. *Path Res Pract* 1986;181:168-174.

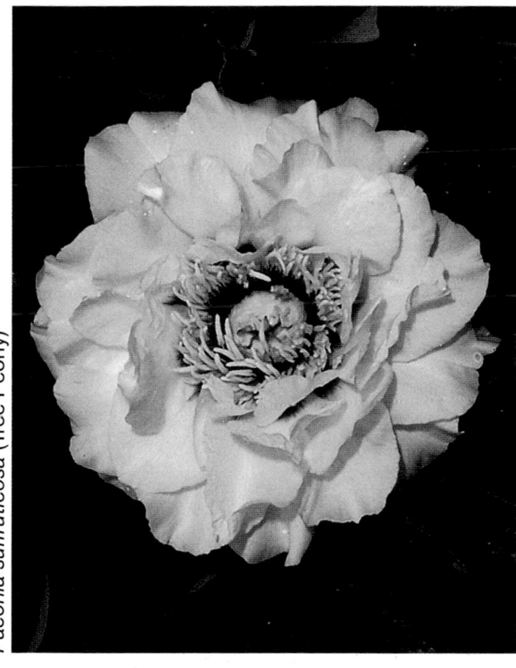
Paeonia suffruticosa (Tree Peony)

Paeonia sp.

Description

Paeonia species have provided useful medicine and attractive ornamental flowers for over 3,000 years in China and at least 500 in Europe.[1] There are four species of this Ranunculaceae family plant that are utilized in traditional Chinese medicine (TCM) under the general rubric of peony: *Paeonia suffruticosa* (tree peony), *Paeonia lactiflora* (Chinese peony), *Paeonia veitchii* (Chinese peony), and *Paeonia obovata* (Chinese peony).

For millennia, peony root has been used to treat wounds, fungal infections, pain, and spasmodic conditions in TCM.[1] In recent times, peony root has received growing research attention, primarily in Japan and China. It has a long history of use in Europe as well, particularly for spasmodic conditions.[2]

All three Chinese peony species are perennial and achieve heights up to nine meters (the tree peony is somewhat larger). They have alternate, elliptical, smooth-edged leaves growing on smooth stems bearing two or more flowers. The large blossoms of the Chinese peony can have a range of color and are generally 4-6 cm in diameter.[1] The roots of all peonies are large, straight, and firm with easily peeled bark that reveals a powdery underlayer when removed.

Active Constituents

Three medicines are produced from peony plants in TCM.[3] *P. suffruticosa* (tree peony) root bark provides *mu dan pi*, referred to below as tree peony. *P. lactiflora*, *P. veitchii* and *P. obovata* root with bark attached provides *chi shao*, referred to below as red peony. The root without the bark of these same three plants provides *bai shao* (white peony), although most often this medicine is derived from *P. lactiflora*. The color designation does not refer to the flowers of these plants (which are most commonly pink, red, purple, or white) but to the color of the root after processing.

White, red, and tree peony contain glycosides (most notably paeoniflorin), flavonoids, proanthocyanidins, tannins, terpenoids, triterpenoids, and complex polysaccharides that may all contribute to its medicinal effects.[3] Paeoniflorin has received the most research attention.

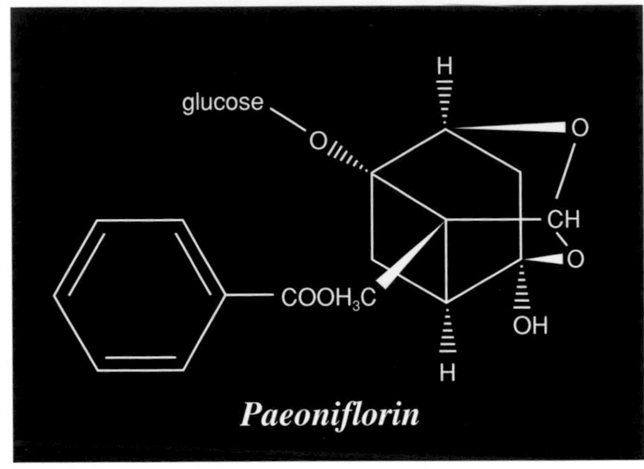

Paeoniflorin

Mechanisms of Action

The exact mechanisms of action of peony constituents have not been determined in their entirety. Paeoniflorin, monoterpenoids, and other constituents in white and red peony have been shown to be spasmolytic. This is in part achieved by interfering with acetylcholine release into neuromuscular junctions (NMJ) associated with gut smooth muscle tissue.[4]

There is a great deal of synergism of activity between white or red peony and licorice (*Glycyrrhiza uralensis*, for which *G. glabra* can be substituted) – the two components of shakuyaku-kanzo-to, a formula commonly used in Japanese and Chinese herbal medicine. One animal study found that peony extracts interfere with acetylcholine release into the NMJ while licorice extracts interfere with acetylcholine's activity in the NMJ.[5] An *in vitro* study found concentrations of paeoniflorin and glycyrrhizin (a major active glycoside in licorice) that individually were too low to inhibit muscle contraction were very active when applied simultaneously.[4]

Other actions possessed by peony extracts and their constituents in preclinical studies include the following: (1) improvement of memory;[6,7] (2) antioxidant activity;[8,9] (3) hepatoprotection;[10] (4) anti-atherosclerotic effects associated with lipid peroxidation inhibition;[11] (5) inhibition of hydrochloric acid secretion;[12] (6) anti-epileptic activity;[13] (7) appetite suppressant and metabolism stimulating activity;[14] (8) antimutagenic properties;[15] (9) protection of endothelium from negative effects of hyperlipidemia;[16] (10) platelet aggregation inhibition;[17] and (11) anticoagulation and fibrinolysis.[18,19] The complex polysaccharides of peony exert immunomodulating effects *in vitro*.[20]

Clinical Indications

Muscle Cramps

The efficacy of white peony for relieving muscle cramps of various types, particularly combined with licorice in the formula shakuyaku-kanzo-to, is supported by several clinical trials. In a double-blind, placebo-controlled trial involving 101 patients with muscle cramps due to hepatic cirrhosis, dried extract of shakuyaku-kanzo-to was significantly superior to placebo in relieving symptoms over a two-week period.[21] The dose in this study – 2.5 g three times daily before meals – was sufficiently high to induce signs of pseudoaldosteronism (edema and weight gain) in five patients (9%) receiving shakuyaku-kanzo-to, due to the high intake of licorice. Other uncontrolled trials have shown that skakuyaku-kanzo-to can help relieve muscle cramps in people with diabetes mellitus,[22] those undergoing dialysis,[23] in alcoholics,[24] and in people with cerebrovascular disease.[25]

Women's Health

Both white and red peony are commonly used for various women's health problems in TCM. There is evidence from preliminary clinical trials supporting their use in dysmenorrhea and polycystic ovary syndrome (PCOS). The TCM formula toki-shakuyaku-san – containing white peony, *Atractylodes lancea* (red atractylodes) rhizome, *Alisma plantago-aquatica* (alisma; water plantain) rhizome, *Poria cocos* (hoelen) sclerotium, *Cnidium monnieri* (cnidium) rhizome, and *Angelica dahurica* (Chinese angelica) radix – has been reported to alleviate pain in patients with primary dysmenorrhea in one double-blind clinical trial.[26] Shakuyaku-kanzo-to reduced dysmenorrhea in 60 percent of women with uterine fibroids in an open trial.[27] Shakuyaku-kanzo-to helped increase fertility in women with PCOS in another open clinical trial.[28] More research is warranted to clarify the exact role and degree of efficacy of white peony by itself and in combination formulae for these and other women's health concerns, particularly luteal dysfunction and menopausal symptoms.[29]

Chronic Viral Hepatitis

Both red and white peony are traditionally utilized in Asia to treat people with chronic viral hepatitis. In one small, open clinical trial using red peony (doses could not be determined but said to be "heavy") over a three-month period, 77 percent of patients with cirrhosis or chronic active hepatitis experienced improvement in liver histology based on repeat biopsy results.[30] A case series also reported the efficacy of this approach.[31] Until more research is conducted to determine effectiveness of red or white peony for chronic hepatitis, these agents should be combined with other, better-established therapies.

Cardiovascular Disorders

Numerous lines of evidence suggest tree, red, and white peony may be beneficial in people with atherosclerosis and/or hypertension. Various extracts and constituents of these herbal medicines have shown antiplatelet and anti-atherosclerotic properties. One open trial found a *Paeonia obovata* extract decreased platelet aggregation in humans.[32] A combination of Chinese angelica and peony was found helpful in an uncontrolled trial of women with pregnancy-induced hypertension.[33] There is also at least one open clinical trial suggesting tree peony can reduce blood pressure in humans.[3] The exact role of peony in atherosclerosis and hypertension remains unknown.

Miscellaneous Indications

There is preclinical evidence suggesting peony might be helpful in people with dementia, Alzheimer's disease, infectious disease, epilepsy, peptic ulcer, obesity, and cancer. However, no clinical trials or reports were found discussing the use of peony for any of these conditions. One review article did suggest an open trial was conducted in Japan showing benefits of toki-shakuyaku-san in Alzheimer's disease patients, but the specifics of this trial could not be located.[29]

Botanical-Drug Interactions

Peony has been shown to reduce sexual dysfunction in men, reportedly caused by neuroleptic-induced hyperprolactinemia.[34,35] Women with dysmenorrhea and/or amenorrhea due to use of the neuroleptic drug risperidone benefited from shakuyaku-kanzo-to according to another report.[36] No published reports suggest any lessening of efficacy of neuroleptics when combined with peony.

Toki-shakuyaku-san has been reported effective in relieving menopausal symptoms as well as frozen shoulder syndrome in some women treated with gonadotropin-releasing hormone superagonists such as leuprolide (Lupron®).[37] Estrogen levels were not affected by the formula. It is unknown if this formula would help men taking these drugs for treatment of prostate cancer.

Toki-shakuyaku-san showed additive effects in improving pregnancy rates in infertile women treated with clomiphene.[38]

When clomiphene was given alone in this uncontrolled trial, 21 percent of study volunteers became pregnant compared to 34 percent who took clomiphene with toki-skakuyaku-san. There was no sign of additive adverse effects.

The anticoagulant and antiplatelet effects of peony suggest it might potentiate anticoagulant drugs such as warfarin and antiplatelet drugs such as aspirin. No published reports have yet appeared confirming this possibility, but caution is warranted.

In a small open trial of cancer patients who suffered muscle pain due to paclitaxel (Taxol®) and carboplatin therapy, adding shakuyaku-kanzo-to to the second course relieved the pain in 7 of 10 patients.[39] In an animal trial, oral shakuyaku-kanzo-to reduced diarrhea due to intravenous cisplatin administration.[40] Further study is warranted on the effect of peony and formulae containing it in cancer patients undergoing chemotherapy.

Finally, peony may not combine well with antibiotics. The gut flora is responsible for cleaving the aglycones of peony glycosides and thereby activating these constituents.[41] Damage to the gut flora by antibiotics might interfere with this process, theoretically decreasing peony's efficacy. Clinical trials will be necessary to determine the importance of this possible interaction.

Side Effects and Toxicity

At the doses indicated below, peony has not been associated with any adverse effects other than occasional gastric upset in susceptible individuals. Shakuyaku-kanzo-to, on the other hand, can cause pseudoaldosteronism with symptoms of hypertension, edema, and weight gain. This is due to the licorice in the formula and is not attributed to peony.

The safety of peony in pregnancy and lactation is unknown. However, as noted above, it has been used without obvious ill effect in one open trial to treat women with pregnancy-induced hypertension.[33]

Until further safety studies have been conducted, caution should be exercised during pregnancy.

Dosage

Peony is generally available as dried crude herb or dried aqueous extract, either in capsules or as powders. The usual dose of white peony is 1.5-4 grams three times daily. The usual dose of red peony and tree peony is 1-3 grams three times daily. The usual dose of the shakuyaku-kanzo-to and toki-shakuyaku-san formulae is 2.5 grams three times daily.

References

1. Foster S, Yue CX. *Herbal Emissaries: Bringing Chinese Herbs to the West.* Rochester, VT: Healing Arts Press; 1992:200-207.
2. Blumenthal M, ed. *The Complete German Commission E Monographs: Therapeutic Guide to Herbal Medicines.* Newton, MA: Integrative Medicine Communications; 1998:364.
3. Bensky D, Gamble A, Kaptchuk T. *Chinese Herbal Medicine Materia Medica*, Revised Edition, Seattle, WA: Eastland Press; 1993:70-71, 277-278, 331-332.
4. Kimura M, Kimura I, Takahashi K, et al. Blocking effects of blended paeoniflorin or its related compounds with glycyrrhizin on neuromuscular junctions in frogs and mice. *Jpn J Pharmacol* 1984;36:275-282.
5. Maeda T, Shinozuka K, Baba K, et al. Effect of shakuyaku-kanzoh-toh, a prescription composed of shakuyaku (*Paeoniae radix*) and kanzoh (*Glycyrrhizae radix*) on guinea pig ileum. *J Pharmacobiodyn* 1983;6:153-160.
6. Hirokawa S, Nose M, Ishige A, et al. Effect of hachimi-jio-gan on scopolamine-induced memory impairment and on acetylcholine content in rat brain. *J Ethnopharmacol* 1996;50:77-84.
7. Ohta H, Ni JW, Matsumoto K, et al. Paeony and its major constituent, paeoniflorin, improve radial maze performance impaired by scopolamine in rats. *Pharmacol Biochem Behav* 1993;45:719-723.
8. Okubo T, Nagai F, Seto T, et al. The inhibition of phenylhydroquinone-induced oxidative DNA cleavage by constituents of moutan cortex and Paeoniae radix. *Biol Pharm Bull* 2000;23:199-203.
9. Zhang WG, Zhang ZS. Anti-ischemia reperfusion damage and anti-lipid peroxidatioin effects of paeonol in rat heart. *Yao Xue Xue Bao* 1994;29:145-148.
10. Qi XG. Protective mechanism of *Salvia miltiorrhiza* and *Paeonia lactiflora* for experimental liver damage. *Zhong Xi Yi Jie He Za Zhi* 1991;11:102-104, 69. [Article in Chinese]
11. Zhang Y. The effects of nifedipine, diltiazem, and *Paeonia lactiflora* Pall on atherogenesis in rabbits. *Zhonghua Xin Xue Guan Bing Za Zhi* 1991;19:100-103. [Article in Chinese]
12. Ono K, Sawada T, Murata Y, et al. Pentagalloylglucose, an antisecretory component of *Paeoniae radix*, inhibits gastric H+, K(+)-ATPase. *Clin Chim Acta* 2000;290:159-167.
13. Tsuda T, Sugaya A, Ohguchi H, et al. Protective effects of peony root extract and its components on neuron damage in the hippocampus induced by the cobalt focus epilepsy model. *Exp Neurol* 1997;146:518-525.
14. Nagasawa H, Iwabuchi T, Inatomi H. Protection by tree-peony (*Paeonia suffruticosa* Andr) of obesity in (SLN x C3H/He) F1 obese mice. *In Vivo* 1991;5:115-118.

15. Sakai Y, Nagase H, Ose Y, et al. Inhibitory action of peony root extract on the mutagenicity of benzo[a]pyrene. *Mutat Res* 1990;244:129-134.

16. Goto H, Shimada Y, Tanaka N, et al. Effect of extract prepared from the roots of *Paeonia lactiflora* on endothelium-dependent relaxation and antioxidant enzyme activity in rats administered high-fat diet. *Phytother Res* 1999;13:526-528.

17. Lin HC, Ding HY, Ko FN, et al. Aggregation inhibitory activity of minor acetophenones from Paeonia species. *Planta Med* 1999;65:595-599.

18. Ishida H, Takamatsu M, Tsuji K, Kosuge T. Studies on active substances in herbs used for oketsu ("stagnant blood") in Chinese medicine. VI. On the anticoagulative principle in *Paeoniae radix*. *Chem Pharm Bull* 1987;35:849-852.

19. Ji LX, Zhang LY, Xu LN. Anticoagulant and fibrinolytic effects of total glycosides of Chi-Shao (*Paeonia lactiflora*) in rats. *Zhongguo Yi Xue Ke Xue Yuan Xue Bao* 1981;3:41-43. [Article in Chinese]

20. Tomoda M, Matsumoto K, Shimizu N, et al. An acidic polysaccharide with immunological activities from the root of *Paeonia lactiflora*. *Biol Pharm Bull* 1994;17:1161-1164.

21. Kumada T, et al. Effect of shakuyaku-kanzo-to (Tsumura TJ-68) on muscle cramps accompanying cirrhosis in a placebo-controlled double-blind parallel study. *J Clin Ther Med* 1999;15:499-523.

22. Yosida M, et al. Effects of shakuyaku-kanzo-to on muscle cramp in diabetics. *Neurol Ther* 1995;12:529-534.

23. Yamashita JI. Effect of Tsumura skakuyaku-kanzo-to on pain at muscle twitch during and after dialysis in the patients undergoing dialysis. *Pain & Kampo Medicine* 1992;2:18-20.

24. Maruyama K, et al. Effectiveness of shakuyaku-kanzo-to on convulsion and pain associated with alcohol dependence. *Kampo Igaku* 1996;20:81-84. [Article in Japanese]

25. Sakamoto T, Hosino M. Effect of shakuyaku-kanzo-to extract granules on convulsion of gastrocnemius muscle in patients with cerebrovascular disorder. *Jpn J Oriental Med* 1995;45:563-568.

26. Kotani N, Oyama T, Hashimoto H, et al. Analgesic effect of a herbal medicine for treatment of primary dysmenorrhea – a double-blind study. *Am J Chin Med* 1997;25:205-212.

27. Sakamoto S, Mitamura T, Iwasawa M, et al. Conservative management for perimenopausal women with uterine leiomyomas using Chinese herbal medicines and synthetic analogs of gonadotropin-releasing hormone. *In Vivo* 1998;12:333-337.

28. Takahashi K, Kitao M. Effect of TJ-68 (shakuyaku-kanzo-to) on polycystic ovarian disease. *Int J Fert Menopausal Studies* 1994;39:69-76.

29. Hagino N. An overview of Kampo medicine: Toki-Shakuyaku-San (TJ-p23). *Phytother Res* 1993;7:391-394.

30. Yang DG. Comparison of pre- and post-treatment hepatohistology with heavy dosage of *Paeonia rubra* on chronic active hepatitis caused liver fibrosis. *Zhongguo Zhong Xi Yi Jie He Za Zhi* 1994;14:207-209, 195. [Article in Chinese]

31. Wang CB, Chang AM. Plasma thromboxane B2 changes in severe icteric hepatitis treated by traditional Chinese medicine – dispelling the pathogenic heat from blood, promoting blood circulation and administrating large doses of radix Paeoniae – a report of 6 cases. Zhong Xi Yi Jie He Za Zhi 1985;5:326-328, 322. [Article in Chinese]

32. Liu J. Effect of *Paeonia obovata* 801 on metabolism of thromboxane B2 and arachidonic acid and on platelet aggregation in patients with coronary heart disease and cerebral thrombosis. *Zhonghua Yi Xue Za Zhi* 1983;63:477-481. [Article in Chinese]

33. Guo TL, Zhou XW. Clinical observations on the treatment of the gestational hypertension syndrome with Angelica and Paeonia powder. *Zhong Xi Yi Jie He Za Zhi* 1986;6:714-716, 707. [Article in Chinese]

34. Yamada K, Kanba S, Murata T, et al. Effectiveness of skakuyaku-kanzo-to in neuroleptic-induced hyperprolactinemia: a preliminary report. *Psychiatr Clin Neurosci* 1996;50:341-342.

35. Yamada K, Kanba S, Yagi G, Asai M. Effectiveness of herbal medicine (skakuyaku-kanzo-to) for neuroleptic-induced hyperprolactinemia. *J Clin Psychopharmacol* 1997;17:234-235.

36. Yamada K, Kanba S, Yagi G, Asai M. Herbal medicine (skakuyaku-kanzo-to) in the treatment of risperidone-induced amenorrhea. *J Clin Psychopharmacol* 1999;19:380-381.

37. Tanaka T. Effects of herbal medicines on menopausal symptoms induced by gonadotropin-releasing hormone agonist therapy. *Clin Exp Obstet Gynecol* 2001;28:20-23.

38. Yasui T, Irahara M, Aono T, et al. Studies on the combination treatment with clomiphene citrate and toki-shakuyaku-san. *Jpn J Fertil Steril* 1995;40:83-91.

39. Yamamoto K, Hoshiai H, Noda K. Effects of shakuyaku-kanzo-to on muscle pain from combination chemotherapy with paclitaxel and carboplatin. *Gynecol Oncol* 2001;81:333-334.

40. Xu JD, Liu ZH, Chen SZ. Effects of Paeonia-glycyrrhiza decoction on changes induced by cisplatin in rats. *Zhongguo Zhong Xi Yi Jie He Za Zhi* 1994;14:673-674. [Article in Chinese]

41. Sung CK, Kang GH, Yoon SS, et al. Glycosidases that convert natural glycosides to bioactive compounds. In: Waller G, Yamasaki K, eds. *Saponins Used in Traditional and Modern Medicine*. New York: Plenum Press; 1996:24.

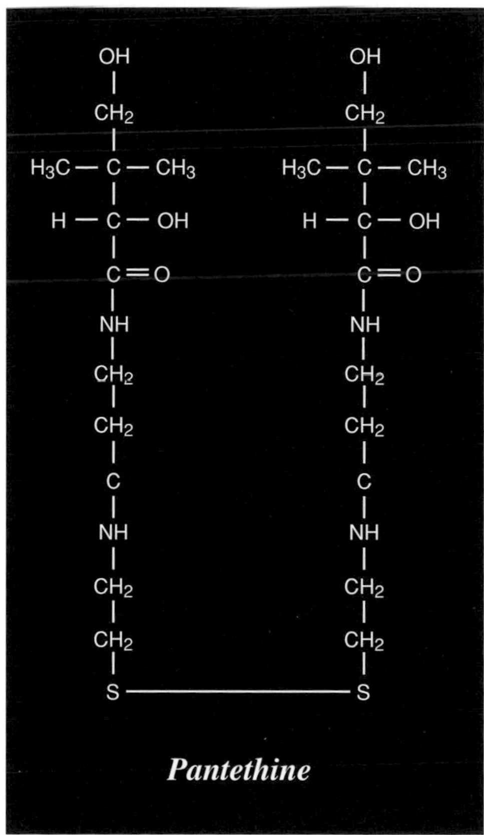

Pantethine

Pantethine

Introduction

Pantethine is the stable disulfate form of pantetheine, the metabolic substrate that constitutes the active part of coenzyme A molecules (CoA) and acyl carrier proteins (ACP). Oral administration of pantethine has consistently shown an ability to favorably impact a variety of lipid risk factors in persons with hypercholesterolemia, arteriosclerosis, and diabetes. Pantethine administration has also been shown to favorably affect parameters associated with platelet lipid composition and cell membrane fluidity. Due to its role in the formation of CoA, pantethine might assist with detoxification of some xenobiotic compounds. Administration also appears to favorably impact adrenal cortex function. In several animal models, preliminary studies have indicated a protective effect against cataract formation.

Biochemistry

The reactive component of both CoA and ACP is not the pantothenic acid molecule, but the sulfhydryl (SH) group donated from cysteine. Although pantothenic acid is commonly known as vitamin B5, pantethine actually contains the SH molecule required for enzyme activity and provides a more metabolically active form of the vitamin.

Mechanism of Action

The metabolic activity of pantethine is probably due to its role in the synthesis of CoA and ACP. CoA is a cofactor in over 70 enzymatic pathways, including fatty acid oxidation, carbohydrate metabolism, pyruvate degradation, amino acid catabolism, heme synthesis, acetylcholine synthesis, and hepatic phase II detoxification acetylations. ACP is an essential component of the fatty acid synthase complex required for fatty acid elongation.

While the exact mechanism of action of pantethine in normalizing parameters associated with dyslipidemia is unknown, several explanations have been proposed. Some authors have suggested pantethine might be capable of directly modulating the action of several enzymes involved in cholesterol synthesis.[1-3] The efficacy of pantethine in normalizing parameters of dyslipidemia might also be due to its ability to increase CoA levels. Theoretically, if pantethine enhances the formation of CoA, the additional CoA might then combine with free acetyl groups to form acetyl-CoA. The acetyl-CoA could then be directed into the TCA cycle or beta-oxidation at the expense of cholesterol formation.

Table 1. Pantethine's reported impact on lipid parameters in patients with Frederickson's type IIa, IIb, and IV dyslipidemia

Type	Clinical Definition	Pantethine's Impact
IIa	total cholesterol elevated LDL elevated triglyceride normal	decrease total cholesterol decrease LDL-cholesterol decrease VLDL-cholesterol decrease triglyceride decrease Apo-A increase HDL-cholesterol increase Apo-A
IIb	total cholesterol elevated LDL elevated VLDL elevated triglyceride elevated	decrease total cholesterol decrease LDL-cholesterol decrease VLDL-cholesterol decrease triglyceride decrease Apo-B
IV	total cholesterol normal VLDL elevated triglyceride elevated	mixed results with total cholesterol mixed results with LDL-cholesterol decrease VLDL-cholesterol decrease triglyceride decrease Apo-B mixed results with HDL-cholesterol increase HDL-cholesterol increase Apo-A

Deficiency States and Symptoms

A deficiency of pantethine is virtually unknown because of its widespread distribution in food.

Clinical Applications

Hyperlipidemia

Oral supplementation with pantethine typically results in a progressive decrease in total cholesterol, triglycerides, low density lipoprotein (LDL) cholesterol, and apolipoprotein B (Apo-B), and an increase in high density lipoprotein (HDL) cholesterol and apolipoprotein A (Apo-A); however, depending on the type of lipidemia, results might vary (Table 1).[4-9]

Platelet Lipid Composition and Fluidity

Pantethine administration has been shown to favorably affect parameters associated with platelet lipid composition and cell membrane fluidity.[10,11] In diabetic patients, composition of platelets is characterized by a derangement in a wide variety of lipid concentrations and a higher microviscosity than in healthy platelets. Administration of pantethine to diabetics is reported to normalize these values to control levels, and result in a concomitant reduction in hyperaggregation.[12,13]

Cataract Protection

Pantethine administration has inhibited cataract formation in several animal models.[14-16]

Detoxification

Acetylation reactions utilizing acetyl-CoA are an important component of the phase II detoxification system. The compounds typically metabolized by acetylation reactions include aliphatic amines (such as histamine and mescaline), aromatic amines (such as sulfonamide), hydrazine and hydrazide, and certain amino acid metabolites (such as phenylcysteine). Because of its biochemical position as the most stable supplemental form of an immediate precursor to CoA, pantethine might be able to play an important role in the metabolism of some xenobiotic compounds.

Adrenal Function

Pantethine appears to exert a positive influence on some indicators of adrenal function. Administration of pantethine to 20 individuals with a variety of clinical conditions was reported to buffer the increase in 24-hour urinary 17-hydroxycorticosteroids and plasma 11-hydroxycorticosteroids stimulated by a loading dose of adrenocorticotropic hormone.[17]

Side Effects and Toxicity

Although digestive disturbances have occasionally been reported in the literature, the majority of researchers have commented on the complete freedom from side effects and subjective complaints experienced by individuals taking pantethine. Doses as high as 10 grams per day in humans produced no toxic manifestations other than occasional diarrhea and minor gastrointestinal disturbances.[18]

Dosage

The most common oral dosage used in the treatment of dyslipidemia has been 300 mg three times per day.

References

1. Ranganathan S, Jackson RL, Harmony JA. Effect of pantethine on the biosynthesis of cholesterol in human skin fibroblasts. *Atherosclerosis* 1982;44:261-273.
2. Cighetti G, Del Puppo M, Paroni R, et al. Effects of pantethine on cholesterol synthesis from mevalonate in isolated rat hepatocytes. *Atherosclerosis* 1986;60:67-77.
3. Cighetti G, Del Puppo M, Paroni R, Galli Kienle M. Modulation of HMG-CoA reductase activity by pantetheine/pantethine. *Biochim Biophys Acta* 1988;963:389-393.
4. Arsenio L, Caronna S, Lateana M, et al. Hyperlipidemia, diabetes and atherosclerosis: efficacy of treatment with pantethine. *Acta Biomed Ateneo Parmense* 1984;55:25-42. [Article in Italian]
5. Maggi GC, Donati C, Criscuoli G. Pantethine: a physiological lipomodulating agent, in the treatment of hyperlipidemias. *Curr Ther Res* 1982;32:380-386.
6. Gaddi A, Descovich GC, Noseda G, et al. Controlled evaluation of pantethine, a natural hypolipidemic compound, in patients with different forms of hyperlipoproteinemia. *Atherosclerosis* 1984;50:73-83.
7. Bertolini S, Donati C, Elicio N, et al. Lipoprotein changes induced by pantethine in hyperlipoproteinemic patients: adults and children. *Int J Clin Pharmacol Ther Toxicol* 1986;24:630-637.
8. Murai A, Miyahara T, Tanaka T, et al. The effects of pantethine on lipid and lipoprotein abnormalities in survivors of cerebral infarction. *Artery* 1985;12:234-243.
9. Binaghi P, Cellina G, Lo Cicero G, et al. Evaluation of the cholesterol-lowering effectiveness of pantethine in women in perimenopausal age. *Minerva Med* 1990;81:475-479.
10. Prisco D, Rogasi PG, Matucci M, et al. Effect of oral treatment with pantethine on platelet and plasma phospholipids in IIa hyperlipoproteinemia. *Angiology* 1987;38:241-247.
11. Gensini GF, Prisco D, Rogasi PG, et al. Changes in fatty acid composition of the single platelet phospholipids induced by pantethine treatment. *Int J Clin Pharmacol Res* 1985;5:309-318.
12. Hiramatsu K, Nozaki H, Arimori S. Influence of pantethine on platelet volume, microviscosity, lipid composition and functions in diabetes mellitus with hyperlipidemia. *Tokai J Exp Clin Med* 1981;6:49-57.
13. Eto M, Watanabe K, Chonan N. Lowering effect of pantethine on plasma B-thromboglobulin and lipids in diabetes mellitus. *Artery* 1987;15:1-12.
14. Hiraoka T, Clark JI. Inhibition of lens opacification during the early stages of cataract formation. *Invest Ophthalmol Vis Sci* 1995;36:2550-2555.
15. Clark JI, Livesey JC, Steele JE. Delay or inhibition of rat lens opacification using pantethine and WR-77913. *Exp Eye Res* 1996;62:75-84.
16. Matsushima H, David LL, Hiraoka T, Clark JI. Loss of cytoskeletal proteins and lens cell opacification in the selenite cataract model. *Exp Eye Res* 1997;64:387-395.
17. Onuki M, Suzawa A. Effect of pantethine on the function of the adrenal cortex. 2. Clinical experience using pantethine in cases under steroid hormone treatment. *Horumon To Rinsho* 1970;18:937-940.
18. Miller DR, Hayes KC. Vitamin excess and toxicity. In: Hathcock JN, ed. *Nutritional Toxicology* Vol 1. New York: Academic Press Inc; 1982:101-116.

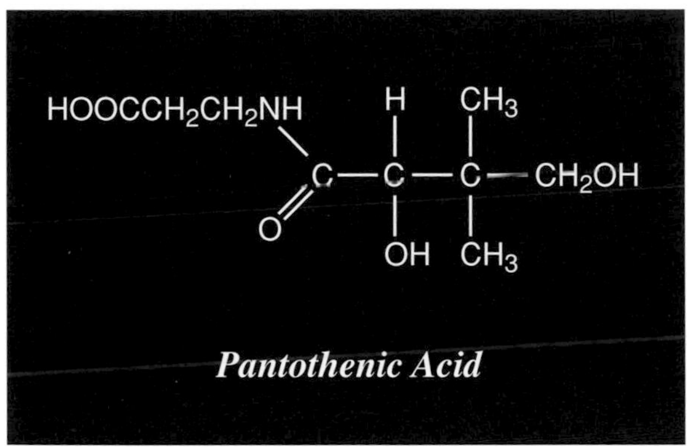

Pantothenic Acid

Pantothenic Acid

Introduction

Pantothenic acid (vitamin B5) is a water-soluble B-complex vitamin that was identified in 1933, isolated in 1938, and synthesized in 1940. Pantothenic acid (from the Greek *panthos*, meaning to be everywhere) was named as such because of its prevalence in food. In dietary supplements it is almost always found in the form of the stable compound calcium pantothenate. A liquid form of the vitamin – D-panthenol – is also available. Proposed clinical uses of pantothenic acid include viral hepatitis, aldehyde detoxification, rheumatoid arthritis, and the effects of chronic stress.

Biochemistry

The metabolic activity of pantothenic acid is assumed to be a result of its role as a precursor of coenzyme A (CoA) and acyl carrier proteins (ACP). Before conversion into these molecules, pantothenic acid must first be converted into the sulfur-containing molecule pantetheine, via the addition of cysteine. The reactive component of both CoA and ACP is not the pantothenic acid molecule, but rather the sulfhydryl group donated from cysteine.

Pharmacokinetics

Pantothenic acid appears to be absorbed rapidly following an oral dose, resulting in increased tissue levels of CoA and other B5 metabolites within six hours.[1] In animals, an intact gut flora is required for pantothenic acid absorption;[2] however, the role of gut flora in the bioavailability of pantothenic acid in humans is not established. After pantothenic acid is absorbed and transported into cells, it can be converted to CoA by undergoing biotransformation via a series of enzymatic reactions requiring magnesium and cysteine as cofactors. In experimental models glucagon increases, while insulin decreases, the incorporation of pantothenic acid into CoA. Glucocorticoids appear to potentiate the effects of glucagon.[3] It appears the cell is equipped to minimize degradation of CoA once it has been formed.[3] Excess pantothenic acid is primarily eliminated by urinary excretion.

Mechanisms of Action

The metabolic activity of pantothenic acid is assumed to be a result of its role in the synthesis of CoA and ACP. CoA is a cofactor in over 70 enzymatic pathways, including fatty acid oxidation, steroid hormone synthesis, cholesterol metabolism, carbohydrate metabolism, pyruvate degradation, amino acid catabolism, heme and bile acid synthesis, acetylcholine synthesis, and hepatic phase II detoxification acetylation. ACP is an essential component of the fatty acid synthase complex required for fatty acid elongation. Pantothenic acid's anti-stress action is thought to be a result of its role in supporting appropriate adrenal cortex function.

Deficiency States and Symptoms

Because pantothenic acid and its derivatives are so widespread in foods, it is generally considered that a dietary deficiency in humans is unlikely; however, deficiency symptoms have been produced in both animals and humans using a pantothenic acid agonist or a semi-synthetic diet virtually free of pantothenic acid, and in animals by antibiotic administration.[2]

Deficient subjects typically complain of headache, listlessness or fatigue, and a sensation of weakness. Other symptoms can include personality changes, depression, sleep disturbances, frequent infections, postural hypotension, rapid heartbeat on exertion, epigastric distress, anorexia, constipation, paresthesias (including numbness and tingling in the hands and feet, and "burning feet syndrome"), and impaired motor coordination.[3,4]

Clinical Indications

Viral Hepatitis A

Calcium pantothenate 300-600 mg, administered for 3-4 weeks as a component of therapy in subjects with viral hepatitis A, produced a favorable immunomodulatory action and an improvement in liver enzymes.[5]

Detoxification and Aldehyde Metabolism

Acetyl-CoA supports acetylation reactions of hepatic phase II detoxification. The compounds metabolized by acetylation reactions include aliphatic amines (such as histamine and mescaline), aromatic amines (such as sulfonamide), hydrazine and hydrazide, and certain amino acid metabolites (such as phenylcysteine).

Pantothenic acid and its derivatives can decrease the acute toxicity of acetaldehyde, as well as the duration of the narcotic action of ethanol in mice and rats.[6] In humans, pantothenic acid combined with vitamin B1 has shown an ability to protect workers engaged in manufacturing of phenol-formaldehyde resins.[7]

Stress

Pantothenic acid has a reputation as an anti-stress vitamin, and appears to be required for optimal adrenal cortex function and hormone production during stressful situations.

Administration of pantethine to 20 humans with a variety of clinical conditions is reported to buffer the increase in 24-hour urinary 17-hydroxycorticosteroids and plasma 11-hydroxycorticosteroids stimulated by a loading dose of adrenocorticotropic hormone.[8]

Men receiving pantothenic acid 10 g per day for six weeks had a less pronounced drop in white blood cell counts and vitamin C levels subsequent to cold-water immersion stress, compared to pre-supplementation values.[9]

Rheumatoid Arthritis

Supplementation of pantothenic acid for two months, beginning at 500 mg per day and increasing to 500 mg four times daily, resulted in slight reductions in pain and morning stiffness in individuals with rheumatoid arthritis.[10]

Rheumatoid arthritis patients may be more likely to have lower whole blood pantothenic acid levels, which may be associated with greater symptom severity. Intramuscular administration of pantothenic acid resulted in improvement of symptoms, which reached a plateau in seven days. After discontinuation of pantothenic acid, blood levels fell to previous levels with a concomitant reappearance of symptoms.[11]

Side Effects and Toxicity

Animal studies have documented the low toxicity and safety of pantothenic acid and its derivatives. Digestive disturbances have occasionally been reported in the literature in subjects taking high doses of pantothenic acid. A single case report mentions development of eosinophilic pleuropericarditis resulting from concomitant use of vitamins B5 and biotin in a 76-year-old woman.[12]

Dosage

A 5 mg daily dose meets 100 percent of the daily supplemental value established by the Food and Nutrition Board; however, therapeutic doses of 500 mg 1-4 times daily are often prescribed, with short-term administration of up to 10 grams per day advocated by some clinicians.

References

1. Moiseenok AG, Tsverbaum EA, Rybalko MA. Pantothenic acid biotransformation in human vitamin deficiency. *Vopr Med Khim* 1981;27:780-784. [Article in Russian]
2. Stein ED, Diamond JM. Do dietary levels of pantothenic acid regulate its intestinal uptake in mice? *J Nutr* 1989;119:1973-1983.

3. Tahiliani AG, Beinlich CJ. Pantothenic acid in health and disease. *Vit Horm* 1991;46:165-227.

4. Chevaux KA, Song WO. Adrenocortical function and cholesterol in pantothenic acid deficiency. *FASEB* 1994;8:2588.

5. Komar VI. The use of pantothenic acid preparations in treating patients with viral hepatitis A. *Ter Arkh* 1991;63:58-60. [Article in Russian]

6. Moiseenok AG, Dorofeev BF, Omel'ianchik SN. The protective effect of pantothenic acid derivatives and changes in the system of acetyl CoA metabolism in acute ethanol poisoning. *Farmakol Toksikol* 1988;51:82-86. [Article in Russian]

7. Skvortsova RI, Pozniakovskii VM. Effect of a therapeutic and prophylactic diet enriched with thiamine and calcium pantothenate on the acetylating capacity of the body of workers engaged in the manufacture of phenol-formaldehyde resins. *Vopr Pitan* 1977;6:40-42. [Article in Russian]

8. Onuki M, Suzawa A. Effect of pantethine on the function of the adrenal cortex. 2. Clinical experience using pantethine in cases under steroid hormone treatment. *Horumon To Rinsho* 1970;18:937-940.

9. Ralli D. NYU Bellevue Med Center, 1952. [abstract]

10. No authors listed. Calcium pantothenate in arthritic conditions. A report from the General Practitioner Research Group. *Practitioner* 1980;224:208-211.

11. Burton-Wright E. The pantothenic acid metabolism of rheumatoid arthritis. *Lancet* 1963;2:862-863. [abstract]

12. Debourdeau PM, Djezzar S, Estival JL, et al. Life-threatening eosinophilic pleuropericardial effusion related to vitamins B5 and H. *Ann Pharmacother* 2001;35:424-426.

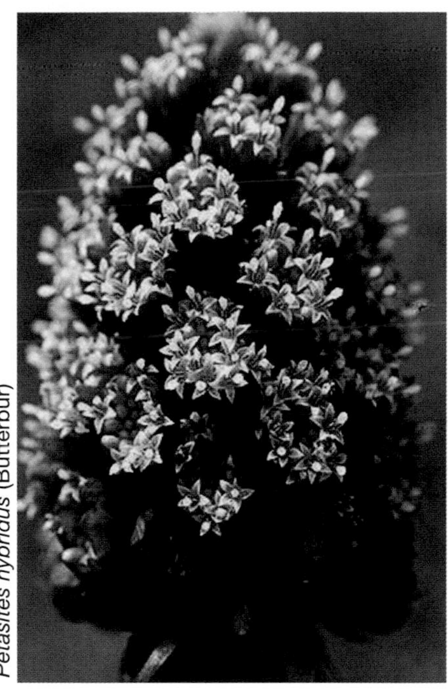
Petasites hybridus (Butterbur)

Petasites hybridus

Description

Petasites hybridus (butterbur) is a perennial shrub that has been used medicinally for centuries and is found throughout Europe as well as parts of Asia and North America. During the Middle Ages butterbur was used to treat plague and fever; in the 17th century its use was noted in treating cough, asthma, and skin wounds.[1,2] The plant can grow to a height of three feet and is usually found in wet, marshy ground, in damp forests, and adjacent to rivers or streams. Its downy leaves can attain a diameter of three feet, making it the largest of all indigenous floras, and their unique characteristics are responsible for the plant's botanical and common names. The genus name, Petasites, is derived from the Greek word petasos, which is the felt hat worn by shepherds.[2] The common name of butterbur is attributed to the large leaves being used to wrap butter during warm weather.[3] Other common names include pestwurz (German), blatterdock, bog rhubarb, and butter-dock.[2] Currently, the primary therapeutic uses for butterbur are for prophylactic treatment of migraines, and as an anti-spasmodic agent for chronic cough or asthma. It has also been used successfully in preventing gastric ulcers, and in treating patients with irritable bladder and urinary tract spasms.[2,4]

Active Constituents

Extracts of *Petasites hybridus* are prepared from the rhizomes, roots, and leaves. The main active constituents are two sesquiterpenes, petasin and isopetasin. Petasin is responsible for the antispasmodic properties of the plant by reducing spasms in smooth muscle and vascular walls, in addition to providing an anti-inflammatory effect by inhibiting leukotriene synthesis. Prostaglandins are important mediators in the inflammatory process and isopetasin's positive impact on prostaglandin metabolism contributes to the effectiveness of Petasites extracts. Extracts of the plant also contain volatile oils, flavonoids, tannins, and pyrrolizidine alkaloids. As these alkaloids are believed to be toxic to the liver and carcinogenic in animals, extracts are available in which the pyrrolizidine alkaloids have been removed.[2]

Mechanisms of Action

The active constituents of Petasites have an antispasmodic effect on vascular walls and appear to have an affinity for cerebral blood vessels. Petasites' ability to reduce smooth muscle spasm suggests it may be a useful therapeutic tool in treating urinary disorders, menstrual cramps, migraine headaches, kidney stone disorders, obstruction of bile flow, as well as other liver or gastrointestinal disorders associated with smooth muscle spasm.[1] The anti-inflammatory properties of butterbur extracts are attributed to inhibition of lipoxygenase activity and down-regulation of leukotriene synthesis, and are primarily due to the petasin content.[5]

Clinical Indications

Migraine Headache

Two clinical studies using 50 mg of a standardized Petasites extract twice daily for 12 weeks demonstrated its effectiveness as a prophylactic treatment for migraines. Both studies were double-blind, placebo controlled, and involved a total of 128 patients. The results of the two studies showed a significant reduction (as much as 60%) in frequency of migraine attacks compared to placebo. Other improvements in the Petasites group included a reduction in the number of days with migraines per month, a decrease in migraine-associated symptoms, and diminished duration and intensity of pain. No adverse reactions were reported in either study. Butterbur extract's high degree of efficacy and excellent tolerability accentuates its value in the prophylactic treatment of migraines.[6,7]

Asthma/Bronchitis

Various parts of the butterbur plant have been used for centuries to treat bronchial asthma and whooping cough, and in folk medicine the leaves of the plant were used as a mucus-reducing cough remedy. Butterbur's ostensible effectiveness in treating upper respiratory disorders such as asthma and bronchitis is attributed to the antispasmodic properties of the petasin constituent. The plant's anti-inflammatory action can also help calm the reactive airways seen in both asthma and bronchitis.[2] A Polish clinical study conducted in 1998 examined the influence of Petasites on lung ventilation and bronchial reactivity in patients suffering from asthma or chronic obstructive bronchitis. The study included three test groups and two control groups. Test Group A exhibited an improvement in forced expiratory volume (FEV1) three hours after an oral dose of 600 mg Petasites extract. Group B experienced a significant decrease in bronchial reactivity two hours after receiving an oral dose of 600 mg Petasites extract. Group C patients were treated for 14 days and received 600 mg of the extract three times daily. Some patients (n=10) were also given corticosteroids due to disease severity. All three groups exhibited a decrease in bronchial reactivity, but the patients in

Group C who received no corticosteroids had the most pronounced results.[8] These results indicate Petasites might be helpful in improving lung ventilation in patients with asthma or chronic obstructive bronchitis.

Gastrointestinal Disorders

Butterbur's use as an antispasmodic for gastrointestinal conditions dates back to the Middle Ages. The leaves and rhizomes were used to treat spasms of the digestive tract associated with colic, plague, and bile flow obstruction.[9,10] A German study conducted in 1993 found ethanolic extracts of *Petasites hybridus* blocked ethanol-induced gastric damage and reduced ulcerations of the small intestine caused by indomethacin, an anti-inflammatory drug used to treat arthritic conditions. The results of this study were attributed to inhibition of lipoxygenase activity and leukotriene biosynthesis.[11]

Side Effects and Toxicity

Until recently, side effects from Petasites extracts had not been reported. In September 2000, a study conducted in Taiwan noted the petasin constituent responsible for many of butterbur's pharmacological properties inhibited the production of testosterone in rat testicular cells, but did not speculate whether this effect would be applicable in humans.[12] The plant's pyrrolizidine alkaloids are thought to cause liver damage and to be carcinogenic in animals; however, extracts are commercially available in which the pyrrolizidine alkaloids have been removed. There are no known interactions with either pharmaceutical or over-the-counter anti-inflammatory agents; however, use of Petasites extracts during pregnancy and lactation is contraindicated.[1]

Dosage

Typically, Petasites extracts are standardized to contain a minimum of 7.5 mg of petasin and isopetasin. The adult dosage ranges from 50-100 mg twice daily with meals. When used to treat migraines, administration is prophylactic and supplementation should be carried out daily for four to six months and then titrated for optimum long-term dosing. Dosage regimens for asthma and gastrointestinal disorders are as yet undefined, dictating the need for further research.

References

1. Eaton J. Butterbur, herbal help for migraine. *Natural Pharmacy* 1998;2:1,23-24.
2. Mauskop A. Petasites hybridus: ancient medicinal plant is effective prophylactic treatment for migraine. *Townsend Lett* 2000;202:104-106.
3. Grieve M. Butterbur. In: Leyel CF, ed. *A Modern Herbal,* electronic version. New York, NY: Dover Publications, Inc.; 1971.

4. Reglin F. A clinical review: Petadolex® (Standardized Butterbur Extract), Praxis-Telegram, Nr. 1/98:13-14.

5. Bickel D, Roder T, Bestmann HJ, Brune K. Identification and characterization of inhibitors of peptido-leukotriene synthesis from *Petasites hybridus*. *Planta Med* 1994;60:318-322.

6. Mauskop A, Grossmann WM, Schmidramsl H. *Petasites hybridus* (butterbur root) extract is effective in the prophylaxis of migraines. Results of a randomized, double-blind trial. *J Head Face Pain* 2000;40:4.

7. Grossmann WM, Schmidramsl H. An extract of *Petasites hybridus* is effective in the prophylaxis of migraine. *Int J Clin Pharmacol Ther* 2000;38:430-435.

8. Ziolo G, Samochowiec L. Study on clinical properties and mechanism of action of Petasites in bronchial asthma and chronic obstructive bronchitis. *Pharmaceutica Acta Helvetica* 1998;72:359-380.

9. Lindauerova T. Palynomorphological investigation of the species *Petasites hybridus* and *Petasites albus*. *Farmaceuticky Obzor* 1981:50:569-574.

10. Blumenthal M, ed. *The Complete German Commission E Monographs*. Austin, TX: American Botanical Council; 1998;183:365.

11. Brune K, Bickel D, Peskar BA. Gastro-protective effects by extracts of *Petasites hybridus*: the role of inhibition of peptido-leukotriene synthesis. *Planta Med* 1993;59:494-496.

12. Lin H, Chien CH, Lin YL, et al. Inhibition of testosterone secretion by S-petasin in rat testicular interstitial cells. *Chin J Physiol* 2000:43:99-103.

DL-Phenylalanine

Introduction

Phenylalanine is a biologically essential amino acid that acts as a precursor to tyrosine and the catecholamines (epinephrine, norepinephrine, dopamine, and tyramine), and is a constituent of many central nervous system neuropeptides. Normal dietary levels of phenylalanine are approximately 1-2 grams daily.[1] As a clinically important amino acid, phenylalanine has been used to treat endogenous depression[2] and attention deficit disorder,[3] and as a potentiator of opiate analgesia in chronic pain.[4]

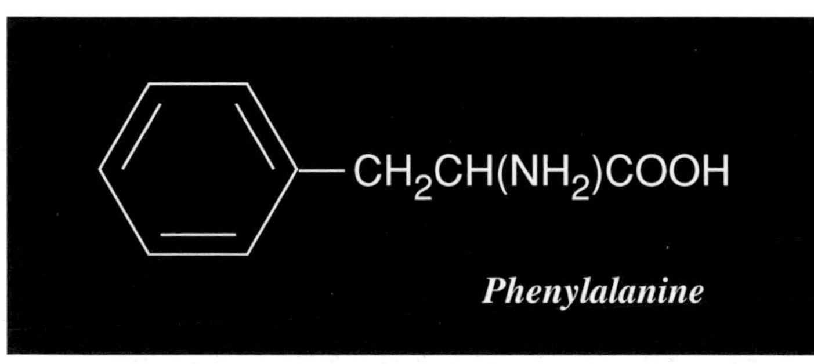

Phenylalanine

Biochemistry

Phenylalanine not needed for tissue synthesis is converted to tyrosine via phenylalanine hydroxylase, an oxygenase enzyme that requires the presence of oxygen and tetrahydrobiopterin (part of the folic acid molecule). The reaction is irreversible, making phenylalanine an essential amino acid and tyrosine a non-essential one.[1] The conversion of phenylalanine to tyrosine is an efficient process; over 95 percent of ingested phenylalanine is converted to tyrosine.[1] When given in a fasting state, phenylalanine can supply 70 percent of the tyrosine appearing in the plasma.[5] Phenylalanine is a precursor to the catecholamines and is also present in several active brain neuropeptides, including somatostatin, vasopressin, melanotropin, ACTH, substance P, enkephalin, angiotensin II, and cholecystokinin.[6]

In phenylkentonuria (PKU), an inborn error of metabolism, either phenylalanine hydroxylase or the cofactor tetrahydrobiopterin are absent. This prevents the production of tyrosine, depresses levels of serotonin in the plasma, and elevates blood and urine levels of phenylalanine.[7] The metabolites of phenylalanine are believed to be responsible for the symptoms of altered mental capacity in children with PKU. Those with untreated PKU have severe retardation and very low IQs. Symptoms include hyperactivity, aggression, convulsions and tremors, light pigmentation, and abnormal posture or gait patterns. Although severe PKU is usually picked up in infancy, mild PKU may not be diagnosed at an early age.[8]

Pharmacokinetics

Phenylalanine is the only amino acid besides methionine in which both isomers, the D- and L-forms, are equally absorbed, due to efficient enzymatic conversion between the isomers. The synthetic isomer (D- form) appears to be absorbed rapidly in humans and converted into the L-form.[9]

Mechanisms of Action

A metabolic end-product of phenylalanine, phenylethylamine (PEA), is metabolized by monoamine oxidase type B to phenylacetic acid (PAA).[10] Tricyclic antidepressants and MAO inhibitors increase PEA levels in the brain.[11] PEA is believed to have amphetamine-like properties, and urine levels have been found to be reduced in patients with depression.[12] Using it as a diagnostic tool, Sabelli found significantly lower levels of PEA in plasma and urine in depressed subjects, compared with normal controls. Treatment with phenylalanine improved mood in 78 percent of depressed subjects.[12]

Phenylalanine has been shown to inhibit enkephalinase and increase levels of met-enkephalin in the brain, producing opiate-mediated analgesia.[13] Enkephalinase-inhibitors are unique analgesia-producing agents that do not show tolerance or dependence. No signs of withdrawal are evident in animal studies when large doses (250-400 mg per kg) are used for long periods of time.[13]

Clinical Indications

Endogenous Depression

Multiple studies indicate a possible role for DL-phenylalanine in the treatment of depression. In an open, uncontrolled trial, 75-200 mg of DL-phenylalanine was administered to 20 patients suffering from endogenous depression. Assessment tools included psychometric testing, including the Hamilton Depression Scale, and psychiatric assessment. At the end of the trial (20 days), 60 percent of patients were asymptomatic and 20 percent were significantly improved and able to be discharged from care.[14]

Other small trials with doses of 50-200 mg DL-phenylalanine reported significant symptom improvement within 13-15 days. Unfortunately, these studies lacked objective diagnostic criteria or depression rating scales.[15,16] In a large trial, 455 patients with depression were given up to 400 mg per day of D-phenylalanine for 2-6 months. Individuals with a diagnosis of endogenous depression showed the most improvement; after 15 days, 73 percent were asymptomatic and 23 percent had significant improvement. In a group of patients with reactive depression, 53 percent recovered and 23 percent had significant improvement of their symptoms. There was no significant effect on patients who had been diagnosed with depression after age 50.[2]

In two double-blind studies comparing equal doses of imipramine to either 100 mg D-phenylalanine or 150-200 mg DL-phenylalanine, improvement in psychometric testing and clinical improvement after 30 days were similar, with the majority of patients improving on either therapy.[2,17]

There are many unanswered questions about the use of phenylalanine in depression. One study using 600 mg D-phenylalanine for one month in 10 depressed individuals had no effect.[18] It is suggested this and other early studies used inadequate dosage levels, and that up to 6 grams DL-phenylalanine may be necessary to normalize PEA levels in treating endogenous depression.[19]

A more recent study attempted using an individualized dosing system of L-phenylalanine with a steady dose of 100 mg pyridoxine in 40 patients with either unipolar or bipolar depression.[12] The authors found maximum dosing levels for symptom alleviation were as high as 14 grams L-phenylalanine daily. In this trial, patients were given 500 mg twice daily as a baseline dose, which was increased by 500 mg daily until therapeutic effects occurred. Complete recovery occurred in 11 patients, and partial recovery in 20. L-phenylalanine reduced suicidal ideation, fatigue, and anhedonia (lack of ability to experience pleasure), and increased self-esteem. Sleep and appetite were not changed, but patients were allowed to continue benzodiazepines for sleep if needed.

An individualized combination trial with 5 mg selegiline (Deprenyl), 100 mg pyridoxine, and 2-6 grams L-phenylalanine was utilized in 10 patients with prior drug-resistant major depressive disorder.[20] L-phenylalanine dosages were increased daily as needed for symptom reduction. Nine of 10 patients experienced mood elevation within hours of taking L-phenylalanine, and six viewed their depression as having terminated within two to three days of starting the regimen. Global Assessment Scale scores were significantly lowered after three days of treatment and remained low on continued treatment for six weeks.

Chronic Pain

In an open study, 78 chronic pain patients were given 750-1,000 mg D-phenylalanine daily. Responses occurred in 50 percent of the study population after one week.[4] In a double-blind, crossover study, 21 patients with chronic intractable pain were given 250 mg D-phenylalanine per day for two weeks; improvement was evident in 30 percent.[21] A small, open study of ten patients with lumbosacral pain receiving 1,000 mg D-phenylalanine resulted in significant improvements in pain relief and analgesic use.[22]

D-phenylalanine has also been used to potentiate acupuncture anesthesia, both in those who were non-responsive and to raise pain thresholds in those who were already responding. The doses used ranged between 2-4 grams.[4,23]

Attention Deficit Disorder

In the only double-blind, crossover study published in this area, dosages of up to 1,200 mg of DL-phenylalanine were used in 19 adults with attention deficit disorder.[3] After 14 days, a significant difference in mood and mood lability was observed in the treatment group. After two to three months, however, those who had improved on the DL-phenylalanine became tolerant to the effect and did not respond to higher doses.

Drug-Nutrient Interactions

Phenylalanine has been shown to compete with levodopa for transport across the blood-brain barrier.[24]

Phenylalanine is a precursor to the catecholamines epinephrine, norepinephrine, dopamine, and tyramine. Theoretically, caution is warranted with the concomitant use of monoamine-oxidase inhibitors and phenylalanine.[25]

Side Effects and Toxicity

LD-50 of D-phenylalanine in mice is more than 10 g/kg. Murine studies of 1 mg/kg body weight per day for six months resulted in no tissue toxicity.[13] Short-term stimulant-type side effects have been reported, including elevation of blood pressure, headache, irritability, aggressiveness, and insomnia. Long-term side effects have not been studied.[26]

Dosage

Dosages vary with the condition; depression responding to intake of 1-14 g daily, and pain management doses ranging from 1-4 g daily.

Warnings and Contraindications

Supplementation of phenylalanine should be avoided in PKU. Phenylalanine can interfere with the absorption and efficacy of levodpa.[24] Contraindications for the use of phenylalanine with schizophrenic patients has also been suggested.[27]

References

1. Wurtman RJ, Caballero B. Control of plasma phenylalanine levels. In: Wurtman RJ, Ritter-Walker E, eds. *Dietary Phenylalanine and Brain Function*. Boston, MA: Birkhauser; 1988:3-12.
2. Heller B. Pharmacological and clinical effects of DL-phenylalanine in the treatment of depression and Parkinson's disease. In: Mosnaim AD, Wolfe ME, eds. *Modern Pharmacology-Toxicology, Noncatecholic Phenylethylamines, Part 1*. New York: Marcel Dekker; 1978:397-417.
3. Wood DR, Reimherr FW, Wender P. Treatment of attention deficit disorder with DL-phenylalanine. *Psychiatry Res* 1985;16:21-26.
4. Balagot RC, Ehrenpreis S, Greenberg J, et al. D-phenylalanine in human chronic pain. In: Ehrenpreis S, Sicuteri F, eds. *Degradation of Endogenous Opioids: Its Relevance in Human Pathology and Therapy.* New York, NY: Raven Press; 1983:207-215.

5. Moldawer LL, Kawamura I, Bistrian BR, Blackburn GL. The contribution of phenylalanine to tyrosine metabolism *in vivo*. Studies in the post-absorptive and phenylalanine-loaded rat. *Biochem J* 1983;210:811-817.

6. Braverman E. *The Healing Nutrients Within.* New Canaan, CT: Keats Publishing; 1997:31.

7. Guroff G. Effects of inborn errors of metabolism on the nutrition of the brain. In: Wurtmann RJ, Wurtmann JJ, eds. *Nutrition and the Brain.* New York, NY: Raven Press; 1979:29-68.

8. Braverman E. *The Healing Nutrients Within.* New Canaan, CT: Keats Publishing; 1997:38.

9. Lehmann WD, Theobald N, Fischer R, Heinrich, HC. Stereospecificity of phenylalanine plasma kinetics and hydroxylation in man following oral application of a stable isotope-labelled pseudo-racemic mixture of L- and D-phenylalanine. *Clin Chim Acta* 1983;128:181-198.

10. Yang H, Neff NH. Monoamine oxidase: A natural substrate for type B enzyme. *Fed Proc* 1973;32:797.

11. Sabelli HC, Mosnaim AD. Phenylethylamine hypothesis of affective behavior. *Am J Psychiatry* 1974;131:695-699.

12. Sabelli HC, Fawcett J, Gusovsky F, et al. Clinical studies on the phenylethylamine hypothesis of affective disorder: urine and blood phenylacetic acid and phenylalanine dietary supplements. *J Clin Psychiatry* 1986;47:66-70.

13. Ehrenpreis S, Bagalot RC, Greenberg J, et al. Analgesic and other pharmacological properties of D-phenylalanine. In: Ehrenpreis S, Sicuteri F, eds. *Degradation of Endogenous Opioids: Its Relevance in Human Pathology and Therapy.* New York, NY: Raven Press; 1983:171-187.

14. Beckmann H, Strauss MA, Ludolph E. DL-phenylalanine in depressed patients: an open study. *J Neural Transm* 1977;41:123-134.

15. Yaryura-Tobias JA, Heller B, Spatz H, et al. Phenylalanine for endogenous depression. *J Orthomol Psychiatry* 1974;3:80-81.

16. Fischer E, Heller B, Nachon M, Spatz H. Therapy of depression by phenylalanine. Preliminary note. *Arzneimittelforschung* 1975;25:132.

17. Beckmann H, Athen D, Olteanu M, Zimmer R. DL-phenylalanine versus imipramine: a double-blind controlled study. *Arch Psychiatr Nervenkr* 1979;227:49-58.

18. Mann J, Peselow ED, Snyderman S, Gershon S. D-phenylalanine in endogenous depression. *Am J Psychiatry* 1980;137:1611-1612.

19. Braverman E. *The Healing Nutrients Within.* New Canaan, CT: Keats Publishing; 1997:40-41.

20. Sabelli HC. Rapid treatment of depression with selegiline-phenylalanine combination. *J Clin Psychiatry* 1991;52:137.

21. Budd K. Use of D-phenylalanine, an enkephalinase inhibitor, in the treatment of intractable pain. In: Bonica JJ, Linblom V, Iggo A, eds. *Advances in Pain Research and Therapy*. New York, NY: Raven Press; 1983:305-308.

22. Godfraind JM, Plaghi L, De Nayer J. A comparative study on the effects of D-phenylalanine, lysozyme and zimelidine in human lumbosacral arachno-epiduritis. A chronic pain state. In: Bromm B, ed. *Pain Measurement in Man: Neurophysiological Correlates of Pain*. New York, NY: Elsevier; 1984:501-511.

23. Kitade T, Minamikawa M, Nawata T, et al. An experimental study on the enhancing effects of phenylalanine on acupuncture analgesia. *Am J Chin Med* 1981;9:243-248.

24. Nutt JG, Woodward WR, Hammerstad JP, et al. The "on-off" phenomenon in Parkinson's disease. Relation to levodopa absorption and transport. *N Engl J Med* 1984;310:483-488.

25. Werbach M. *Textbook of Nutritional Medicine.* Tarzana, CA: Third Line Press; 1999:175-178.

26. Simonson M. L-phenylalanine. *J Clin Psychiatry* 1985;46:355. [Letter]

27. Yaryura-Tobias JA, Neziroglu F. Phenylethylamine and glucose in true depression. *J Orthomol Psychiatry* 1976;5:199-202.

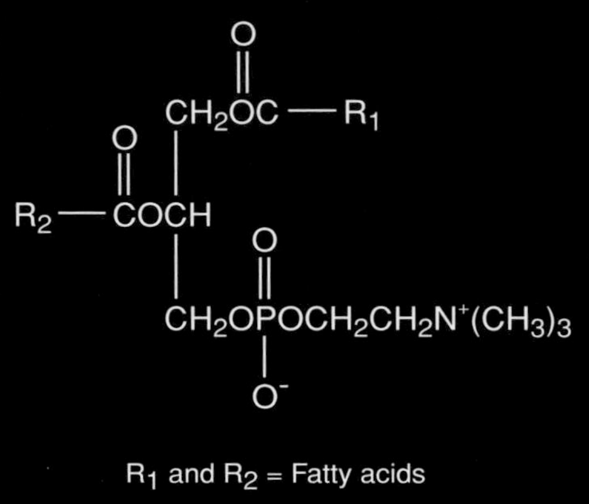

R_1 and R_2 = Fatty acids

Phosphatidylcholine

Phosphatidylcholine

Introduction

Phosphatidylcholine (PC) is a phospholipid, one of a primal class of substances ubiquitous among life forms.[1] PC is the predominant phospholipid of all cell membranes and of the circulating blood lipoproteins. It is the main functional constituent of the natural surfactants, and the body's foremost reservoir of choline, an essential nutrient.[2] PC is a normal constituent of the bile that facilitates fat emulsification, absorption, and transport, and is recycled via enterohepatic circulation.

Until recently the nomenclature of PC was confused with lecithin, a complex mixture of phospholipids and other lipids. Lecithin preparations enriched in PC at or above 30 percent by weight are considered PC concentrates.

Pharmacokinetics and Metabolism

Chemically, PC is a glycerophospholipid,[3] built on glycerol (CH_2OH-CHOH-CH_2OH) and substituted at all three carbons. Carbons 1 and 2 are substituted by fatty acids and carbon 3 by phosphorylcholine. Simplistically, the PC molecule consists of a head-group (phosphorylcholine), a middle piece (glycerol), and two tails (the fatty acids, which vary). Variations in the fatty acids in the tails account for the great variety of PC molecular species in human tissues.

In vivo, PC is produced via two major pathways.[4] In the predominant pathway, two fatty acids (acyl "tails") are added to glycerol phosphate (the "middle piece"), to generate phosphatidic acid (PA). Next, PA is converted to diacylglycerol, after which phosphocholine (the "head-group") is added on from CDP-choline. The second, minor pathway is phosphatidylethanolamine (PE) methylation, in which the phospholipid PE has three methyl groups added to its ethanolamine head-group, thereby converting it into PC.

Taken orally, PC is very well absorbed, up to 90 percent per 24 hours when taken with meals. Postprandially, PC enters the blood gradually and its levels peak over 8-12 hours. During the digestive process, the position-2 fatty acid becomes detached (de-acylation) in the majority of the PC molecules.[5] The resulting lyso-PC readily enters intestinal lining cells, and is subsequently re-acylated at position 2. The position-2 fatty acid contributes to membrane fluidity (along with position 1), but is preferentially available for eicosanoid generation and signal transduction. The omega-6/omega-3 balance of the PC fatty acids is subject to adjustment via dietary fatty acid intake.[6,7]

Choline is most likely an essential nutrient for humans,[8] and dietary choline is ingested predominantly as PC. Greater than 98 percent of blood and tissue choline is sequestered in PC,[2] and dietary PC serves as a "slow-release" blood choline source.[9] Malnourished individuals with lowered blood choline frequently display liver steatosis and related dysfunctions; these often respond favorably to PC supplementation.[10]

Methyl group ($-CH_3$) availability is crucial for protein and nucleic acid synthesis and regulation, phase-two hepatic detoxification, and numerous other biochemical processes involving methyl donation.[11] Methyl deficiency induced by restricted choline intake is linked to liver steatosis in humans, and to increased cancer risk in many mammals. PC is an excellent source of methyl groups, supplying up to three per PC molecule.

Mechanisms of Action

PC is the main structural support of cell membranes, the dynamic molecular sheets on which most life processes occur.[1] Comprising 40 percent of total membrane phospholipids, PC's presence is important for homeostatic regulation of membrane fluidity. The PC molecules of the outermost cell membrane deliver fatty acids on demand for prostaglandin/eicosanoid cellular messenger functions, and support signal transduction from the cell's exterior to its interior.[6]

PC is the main lipid constituent of the lipoprotein particles circulating in the blood. The amphipathic properties of PC render it an obligatory micellizing constituent of bile.[12,13] PC has surfactant (surface-active) properties that substantially protect the epithelial-luminal interfaces of the lungs and GI tract.[14,15]

Biochemically, PC is the preferred precursor for certain phospholipids and other biologically important molecules.[4] PC also provides antioxidant protection *in vivo*.[16] In animal and human studies, PC protected against a variety of chemical toxins and pharmaceutical adverse effects.[1]

Clinical Indications

The best-documented clinical success with PC to date is its significant amelioration of liver damage, probably because liver recovery following damage requires substantial replacement of cell membrane mass. The findings from eight double-blind trials and numerous other clinical reports[1,7] indicate consistently significant clinical benefit, including improvement of enzymatic and other biochemical indicators, faster functional and structural rebuilding of liver tissue, accelerated restoration of subjects' overall well-being, and improved survival following PC treatment.

Alcoholic Hepatic Steatosis and Inflammation

Knuechel conducted a double-blind trial on 40 male subjects with hepatic steatosis (fatty liver) and inflammation linked to alcohol intake.[17] Subjects were taken off pharmaceuticals and randomized into two groups; one group received placebo, the other 1,350 mg PC per day by mouth (fortified with B vitamins). Benefits from PC were evident at two weeks, and by the eighth week a wide variety of biochemical liver function measures were significantly improved over placebo.

Three subsequent double-blind trials corroborated these findings. Schuller Perez and San Martin concluded, "It is our view that the use of highly-unsaturated phosphatidylcholine for therapy of alcohol-dependent steatoses is very productive."[18] Buchman et al administered PC double blind to 15 subjects with fatty liver as part of a total parenteral nutrition intravenous feeding regimen, and also obtained significant benefit.[19] Other researchers report that subjects with mild to moderate hepatic inflammation benefit the most from PC supplementation.[20]

In an animal study, baboons were placed on a daily alcohol regimen for up to eight years. Following a blinded trial design, PC was added to the diet of some of the animals. After several years, baboons fed alcohol without PC had progressed to advanced fibrosis, while the PC-supplemented baboons developed fatty liver and mild fibrosis, but did not progress further. After three of the animals were taken off PC and kept on alcohol, they rapidly progressed to extensive, life-terminating liver fibrosis.[21]

Drug-Induced Liver Damage

In a double-blind trial, 101 tuberculous subjects who had suffered liver damage from rifampin and two other anti-tuberculosis pharmaceuticals received placebo or 1,350 mg of fortified PC daily. After three months, the PC group had significantly lower SGOT and SGPT enzyme levels.[22]

Hepatitis B

In a double-blind trial of 30 subjects with progressing liver damage from chronic hepatitis B virus infection (negative for HBsAg), standard immunosuppressive therapy was retained and subjects received either PC (2,300 mg per day) or placebo. At one year, the PC group had clinically stabilized, with significant improvement of liver structure, whereas the placebo group had worsened.[23]

Sixty subjects positive for hepatitis B (HBsAg-positive) were placed in a fortified PC group (1,350 mg per day) or a placebo group for 60 days. From 30 days onward the PC group was clinically improved over placebo, with 50 percent becoming HbsAg-negative, compared to 25 percent of the placebo group.[24]

In a double-blind trial of 50 subjects, all HBsAg-positive and manifesting extremely severe liver damage verified by biopsy and immunologic testing, the PC group (1,350 mg fortified PC per day) benefited considerably more ($p<0.001$) than placebo. In the PC group, 80 percent (20 of 25) were judged greatly improved, while 24 percent (6 of 25) moderately improved in the placebo group. Cell-structure, biochemical, immunologic, and hematologic parameters were significantly improved over placebo. Clinical improvement continued well past the end of the one-year trial.[25]

Hepatitis C

In a multicenter, double-blind trial, 176 patients with chronic viral hepatitis (B or C) were begun on interferon alpha for 24 weeks then randomized to PC (1.8 g/day) or placebo for 24 weeks. Significantly more patients responded to PC, particularly in the hepatitis C subgroup. In addition, PC supplementation sustained a longer-term improvement from hepatitis C over another 24 weeks.[26]

A long-term, multicenter, double-blind trial of PC for liver disease is ongoing; its results could signal a breakthrough in nutritional management of this life-threatening disease.[27]

Respiratory Distress Syndrome

The surfactant of premature babies is abnormally low in PC. Treatment with exogenous, mature-profile surfactant (with PC 70-80% of the total phospholipids) is the standard therapy for infants with, or at risk of having, respiratory distress syndrome (RDS). A meta-analysis of clinical trials suggests improved survival and overall better outcome from natural surfactant over synthetic forms.[28] In another randomized trial with 78 RDS babies, natural surfactant proved superior after six hours, and by 24 hours normalized the surfactant PC profile.[14]

Necrotizing Enterocolitis, Gastrointestinal Protection

As the major intrinsic surfactant of the gastrointestinal tract, PC helps maintain the acid barrier properties of the gastric epithelium. Animal research suggests PC helps protect against the adverse GI effects of aspirin and other non-steroidal anti-inflammatory drugs without blocking their efficacy.[15,29,30] Carlson et al reported a lower incidence of necrotizing enterocolitis in pre-term infants fed with formula high in PC and other phospholipids.[31]

Central Nervous System Cholinergic Imbalances

In contrast to persistent anecdotal claims, PC failed to benefit cognition in ten double-blind, placebo-controlled trials.[32] There are indications the "therapeutic window" for PC might be very narrow,[33] which could also explain the disappointing trial results against ataxias, tardive dyskinesia, and other CNS conditions that feature cholinergic imbalances.

Side Effects and Toxicity

PC is freely compatible with other nutrients, and when co-administered may enhance their absorption. Standard toxicological assessments indicate no significant acute or chronic toxicity from PC, as well as no mutagenicity and no teratogenicity. PC is well tolerated at daily intakes of up to 18 grams.[7] Symptoms of intolerance are almost exclusively restricted to GI discomfort – diarrhea, excessive fullness, and nausea.

Dosage

The therapeutic range of intake is 800-2,400 mg daily, and 4.6 grams or higher for liver salvage. For subjects with severe liver damage, best results may be obtained by initiating therapy with intravenous and oral PC, then maintaining on oral supplementation after improvement has begun. In cases of liver damage from deathcap mushroom poisoning this procedure has proved lifesaving.[34]

References

1. Kidd PM. Dietary phospholipids as anti-aging nutraceuticals. In: Klatz RA, Goldman R, eds. *Anti-Aging Medical Therapeutics*. Chicago, IL: Health Quest Publications; 2000:283-301.
2. Zeisel SH, Blusztajn JK. Choline and human nutrition. *Annu Rev Nutr* 1994;14:269-296.
3. Schneider M. Phospholipids. In: Gunstone FD, Padley FB, eds. *Lipid Technologies and Applications*. New York, NY: Marcel Dekker; 1997:15-30.
4. Kent C. Eukaryotic phospholipid biosynthesis. *Annu Rev Biochem* 1995;64:315-343.
5. Zierenberg O, Grundy SM. Intestinal absorption of polyenephosphatidylcholine in man. *J Lipid Res* 1982;23:1136-1142.
6. Kidd PM. Cell membranes, endothelia, and atherosclerosis – the importance of dietary fatty acid balance. *Altern Med Rev* 1996;1:148-167.
7. Kidd PM. Phosphatidylcholine, a superior protectant against liver damage. *Altern Med Rev* 1996;1:258-274.
8. Zeisel SH, Da Costa K, Franklin PD, et al. Choline, an essential nutrient for humans. *FASEB* 1991;5:2093-2098.
9. Wurtman RJ, Hirsch MJ, Growdon JH. Lecithin consumption raises serum free choline levels. *Lancet* 1977;ii:68-69.
10. Buchman AL, Dubin MD, Moukarzel AA, et al. Choline deficiency: a cause of hepatic steatosis during parenteral nutrition that can be reversed with intravenous choline supplementation. *Hepatology* 1995;22:1399-1403.
11. Ghyczy M, Boros M. Electrophilic methyl groups present in the diet ameliorate pathological states induced by reductive and oxidative stress: a hypothesis. *Brit J Nutr* 2001;85:409-414.
12. Thistle JL, Schoenfield LJ. Bile acid, lecithin, and cholesterol in repeated human duodenal biliary drainage: effect of lecithin feeding. *Clin Res* 1968;16:450.
13. Toouli J, Jablonski P, Watts JM. Gallstone dissolution in man using cholic acid and lecithin. *Lancet* 1975;ii:1124-1126.
14. Lloyd J, Todd DA, John E. Serial phospholipid analysis in preterm infants: comparison of Exosurf and Survanta. *Early Human Dev* 1999;54:157-168.

15. Dunjic BS, Axelson J. Gastroprotective capability of exogenous phosphatidylcholine in experimentally induced chronic gastric ulcers in rats. *Scand J Gastroenterol* 1993;28:89-94.
16. Lieber CS, Leo MA. Polyenylphosphatidylcholine decreases alcohol-induced oxidative stress in the baboon. *Alcoholism Clin Exp Res* 1997;21:375-379.
17. Knuchel F. Double blind study in patients with alcohol-toxic fatty liver. *Med Welt* 1979;30:411-416.
18. Schuller-Perez A, San Martin FG. Controlled study using multiply-unsaturated phosphatidylcholine in comparison with placebo in the case of alcoholic liver steatosis. *Med Welt* 1985;72:517-521.
19. Buchman AL, Dubin M, Jenden D, et al. Lecithin increases plasma free choline and decreases hepatic steatosis in long-term total parenteral nutrition patients. *Gastroenterology* 1992;102:1363-1370.
20. Panos MZ, Polson R, Johnson R, et al. Activity of polyunsaturated phosphatidylcholine in HBsAg negative (autoimmune) chronic active hepatitis and in acute alcoholic hepatitis. In: Gundermann KJ, Schumacher R, eds. *50th Anniversary of Phospholipid Research (EPL)*. Bingin-Rhein, Germany: wbn-Verlag; 1990:103-110.
21. Lieber CS, Robins SJ, Li J, et al. Phosphatidylcholine protects against fibrosis and cirrhosis in the baboon. *Gastroenterology* 1994;106:152-159.
22. Marpaung B, Tarigan P, Zein LH, et al. Tuberkulostatische kombinations therapie aus INH, RMP und EMB. *Therapiewoche* 1988;38:734-740.
23. Jenkins PJ, Portmann BP. Use of polyunsaturated phosphatidyl choline in HBsAg negative chronic active hepatitis: results of prospective double-blind controlled trial. *Liver* 1982;2:77-81.
24. Visco G. Polyunsaturated phosphatidylcholine (EPL) associated with vitamin B-complex in the treatment of acute viral hepatitis-B. *La Clinica Terapeutica* 1985;114:183-188.
25. Ilic V, Begic-Janev A. Therapy for HBsAg-positive chronically active hepatitis. *Med Welt* 1991;42:523-525.
26. Niederau C, Strohmeyer G, Heintges T, et al. Polyunsaturated phosphatidylcholine and interferon alpha for treatment of chronic hepatitis B and C: a multicenter, double-blind, placebo-controlled trial. *Hepatogastroenterol* 1998;45:797-804.
27. Schenker S. Polyunsaturated lecithin and alcoholic liver disease: a magic bullet? *Alcoholism Clin Exp Res* 1994;18:1286-1288.
28. Halliday HL. Natural vs synthetic surfactants in neonatal respiratory distress syndrome. *Drugs* 1996;51:226-237.
29. Leyck S, Dereu N, Etschenberg E, et al. Improvement of the gastric tolerance of non-steroidal anti-inflammatory drugs by polyene phosphatidylcholine (Phospholipon 100). *Eur J Pharmacol* 1985;117:35-42.
30. Swarm RA, Ashley SW, Soybel DI, et al. Protective effect of exogenous phospholipid on aspirin-induced gastric mucosal injury. *Am J Surg* 1987;153:48-53.
31. Carlson SE. Lower incidence of necrotizing enterocolitis in infants fed a preterm formula with egg phospholipids. *Pediatr Res* 1998;44:491-495.
32. Kidd PM. Unpublished analysis. 1998; El Cerrito, California, USA: drkidd@aol.com.
33. Little A, Levy R, Chuaqui-Kidd P, et al. A double-blind, placebo controlled trial of high-dose lecithin in Alzheimer's disease. *J Neurol Neurosurg Psychiatr* 1985;48:736-742.
34. Esslinger F. Death cap mushroom poisoning: report of clinical experience. *Med Welt* 1966;19:1057-1063.

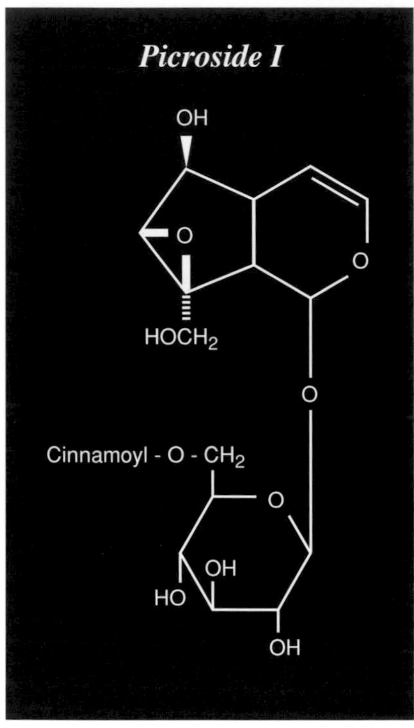

Picrorhiza kurroa

Description

Picrorhiza kurroa is a well-known herb in the Ayurvedic system of medicine and has traditionally been used to treat disorders of the liver and upper respiratory tract, reduce fevers, and to treat dyspepsia, chronic diarrhea, and scorpion sting. It is a small perennial herb from the Scrophulariaceae family, found in the Himalayan region growing at elevations of 3,000-5,000 meters. *Picrorhiza kurroa* has a long, creeping rootstock that is bitter in taste, and grows in rock crevices and moist, sandy soil. The leaves of the plant are flat, oval, and sharply serrated. The flowers, which appear June through August, are white or pale purple and borne on a tall spike; manual harvesting of the plant takes place October through December. The active constituents are obtained from the root and rhizomes. The plant is self-regenerating but unregulated over-harvesting has caused it to be threatened. Current research on *Picrorhiza kurroa* has focused on its hepatoprotective, anticholestatic, antioxidant, and immune-modulating activity.[1,2]

Active Constituents

Kutkin is the active principal of *Picrorhiza kurroa* and is comprised of kutkoside and the iridoid glycoside picrosides I, II, and III. Other identified active constituents are apocynin, drosin, and nine cucurbitacin glycosides.[3,4] Apocynin is a catechol that has been shown to inhibit neutrophil oxidative burst in addition to being a powerful anti-inflammatory agent,[5] while the curcubitacins have been shown to be highly cytotoxic and possess anti-tumor effects.[6]

Mechanisms of Action

The hepatoprotective action of *Picrorhiza kurroa* is not fully understood but may be attributed to Picrorhiza's ability to inhibit the generation of oxygen anions and to scavenge free radicals.[7] Picrorhiza's antioxidant effect has been shown to be similar to that of superoxide dismutase, metal-ion chelators, and xanthine oxidase inhibitors.[8] In rats infected with malaria, Picrorhiza restored depleted glutathione levels, thereby enhancing detoxification and antioxidation, and helping maintain a normal oxidation-reduction balance.[9] In this same animal model, Picrorhiza also demonstrated an anti-lipid peroxidative effect.[10] Like silymarin, Picrorhiza has demonstrated liver regeneration in rats, possibly via stimulation of nucleic acid and protein synthesis.[11] Picrorhiza's anti-inflammatory action is attributed to the apocynin constituent, which has potent anti-inflammatory properties, in addition to inhibiting oxidative burst in neutrophils.[5] Although the mechanism is unclear, animal studies indicate Picrorhiza's constituents exhibit a strong anticholestatic activity against a variety of liver-toxic substances, appearing to be even more potent than silymarin. Picrorhiza also exhibits a dose-dependent choleretic activity, evidenced by an increase in bile salts and acids, and bile flow.[12]

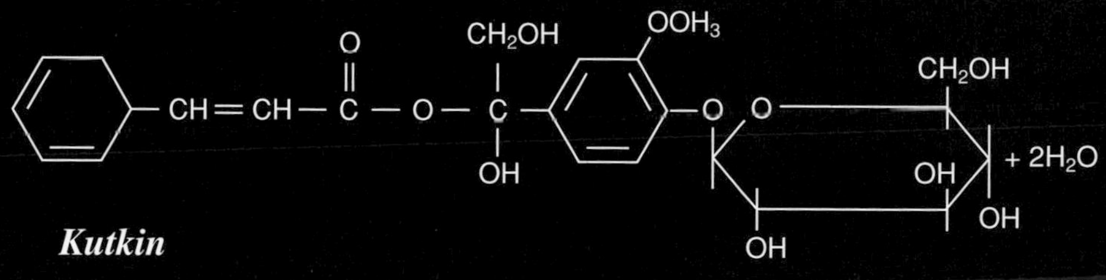

Clinical Indications

Hepatic Insult and Damage

Numerous animal studies, primarily in rats, have established the active constituents of *Picrorhiza kurroa* are effective at preventing liver toxicity and the subsequent biochemical changes caused by numerous toxic agents. Hepatocytes damaged by exposure to galactosamine, thiocetamide, and carbon tetrachloride were incubated with Picrorhiza constituents, and a concentration-dependent restorative effect was observed in regard to normal hepatocyte function.[13] A similar effect was seen when 25 mg/kg/day oral Picrorhiza extract was administered to rats poisoned by aflatoxin B1; biochemical changes normally induced by aflatoxin B1 were prevented.[14] Picrorhiza extract, when given at a dose of 3-12 mg/kg orally for 45 days, was also effective in reversing ethanol-induced liver damage in rats.[15] In an animal model of hepatic ischemia, rats given Picrorhiza orally at 12 mg/kg daily for seven days, prior to induced ischemia, demonstrated improved hepatocyte glycogen preservation and reduced apoptosis, compared to control animals.[16] Picrorhiza was also effective in treating Amanita mushroom poisoning in an *in vivo* animal model.[17] An *in vitro* study demonstrated Picrorhiza's antioxidant activity by subjecting human Glioma and Hep 3B cells to a hypoxic state. Picrorhiza treatment reduced cellular damage cause by hypoxia, indicating Picrorhiza constituents may protect against hypoxia/reoxygenation-induced injuries.[18]

Viral Hepatitis

Studies indicate Picrorhiza extracts may be of therapeutic value in treating viral hepatitis. An *in vitro* study investigated anti-hepatitis B-like activity of Picrorhiza and found it to have promising anti-hepatitis B surface antigen activity.[19] In a randomized, double-blind, placebo-controlled trial of 33 patients diagnosed with acute viral hepatitis, 375 mg Picrorhiza root powder was given three times daily for two weeks. The treatment group was comprised of 15 patients; the remaining 18 subjects acted as controls and received placebo. Bilirubin, SGOT, and SGPT values were significantly lower in the treatment group, and the time required for bilirubin values to drop to 2.5 mg/dL was 27.4 days in the treatment group versus 75.9 days for the placebo group.[20]

Asthma and Allergy

In vivo studies of bronchial obstruction indicate the drosin constituent of *Picrorhiza kurroa* prevented allergen- and platelet activating factor-induced bronchial obstruction when given to guinea pigs via inhalant and oral routes. *In vitro* histamine release was also inhibited by the plant extract.[21] Picrorhiza extract given orally at 25 mg/kg to mice and rats resulted in a concentration-dependent decrease in mast cell degranulation. However, induced bronchospasm was not prevented, indicating a lack of direct post-synaptic histamine receptor blocking activity.[22]

Side Effects and Toxicity

Picrorhiza root extracts are widely used in India with no adverse effects having been reported. The LD_{50} of kutkin is greater than 2,600 mg/kg in rats, with no data available for humans.[23]

Dosage

Picrorhiza is not readily water-soluble and is therefore not usually taken as a tea. While it is ethanol soluble, its bitter taste makes tinctures unpalatable, so it is therefore usually administered as a standardized (4% kutkin) encapsulated powder extract. Typical adult dosage is 400 to 1,500 mg/day, with dosages up to 3.5 g/day sometimes being recommended for fevers.

References

1. Atal CK, Sharma ML, Kaul A, Khajuria A. Immunomodulating agents of plant origin. I: preliminary screening. *J Ethnopharmacol* 1986;18:133-141.
2. Subedi BP. Plant profile: Kutki (*Picrorhiza scrophulariiflora*). *Himalayan Bioresources* 2000;4.
3. Weinges K, Kloss P, Henkels WD. Natural products from medicinal plants. XVII. picroside-II, a new 6-vanilloyl-catapol from *Picrorhiza kuroa* Royle and Benth. *Justus Liebigs Ann Chem* 1972;759:173-182. [Article in German]
4. Stuppner H, Wagner H. New cucurbitacin glycosides from *Picrorhiza kurroa. Planta Med* 1989;55:559-563.
5. Simons JM, 't Hart BA, Ip Vai Ching TR, et al. Metabolic activation of natural phenols into selective oxidative burst agonists by activated human neutrophils. *Free Radic Biol Med* 1990;8:251-258.
6. Stuppner H, Wagner H. New cucurbitacin glycosides from *Picrorhiza kurroa. Planta Med* 1989;55:559.
7. Russo A, Izzo AA, Cardile V, et al. Indian medicinal plants as antiradicals and DNA cleavage protectors. *Phytomedicine* 2001;8:125-132.
8. Chander R, Kapoor NK, Dhawan BN. Picroliv, picroside-I and kutkoside from *Picrorhiza kurroa* are scavengers of superoxide anions. *Biochem Pharmacol* 1992;44:180-183.
9. Chander R, Kapoor NK, Dhawan BN. Effect of picroliv on glutathione metabolism in liver and brain of *Mastomys natalensis* infected with *Plasmodium berghei. Indian J Exp Biol* 1992;30:711-714.
10. Chander R, Singh K, Visen PK, et al. Picroliv prevents oxidation in serum lipoprotein lipids of *Mastomys coucha* infected with *Plasmodium berghei. Indian J Exp Biol* 1998;36:371-374.
11. Singh V, Kapoor NK, Dhawan BN. Effect of picroliv on protein and nucleic acid synthesis. *Indian J Exp Biol* 1992;30:68-69.
12. Shukla B, Visen PK, Patnaik GK, et al. Choleretic effect of picroliv, the hepatoprotective principle of *Picrorhiza kurroa. Planta Med* 1991;57:29-33.
13. Visen PK, Saraswat B, Dhawan BN. Curative effect of picroliv on primary cultured rat hepatocytes against different hepatotoxins: an *in vitro* study. *J Pharmacol Toxicol Methods* 1998;40:173-179.
14. Rastogi R, Srivastava AK, Rastogi AK. Biochemical changes induced in liver and serum aflatoxin B1-treated male wistar rats: preventive effect of picroliv. *Pharmacol Toxicol* 2001;88:53-58.
15. Saraswat B, Visen PK, Patnaik GK, Dhawan BN. *Ex vivo* and *in vivo* investigations of picroliv from *Picrorhiza kurroa* in an alcohol intoxication model in rats. *J Ethnopharmacol* 1999;66:263-269.
16. Singh AK, Mani H, Seth P. Picroliv preconditioning protects the rat liver against ischemia-reperfusion injury. *Eur J Pharmacol* 2000;395:229-239.
17. Dwivedi Y, Rastogi R, Garg NK, Dhawan BN. Effects of picroliv, the active principle of *Picrorhiza kurroa*, on biochemical changes in rat liver poisoned by *Amanita phalloides. Zhongguo Yao Li Xue Bao* 1992;13:197-200.
18. Gaddipati JP, Madhavan S, Sidhu GS, et al. Picroliv – a natural product protects cells and regulates the gene expression during hypoxia/reoxygenation. *Mol Cell Biochem* 1999;194:271-281.
19. Mehrotra R, Rawat S, Kulshreshtha DK, et al. *In vitro* studies on the effect of certain natural products against hepatitis B virus. *Indian J Med Res* 1990;92:133-138.
20. Vaidya AB, Antarkar DS, Doshi JC, et al. *Picrorhiza kurroa* (Kutaki) Royle ex Benth as a hepatoprotective agent – experimental and clinical studies. *J Postgrad Med* 1996;42:105-108.
21. Dorsch W, Wagner H. New antiasthmatic drugs from traditional medicine? *Int Arch Allergy Appl Immunol* 1991;94:262-265.
22. Baruah CC, Gupta PP, Nath A, et al. Anti-allergic and anti-anaphylactic activity of picroliv – a standardised iridoid glycoside fraction of *Picrorhiza kurroa. Pharmacol Res* 1998;38:487-492.
23. Annual Report, Regional Research Laboratory, Council for Scientific and Industrial Research, India. 1989-1990.

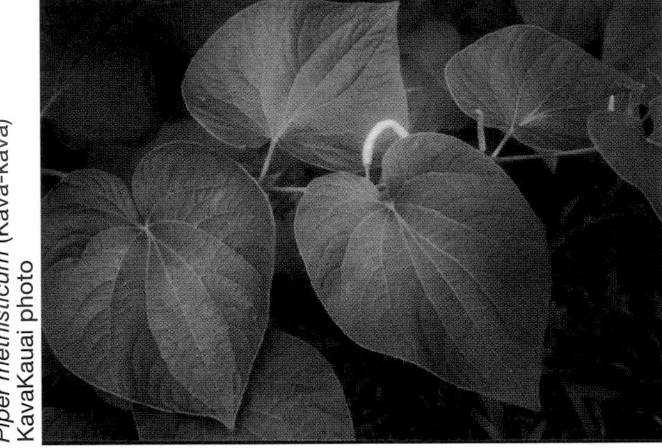
Piper methisticum (Kava-kava)
KavaKauai photo

Piper methysticum

Description

Piper methysticum G. Forst. (kava kava) is a perennial plant native to the Pacific islands. A member of the Piperaceae family, kava grows best in stony ground with good sun exposure. Although it can reach a height of 20 feet, it is usually harvested at 7 to 8 feet. Modern kava preparations primarily use the dried rhizome or rootstock for extraction.[1]

The history of kava and its use in traditional ceremonies of the Pacific islands has been the subject of many lengthy anthropological reports and textbooks. An excellent overview of the plant's origins, traditional use, and chemical constituents is the book by Vincent Lebot, Mark Merlin, and Lamont Lindstrom entitled *Kava: The Pacific Drug* (Yale University Press, 1992).

A nonalcoholic drink made from kava root has played a role in a variety of social and ceremonial rituals in the Pacific islands.[2] Kava ceremonies were a key event to welcome visiting royalty or highly honored guests, and were first described to the western world by a botanist and artist who accompanied Captain James Cook on his first voyage in the Endeavor (1768-1771).

Active Constituents

The active constituents consist of a group of lactones, organized around an arylethylene-alpha-pyrone skeleton.[3] To date, 15 kava lactones (also called kava pyrones) have been identified. Found in the fat-soluble portion of the rhizome and root, high quality kava rhizome contains 3.5-15 percent kava lactones.[4] Modern kava extracts commercially available in North America and Europe contain 30-70 percent kava lactones, depending on the extraction process employed.

Mechanisms of Action

CNS Effects

Kava's exact mechanism of action on the central nervous system has not been fully elucidated. One hypothesis is that kava lactones potentiate GABA receptors. In both *in vivo* and *in vitro* studies, only weak GABA-binding activity was observed.[5] However, another *in vitro* study found GABA-binding to be a mechanism for some of kava's sedative effects.[6]

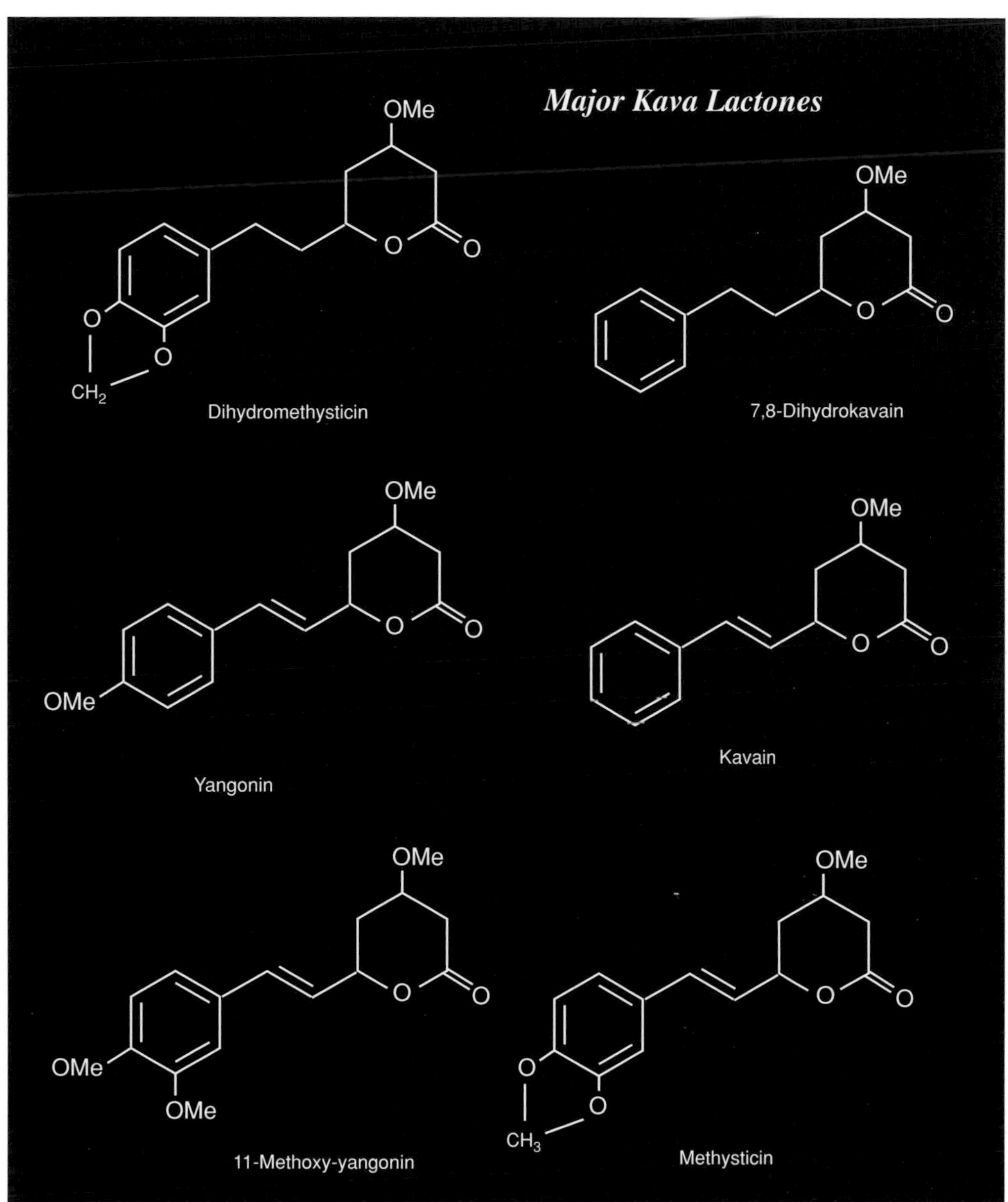
Major Kava Lactones
OMe
O
O
O
O
CH2
Dihydromethysticin
7,8-Dihydrokavain
OMe
Yangonin
Kavain
11-Methoxy-yangonin
CH3
Methysticin

In vitro studies have found that, while kava lactones were not found to efficiently block uptake of serotonin, inhibition of noradrenaline uptake was demonstrated by three lactones, providing another possible mechanism of action.[7]

Human pharmacology studies have found kava and the kava lactone kavain creates brain activity changes (measured by EEG) typical of anxiolytic drugs but without their sedative or hypnotic effects.[8,9] Two studies with healthy volunteers found kava extract actually improved reaction time and performance on a word recognition test compared to a decrease in performance and reaction time in persons taking oxazepam.[10,11]

In animal models, kava is known to inhibit experimentally induced convulsions.[12-14] Research indicates this anticonvulsant effect may be mediated by Na^+ channel receptor sites, a common target of anti-epileptic drugs.[15-17]

Analgesic/Anesthetic Effects

Four lactones from kava (kavain, dihydrokavain, methysticin, and dihydromethysticin) have been found to possess significant analgesic effects in animal studies. The analgesia appears to be via non-opiate pathways.[18] A dose of 120 mg/kg of either dihydromethysticin or dihydrokavain was equivalent to 2.5 mg/kg morphine.[19]

Kavain appears to be an effective surface anesthetic, comparable to cocaine in strength and duration of action.[20] Subcutaneous injections provide anesthesia from several hours to several days. Too high a dose, however, can induce temporary paralysis, rendering it not the most suitable local anesthetic.[21] To date, none of these analgesic or anesthetic actions has been tested in humans.

Clinical Indications

Anxiety

Kava extracts have been found to be effective anxiolytic agents and are approved in the German Commission E for the treatment of "conditions of nervous anxiety, stress, and restlessness."[22] Clinical research suggests the extract be used primarily for treating milder forms of anxiety.[23] The extract used in most published clinical trials testing kava for anxiety is standardized to 70-percent kava lactones.

Four randomized, placebo-controlled trials found 100 mg of the above-mentioned 70-percent kava lactone extract (delivering 70 mg of kava lactones per dose) administered three times per day significantly reduced anxiety according to the Hamilton Anxiety Scale (HAMA) in persons with mild to moderate anxiety.[24-27] One of the trials focused on anxiety associated with menopause.[25] Notable among the four studies is a 25-week trial of 101 patients; from week eight until the end of the trial, HAMA scores were significantly reduced in persons taking kava compared to those taking placebo.[26]

A six-week trial of kava (at the same dosage as above) in 172 patients with anxiety, agitation, and tension of non-psychotic origin found kava was as effective as oxazepam (5 mg/day) or bromazepam (3 mg/day) in the treatment of anxiety.[28]

Side Effects and Toxicity

Use of kava extract at dosages used in clinical trials has been associated with mild side effects such as fatigue, pruritis, and nausea. The most common side effect of heavy kava consumption is a skin rash known as "kava dermopathy," an ichthyosiform skin rash with onset typically beginning in the face.[29] Ocular photosensitivity also sometimes accompanies the rash. This type of rash is typically seen only in heavy long-term consumption of the beverage, such as is seen in Polynesia. However, doses of 300-800 mg daily of the isolated lactone, dihydromethysticin, have been known to cause the rash.[30] According to some case studies, kava extract may cause a sebotropic reaction[31] and has been rarely associated with allergic skin reactions.[32] At the recommended dosages kava does not appear to be addictive.

Kava is contraindicated during pregnancy and lactation.[22] It does not appear to impair reaction time while driving.[33] Recently, concern has been expressed about the possible association of kava intake and hepatotoxicity due to 25 cases reported in the European literature.[34] While one case of necrotizing hepatitis[35] and one case of fulminant hepatic failure[36] might have been linked to kava intake, these cases are rare in light of the safety associated with standardized kava extract use in Europe. However, it is probably prudent to regularly test liver enzymes in patients taking kava long-term.

The German Commission E monograph warns against concomitant use with alcohol, barbiturates, antidepressants, anxiolytics, or any other drugs that may work on the CNS.[22] Kava has been reported to interact with alprazolam, resulting in grogginess and oversedation in one case.[37] There are also scattered reports of extrapyramidal dystonic reactions and worsening of Parkinson's disease with kava use.[38] Therefore, persons with Parkinson's disease should probably avoid kava. Finally, because kava extracts have been found to inhibit monoamine oxidase B in vitro, people taking selegiline (L-deprenyl, an MAO-B inhibitor) should probably avoid kava.

Dosage

The use of kava extract as an anxiolytic is typically based on kava lactones. While the German Commission E recommends that extracts supply 60-120 mg of kava lactones per day, clinical studies suggest daily kava lactone dosage may need to approach 210 mg for efficacy.

References

1. Singh YN. Kava: an overview. *J Ethnopharmacol* 1992;37:13-45.
2. Newell WH. The kava ceremony in Tonga. *J Polynesian Society* 1947;56:364-414.
3. Shulgin AT. The narcotic pepper–the chemistry and pharmacology of *Piper methysticum* and related species. *Bull Narc* 1973;25:59-74.
4. Leung A, Foster S. *Encyclopedia of Common Natural Ingredients Used in Food, Drugs, and Cosmetics*. New York: John Wiley and Sons; 1996:330-331.
5. Davies LP, Drew CA, Duffield P, et al. Kava pyrones and resin: studies on GABAA, GABAB and benzodiazepine binding sites in rodent brain. *Pharmacol Toxicol* 1992;71:120-126.
6. Keledjian J, Duffield PH, Jamieson DD, et al. Uptake into mouse brain of four compounds present in the psychoactive beverage kava. *J Pharm Sci* 1988;77:1003-1006.
7. Seitz U, Schule A, Gleitz J. [3H]-monoamine uptake inhibition properties of kava pyrones. *Planta Med* 1997;63:548-549.
8. Johnson D, Frauendorf A, Stecker K, Stein U. Neurophysiological active profile and tolerance of kava extract WS 1490. *TW Neurologie Psychiatr* 1991;5:349-354.
9. Saletu B, Gr¸nberger J, Linzmayer L, Anderer P. EEG brain-mapping, psychometric and psychophysiological studies on the central effects of kavain–a kava plant derivative. *Human Psychopharmacol* 1989;4:169-190.
10. Munte TF, Heinze HJ, Matzke M, Steitz J. Effects of oxazepam and an extract of kava roots (*Piper methysticum*) on event-related potentials in a word recognition task. *Neuropsychobiology* 1993;27:46-53.
11. Heinze HJ, Munthe TF, Steitz J, Matzke M. Pharmacopsychological effects of oxazepam and kava-extract in a visual search paradigm assessed with event-related potentials. *Pharmacopsychiatry* 1994;27:224-230.
12. Klohs MW, Keller F, Willimas RE, et al. A chemical and pharmacological investigation of *Piper methysticum* Forst. *J Medication Pharm Chem* 1959;1:95-103.
13. Kretzschmar R, Meyer HJ. Comparative studies on the anticonvulsant activity of the pyrone compounds of *Piper methysticum* Forst. *Arch Int Pharmacodyn* 1969;177:261-267. [Article in German]
14. Meyer HJ. Pharmacology of kava. In: Efron DH, Holmsted B, Kline NS, eds. *Ethnopharmacologic Search for Psychoactive Drugs*. New York: Raven Press; 1979:133.
15. Gleitz J, Friese J, Beile A, et al. Anticonvulsive action of (+/-)-kavain estimated from its properties on stimulated synaptosomes and Na^+ channel receptor sites. *Eur J Pharmacol* 1996;315:89-97.
16. Gleitz J, Beile A, Peters T. (+/-)-Kavain inhibits veratridine-activated voltage-dependent Na(+)-channels in synaptosomes prepared from rat cerebral cortex. *Neuropharmacology* 1995;34:1133-1138.
17. Gleitz J, Beile A, Peters T. (+/-)-kavain inhibits the veratridine- and KCl-induced increase in intracellular Ca^{2+} and glutamate-release of rat cerebrocortical synaptosomes. *Neuropharmacology* 1996;35:179-186.
18. Jamieson DD, Duffield PH. The antinociceptive actions of kava components in mice. *Clin Exp Pharmacol Physiol* 1990;17:495-507.
19. Bruggemann F, Meyer HJ. Die analgetische wirkung der kawa-inhaltsstoffe dihydrokawain und dihydromethistizin. *Arzneimittelforschung* 1963;13:407-409.
20. Lebot V, Merlin M, Linstrom L. *Kava the Pacific Drug*. New Haven, CT: Yale University Press; 1992:10.
21. Baldi D. Sulle proprieta farmacologische del *Piper methysticum*. *Terapia Moderna* 1980:359-364.
22. Blumenthal M, Busse WR, Goldberg A, et al, eds. *The Complete Commission E Monographs*. Boston, MA: Integrative Medicine Communications; 1998:156-157.
23. Pittler M, Ernst E. Efficacy of kava extract for treating anxiety: systematic review and meta-analysis. *J Clin Psychopharmacol* 2000;20:84-89.

24. Kinzler E, Kromer J, Lehmann EE. Effect of a special kava extract in patients with anxiety-, tension-, and excitation states of non-psychotic genesis. Double blind study with placebos over 4 weeks. *Arzneimittelforschung* 1991;41:584-588. [Article in German]

25. Warnecke G. Psychosomatic dysfunctions in the female climacteric. Clinical effectiveness and tolerance of Kava Extract WS 1490. *Fortschr Med* 1991;109:119-122. [Article in German]

26. Lehmann EE, Kinzler J, Friedmann J. Efficacy of a special kava extract *(Piper methysticum)* in patients with states of anxiety, tension and excitedness of non-mental origin. A double-blind placebo-controlled study of four weeks treatment. *Phytomedicine* 1996;3:113-119.

27. Volz HP, Kieser M. Kava-kava extract WS 1490 versus placebo in anxiety disorders–a randomized placebo-controlled 25-week outpatient trial. *Pharmacopsychiatry* 1997;30:1-5.

28. Woelk H, Kapoula S, Lehrl S, et al. Treatment of patients suffering from anxiety–double-blind study: Kava special extract versus benzodiazepines. *Z Allgemeinmed* 1993;69:271-277.

29. Ruze P. Kava-induced dermopathy: a niacin deficiency? *Lancet* 1990;335:31-39.

30. Keller F, Klohs MW. A review of the chemistry and pharmacology of the constituents of *Piper methysticum*. *Lloydia* 1963;26:1-15.

31. Jappe U, Franke I, Reinhold D, Gollnick HPM. Sebotropic drug reaction resulting from kava-kava extract therapy: a new entity? *J Amer Acad Dermatol* 1998;38:104-106.

32. Schmidt P, Boehncke WH. Delayed-type hypersensitivity reaction to kava-kava extract. *Contact Derm* 2000;42:363-364.

33. Herberg KW. Driving ability after intake of kava special extract WS 1490. *Z Allgemeinmed* 1991;67:842–846.

34. Stoller R. Liver damage and kava extracts. *Schweizerische frtzeitung* 2000;81:1335-1336.

35. Strahl S, Ehret V, Dahm HH, Maier KP. Necrotizing hepatitis after taking herbal medication. *Dtsch Med Wochenschrr* 1998;123:1404-1414. [Article in German]

36. Escher M, Desmeules J. Hepatitis associated with kava, a herbal remedy for anxiety. *BMJ* 2001;322:139. [letter]

37. Almeida JC, Grimsley EW. Coma from the health food store: interaction between kava and alprazolam. *Ann Intern Med* 1996;125:940-941.

38. Schelosky L, Raffauaf C, Jendroska K, Poewe W. Kava and dopamine antagonism. *J Neurol Neurosurg Psychiatr* 1995;58:639-640. [letter]

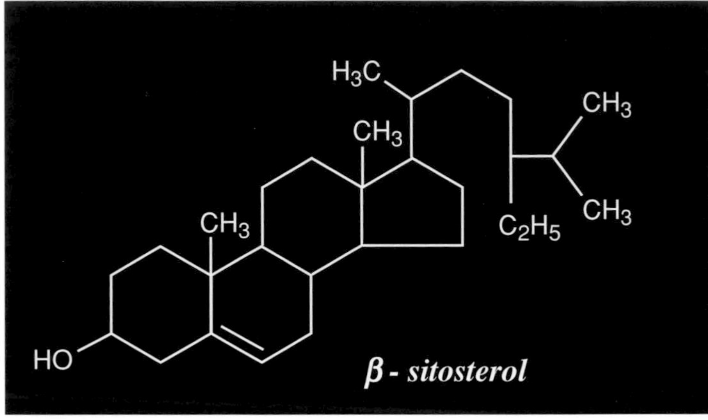

Plant Sterols and Sterolins

Introduction

Sterols and sterolins, also known as phytosterols, are fats present in all plants, including fruits and vegetables. Although they are chemically similar to the animal fat, cholesterol, they have been shown to exert significant unique biochemical effects in both animals and humans. Because they are bound to the fibers of the plant, they are difficult to absorb during the transit of digested food through the gut, particularly in individuals with impaired digestive function.[1] For this reason, and because much of the modern diet is over-processed and low in fresh plant materials, sterols and sterolins appear in the serum and tissue of healthy humans at 800-1000 times lower concentrations than that of cholesterol. Beta-sitosterol (BSS) is the major phytosterol in higher plants along with its glycoside, beta-sitosterolin (BSSG). Animal studies have demonstrated BSS and BSSG possess anti-inflammatory, antipyretic, antineoplastic, and immune-modulating properties. In other *in vitro*, animal, and human studies, a proprietary BSS:BSSG mixture has shown promise in normalizing T-cell function, dampening overactive antibody responses, and normalizing DHEA:cortisol ratios. Research has shown plant oils contain the highest concentration of phytosterols, nuts and seeds contain moderate amounts, and fruits and vegetables generally contain the lowest phytosterol concentrations.[2] Because only low levels of these substances are found in humans, increased dietary intake of unprocessed fruits and vegetables or supplementation with commercial phytosterols may be of benefit in re-establishing optimal immune parameters. Restoring balance to the immune system may be of therapeutic benefit in disease processes such as chronic viral infections, stress-induced immune suppression, tuberculosis, allergies, cancer, and rheumatoid arthritis and other autoimmune conditions.[3,4]

Pharmacokinetics

Beta-sitosterol is not synthesized endogenously in man, and several animal studies over the last 70 years[5-7] have demonstrated its intestinal absorption in mammals is minimal, possibly as little as five percent of total dietary beta-sitosterol consumed. By comparison, intestinal absorption of cholesterol is 45-54 percent of intake. Unlike cholesterol, beta-sitosterol is rapidly secreted into the bile and is esterified outside the intestinal wall at a much slower rate.[8] Beta-sitosterol is secreted into the bile, stored in the gallbladder, released intermittently into the duodenum, and subsequently incorporated into feces.

Mechanisms of Action

Anti-inflammatory/Antipyretic Agent

Animal research on plant sterols given to rats demonstrated potent anti-inflammatory properties similar to cortisone. A proprietary blend of sterols and sterolins was capable of reducing the secretion of pro-inflammatory cytokines and tumor necrosis factor-alpha.[1,9,10] Phytosterols also reduced experimentally-induced edema. Animal research found antipyretic effects of phytosterols was comparable to that of aspirin.[9]

Immune Modulation

In vitro, animal, and human studies have shown that a 100:1 BSS:BSSG mixture is capable of enhancing several aspects of the immune response. By selectively enhancing activity of T-Helper-1 (T_H1) cells and leaving unchanged or dampening the effect of T_H2 cells, administration results in a significant rise in interleukin 2 (IL-2) and gamma interferon (IFN-γ) which enhance direct natural killer (NK) cell activity. Dampening of T_H2 leads to decreased levels of interleukins (IL-4, IL-6, IL-10) involved in B-lymphocyte differentiation and inflammation. This combination also resulted in maintenance of cortisol and elevation of DHEA levels, thereby decreasing cortisol:DHEA ratios and buffering negative stress responses.[10]

Blood Sugar Control

The hypoglycemic properties of phytosterols were elucidated in an animal study using normo- and hyperglycemic rats. Results demonstrated that when either BSS or BSSG were given orally, fasting glucose levels were lowered and fasting insulin levels increased. This research also found beta-sitosterol was more effective over time in moderating glucose levels than its glycoside, beta-sitosterolin. It is thought phytosterol administration increases circulating insulin levels via stimulation of insulin secretion from pancreatic beta cells.[11]

Clinical Indications

Rheumatoid Arthritis

Rheumatoid arthritis (RA) is an inflammatory disease characterized by dysregulation of the immune system. B-lymphocytes become overactive and secrete antibodies that destroy synovial tissues of the joint. A BSS:BSSG combination was shown to increase the levels of T_H1 cells, down-regulating antibody production by B-lymphocytes. The phytosterol mixture also decreased secretion of proinflammatory cytokines by macrophages, thereby decreasing inflammation. Most conventional RA treatments involve the use of drugs with significant side effects that are designed to control pain and suppress the entire immune response of the body, without addressing the actual immune dysfunction. By selectively activating or inhibiting certain aspects of the immune response, BSS:BSSG compounds can effectively regulate and control the overactive immune response seen in RA and other autoimmune diseases.[1]

HIV/FIV Infection

Animal and human research conducted in South Africa studied the effects of BSS:BSSG on disease progression of Feline Immunodeficiency Virus (FIV) and Human Immunodeficiency Virus (HIV). The initial positive studies were performed on cats infected with FIV (a feline retrovirus essentially equivalent to HIV) and prompted subsequent research on human subjects with HIV infection. Subjects given the sterol/sterolin mixture were able to maintain stable CD4 cell counts, and apoptosis of CD4 lymphocytes declined slightly, thereby slowing disease progression. These studies also demonstrated a significant decrease in IL-6 levels, possibly slowing viral replication rates in infected cells and thereby decreasing viral load.[12]

Cancer

A lack of secretion of IL-2 and IFN-γ by T_H1 cells leads to NK cells that are not capable of recognizing structures on the surface of tumor cells. Sterols and sterolins are known to increase secretion of IL-2 and IFN-γ, enhancing NK cell activity and decreasing inflammation. A double-blind, placebo-controlled study of patients with cervical lesions (CIN III) caused by Human Papilloma Virus (HPV) was conducted over a nine-month period. Fifty-percent of patients experienced remission of lesions, compared to the placebo group that either experienced no remission or disease progression.[13]

Benign Prostatic Hypertrophy (BPH)

Two randomized, placebo-controlled, clinical studies were conducted on 350 men diagnosed with benign prostatic hypertrophy. Both studies lasted six months and dosages ranged from 60-130 mg beta-sitosterol daily. Although the exact mechanism is still unclear, beta-sitosterol administration resulted in improved peak urinary flow rate in both studies, as well as an improvement in subjective symptoms of BPH. Herbal remedies for BPH include saw palmetto, *Pygeum africanus*, and pumpkin seeds, and their effectiveness may be due to their phytosterol content. An herbal preparation for the treatment of BPH called Harzol, which contains beta-sitosterol and other phytosterols, has been available in Germany for the past 20 years.[14,15]

Immunosuppression in Endurance Athletes

Marathon runners and endurance athletes often exhibit an increased inflammatory response to injury, as well as an immune suppression characterized by frequent bacterial and viral respiratory infections, all a result of high-intensity training. A double-blind study of marathon runners given a 100:1 BSS/BSSG mixture found improved maintenance of normal hematologic parameters, normalization of cortisol:DHEA ratios, and a decreased inflammatory response. This study indicates the phytosterol mixture acted to buffer cortisol release and its immunosuppressive effects.[10]

Diabetes

Animal research found that in an oral glucose tolerance test BSS and BSSG protected test animals from an excessive rise in serum glucose levels due to glucose loading. This may be attributable to the fact that these phytosterols are capable of stimulating insulin secretion and thereby raising circulating insulin levels for better blood sugar control. The hypoglycemic effect of BSS and BSSG in animals indicates it might be an effective therapeutic tool for humans with diabetic and pre-diabetic conditions.[11] Also, due to their potential to down-regulate antibody production, this combination of sterols and sterolins may intervene in the inflammatory process associated with early-stage type 1 diabetes, protecting pancreatic beta cells from destruction. Further research in this area is warranted.

Pulmonary Tuberculosis

A double-blind, randomized, placebo-controlled trial was conducted with 47 culture-positive pulmonary tuberculosis patients. Patients were divided into two groups, hospitalized throughout the six-month long treatment, and treated with a standard regimen of isoniazid, rifampicin, and pyrazinamide. The test group also received a BSS:BSSG mixture. While several disease markers showed similar results between placebo and test groups, patients given the sterol/sterolin mixture showed a significantly faster weight recovery compared to the placebo group. Patients in the phytosterol group also exhibited notable differences in certain hematological parameters, including increased lymphocyte, eosinophil, and monocyte counts. The results of this study suggest the immune modulating activity of phytosterols might be of therapeutic value in cases of multi-drug-resistant tuberculosis.[16]

Side Effects and Toxicity

Phytosterols are non-toxic, do not result in general immune suppression, and are rarely associated with side effects. Their high margin of safety make them an attractive therapeutic tool for a variety of conditions.

Dosage

The research has been conducted on a 100:1 BSS:BSSG formula containing 20 mg beta-sitosterol and 200 mcg beta-sitosterolin per capsule. A loading dose of two capsules three times daily should be given for one month, at which time this can be decreased to one capsule three times daily. Phytosterols work best if taken on an empty stomach, one hour before meals. They should not be taken with animal fats (including milk) as these foods inhibit absorption.

Warnings and Contraindications

Although many autoimmune diseases are TH-2 dominant, a few may exhibit excessive TH-1 activity. Multiple sclerosis is in this category, and, although there have been anecdotal reports of plant sterols being beneficial for MS patients, some patients may experience worsening of their condition. Therefore, caution should be used in patients with MS.

References

1. Bouic, PJD. Sterols/Sterolins: the natural, nontoxic immuno-modulators and their role in the control of rheumatoid arthritis. *The Arthritis Trust* 1998;Summer:3-6.
2. Weihrauch JL, Gardner JM. Sterol content of foods of plant origin. *J Am Diabetes Assoc* 1978;73:39-47.
3. Pegel KH. The importance of sitosterol and sitosterolin in human and animal nutrition. *S A J Sci* 1997;93:263-268.
4. Dwyer JT. Health aspects of vegetarian diets. *Am J Clin Nutr* 1988;48:712-738.
5. Schonheimer R. New contributions in sterol metabolism. *Science* 1931:74:579.
6. Gould RG. Absorbability of beta-sitosterol. *Trans NY Acad Sci* 1955;18:129.
7. Borgstrom B. Quantitative aspects of the intestinal absorption and metabolism of cholesterol and β-sitosterol in the rat. *J Lipid Res* 1968;9:473.
8. Swell L, Boiter TA, Field H, Treadwell CR. The absorption of plant sterols and their effect on serum and liver sterol levels. *J Nutr* 1956;58:385.
9. Gupta MB, Nath R, Srivastava N, et al. Anti-inflammatory and antipyretic activities of B-sitosterol. *Planta Medica* 1980;39:157-163.
10. Bouic PJD, Etsebeth S, Liebenberg RW, et al. Beta-sitosterol and beta-sitosterol glycoside stimulate human peripheral blood lymphocyte proliferation: implications for their use as an immunomodulatory vitamin combination. *Int J Immunopharmacol* 1996:18:693-700.
11. Ivorra MD, D'Ocon MP, Paya M, Villar A. Antihyperglycemic and insulin-releasing effects of B-sitosterol 3-B-D-Glucoside and its aglycone, B-sitosterol. *Archives of the International Pharmacodyn Ther* 1988;296:224-231.
12. Bouic PJD. Immunomodulation in HIV/AIDS: The Tygerberg/Stellenbosch University Experience. *AIDS Bulletin* 1997;6:18-20.
13. Bouic PJD. Moducare®, the Mixture of Plant Sterols/Sterolins: From Laboratory to Bedside. Lecture, American Association of Naturopathic Physicians Annual Convention, September 15th, 2000. Bellevue, WA.
14. Klippel KF, Hiltl DM, Schipp B. A multicentric, placebo-controlled, double-blind clinical trial of beta-sitosterol (phytosterol) for the treatment of benign prostatic hypertrophy. *Br J Urol* 1997;80:427-432.
15. Berges RR, Windeler J, Trampisch TH, Senge TH. Randomized, placebo-controlled, double-blind clinical trial of beta-sitosterol in patients with benign prostatic hypertrophy. *Lancet* 1995;345:1529-1532.
16. Donald PR, Lamprecht JH, Freestone M, et al. A randomized placebo-controlled trial of the efficacy of beta-sitosterol and its glycoside as adjuvants in the treatment of pulmonary tuberculosis. *Int J Tuberc Lung Dis* 1997;1:518-522.

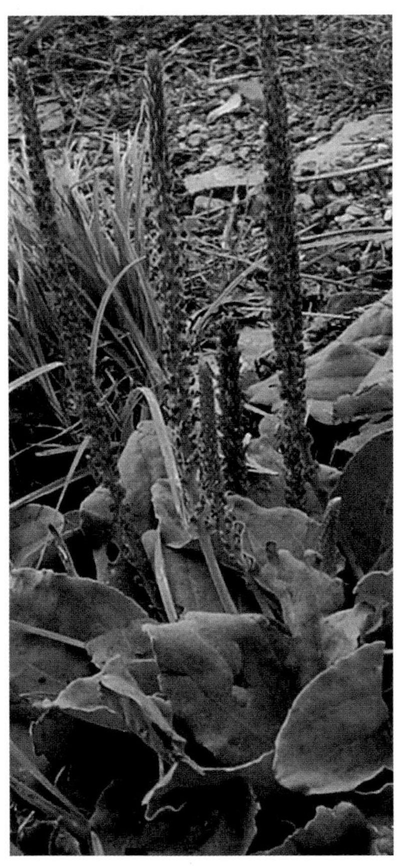

Plantago ovata

Description

Although true psyllium comes from the plant *Plantago psyllium*, the husk and seed of *Plantago ovata* (Plantaginaceae) is commonly referred to as psyllium. Psyllium is widely used as a fiber supplement for the treatment of constipation. Psyllium husk is obtained by milling the seed of *P. ovata* to remove the hulls. In some studies the seed has been used instead of the husk, and is also commercially available.

Active Constituents

Psyllium husk contains a high proportion of hemicellulose, composed of a xylan backbone linked with arabinose, rhamnose, and galacturonic acid units (arabinoxylans). The seed consists of 35-percent soluble and 65-percent insoluble polysaccharides (cellulose, hemicellulose, and lignin). Psyllium is classified as a mucilaginous fiber due to its powerful ability to form a gel in water. This ability comes from its role as the endosperm of the *P. ovata* seed, where it functions to retain water in order to prevent the seed from drying out.

Mechanisms of Action

Many studies have shown dietary fiber shortens gastrointestinal transit time and increases stool weight.[1] When given to healthy volunteers, 18 grams daily of psyllium husk increased fecal weight and the production of short chain fatty acids.[2] Most of the psyllium was shown to reach the cecum four hours after ingestion in an intact and highly polymerized form. The husk appears to be relatively resistant to fermentation. Psyllium husks also significantly increase the level of stool moisture, as well as wet and dry stool weight.[3]

Anaerobic fermentation of the soluble non-starch polysaccharides from psyllium seed results in the production of the short-chain fatty acids acetate, propionate, and butyrate in the intestines.[4] Psyllium husk contains only the epidermis of the seed, while the actual seed has a higher amount of fermentable fiber. Because of this fiber content, psyllium seed degrades more slowly than pectin and produces fairly large amounts of butyrate and acetate. Butyric acid exhibits antineoplastic activity against colorectal cancer, is the preferred oxidative substrate for colonocytes, and may be helpful in the treatment of ulcerative colitis. In a study of resected colorectal cancer patients, those given 20 grams of psyllium seed daily for three months exhibited an average increase of butyric acid production of 42 percent, which decreased to pretreatment levels within two months of cessation of supplementation.[5]

Psyllium also has hypocholesterolemic effects, although the exact mechanism by which psyllium husk brings about a reduction of cholesterol is not totally clear. Animal studies have shown psyllium increases the activity of cholesterol 7 alpha-hydroxylase (the rate-limiting enzyme in bile acid synthesis also referred to as cytochrome 7A [CYP7A]) more than twice that of cellulose or oat bran, but less than cholestyramine.[6] In animals fed a high-fat diet, psyllium increased the activity of cholesterol 7 alpha-hydroxylase and HMG-CoA reductase.[7] This animal study also noted both pectin and psyllium reduced Apo B secretion and that LDL catabolic rates were 100-percent faster in animals fed psyllium. In a human study, psyllium lowered LDL cholesterol, decreased cholesterol absorption, and increased the fractional turnover of both chenodeoxycholic and cholic acids.[8] The authors' conclusion was that psyllium lowered LDL cholesterol primarily via stimulation of bile acid synthesis. Further research might show this action to be through the stimulation of cholesterol 7 alpha-hydroxylase in humans as well.

Clinical Indications

Constipation

The effectiveness of fiber, and psyllium in particular, on constipation depends on the main cause of the constipation. In a study of 149 patients with chronic constipation, the consumption of 15-30 grams daily of a psyllium seed preparation provided bowel relief in 85 percent of participants who had no known pathological cause for their constipation. Only 20 percent of individuals with slow transit responded to psyllium. A slightly greater percentage (37%) of those with disorders of defecation – including rectocele, internal prolapse, anismus, and rectal hyposensitivity – found improvement.[9]

Fecal Incontinence

Because of its ability to retain water, psyllium has also been shown to benefit individuals with fecal incontinence from liquid stools or diarrhea. A placebo-controlled trial of persons with liquid stool fecal incontinence was performed in which supplementation with both gum arabic and psyllium showed approximately a 50-percent decrease in the occurrence of incontinent stools. The psyllium group had the highest water-holding capacity of water-insoluble solids and total water-holding capacity of the stool.[10]

Hemorrhoids

With the known benefit of psyllium for both constipation and loose stools, it is not surprising it would also be of benefit for hemorrhoids. Fifty persons with internal bleeding hemorrhoids were given either a placebo of B vitamins or 11.6 grams of Metamucil® daily for 40 days. Individuals in the psyllium group had significant improvement in reduction of bleeding and a dramatic reduction of congested hemorrhoidal cushions. Bleeding on contact stopped after treatment in the psyllium group, while those in the control group experienced no difference.[11] It also appears psyllium treatment for this problem must be done for a minimum of one month, as a study of 30-day fiber supplementation failed to show improvement;[12] whereas, when taken for 40 days significant improvement was noted.[13]

Ulcerative Colitis

In an open label, randomized, multi-center trial of persons with ulcerative colitis, psyllium seed supplementation (10 grams twice daily) was as effective as mesalamine in maintaining remission.[14] This effect may likely be due to increased levels of butyric acid with psyllium supplementation.

Appetite

Psyllium may also have an effect on appetite. A triple-blind study on 17 women looked at the effect of taking 20 grams of psyllium seed three hours pre-meal and again immediately post-meal during three 3-day study periods. The subjects reported significantly increased feelings of fullness one hour after meals with the psyllium, and exhibited a significantly lower fat intake with those meals.[15]

Hyperlipidemia

Psyllium has been shown to reduce total cholesterol and LDL cholesterol in animals[16-18] and in humans. Sprecher et al demonstrated a 3.5-percent reduction in total cholesterol and a 5.1-percent reduction in LDL levels after consuming 5.1 grams of psyllium husk twice daily for eight weeks.[19] Another study began with individuals on the American Heart Association Step-1 diet, then added eight weeks of psyllium, resulting in decreased total cholesterol (4.8%) and LDL (8.8%).[20] A meta analysis was performed on eight trials of psyllium husk in conjunction with a low-fat diet in the treatment of hypercholesterolemia. After an initial eight-week, low-fat diet run-in, 10.2 g psyllium was given per day, resulting in a four-percent reduction in serum total cholesterol and a seven-percent reduction in LDL cholesterol, compared to diet and placebo. A six-percent reduction in the ratio of apolipoprotein (apo) B to apo A-I was also noted.[21] Longer trials (16 weeks[22] and 26 weeks[23]) mirrored the above results.

A meta-analysis of 12 studies of psyllium-enhanced cereal product consumption on total and LDL cholesterol in 404 adults with mild to moderate hypercholesterolemia demonstrated a reduction of total cholesterol and LDL cholesterol of five- and nine-percent, respectively.[24] Researchers studied the effect of fiber-enhanced cookies on blood lipids in hypercholesterolemic men, using wheat bran-, psyllium-, or oat bran-containing cookies (wheat bran was used as the placebo since it has no demonstrated cholesterol-lowering effect). At the end of the eight-week study, plasma LDL cholesterol had decreased 22.6-percent in the psyllium group and 26-percent in the oat bran group.[25]

A four-month study of 12 elderly patients showed psyllium husk reduced total serum cholesterol by 20 percent, a figure much higher than the above-mentioned studies.[26] In another study, a significant reduction in total serum cholesterol was noted in 176 elderly persons who used psyllium for one year.[27] The authors found for every one-gram increase in daily psyllium dose there was a 0.022-mmol/liter (0.84mg/dl) decrease in serum total cholesterol concentration.

In the first study to examine age and gender differences in the effect of psyllium on blood lipids, men and pre- and postmenopausal women were given psyllium (15 grams daily) or placebo. Psyllium lowered plasma LDL cholesterol by 7-9 percent in all groups. Triglyceride levels were lowered by 17 percent in men, but were increased by 16 percent in postmenopausal women. Premenopausal women displayed no significant shift in triglycerides.[28]

Diabetes Mellitus

The effect of psyllium husk was studied in 34 men with type 2 diabetes and hypercholesterolemia given either placebo or 5.1 g psyllium twice daily for eight weeks. Total cholesterol was lower by 8.9 percent and LDL by one percent. In addition, the postprandial rise of glucose was significantly reduced.[29]

Drug-Botanical Interactions

Changes in plasma drug levels have not been noted. One study in female rabbits showed that while guar gum reduced the absorption of ethinylestradiol, psyllium actually slightly increased the total absorption, but caused a slower absorption rate.[30]

Side Effects and Toxicity

No adverse effects of supplementation with either psyllium seed or husk were noted in any clinical studies noted in this paper. In many of the studies there were greater levels of adverse effects with the placebo. No changes in blood indices or in vitamin or mineral content were found in any of those studies (including both meta-analyses). A 52-week study of 93 healthy individuals did find there were some small but statistically significant changes in some measurements of mineral and vitamin levels and in some hematological and biochemical parameters. But the authors note that none were of clinical significance with the possible exception of reduced levels of vitamin B12.[31]

Dosage

Based on the above studies, the recommended dosage for psyllium husk ranges from 10-30 grams daily, in divided doses. Starting with a lower dose and increasing gradually is often recommended. Keeping well hydrated while taking psyllium will prevent constipation.

Warnings and Contraindications

Several cases have been published of individual allergic and anaphylactic reactions to psyllium,[32-35] mostly in individuals who inadvertently inhaled the powder while preparing it, so caution must be exercised in this regard.

References

1. Devroede G. Constipation. In: Sleisinger MH, Fordtran JS, eds. *Gastrointestinal Disease: Pathophysiology, Diagnosis, Management*. Philadelphia, PA: WB Saunders; 1993:837-887.
2. Marteau P, Flourie B, Cherbut C, et al. Digestibility and bulking effect of ispaghula husks in healthy humans.*Gut* 1994;35:1747-1752.
3. Marlett JA, Kajs TM, Fischer MH. An unfermented gel component of psyllium seed husk promotes laxation as a lubricant in humans. *Am J Clin Nutr* 2000;72:784-789.
4. Mortensen PB, Nordgaard-Andersen I. The dependence of the *in vitro* fermentation of dietary fibre to short-chain fatty acids on the contents of soluble non-starch polysaccharides. *Scan J Gastroenterol* 1993;28:418-422.
5. Nordgaard I, Hove H, Clausen MR, Mortensen PB. Colonic production of butyrate in patients with previous colonic cancer during long-term treatment with dietary fibre (*Plantago ovata* seeds). *Scand J Gastroenterol* 1996;31:1011-1020.
6. Matheson HB, Colon IS, Story JA. Cholesterol 7 alpha-hydroxylase activity is increased by dietary modification with psyllium hydrocolloid, pectin, cholesterol and cholestyramine in rats. *J Nutr* 1995;125:454-458.
7. Vergara-Jimenez M, Conde K, Erickson SK, Fernandez ML. Hypolipidemic mechanisms of pectin and psyllium in guinea pigs fed high fat-sucrose diets: alterations on hepatic cholesterol metabolism. *J Lipid Res* 1998;39:1455-1465.
8. Everson GT, Daggy BP, McKinley C, Story JA. Effects of psyllium hydrophilic mucilloid on LDL-cholesterol and bile acid synthesis in hypercholesterolemic men. *J Lipid Res* 1992;33:1183-1192.
9. Voderholzer WA, Schatke W, Muhldorfer BE, et al. Clinical response to dietary fiber treatment of chronic constipation. *Am J Gastroenterol* 1997;92:95-98.
10. Bliss DZ, Jung HJ, Savik K, et al. Supplementation with dietary fiber improves fecal incontinence. *Nurs Res* 2001;50:203-213.
11. Perez-Miranda M, Gomez-Cedenilla A, Leon-Colombo T, et al. Effect of fiber supplements on internal bleeding hemorrhoids. *Hepatogastroenterology* 1996;43:1504-1507.
12. Broader JH, Gunn IF, Alexander-Williams J. Evaluation of a bulk-forming evacuant in the management of hemorrhoids. *Br J Surg* 1974;61:142-144.
13. Webster DJ, Pugh DC, Craven JL. The use of bulk evacuant in patients with hemorrhoids. *Br J Surg* 1978;65:291-292.

14. Fernandez-Banares F, Hinojosa J, Sanchez-Lombrana JL, et al. Randomized clinical trial of *Plantago ovata* seeds (dietary fiber) as compared with mesalamine in maintaining remission in ulcerative colitis. *Am J Gastroenterol* 1999;94:427-433.
15. Turnbull WH, Thomas HG. The effect of *Plantago ovata* seed containing preparation on appetite variables, nutrient and energy intake. *Int J Obes Relat Metab Disord* 1995;19:338-342.
16. Fernandez ML. Distinct mechanisms of plasma LDL lowering by dietary fiber in the guinea pig: specific effects of pectin, guar gum, and psyllium. *J Lipid Res* 1995;36:2394-2404.
17. Fernandez ML, Ruiz LR, Conde AK, et al. Psyllium reduces plasma LDL in guinea pigs by altering hepatic cholesterol homeostasis. *J Lipid Res* 1995;36:1128-1138.
18. Terpstra AH, Lapre JA, de Vries HT, Beynen AC. Hypocholesterolemic effect of dietary psyllium in female rats. *Ann Nutr Metab* 2000;44:223-228.
19. Sprecher DL, Harris BV, Goldberg AC, et al. Efficacy of psyllium in reducing serum cholesterol levels in hypercholesterolemic patients on high- or low-fat diets. *Ann Intern Med* 1993;119:545-554.
20. Bell LP, Hectorne K, Reynolds H, Hunninghake DB. Cholesterol-lowering effects of psyllium hydrophilic mucilloid. *JAMA* 1989;261:3419-3423.
21. Anderson JW, Allgood LD, Lawrence A, et al. Cholesterol-lowering effects of psyllium intake adjunctive to diet therapy in men and women with hypercholesterolemia: meta-analysis of 8 controlled trials. *Am J Clin Nutr* 2000;71:472-479.
22. Levin EG, Miller VT, Muesing RA, et al. Comparison of psyllium hydrophilic mucilloid and cellulose as adjuncts to a prudent diet in the treatment of mild to moderate hypercholesterolemia. *Arch Intern Med* 1990;150:1822-1827.
23. Anderson JW, Davidson MH, Blone L, et al. Long-term cholesterol-lowering effects of psyllium as an adjunct to diet therapy in the treatment of hypercholesterolemia. *Am J Clin Nutr* 2000;71:1433-1438.
24. Olson BH, Anderson SM, Becker MP, et al. Psyllium-enriched cereals lower blood total cholesterol and LDL cholesterol, but not HDL cholesterol, in hypercholesterolemic adults: results of a meta-analysis. *J Nutr* 1997;127:1973-1980.
25. Romero AL, Romero JE, Galviz S, Fernandez ML. Cookies enriched with psyllium or oat bran lower plasma LDL cholesterol in normal and hypercholesterolemic men from Northern Mexico. *J Am Coll Nutr* 1998;17:601-608.
26. Burton R, Manninen V. Influence of a psyllium-based fibre preparation on faecal and serum parameters. *Acta Med Scand* 1982;668:S91-S94.
27. Stewart RB, Hale WE, Moore MT, et al. Effect of psyllium hydrophilic mucilloid on serum cholesterol in the elderly. *Dig Dis Sci* 1991;36:329-334.
28. Vega-Lopez S, Vidal-Quintanar RL, Fernandez ML. Sex and hormonal status influence plasma lipid responses to psyllium. *Am J Clin Nutr* 2001;74:435-441.
29. Anderson JW, Allgood LD, Turner J, et al. Effects of psyllium on glucose and serum lipid responses in men with type 2 diabetes and hypercholesterolemia. *Am J Clin Nutr* 1999;70:466-473.
30. Garcia JJ, Fernandez N, Diez MJ, et al. Influence of two dietary fibers in the oral bioavailability and other pharmacokinetic parameters of ethinyloestradiol. *Contraception* 2000;6:253-257.
31. Oliver SD. The long-term safety and tolerability of ispaghula husk. *J R Soc Health* 2000;120:107-111.
32. Lantner RR, Espiritu BR, Zumerchik P, Tobin MC. Anaphylaxis following ingestion of a psyllium-containing cereal. *JAMA* 1990;264:2534-2536.
33. James JM, Cooke SK, Barnett A, Sampson HA. Anaphylactic reactions to a psyllium-containing cereal. *J Allergy Clin Immunol* 1991;88:402-408.
34. Suhonen R, Kantola I, Bjorksten F. Anaphylactic shock due to ingestion of psyllium laxative. *Allergy* 1983;38:363-365.
35. Freeman GL. Psyllium hypersensitivity. *Ann Allergy* 1994;73:490-492.

Saccharum offinarum (Sugar cane) Harold St. John photo

Octacosanol

$$CH_3 - (CH_2)_{27} - OH$$

Policosanol

Introduction

Policosanol, an extract from sugar cane (*Saccharum officinarum* L), has been heavily researched in Cuba for its cholesterol-lowering properties in several different human populations. In addition to improving serum lipids, policosanol reduces LDL oxidation, decreases platelet aggregation, decreases smooth muscle proliferation, and improves symptoms of cardiovascular disease. Side effects are virtually non-existent.

Biochemistry

Cuban-manufactured policosanol is a mixture of alcohols isolated and purified from sugar cane, and consists of 66-percent octacosanol (CH_3-CH_2(26)-CH_2-OH), 12-percent triacontanol, and 7-percent hexacosanol. Other alcohols (15%), namely tetracosanol, heptacosanol, nonacosanol, dotriacontanol and tetratriacontanol, are minor components.[1]

Mechanisms of Action

Policosanol appears to cause decreased synthesis and increased degradation of 3-hydroxy-3-methylglutaryl Coenzyme A (HMG-CoA) reductase, the rate-limiting step in cholesterol synthesis.[2,3] This is different than the mechanism of action of statin drugs, which work by competitively inhibiting HMG-CoA reductase. Policosanol has also demonstrated improvement in LDL metabolism by increasing LDL binding, uptake, and degradation in human fibroblasts.[4]

LDL oxidation is thought to be a necessary step in the development of atherosclerosis. Studies on humans and rats show policosanol decreases *in vitro* LDL oxidation using multiple oxidation models.[5,6] Another step in the formation of atherosclerotic plaques is an increase in smooth muscle proliferation. In rabbits, policosanol decreased neointimal formation, indicating decreased smooth muscle cell proliferation.[7] In a comparative study, policosanol demonstrated a greater effect on neointimal formation than lovastatin.[8]

Policosanol decreases platelet aggregation by decreasing the synthesis of platelet-aggregating thromboxane B2 (TXB2), with no effect on prostacyclin (PGI2).[9] Studies show policosanol reduces platelet aggregation induced by a number of experimental substances,[9-14] with dose-dependent increases from 10-50 mg/day. Policosanol alone at 20 mg/day was more effective than 100 mg aspirin at reducing platelet aggregation induced by ADP, and equal when induced by epinephrine and collagen.[13] Despite decreased platelet aggregation, there was no increase in coagulation time when policosanol was taken alone; however, when combined with 100 mg/day aspirin, coagulation time increased.

Clinical Indications

Hypercholesterolemia

The majority of policosanol research is on patients with type II hypercholesterolemia. Fourteen randomized, placebo-controlled, double-blind studies have shown positive results.[15-28] Significant decreases in total cholesterol (8-23%), LDL (11.3-27.5%), LDL/HDL (15.3-38.3%), and TC/HDL (9.1-30.5%) were seen in all 14 trials. Of the 13 trials measuring HDL, seven showed significant increases and in six HDL was unchanged. Doses ranged from 2-40 mg/day, with decreases in TC, LDL, LDL/HDL, and TC/HDL and increases in HDL being dose-dependent up to 20 mg/day, with no further benefit at 40 mg/day. However, 40 mg/day significantly decreased triglycerides (TG), which was not seen with lower doses.[28]

Policosanol was effective in three studies on patients with type 2 diabetes mellitus and hypercholesterolemia.[29-31] All three trials used 5 mg twice daily for 12 weeks. Total cholesterol was reduced by 14-29 percent, LDL was reduced by 20-44 percent, LDL/HDL ratio by 24-52 percent, and HDL was increased by 8-24 percent. No adverse effect on glycemic control was noted in any of the studies. In a trial comparing policosanol with lovastatin (20 mg/day), policosanol performed significantly better at raising HDL and lowering the LDL/HDL ratio.[31]

Two studies with at total of 300 patients showed policosanol to be effective in postmenopausal women with hyperlipidemia.[32,33] Both studies started with 5 mg per day, which was later increased (at week eight in one study[32] and week 12 in the other[33]) to 10 mg per day for a period of eight or 12 more weeks. At the end of the 5 mg portion, TC, LDL, LDL/HDL, and TC/HDL decreased by 13-20 percent, 17-18 percent, 17.0-17.2 percent, and 16.3-16.7 percent, respectively, whereas HDL was unchanged in one trial and increased by 16.5 percent in the other. At the end of the 10 mg/day period policosanol supplementation resulted in decreased TC, LDL, LDL/HDL, and TC/HDL by 17-20 percent, 25-28 percent, 27-30 percent, and 21-27 percent, respectively, and increased HDL 7-29 percent. Significantly more side effects were seen in the placebo group in each trial.

In comparative trials, policosanol improved lipid profiles to a statistically equal or greater extent than simvastatin,[34,35] pravastatin,[10,36] lovastatin,[31,37] probucol,[38] and acipimox.[39] Two trials on patients with type II hypercholesterolemia, comparing low dose simvastatin (5 or 10 mg/day) and moderate dose policosanol (5 or 10 mg/day), demonstrated that both substances greatly improved lipid profiles, with no significant differences between the groups.[34,35] Furthermore, there were no differences in side effects between these groups. Policosanol (10 mg/day) compared favorably to low-dose pravastatin (10 mg/day) in patients with type II hypercholesterolemia in two studies.[10,36] In one trial, policosanol-treated patients had significantly greater decreases in LDL, LDL/HDL, TC/HDL and increases in HDL,[36] while in another trial policosanol-treated patients had significantly greater increases in HDL.[10] The pravastatin group had more side effects in both studies.

Comparing policosanol to lovastatin on patients with type 2 diabetes and hypercholesterolemia (type II) found policosanol (10 mg/day) is more effective at lowering LDL/HDL and increasing HDL than 10 mg/day lovastatin, with significantly fewer side effects.[31] Additionally, in patients with type II hypercholesterolemia and concomitant coronary risk factors, policosanol (10 mg/day) decreased LDL/HDL and increased HDL more effectively than 20 mg/day lovastatin, with fewer side effects.[37]

Policosanol (5 mg twice daily) also compared favorably to probucol (500 mg twice daily) at reducing TC, LDL, and TG in patients with type II hypercholesterolemia.[38]

Finally, policosanol (10 mg/day) compared favorably to acipimox (750 mg/day), a niacin derivative, in regards to TC, LDL, LDL/HDL, TC/HDL, and HDL, with fewer side effects.[39]

In contrast to statin drugs, policosanol has shown no adverse effects on the liver and may even reduce liver damage. In a trial to determine whether policosanol could safely be used on patients with altered liver function tests, 46 patients with primary hypercholesterolemia and elevated liver enzymes were treated with policosanol (5 or 10 mg/day) or placebo for 12 weeks. Both 5 and 10 mg significantly lowered lipids and reduced serum levels of alanine aminotransferase (ALT), suggesting improvement in liver function.[40]

Intermittent Claudication

Two studies showed positive results using policosanol on patients with intermittent claudication. In 62 patients treated with 10 mg policosanol twice per day for six months, the distance individuals could walk on a treadmill before noticing claudication symptoms was increased by 63.1 percent, and absolute distance to not being able to walk anymore was increased by 65.1 percent, while placebo had no effect on walking distances. Policosanol also improved lower extremity symptoms of coldness and pain compared to placebo.[41] In a two-year follow-up study with 56 patients, improvements were progressive throughout the study, with the distance walked before initial claudication symptoms improving by 60.1 percent after six months and 187.8 percent after 24 months. Absolute walking distance increased by 81 percent after six months and 249 percent after 24 months. Policosanol also significantly decreased symptoms of claudication and increased the ankle/arm pressure ratio at 12 and 24 months. Even more impressive, significantly more patients in the placebo group had serious vascular events (8 patients with 10 total serious adverse events), while none did in the policosanol group.[42]

Ischemic Heart Disease

Forty-five patients with documented ischemic heart disease were placed on 5 mg policosanol twice daily, 5 mg policosanol twice daily plus 125 mg aspirin (ASA), or 125 mg ASA for 20 months.[43] The policosanol groups showed an insignificantly lower percentage of patients with functional progression of ischemia and a significantly greater partial regression of ischemia. Furthermore, exercise capacity and left ventricular function improved significantly in the policosanol groups compared to the ASA-only group. Both policosanol groups were more effective than ASA alone, but policosanol plus aspirin therapy was more effective than policosanol alone. There were four vascular events in ASA alone (1 fatal myocardial infarction (MI), 2 unstable angina, 1 cardiac failure), one in the group taking policosanol alone (non-fatal MI), and none in the combined group. A follow-up study on the same patients examined treadmill exercise ECG testing performance.[44] Those taking policosanol demonstrated decreases in cardiovascular functional class, rest- and exercise-induced angina, cardiac events, and ischemic ST-segment response. These benefits were greatest in the policosanol plus aspirin group. Additionally, policosanol showed an increase in maximum oxygen uptake, a decline in double product (peak heart rate times peak systolic blood pressure), and an increase in aerobic functional capacity compared to placebo.

Atherosclerotic lesions in patients with carotid-vertebral atherosclerosis improved when given policosanol in 22 patients using 10 mg/day policosanol for 1 year.[45] Carotid-vertebral atherosclerosis assessed using Doppler-ultrasound showed progression of disease in 3/11 patients on placebo and 0/11 patients on policosanol. Disease regression occurred in 6/11 on policosanol and 1/11 on placebo. Neither of these values reached statistical significance; however, when a progression/regression ratio was calculated it did reach statistical significance for improvement with policosanol.

Policosanol (2 mg/day) improved abnormal rest and stress ECG patterns, and decreased symptoms of angina in a single-blind, 14-month, placebo-controlled trial in 23 middle-aged patients with primary or marginal hypercholesterolemia. No patient had a new coronary event, but significantly more patients (5/12) in the policosanol group with stable angina or silent ischemia had improved coronary symptoms and/or rest and stress ECG patterns, compared to placebo (0/11). Policosanol-treated patients also had no deterioration in symptoms or ECG patterns, while 3/11 placebo-treated patients deteriorated.[25]

Drug-Nutrient Interactions

Policosanol inhibits platelet aggregation, and may enhance the effect of other anticoagulant medications. When combined with aspirin, policosanol increased coagulation time in humans.[13]

Side Effects and Toxicity

In post-marketing studies looking at 27,879 patients, the most significant adverse effects were weight loss (0.07%), polyuria (0.07%), insomnia (0.05%), or polyphagia (0.05%).[46] Only 22 patients had to discontinue treatment because of side effects. In clinical trials there was either no significant difference in adverse events or significantly more adverse events in placebo groups, compared to policosanol.

Toxicity studies in rats, dogs, mice, and monkeys have shown policosanol to be non-toxic and not carcinogenic at doses 1,500 times normal human dosage.[47-51] Reproductive studies on rats and mice show policosanol at 1,500 times the normal human dose has no adverse effect on fertility, reproduction, teratogenesis, or development.[52-54]

Dosage

Significant reduction in cholesterol can be achieved with doses as low as 2 mg/day; however, maximum reductions should be seen at 5-20 mg/day. Greater than 20 mg/day seems to offer no further benefit. A prudent recommendation would be to start with 5 mg per day and increase to 10 mg twice daily if needed.

References

1. Arruzazabala ML, Noa M, Menendez R, et al. Protective effect of policosanol on atherosclerotic lesions in rabbits with exogenous hypercholesterolemia. *Braz J Med Biol Res* 2000;33:835-840.
2. Menendez R, Amor AM, Gonzalez R, et al. Effect of policosanol on the hepatic cholesterol biosynthesis of normocholesterolemic rats. *Biol Res* 1996;29:253-257.
3. Menendez R, Amor AM, Rodeiro I, et al. Policosanol modulates HMG-CoA reductase activity in cultured fibroblasts. *Arch Med Res* 2001;32:8-12.
4. Menendez R, Fernandez SI, Del Rio A, et al. Policosanol inhibits cholesterol biosynthesis and enhances low density lipoprotein processing in cultured human fibroblasts. *Biol Res* 1994;27:199-203.
5. Menendez R, Fraga V, Amor MA, et al. Oral administration of policosanol inhibits *in vitro* copper ion-induced rat lipoprotein peroxidation. *Physiol Behav* 1999;67:1-7.
6. Menendez R, Mas R, Amor MA, et al. Effects of policosanol treatment on the susceptibility of low density lipoprotein (LDL) isolated from healthy volunteers to oxidative modification *in vitro*. *Br J Clin Pharmacol* 2000;50:255-262.
7. Noa M, Mas R, Mesa R. Effect of policosanol on intimal thickening in rabbit cuffed carotid artery. *Int J Cardiol* 1998;67:125-132.
8. Noa M, Mas R, Mesa R. A comparative study of policosanol vs. lovastatin on intimal thickening in rabbit cuffed carotid artery. *Pharmacol Res* 2001;43:31-37.
9. Carbajal D, Arruzazabala ML, Valdes S, Mas R. Effect of policosanol on platelet aggregation and serum levels of arachidonic acid metabolites in healthy volunteers. *Prostaglandins Leukot Essent Fatty Acids* 1998;58:61-64.

10. Castano G, Mas R, Arruzazabala M, Noa M, et al. Effects of policosanol and pravastatin on lipid profile, platelet aggregation and endothelemia in older hypercholesterolemic patients. *Int J Clin Pharmacol Res* 1999;29:105-116.

11. Valdes S, Arruzazabala MI, Fernandez L, et al. Effect of policosanol on platelet aggregation in healthy volunteers. *Int J Clin Pharmacol Res* 1996;16:67-72.

12. Arruzazabala ML, Valdes S, Mas L, et al. Effect of policosanol successive dose increase on platelet aggregation in healthy volunteers. *Pharmacol Res* 1996;34:181-185.

13. Arruzazabala ML, Valdes S, Mas R, et al. Comparative study of policosanol, and the combination therapy policosanol-aspirin on platelet aggregation in healthy volunteers. *Pharmacol Res* 1997;36:293-297.

14. Arruzazabala ML, Mas R, Molina V, et al. Effect of policosanol on platelet aggregation in type II hypercholesterolemic patients. *Int J Tissue React* 1998;20:119-124.

15. Pons P, Mas R, Illnait J, et al. Efficacy and safety of policosanol in patients with primary hypercholesterolemia. *Curr Ther Res Clin Exp* 1992;52:507-513.

16. Aneiros E, Calderon B, Mas R, et al. Effect of successive dose increases of policosanol on the lipid profile and tolerability of treatment. *Curr Ther Res Clin Exp* 1993;54:304-312.

17. Pons P, Rodriguez M, Mas R, et al. One-year efficacy and safety of policosanol in patients with type II hypercholesterolemia. *Curr Ther Res Clin Exp* 1994;55:1084-1092.

18. Pons P, Rodriquez M, Robaina C, et al. Effects of successive dose increases of policosanol on the lipid profile of patients with type II hypercholesterolemia and tolerability to treatment. *Int J Clin Pharmacol Res* 1994;14:27-33.

19. Canetti M, Moreira M, Illnait J, et al. One-year study of the effect of policosanol on lipid profile in patients with type II hypercholesterolemia. *Adv Ther* 1995;12:245-254.

20. Aneiros E, Mas R, Calderon B, et al. Effect of policosanol in lowering cholesterol levels in patients with type II hypercholesterolemia. *Curr Ther Res Clin Exp* 1995;56:176-182.

21. Castano G, Mas R, Nodarse M, et al. One-year study of the efficacy and safety of policosanol (5 mg twice daily) in the treatment of type II hypercholesterolemia. *Curr Ther Res Clin Exp* 1995;56:296-304.

22. Canetti M, Moreira M, Mas R, et al. A two-year study on the efficacy and tolerability of policosanol in patients with type II hyperlipoproteinemia. *Int J Clin Pharmacol Res* 1995;15:159-165.

23. Castano G, Canetti M, Moreira M, et al. Efficacy and tolerability of policosanol in elderly patients with type II hypercholesterolemia: a 12-month study. *Curr Ther Res Clin Exp* 1995;56:819-827.

24. Castano G, Tula L, Canetti M, et al. Effects of policosanol in hypertensive patients with type II hypercholesterolemia. *Curr Ther Res Clin Exp* 1996;57:691-699.

25. Batista J, Stusser R, Saez F, Perez B. Effect of policosanol on hyperlipidemia and coronary heart disease in middle-aged patients. A 14-month pilot study. *Int J Clin Pharmacol Ther* 1996;34:134-137.

26. Mas R, Castano G, Illnait J, et al. Effects of policosanol in patients with type II hypercholesterolemia and additional coronary risk factors. *Clin Pharmacol Ther* 1999;65:439-447.

27. Castano G, Mas R, Fernandez JC, et al. Effects of policosanol in older patients with type II hypercholesterolemia and high coronary risk. *J Gerontol* 2001;56A:M186-M192.

28. Castano G, Mas R, Fernandez L, et al. Effects of policosanol 20 versus 40 mg/day in the treatment of patients with type II hypercholesterolemia: a 6-month double-blind study. *Int J Clin Pharmacol Res* 2001;21:43-57.

29. Crespo N, Alvarez, R, Mas R, et al. Effects of policosanol on patients with non-insulin-dependent diabetes mellitus and hypercholesterolemia: a pilot study. *Curr Ther Res Clin Exp* 1997;58:44-51.

30. Torres O, Agramonte A, Illnait J, et al. Treatment of hypercholesterolemia in NIDDM with policosanol. *Diabetes Care* 1995;18:393-397.

31. Crespo N, Illnait J, Mas R, et al. Comparative study of the efficacy and tolerability of policosanol and lovastatin in patients with hypercholesterolemia and noninsulin dependent diabetes mellitus. *Int J Clin Pharmacol Res* 1999;29:117-127.

32. Castano G, Mas R, Fernandez L, et al. Effects of policosanol on postmenopausal women with type II hypercholesterolemia. *Gynecol Endocrinol* 2000;14:187-195.

33. Mirkin A, Mas R, Martinto M, et al. Efficacy and tolerability of policosanol in hypercholesterolemic postmenopausal women. *Int J Clin Pharmacol Res* 2001;21:31-41.

34. Ortensi G, Gladstein J, Valli H, Tesone PA. A comparative study of policosanol versus simvastatin in elderly patients with hypercholesterolemia. *Curr Ther Res Clin Exp* 1997;58:390-401.

35. Illnait J, Castano G, Mas R, Fernandez JC. A comparative study on the efficacy and tolerability of policosanol and simvastatin for treating type II hypercholesterolemia. *Can J Cardiol* 1997;13:342B.

36. Benitez M, Romero C, Mas R, et al. A comparative study of policosanol versus pravastatin in patients with type II hypercholesterolemia. *Curr Ther Res Clin Exp* 1997;58:859-867.

37. Castano G, Mas R, Fernandez JC, et al. Efficacy and tolerability of policosanol compared with lovastatin in patients with type II hypercholesterolemia and concomitant coronary risk factors. *Curr Ther Res Clin Exp* 2000;61:137-146.

38. Pons P, Illnait J, Mas R, et al. A comparative study of policosanol versus probucol in patients with hypercholesterolemia. *Curr Ther Res Clin Exp* 1997;58:26-35.

39. Alcocer L, Fernandez L, Compos E, Mas R. A comparative study of policosanol versus acipimox in patients with type II hypercholesterolemia. *Int J Tissue React* 1999;21:85-92.

40. Zardoya R, Tula L, Castano G, et al. Effects of policosanol on hypercholesterolemic patients with abnormal serum biochemical indicators of hepatic function. *Curr Ther Res Clin Exp* 1996;57:568-577.

41. Castano G, Mas R, Roca J, et al. A double-blind, placebo-controlled study of the effects of policosanol in patients with intermittent claudication. *Angiology* 1999;50:123-130.

42. Castano G, Mas R, Fernandez L, et al. A long-term study of policosanol in the treatment of intermittent claudication. *Angiology* 2001;52:115-125.

43. Batista J, Strusser R, Padron R, et al. Functional improvement in coronary artery disease after 20 months of lipid-lowering therapy with policosanol. *Adv Ther* 1996;13:137-148.

44. Strusser R, Batista J, Padron R, et al. Long-term therapy with policosanol improves treadmill exercise-ecg testing performance of coronary heart disease patients. *Int J Clin Pharmacol Ther* 1998;36:469-473.

45. Batista J, Stusser R, Penichet M, Uguet E. Doppler-ultrasound pilot study of the effects of long-term policosanol therapy on carotid-vertebral atherosclerosis. *Curr Ther Res Clin Exp* 1995;56:906-914.

46. Fernandez L, Mas R, Illnait J, Fernandez JC. Policosanol: results of a postmarketing surveillance study of 27,879 patients. *Curr Ther Res Clin Exp* 1998;59:717-722.

47. Celia AL, Mas R, Hernandez C, et al. A 12-month study of policosanol oral toxicity in Sprague Dawley rats. *Toxicol Lett* 1994;70:77-87.

48. Aleman CL, Mas R, Noa M, et al. Carcinogenicity of policosanol in Sprague Dawley rats: a 24 month study. *Teratog Carcinog Mutagen* 1994;14:239-249.

49. Mesa AR, Mas R, Noa M, et al. Toxicity of policosanol in beagle dogs: one-year study. *Toxicol Lett* 1994;73:81-90.

50. Rodreguez-Echenigue C, Mesa R, Mas R, et al. Effects of policosanol chronically administered in male monkeys (*Macaca arctoides*). *Food Chem Toxicol* 1994;32:565-575.

51. Aleman CL, Noa M, Elias EC, et al. Carcinogenicity of policosanol in mice: an 18-month study. *Food Chem Toxicol* 1995;33:573-578.

52. Rodriguez MD, Garcia H. Evaluation of peri- and post-natal toxicity of policosanol in rats. *Teratog Carcinog Mutagen* 1998;18:1-7.

53. Rodriguez MD, Carcia H. Teratogenic and reproductive studies of policosanol in the rat and rabbit. *Teratog Carcinog Mutagen* 1994;14:107-113.

54. Rodriguez MD, Sanchez M, Garcia H. Multigeneration reproduction study of policosanol in rats. *Toxicol Lett* 1997;90:97-106.

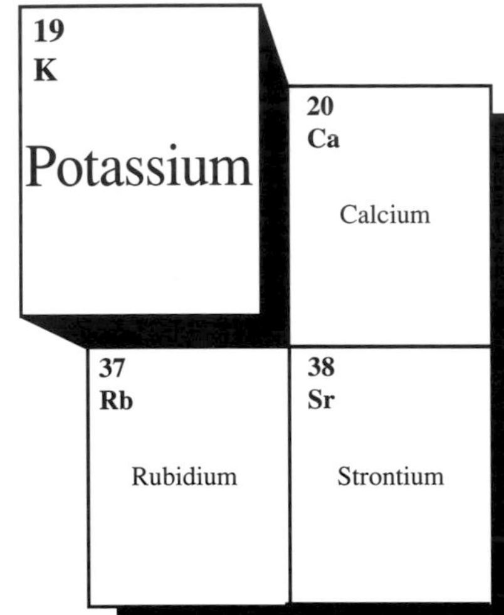

Potassium

Introduction

Potassium is the main cation (i.e., a positively charged electrolyte) in intracellular fluid, with a concentration approximately 30-fold greater than found in extracellular fluids.

In contrast to potassium's role as an intracellular cation, sodium acts as the primary extracellular cation. Together, these two cations maintain the electrical potential across cell membranes; however, to accomplish this physiological task, an appropriate balance of potassium and sodium is required. Potassium researchers recommend a diet that maintains an optimal sodium-to-potassium ratio of 1:5 or less.[1] Otherwise, a chronic state of cation imbalance exists in an individual.

In addition to this role in maintaining cell membrane electrical gradients, potassium plays a role in energy metabolism and fluid and acid-base balance; is required for optimal cardiac, adrenal, and renal function; and promotes muscular and neurological function.[2]

Potassium supplementation has been shown to be effective in treating hypertension and in the prevention of recurrent nephrolithiasis.

Pharmacokinetics

Dietary and supplemental potassium are well absorbed in the gastrointestinal tract. Potassium transport into cells is promoted by insulin and catecholamines. Most potassium is excreted via the kidneys, although some is eliminated via the gastrointestinal tract.[3]

Mechanisms of Action

Potassium's mechanism of action is primarily related to its role in maintaining membrane charge potentials, osmotic balance, and acid/base balance.

Potassium's mechanism of action in hypertension is thought to be a consequence of impacting sodium elimination and the renin-angiotension system, having a vasodilatory effect, improving baroreceptor and possibly insulin sensitivity, and enhancing catecholamine function and metabolism.

Deficiency States and Symptoms

Potassium is responsible for normal electrical excitability of muscle tissue. Many of the signs and symptoms of potassium deficiency can be related to the role of potassium in membrane excitability: muscle weakness, arrhythmias, autonomic insufficiency, continuous thirst, vertigo, nervous disorders, and constipation.[4,5] Because potassium is necessary in normal skeletal muscle function, hypokalcmia will manifest as a vague type of myalgia, an aching sensation often alleviated by positional changes; however, the symptoms return quickly – similar to symptoms of restless leg syndrome. Cramping may be prominent, along with localized muscular swelling and stiffness.[2]

Potassium's role in acid/base balance can influence kidney function. Potassium deficiency causes intracellular acidosis and ammonium ions are formed in the urine, causing tissue damage and increasing protein needs. If protein intake is low, potassium deficiency will cause muscle atrophy because skeletal muscle will be catabolized to provide nitrogen for ammonia production in the kidney. Urinary tract infections may occur in potassium deficiency as a result of acidification with ammonia in the renal medulla. Chronic elevation of renal ammonia as a result of chronic potassium deficiency has also been shown to damage the kidney.[4]

A number of conditions induce potassium deficiency, including prolonged fluid loss from perspiration, vomiting, or diarrhea; hypothermia; protein-modified fasts; diabetic ketoacidosis; insulin shock; alcoholism; excessive caffeine, salt, or sugar consumption; villous adenoma; and anorexia and bulimia.[2]

Clinical Indications

Hypertension

Epidemiological studies have shown a correlation with high potassium diets and lowered risk of stroke and hypertension.[6] Multiple studies have shown potassium supplementation of 2.5-5.0 grams daily has a significant effect on hypertension.[7-10] A recent meta-analysis of 33 randomized, controlled studies of potassium supplementation in 2,609 hypertensive subjects revealed supplementation had a significant effect in lowering both systolic and diastolic pressures.[11] Even though the effect was small, -3.11 mmHg systolic and -1.97 mmHg diastolic, the effect was consistent throughout the meta-analysis and the authors conclude increased potassium intake is recommended for both preventive and therapeutic approaches to hypertension, especially in those unable to reduce sodium intake. Recent studies in elderly subjects taking 2.5 grams potassium chloride daily had even greater effects – a drop of 12-15 points in systolic pressure in four weeks of treatment.[8,9] These studies compare favorably with results of antihypertensive medications in elderly populations.[10]

In several trials, a blood-pressure lowering effect of potassium chloride could be demonstrated. However, it is not known whether other potassium salts are also effective. In a randomized, cross-over trial, 12 patients with essential hypertension were treated for eight weeks with placebo and 120 mMol potassium per day. Potassium was given together with 50-percent citrate and 50-percent bicarbonate as anions. Urinary potassium excretion rose from 61.8 ± 8.1 to 166.7 ± 21.2 mMol/24 hours during potassium supplementation. However, blood pressure and heart rate remained unchanged when compared to placebo. Non-chloride potassium salts may not be effective in lowering blood pressure in essential hypertension.[12]

Urinary Tract Infections

Alkalinizing the urine using potassium or sodium citrate is an established effective treatment to alleviate the symptoms of a urinary tract infection (UTI).[13] Although acidifying the urine is theoretically an effective bacteriostatic treatment, the use of supplemental ascorbic acid or cranberry juice at dosages commonly prescribed is ineffective at altering urinary pH.[14] The efficacy of cranberry juice in treating urinary tract infections appears to be through mechanisms other than acidifying the urine.[15] In a clinical trial of recurrent UTI in 59 children, potassium citrate was prescribed along with salt, protein, and calcium restriction due to hypercalciuria.[16] In 95 percent of the children, no further episodes of UTI occurred once normocalciuria was achieved. The authors hypothesize hypercalciuria may play a predisposing role for recurrent UTIs in children by promoting the formation of microcrystals that damage the uroepithelium.

Kidney Stones

Potassium has therapeutic benefit in the prevention and treatment of kidney stones by decreasing urinary calcium excretion[17,18] and increasing urinary citrate.[17] Potassium chloride and potassium bicarbonate have been found to decrease thiazide-induced hypercalciuria, with greater effect from potassium bicarbonate.[19] Results of another study found increased urinary potassium excretion correlated with a decreased risk of stone formation in post-lithotripsy patients.[20]

Supplementing potassium in the form of potassium citrate may provide added benefit. The efficacy of citrate in the treatment of calcium oxalate and urate kidney stones has been well documented.[21] As a potassium salt, citrate raises the pH of urine and increases uric acid dissociation, thus inhibiting uric acid stone formation. Potassium citrate also decreases urinary excretion of calcium and inhibits growth and precipitation of calcium phosphate and calcium oxalate crystals in the urine.[22] A recent study assessed the effect of potassium citrate in preventing recurrences of kidney stones in 64 patients, who were followed 24-60 months after initial incident.[23] Compared to a control group who received no prophylaxis (46.2% recurrence), or a group with intermittent prophylaxis (30% recurrence), those on potassium citrate had only a 7.8-percent recurrence rate.

Potassium citrate has also been found to be effective in prevention of stone formation in patients with renal polycystic disease, in children with distal renal tubular acidosis complicated by hypercalciuria, and the prevention of renal complications at the time of glaucoma treatment with acetazolamide.[24] In other studies with potassium citrate, inhibition of recurrent stone formation was seen in 70-75 percent of patients.[24] In combination with magnesium citrate, potassium citrate has been shown to be even more effective in promoting an alkaline pH in the urine.[25]

Congestive Heart Failure

Tissue potassium deficiency is well documented in congestive heart failure.[26] However, due to concomitant magnesium deficiency, potassium replacement alone might not correct potassium deficiency in this condition.[27] Similar to chronic electrolyte depletion resulting from body fluid loss or malnutrition, magnesium repletion is necessary to correct tissue potassium deficits.[28]

Insulin Resistance

Evidence suggests a diet inducing potassium depletion results in a resistance to insulin action at post-receptor sites, a resistance that is reversed when potassium is resupplied.[29]

Currently no information is available on potassium supplementation under other circumstances; however, this mineral appears to have a close association with insulin resistance and merits future investigation.

Drug-Nutrient Interactions

Medications that induce potassium depletion include aspirin, bisacodyl, choline magnesium trisalicylate, colchicine, corticosteroids, non-potassium sparing diuretics (such as thiazide diuretics), laxatives, and sodium bicarbonate.[5]

The botanical *Glycyrrhiza glabra* may also result in potassium loss. While it more commonly occurs with long-term use of more than 1 g glycyrrhizin daily, some people experience signs of potassium loss with lower doses.

ACE inhibitors (captopril, enalapril, ramipril, etc.) produce potassium retention by inhibiting aldosterone. Potassium supplementation with ACE inhibitors and potassium-sparing diuretics (spironolactone, amilroide, triamterene, etc.) should be approached with caution to prevent hyperkalemia.[3]

Side Effects and Toxicity

Side effects of excessive doses may include gastrointestinal problems (nausea, stomach pain, vomiting, diarrhea, flatulence), bradycardia, hyperkalemia and consequences thereof, and respiratory problems, including difficulty breathing.

Potassium intolerance may be aggravated by concomitant use of beta-blockers, digitalis, medications that suppress aldosterone production (NSAIDs, angiotensin-converting enzyme inhibitors), potassium-sparing diuretics, and other medications that interfere with aldosterone or renin.[4]

Toxic effects include muscle weakness, lethargy, gastric hypomotility, paralysis, arrhythmias, cardiac conduction disturbances, and even death.

Dosage

Potassium chloride dosages used in treating hypertension usually range from 2.5-5.0 g daily. Potassium citrate dosages in kidney stone prevention range from 1.1-3.3 g daily.[2] The estimated safe and adequate daily dietary intake of potassium for adults, according to the Committee on Recommended Daily Allowances, is 1.9-5.6 grams. Current guidelines do not recommend increasing potassium above the safe and adequate dietary potassium intake during pregnancy or lactation.

Oral doses greater than 18 grams daily may lead to severe hyperkalemia in people with normal kidney function.[3] One milliequivalent or millimole is equal to 39.09 mg.

Warnings and Contraindications

Use with caution in subjects with renal insufficiency, since disrupted renal function might inhibit potassium elimination and result in hyperkalemia. Potassium citrate is contraindicated in struvite (magnesium ammonium phosphate) renal stone disease, peptic ulcer, gastritis, gastrointestinal bleeding, disorders of coagulation, and metabolic alkalosis.[23]

Care should be taken in prescribing potassium to elderly people since evidence has demonstrated the elderly to be at increased risk for hyperkalemia. This is probably a result of impaired renal elimination and deterioration of cell membrane health/function resulting in a higher amount of extracellular potassium.

Potassium supplementation with ACE inhibitors and potassium-sparing diuretics should be approached with caution to prevent hyperkalemia.

References

1. Murray M, Pizzorno J. Nutritional medicine. In: Pizzorno J, Murray M, eds. *Textbook of Natural Medicine, Volume 1*, 2nd ed. New York, NY: Churchill Livingstone; 1999:376.
2. Schuster VL. Potassium deficiency: pathogenesis and treatment. In: Seldin DW, Giebisch G, eds. *The Regulation of Potassium Balance*. New York, NY: Raven Press; 1989:241-267.
3. Hendler SS, Rorvik D. *PDR for Nutritional Supplements*, 1st ed. Des Moines, IA: Medical Economics – Thompson Healthcare; 2001.
4. Knochel JP. Clinical expression of potassium disturbances. In: Seldin DW, Giebisch G, eds. *The Regulation of Potassium Balance*. New York, NY: Raven Press; 1989:207-240.

5. Pelton R, LaValle JB, Hawkins EB, Krinsky DL. *Drug-Induced Nutrient Depletion Handbook.* Hudson, OH: Lexi-Comp; 1999:256-257.

6. Rouse IL, Berlin LJ, Mahoney DP, et al. Vegetarian diet and blood pressure. *Lancet* 1983;2:742-743.

7. Patki PS, Singh J, Gokhale SV, et al. Efficacy of potassium and magnesium in essential hypertension: a double-blind, placebo controlled, crossover study. *BMJ* 1990;301:521-523.

8. He J, Whelton P. Potassium, blood pressure and cardiovascular disease. *Cardiol Rev* 1997;5:255-260.

9. Fotherby MD, Potter JF. Long-term potassium supplementation lowers blood pressure in elderly hypertensive patients. *Int J Clin Pract* 1997;51:219-222.

10. Fotherby MD, Potter JF. Potassium supplementation reduces clinic and ambulatory blood pressure in elderly hypertensive patients. *J Hypertens* 1992;10:1403-1408.

11. Thijs L, Amery A, Birkenhager W, et al. Age-related effects of placebo and active treatment in patients beyond the age of 60 years: the need for a proper control group. *J Hypertens* 1990;8:997-1002.

12. Overlack A, Conrad H, Stumpe KO. The influence of oral potassium citrate/bicarbonate on blood pressure in essential hypertension during unrestricted salt intake. *Klin Wochenschr* 1991;69:79-83.

13. Kahn HD, Panariello VA, Saeli J, et al. Effect of cranberry juice on urine. *J Am Diet Assoc* 1967;51:251-254.

14. Bodel PT, Cotran R, Kass EH. Cranberry juice and the antibacterial action of hippuric acid. *J Lab Clin Med* 1959;54:881.

15. Munday PE, Savage S. Cymalon in the management of urinary tract symptoms. *Genitourin Med* 1990;66:461.

16. Lopez MM, Castillo LA, Chavez JB, Ramones C. Hypercalciuria and recurrent urinary tract infection in Venezuelan children. *Pediatr Nephrol* 1999;13:433-437.

17. Martini LA, Cuppari L, Cunha MA, et al. Potassium and sodium intake and excretion in calcium stone forming patients. *J Ren Nutr* 1998;8:127-131.

18. Lemann J Jr. Relationship between urinary calcium and net acid excretion as determined by dietary protein and potassium: a review. *Nephron* 1999;81:18-25.

19. Frassetto LA, Nash E, Morris RC Jr, Sebastian A. Comparative effects of potassium chloride and bicarbonate on thiazide-induced reduction in urinary calcium excretion. *Kidney Int* 2000;58:748-752.

20. Pierratos A, Dharamsi N, Carr LK, et al. Higher urinary potassium is associated with decreased stone growth after shock wave lithotripsy. *J Urol* 2000;164:1486-1489.

21. Pak CY, Sakhaee K, Fuller C. Successful management of uric acid nephrolithiasis with potassium citrate. *Kidney Int* 1986;30:422-428.

22. Sakhaee K, Nicar M, Hill K, Pak CY. Contrasting effects of potassium citrate and sodium citrate therapies on urinary chemistries and crystallization of stone-forming salts. *Kidney Int* 1983;24:348-352.

23. Lee YH, Huang WC, Tsai JY, Huang JK. The efficacy of potassium citrate based medical prophylaxis for preventing upper urinary tract calculi: a midterm followup study. *J Urol* 1999;161:1453-1457.

24. Zmonarski SC, Klinger M, Puziewicz-Zmonarska A. Therapeutic use of potassium citrate. *Przegl Lek* 2001;58:82-86. [Article in Polish]

25. Koenig K, Padalino P, Alexandrides G, Pak CY. Bioavailability of potassium and magnesium and citrauric response from potassium-magnesium citrate. *J Urol* 1991;145:330-334.

26. Packer M. Potential role of potassium as a determinant of morbidity and mortality in patients with systemic hypertension and congestive heart failure. *Am J Cardiol* 1990;65:45E-51E.

27. Wester PO, Dyckner T. Intracellular electrolytes in cardiac failure. *Acta Med Scand Suppl* 1986;707:33-36.

28. Altura BM, Altura BT. Biochemistry and pathophysiology of congestive heart failure: is there a role for magnesium? *Magnesium* 1986;5:134-143.

29. Norbiato G, Bevilacqua M, Meroni R, et al. Effects of potassium supplementation on insulin binding and insulin action in human obesity: protein-modified fast and refeeding. *Eur J Clin Invest* 1984;14:414-419.

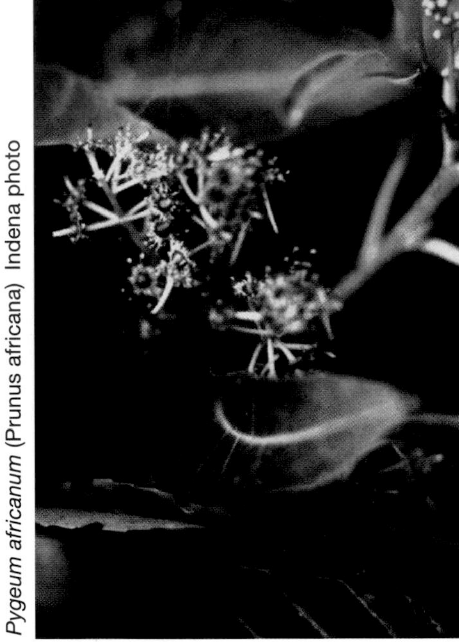
Pygeum africanum (Prunus africana) Indena photo

Pygeum africanum

Description

Pygeum africanum (also known as *Prunus africana* and African plum tree), a member of the Rosaceae family, is an evergreen species found across the entire continent of Africa at altitudes of 3,000 feet or higher. It grows up to 150 feet tall. Interest in the species began in the 1700s when European travelers learned from South African tribes how to soothe bladder discomfort and treat "old man's disease" with the bark of *P. africanum*.[1] Pygeum bark extract has been used in Europe since the mid-1960s to treat men suffering from benign prostatic hyperplasia (BPH).[2] Currently, Pygeum is the most commonly used medicine in France for BPH, backed by many double-blind studies pointing to its efficacy for reducing its symptoms.[3,4]

Active Constituents

The active constituents of Pygeum extract include phytosterols (e.g., beta-sitosterol) that have anti-inflammatory effects by inhibiting production of pro-inflammatory prostaglandins in the prostate. Pygeum also contains pentacyclic triterpenes (ursolic and oleanic acids) that have anti-edema properties, and ferulic acid esters (n-docosanol and tetracosanol) that reduce prolactin levels and block the accumulation of cholesterol in the prostate. Prolactin is purported to increase the uptake of testosterone by the prostate, and cholesterol increases binding sites for dihydrotestosterone (DHT).[1,5]

Mechanisms of Action

Although Pygeum's exact mechanism of action is still unclear, in animal models Pygeum has been shown to modulate bladder contractility by reducing the sensitivity of the bladder to electrical stimulation, phenylephrine, adenosine triphosphate, and carbachol.[4] Pygeum also has anti-inflammatory activity, by decreasing production of prostaglandins, as well as leukotrienes and other 5-lipoxygenase metabolites [6] Furthermore, Pygeum inhibits fibroblast production, increases adrenal androgen secretion, and restores the secretory activity of prostate and bulbourethral epithelium.[4,7]

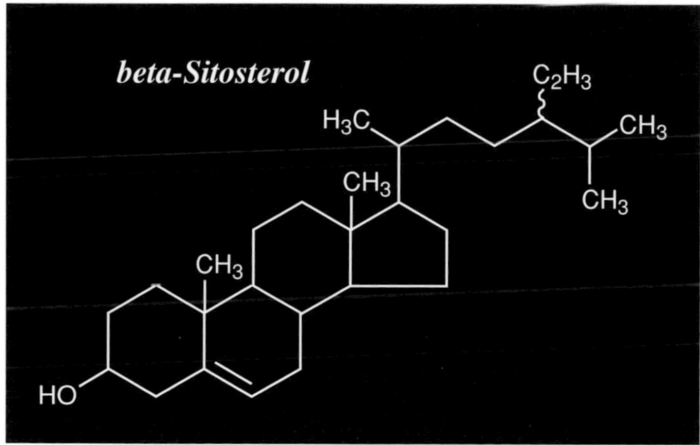

Basic fibroblast growth factor (bFGF) is hypothesized to play a role in the development of BPH and Pygeum has been shown to have a significant inhibitory effect on cell proliferation induced by bFGF.[7-9] Furthermore, in patients with abnormally low prostatic acid phosphatase activity, *P. africanum* extract can restore acid phosphatase activity and total protein secretion, although it is more effective in patients without prostatic inflammation.[10]

Clinical Indications

Benign Prostatic Hypertrophy

In a large, placebo-controlled, double-blind study (n=263), Pygeum administered at a dosage of 100 mg per day for 60 days improved urinary maximum flow by 17.2 percent, increased voided volume by 12 percent, decreased residual volume by 24.5 percent, decreased nocturia by 31 percent, decreased daytime frequency by 19.4 percent, and resulted in overall improvement of 50 percent. Sixty-five percent of the subjects reported an improvement in this study as compared to 31 percent in the placebo group.[11]

A recent literature review analyzed studies from 1966-2000 containing a total of 18 randomized, controlled trials involving 1,562 men. Compared with placebo, the combined outcome of urological symptoms and flow measures were significantly improved with *P. africanum* use. In addition, subjects taking Pygeum extract were more than twice as likely to report an improvement in overall symptoms; nocturia was reduced by 19 percent, residual urine volume by 24 percent; and peak urine flow was increased by 23 percent.[3]

A lengthy 1995 literature review of the use of Pygeum extract for BPH also yielded positive findings for its efficacy. Twelve double-blind, placebo-controlled studies of *P. africanum* extract were analyzed, in which 358 patients received *P. africanum* extract and 359 received placebo. Taken as a whole, the results show a statistically significant benefit for *P. africanum* extract over placebo. Unfortunately, most of the studies had small patient numbers, although one study with 126 subjects showed a statistically significant benefit for Pygeum extract in maximum urinary flow rate, voided volume, residual volume, nocturia, daytime frequency, and impression of improvement scored by physicians and patients.[4]

In an experiment with 209 subjects with BPH using a parallel-group, double-blind, comparative phase (group A, 50 mg twice daily; group B, 100 mg once daily) and a ten-month open phase (100 mg once daily), the average International Prostate Symptom Score (IPSS) improved by 38 percent in group A and 35 percent in group B. Furthermore, the quality of life (QOL) index improved 28 percent in both groups, and the maximum urinary flow rate (Qmax) increased 16 percent in group A and 19 percent in group B.[12] After 12 months, the IPSS decreased an average of 46 percent and the Qmax increased 15 percent. In another open phase trial testing the efficacy of Tadenan®, a plant extract from Pygeum, 85 patients had significant improvements in IPSS (40%), QOL (32%), and nocturnal frequency (32%). Improvements in Qmax, average urinary flow, and urine volume were also statistically significant.[13]

In four relatively small studies, *P. africanum* was compared with: (1) sitosterin (n=53), (2) Urticae urtae radix extract (n=42), (3) non-steroidal anti-inflammatory or anti-infective treatment (n=39), or (4) non-steroidal anti-inflammatory treatment only (n=49). Although the results favored *P. africanum* extract over the other treatment groups, only a small number of patients were studied, and no statistical comparisons were made among treatments.[4]

Chronic Prostatitis

P. africanum extract (100 mg/d for 5-7 weeks) was used to treat 47 patients with chronic prostatitis (8 septic, 39 non-septic) in an open-label study. Eighty-nine percent of patients experienced complete remission of symptoms; whereas, there were no improvements in three septic patients and two non-septic patients.[4] In another study, *P. africanum* extract (200 mg/d for 60 days) was used either alone or in combination with antibiotics to treat 18 patients suffering from sexual disturbances due to either BPH or chronic prostatitis. Pygeum improved all the urinary parameters investigated by medical history and prostatic transrectal echography, and improved sexual function despite the fact there were no significant differences found between hormonal levels and nocturnal penile tumescence and rigidity monitoring before and after therapy. The authors stated that the results should be confirmed by other investigators but suggested *P. africanum* extract may be beneficial in the treatment of patients with sexual and/or reproductive dysfunction.[14]

Obstruction-induced Contractile Dysfunction

The obstructive component of the enlarged prostate often results in bladder outlet obstruction (BOO) due to increased outlet resistance. BOO results in detrusor muscle hypertrophy, hyperplasia, and instability, as well as collagen deposition. Tadenan was tested in four groups of New Zealand white rabbits to determine its ability to protect the bladder from contractile dysfunction caused by experimentally-induced BOO. In this study, Tadenan had a significant outcome of reducing the effect of BOO on bladder mass and reversing the contractile response secondary to urethral obstruction. These improvements were associated with Pygeum's ability to alter the expression of myosin isoforms (the contractile proteins in muscle fibers).[15] A similar study also found Tadenan was able to reverse bladder dysfunction induced by mild BOO and improve bladder function with severe BOO.[16] This extract also exerted a protective effect when administered as a pretreatment to rabbits prior to experimentally-induced BOO.[17]

Side Effects and Toxicity

The majority of the studies report an absence of any significant adverse effects of Pygeum, although there have been rare complaints of diarrhea, constipation, dizziness, gastric pain, and visual disturbances.[4,5] One study demonstrated continued satisfactory safety profiles in 174 human subjects after 12 months of 100 mg daily doses.[12] Toxicological studies have likewise shown very good tolerability after oral administration. Administration of Pygeum to dog and rat subjects equivalent to 560 times the therapeutic dose for six-month periods resulted in no adverse effects on hematological, biochemical, or anatomical/pathological parameters. The extract had no effect on fertility in male rats and rabbits at doses up to 80 mg/kg/day – a safety margin of 50 times the therapeutic dose. Furthermore, *in vivo* and *in vitro* mutagenicity studies showed a complete absence of mutagenic or clastogenic potential. In fact, many of the constituents of Pygeum have anticarcinogenic and antimutagenic properties *in vitro* and *in vivo*.[3]

Dosage

P. africanum extract is usually administered at a dose (standardized to contain 14 percent triterpenes including beta-sitosterol and 0.5percent n-docosanol) of 50-100 mg twice daily.[18] The efficacy of Pygeum extract at 50 mg twice daily and 100 mg once daily has been shown to have equivalent effectiveness.[12]

References

1. Simons AJ, Dawson IK, Dugumba B, Tchoundjeu Z. Passing problems: prostate and prunus. *HerbalGram* 1998;43:49-53.
2. Isaacs JT. Importance of the natural history of benign prostatic hyperplasia in the evaluation of pharmacologic intervention. *Prostate* 1990:3:1-7.
3. Ishani A, MacDonald R, Nelson D, et al. *Pygeum africanum* for the treatment of patients with benign prostatic hyperplasia: a systematic review and quantitative meta-analysis. *Am J Med* 2000;109:654-664.
4. Andro MC, Riffaud JP. *Pygeum africanum* extract for the treatment of patients with benign prostatic hyperplasia: a review of 25 years of published experience. *Curr Ther Res* 1995;56:796-817.
5. Murray MT. *The Healing Power of Herbs*. Rocklin, CA: Prima Publishing; 1995:286-293.
6. Paubert-Braquet M, Cave A, Hocquemiller R, et al. Effect of *Pygeum africanum* extract on A23187-stimulated production of lipoxygenase metabolites from human polymorphonuclear cells. *J Lipid Mediat Cell Signal* 1994;9:285-290.

7. Robinette CL. Sex-hormone induced inflammation and fibromuscular proliferation in the rat lateral prostate. *Prostate* 1988;12:271-286.
8. Paubert-Braquet M, Monboisse JC, Servent-Saez N, et al. Inhibition of bFGF and EGF-induced proliferation of 3T3 fibroblasts by extract of *Pygeum africanum* (Tadenan*). Biomed Pharmacother* 1994;48:43-47.
9. Desgrandchamps F. Clinical relevance of growth factor antagonists in the treatment of benign prostatic hyperplasia. *Eur Urol* 1997;32:28-31.
10. Luchetta G, Weill A, Becker N, et al. Reactivation of the secretion from the prostatic gland in cases of reduced fertility. Biological study of the seminal fluid modifications. *Urol Int* 1984;39:222-224.
11. Barlet A, Albrecht J, Aubert A, et al. Efficacy of *Pygeum africanum* extract in the medical therapy of urination disorders due to benign prostatic hyperplasia: evaluation of objective and subjective parameters. A placebo controlled double-blind multicenter study. *Wien Klin Wochenschr* 1990;102:667-673. [Article in German]
12. Chatelain C, Autet W, Brackman F. Comparison of once and twice daily dosage forms of *Pygeum africanum* extract in patients with benign prostatic hyperplasia: a randomized, double-blind study, with long-term open label extension. *Urol* 1999;54:473-478.
13. Breza J, Dzurny O, Borowka A, et al. Efficacy and acceptability of Tadenan (*Pygeum africanum* extract) in the treatment of benign prostatic hyperplasia (BPH): a multicentre trial in central Europe. *Curr Med Res Opin* 1998;14:127-139.
14. Carani C, Salvioli V, Scuteri A, et al. Urological and sexual evaluation of treatment of benign prostatic disease using *Pygeum africanum* at high doses. *Arch Ital Urol Nefrol Androl* 1991;63:341-345. [Article in Italian]
15. Gomes CM, Disanto ME, Horan P, et al. Improved contractility of obstructed bladders after Tadenan treatment is associated with reversal of altered myosin isoform expression. *J Urol* 2000;163:2008-2013.
16. Levin RM, Das AK, Haugaard N, et al. Beneficial effects of Tadenan therapy after two weeks of partial obstruction in the rabbit. *Neurourol Urodyn* 1997;16:583-599.
17. Levin RM, Riffaud JP, Bellamy F, et al. Protective effect of Tadenan on bladder function secondary to partial outlet obstruction. *J Urol* 1996;155:1466-1470.
18. Murray M, Pizzorno J. *Encyclopedia of Natural Medicine.* Rocklin, CA: Prima Publishing; 1998:762.

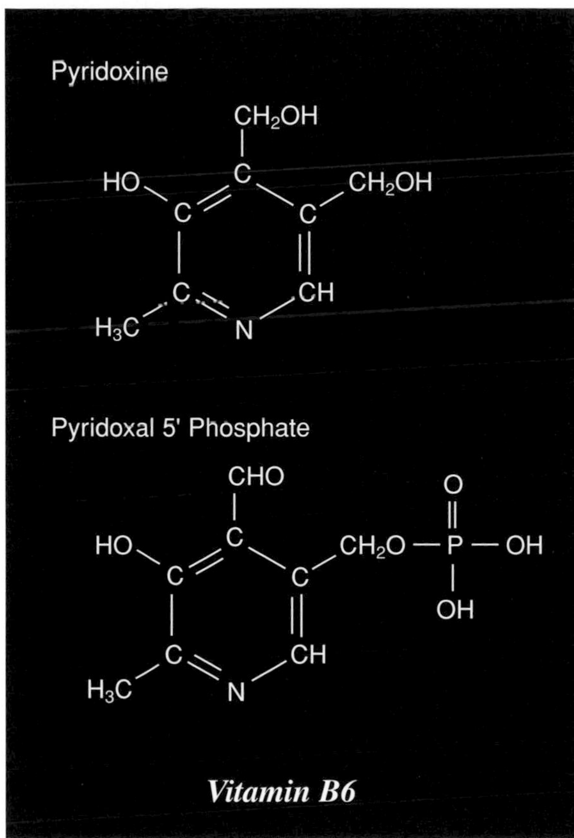

Vitamin B6

Pyridoxine and Pyridoxal 5'-Phosphate

Introduction

Vitamin B6 (also know as Pyridoxine and Pyridoxal 5'-phosphate) was first isolated in 1934 and named by Albert Szent-Gyorgy.[1] Vitamin B6 consists of three related pyrimidine vitamer derivates: pyridoxine, pyridoxal, and pyridoxamine, and their phosphate esters. The metabolically active coenzyme form of vitamin B6 is pyridoxal 5'-phosphate (P5P),[1] which is the main circulating form exported from the liver and is considered the most relevant direct measure of vitamin B6 status.[2] The standard B6 vitamin supplement is pyridoxine hydrochloride (HCl), which is the least expensive to produce commercially;[3] however, P5P is the only form that can be used by enzymes involved in numerous biochemical processes.[4]

Pharmacokinetics

Pyridoxine is water soluble and stable in heat and acid mediums, while it is unstable in alkaline solutions and light.[5] Pyridoxine and its vitamers are absorbed in the upper small intestine by simple diffusion and transported to the liver for biotransformation into the active coenzyme P5P. B6 vitamers are first oxidized to pyridoxal, and rapidly phosphorylated to P5P in the liver,[6] then exported from the liver bound to albumin. Uptake into tissue is by extracellular de-phosphorylation, followed by metabolic trapping intracellularly as P5P.[7]

Plasma P5P levels were found to be significantly lower than normal in 22 out of 31 patients with impaired liver function, which reflects the liver's importance in B6 conversion. In patients receiving intravenous pyridoxine HCl, only 33 percent responded with an increase in plasma P5P, while all of the patients receiving P5P responded with an increase.[8]

P5P-dependent enzymes are involved in the following reactions:[7]

- decarboxylation of amino acids to yield amines, many of which are important neurotransmitters and hormones.
- transamination of amino acids to keto-acids, which are then oxidized and used as metabolic fuel.
- phosphorolytic cleavage of glycogen (from liver and muscle) to glucose-one-phosphate.
- formation of alpha aminolevulinic acid, a precursor to heme.
- decarboxylation of phosphatidylserine to phosphatidylethanolamine in phospholipid synthesis.
- as a co-factor in a variety of reactions involving side-chain cleavage, including cystathionine synthase and cystathionase.

Deficiency States and Symptoms

Overt vitamin B6 deficiency can manifest in a variety of symptoms including: seborrheic dermatitis, glossitis, chelosis, peripheral neuropathy, lymphopenia, and anemia. In infants, B6 deficiency can also cause convulsions.

Clinical Indications

Anemia

P5P is necessary for the activation of glycine in the initial stages of heme production. Several cases of B6-responsive anemia have shown no response to pyridoxine and prompt response to P5P. This suggests an enzymatic deficiency or inhibition of pyridoxal kinase.[9] In another study, excessive alcohol produced bone marrow sideroblastic changes that were responsive to P5P, while no response was achieved from pyridoxine or folic acid.[10] From a therapeutic point of view, P5P should be tried in all cases of symptomatic primary sideroblastic anemia that have shown no response to pyridoxine.[9]

In 16 patients with sickle cell anemia, plasma P5P concentrations were significantly lower than in 16 controls. Oral supplementation of five of the patients with 50 mg pyridoxine twice daily for two months resulted in increased plasma P5P levels.[11] Since pyridoxine and P5P have been shown to have anti-sickling properties *in vitro*,[12,13] these studies suggest P5P supplementation may also be of therapeutic benefit *in vivo* in sickle cell anemia.[11]

Carpal Tunnel Syndrome

Researchers have found a direct correlation between carpal tunnel syndrome (CTS) and a deficiency in P5P, and that treatment with 100-200 mg pyridoxine daily for at least 12 weeks was highly beneficial in reducing both the symptomatology and a P5P deficiency associated with CTS.[14-16] A few studies have shown no clinical benefit from pyridoxine HCl supplementation,[17-19] with most of the reports of beneficial effects coming from Ellis et al.[15,20-23] A 1996 literature review of clinical trials using pyridoxine to treat CTS concluded that the evidence for the use of pyridoxine as the sole treatment for CTS is weak, but that it may be valuable as an adjunctive treatment through its effect on altered perception of pain and increased pain threshold.[24]

Premenstrual Syndrome (PMS)

Vitamin B6 nutritional status has a significant and selective modulatory impact on central production of both serotonin and GABA – neurotransmitters that control depression, pain perception, and anxiety.[25] P5P is a cofactor in the synthesis of these neurotransmitters.[26] Authors of a 1999 review of published and unpublished randomized placebo-controlled trials of the effectiveness of vitamin B-6 in the management of PMS concluded that the pooled data of nine trials representing 940 patients suggests doses of pyridoxine up to 100 mg/day are likely to be of benefit in treating premenstrual symptoms, including premenstrual depression.[27]

Hyperhomocysteinemia

High levels of plasma homocysteine are considered an independent risk factor for atherosclerotic disease and venous thrombosis. Homocysteine, an intermediate in methionine metabolism, can be re-methylated to methionine, or be channeled through the trans-sulfuration pathway to cysteine, which requires two P5P-dependent enzymes: cystathionine synthase and cystathionase.[7]

A study of 1,160 elderly subjects (67-96 years) correlated high homocysteine levels with low folate and B6.[28] Results of the 1998 Nurses' Health Study showed cardiovascular disease risk was lowest among those women with the highest intakes of folate and B6.[29] Vitamin therapy – a combination of folic acid (500 mcg) and pyridoxine (100 mg) – in 49 hyperhomocysteinemic individuals significantly reduced fasting plasma homocysteine concentrations (median 13.9 to 9.3 mM/L, reduction 32%) and post-methionine load concentrations (median 55.2 to 36.5 mM/L, reduction 30%).[30]

Other Clinical Indications

A double-blind trial using pyridoxine (25 mg every eight hours for three days) in the treatment of morning sickness resulted in a significant reduction in vomiting, and an improvement in nausea in those who initially reported severe nausea.[31]

Researchers in Japan published animal studies suggesting that B6 deficiencies impair conversion of alpha-linolenic acid to EPA and DHA, with the most pronounced reduction in production of DHA.[32]

P5P has also been shown to protect rat kidneys from the nephrotoxicity of aminoglycoside antibiotics.[33] Pyridoxine in low doses (10 mg/day) is also of therapeutic value for hyperoxaluric kidney stone formers.[34]

There are many more proposed indications for P5P such as asthma, autism, acne, diabetes mellitus, depression, toxemia of pregnancy, and side effects of oral contraceptives, which are less clinically and experimentally documented.[35-41]

Drug-Nutrient Interactions

- The anti-tuberculosis drug isoniazid can result in a functional vitamin B6 deficiency.[42]
- Anti-Parkinsonian drugs benserazide and carbidopa cause vitamin B6 depletion by forming hydrazones.[43]
- Pyridoxine will reduce the efficacy of levodopa in controlling Parkinsonian symptoms, the magnitude of the effect proportional to the dose of pyridoxine.[44]
- There have been many reports of abnormal tryptophan metabolism in women taking either oral contraceptive or menopausal hormone replacement therapy, which have been interpreted as indicating estrogen-induced vitamin B6 deficiency or depletion.[7]

Side Effects and Toxicity

The use of supplemental P5P has not been associated with toxicity, although the inactive form, pyridoxine, has been associated with reports of peripheral neuropathy.[45] One hypothesis is that pyridoxine toxicity is caused by exceeding the liver's ability to phosphorylate pyridoxine to P5P, yielding high serum levels of pyridoxine which may be directly neurotoxic or may compete with P5P for binding sites, resulting in a relative deficiency.[46]

Mpofu et al reported electrophysiological and neurological examination of 17 homocystinuric patients who had been treated with 200-500 mg pyridoxine HCl daily for 10-24 years, and found no evidence of neuropathy.[47] Most reported cases of neuropathy associated with pyridoxine supplementation have involved intake of at least 500 mg/day for two years or more.[48] While there is little doubt that vitamin B6 can be neurotoxic in gross excess, there is considerable controversy over the way in which toxicological data have been translated into advised limits.[7]

Dosage

While the RDA for adults is 2-4 mg daily, the typical therapeutic dose is 50-200 mg/day.

References

1. Oka T. Vitamin B6. *Nippon Rinsho* 1999;57:2199-2204. [Article in Japanese]
2. Leklem JE. Vitamin B6: a status report. *J Nutr* 1990;120:1503-1507.
3. Haas E. *Staying Healthy with Nutrition. The Complete Guide to Diet and Nutritional Medicine*. Berkeley, CA: Celestial Arts Publishing; 1992:122.
4. Parker TH, Marshall JP 2d, Roberts RK, et al. Effect of acute alcohol ingestion on plasma pyridoxal 5'-phosphate. *Am J Clin Nutr* 1979;32:1246-1252.
5. Marz R. *Medical Nutrition from Marz. A Textbook in Clinical Nutrition*. Portland, OR: Omni Press; 1997:211.
6. Merrill AH Jr, Henderson JM. Vitamin B6 metabolism by human liver. *Ann N Y Acad Sci* 1990;585:110-117.
7. Bender D. Non-nutritional uses of vitamin B6. *Br J Nutr* 1999;81:7-20.
8. Labadarios D, Rossouw JE, McConnell JB, et al. Vitamin B6 deficiency in chronic liver disease – evidence for increased degradation of pyridoxal-5-phosphate. *Gut* 1977;18:23-27.
9. Mason DY, Emerson PM. Primary acquired sideroblastic anemia: response to treatment with pyridoxal-5-phosphate. *Br Med J* 1973;1:389-390.
10. Hines JD, Cowan DH. Studies on the pathogenesis of alcohol-induced sideroblastic bone-marrow abnormalities. *N Engl J Med* 1970;283:441-446.
11. Natta CL, Reynolds RD. Apparent vitamin B6 deficiency in sickle cell anemia. *Am J Clin Nutr* 1984;40:235-239.
12. Kark JA, Kale MP, Tarassoff PG, et al. Inhibition of erythrocyte sickling *in vitro* by pyridoxal. *J Clin Invest* 1978;62:888-891.
13. Kark JA, Tarassoff PG, Bongiovanni R. Pyridoxal phosphate as an antisickling agent *in vitro*. *J Clin Invest* 1983;71:1224-1229.
14. Fuhr JE, Farrow A, Nelson HS Jr. Vitamin B6 levels in patients with carpal tunnel syndrome. *Arch Surg* 1989;124:1329-1330.
15. Ellis JM. Treatment of carpal tunnel syndrome with vitamin B6. *South Med J* 1987;80:882-884.
16. Ellis J, Folkers K, Watanabe T, et al. Clinical results of a cross-over treatment with pyridoxine and placebo of the carpal tunnel syndrome. *Am J Clin Nutr* 1979;32:2040-2046.
17. Spooner GR, Desai HB, Angel JF, et al. Using pyridoxine to treat carpal tunnel syndrome. Randomized control trial. *Can Fam Physician* 1993;39:2122-2127.
18. Stransky M, Rubin A, Lava NS, Lazaro RP. Treatment of carpal tunnel syndrome with vitamin B6: a double blind study. *South Med J* 1989;82:841-842.
19. Franzblau A, Rock CL, Werner RA, et al. The relationship of vitamin B6 status to median nerve function and carpal tunnel syndrome among active industrial workers. *J Occup Environ Med* 1996;38:485-491.
20. Ellis JM, Azuma J, Watanabe T, et al. Survey and new data on treatment with pyridoxine of patients having a clinical syndrome including the carpal tunnel and other defects. *Res Commun Chem Pathol Pharmacol* 1977;17:165-177.
21. Ellis JM, Folkers K. Clinical aspects of treatment of carpal tunnel syndrome with vitamin B6. *Ann N Y Acad Sci* 1990;585:302-320.
22. Ellis JM, Folkers K, Levy M, et al. Response of vitamin B-6 deficiency and the carpal tunnel syndrome to pyridoxine. *Proc Natl Acad Sci U S A* 1982;79:7494-7498.
23. Ellis JM, Kishi T, Azuma J, Folkers K. Vitamin B6 deficiency in patients with a clinical syndrome including the carpal tunnel defect. Biochemical and clinical response to therapy with pyridoxine. *Res Commun Chem Pathol Pharmacol* 1976;13:743-757.
24. Jacobson MD, Plancher KD, Kleinman WB. Vitamin B6 (pyridoxine) therapy for carpal tunnel syndrome. *Hand Clin* 1996;12:253-257.

25. McCarty MF. High-dose pyridoxine as an 'anti-stress' strategy. *Med Hypotheses* 2000;54:803-807.

26. Head KA. Premenstrual syndrome: nutritional and alternative approaches. *Altern Med Rev* 1997;2:12-25.

27. Wyatt KM, Dimmock PW, Jones PW, Shaughn O'Brien PM. Efficacy of vitamin B6 in the treatment of premenstrual syndrome: systematic review. *BMJ* 1999;318:1375-1381.

28. Selhub J, Jacques PF, Wilson PW, et al. Vitamin status and intake as primary determinants of homocysteinemia in an elderly population. *JAMA* 1993;270:2693-2698.

29. Rimm EB, Willett WC, Hu FB, et al. Folate and vitamin B6 from diet and supplements in relation to risk of coronary heart disease among women. *JAMA* 1998;279:359-364.

30. Van der Griend R, Haas FJ, Biesma DH, et al. Combination of low-dose folic acid and pyridoxine for treatment of hyperhomocysteinaemia in patients with premature arterial disease and their relatives. *Atherosclerosis* 1999;143:177-183.

31. Sahakian V, Rouse D, Sipes S, et al. Vitamin B6 is effective therapy for nausea and vomiting of pregnancy: a randomized, double-blind placebo-controlled study. *Obstet Gynecol* 1991;78:33-36.

32. Tsuge H, Hotta N, Hayakawa T. Effects of vitamin B-6 on (n-3) polyunsaturated fatty acid metabolism. *J Nutr* 2000;130:333S-334S.

33. Kojima R, Ito M, Suzuki Y. Studies on the nephrotoxicity of aminoglycoside antibiotics and protection from these effects (8): Protective effect of pyridoxal-5'-phosphate against tobramycin nephrotoxicity. *Jpn J Pharmacol* 1990;52:11-21.

34. Murthy MS, Farooqui S, Talwar HS, et al. Effect of pyridoxine supplementation on recurrent stone formers. *Int J Clin Pharmacol Ther Toxicol* 1982;20:434-437.

35. Sur S, Camara M, Buchmeier A, et al. Double-blind trial of pyridoxine (vitamin B6) in the treatment of steroid-dependent asthma. *Ann Allergy* 1993;70:147-152.

36. Rimland B, Calloway E, Dreyfus P. The effect of high doses vitamin B6 on autistic children: a double-blind crossover study. *Am J Psychiatry* 1978;135:472-475.

37. Snider BL, Dieteman DF. Pyridoxine therapy for premenstrual acne flare. *Arch Dermatol* 1974;110:130-131. [Letter]

38. Spellacy WN, Buhi WC, Birk SA. Vitamin B6 treatment of gestational diabetes mellitus: studies of blood glucose and plasma insulin. *Am J Obstet Gynecol* 1977;127:599-602.

39. Russ CS. Vitamin B6 status of depressed and obsessive-compulsive patients. *Nutr Rep Int* 1983;27:867-873.

40. Wachstein G. Influence of B6 on the incidence of pre-eclampsia. *Gynecol* 1956;8:177.

41. Adams PW, Wynn V, Folkard J, et al. Influence of oral contraceptives, pyridoxine, and tryptophan on carbohydrate metabolism. *Lancet* 1975;1:759-764.

42. Standal BR, Kao-Chen SM, Yang GY, Char DF. Early changes in pyridoxine status of patients receiving isoniazid therapy. *Am J Clin Nutr* 1974;27:479-484.

43. Bender DA. Effects of benserazide, carbidopa and isoniazid administration on tryptophan-nicotinamide nucleotide metabolism in the rat. *Biochem Pharmacol* 1980;29:2099-2104.

44. Hunter KR, Stern GM, Laurence DR. Use of levodopa with other drugs. *Lancet* 1970;2:1283-1285.

45. Schaumburg H, Kaplan J, Windebank A, et al. Sensory neuropathy from pyridoxine abuse. A new megavitamin syndrome. *N Engl J Med* 1983;309:445-448.

46. Parry GJ, Bredesen DE. Sensory neuropathy with low-dose pyridoxine. *Neurology* 1985;35:1466-1468.

47. Mpofu C, Alani SM, Whitehouse C, et al.. No sensory neuropathy during pyridoxine treatment in homocystinuria. *Arch Dis Child* 1991;66:1081-1082.

48. Bendich A, Cohen M. Vitamin B6 safety issues. *Ann N Y Acad Sci* 1990;585:321-330.

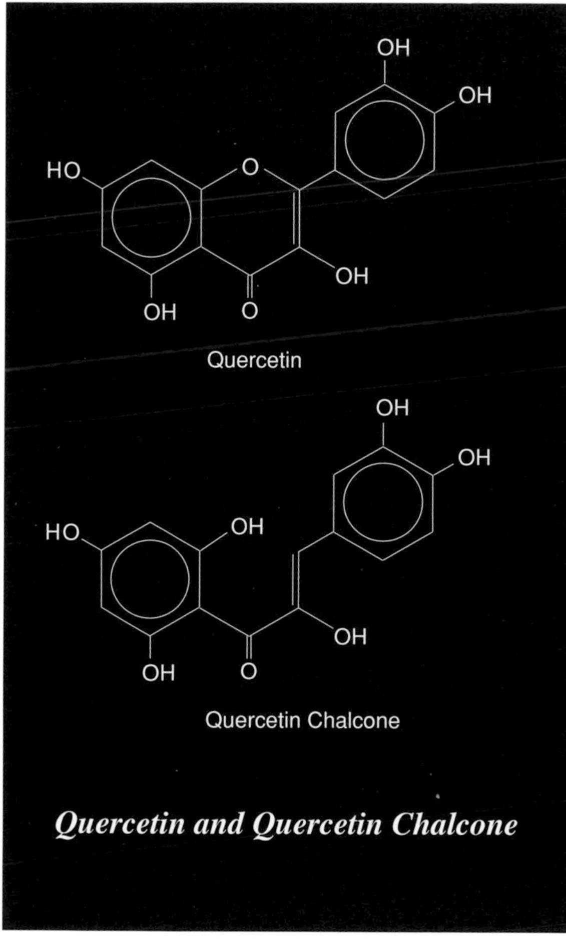

Quercetin and Quercetin Chalcone

Quercetin

Introduction

Quercetin is widely distributed in the plant kingdom and is the most abundant of the flavonoid molecules. It is found in many often-consumed foods, including apple, onion, tea, berries, and brassica vegetables, as well as many seeds, nuts, flowers, barks, and leaves. It is also found in medicinal botanicals, including *Ginkgo biloba*, *Hypericum perforatum* (St. John's Wort), *Sambucus canadensis* (Elder), and many others, and is often a component of the medicinal activity of the plant. Quercetin appears to have many beneficial effects on human health, including cataract prevention, cardiovascular protection, as well as anti-cancer, anti-ulcer, anti-allergy, antiviral, and anti-inflammatory activity.

All flavonoids have the same basic chemical structure – a three-ringed molecule with hydroxyl (OH) groups attached. A multitude of other substitutions can occur, giving rise to more than 4,000 identified flavonoids. Flavonoids often occur in foods as a glycoside – with a sugar molecule (rhamnose, glucose, galactose, etc.) attached to the C ring. Quercetin is the aglycone (without the sugar molecule) of a number of other flavonoids, including rutin, quercetrin, isoquercetin, and hyperoside. These molecules have the same structure as quercetin except they have a specific sugar molecule in place of one of quercetin's hydroxyl groups on the C ring. This difference can dramatically change the activity of the molecule, as activity comparison studies have identified other flavonoids as often having similar effects as quercetin, but quercetin usually having the greatest activity.

Pharmacokinetics

Few human quercetin absorption studies exist. It appears only a small percentage of quercetin is absorbed after an oral dose; only two percent according to one study.[1] A study of quercetin absorption in ileostomy patients revealed absorption of 24 percent of the pure aglycone and 52 percent of quercetin glycosides from onions;[2] however, no intestinal permeability values were obtained in this group, and thus the results might not be reliable. Absorbed quercetin is transported to the liver bound to albumin,[3] where some may be metabolized via hydroxylation, methylation, sulphation, or conjugation.[4] Unabsorbed quercetin undergoes bacterial metabolism in the intestinal tract, where it is converted into phenolic acids.

Mechanisms of Action

Flavonoids, as a rule, are antioxidants, and a number of quercetin's effects appear to be due to its antioxidant activity. Quercetin scavenges oxygen radicals,[5,6] inhibits xanthine oxidase,[7,8] and inhibits lipid peroxidation *in vitro*.[9,10] As another indicator of its antioxidant effects, quercetin inhibits oxidation of LDL cholesterol *in vitro*,[11,12] probably by inhibiting LDL oxidation itself, by protecting vitamin E in LDL from being oxidized or by regenerating oxidized vitamin E.[13] By itself, and paired with ascorbic acid, quercetin reduced the incidence of oxidative damage to human lymphocytes and neurovasculature structures in skin, and inhibited damage to neurons caused by experimental glutathione depletion.[14,15]

Quercetin's anti-inflammatory activity appears to be due to its antioxidant capacity, its inhibitory effects on inflammation-producing enzymes (cyclooxygenase, lipoxygenase), and the subsequent inhibition of inflammatory mediators including leukotrienes and prostaglandins.[16-18] Inhibition of histamine release by mast cells and basophils[19-21] also contributes to quercetin's anti-inflammatory activity.

Aldose reductase, the enzyme that catalyzes the conversion of glucose to sorbitol, is especially important in the eye and plays a part in the formation of diabetic cataracts. Quercetin is a strong inhibitor of aldose reductase in the human lens.[22]

Quercetin exerts antiviral activity against reverse transcriptase of HIV[23] and other retroviruses, and was shown to reducc the infectivity and cellular replication of herpes simplex virus type 1, polio-virus type 1, parainfluenza virus type 3, and respiratory syncytial virus (RSV).[24]

Clinical Indications

Allergies

Quercetin's mast cell-stabilizing effects make it an obvious choice for use in preventing histamine release in allergy cases, similar to the use of the synthetic flavonoid analogue cromolyn sodium. Studies show quercetin's ability to inhibit histamine release stimulated by IgE-dependent ligands.[21] Absorption of the pure aglycone quercetin is poor; however, much of quercetin's anti-allergy effects may be due to anti-inflammatory and anti-histaminic effects in the gut.

Cardiovascular Disease Prevention

Quercetin's cardiovascular effects center on its antioxidant and anti-inflammatory activity, and possibly by its ability to inhibit platelet aggregation.[25]

The Zutphen Elderly Study investigated dietary flavonoid intake and risk of coronary heart disease.[26] The risk of heart disease mortality decreased significantly as flavonoid intake increased. Individuals in the upper 25 percent of flavonoid intake had a relative risk of 0.42 compared to the lowest 25 percent in this five-year follow-up study of men ages 65-84. The flavonoid-containing foods most commonly eaten in this study contained a high amount of quercetin (tea, onions, apples). In a cohort of the same study, dietary intake of flavonoids (mainly quercetin) was inversely associated with stroke incidence.[27] In a clinical trial of quercetin supplementation in healthy subjects, a marked increase in plasma quercetin levels was seen; however, no improvements were noted in selected risk factors for cardiovascular disease or thrombogenesis.[28]

Inflammation

Quercetin is indicated in inflammatory conditions, as it inhibits formation of prostaglandins and leukotrienes, as well as histamine release. This may be especially helpful in asthma, as leukotriene B4 is a potent bronchoconstrictor. Patients suffering from chronic inflammatory conditions such as chronic prostatitis and interstitial cystitis show significant symptomatic improvement with oral quercetin supplementation (500 mg BID for one month).[29,30]

Ulcer/Gastritis

Animal studies have shown quercetin to be protective of gastric ulceration caused by ethanol, probably by inhibiting lipid peroxidation of gastric cells[31,32] and/or by inhibition of gastric acid secretion.[33] An interesting aspect of quercetin's anti-ulcer effect is that it has been shown to inhibit growth of *Helicobacter pylori* in a dose-dependent manner *in vitro*.[33]

Cancer

Quercetin has been investigated in a number of animal models and human cancer cell lines, and has been found to have antiproliferative effects in numerous cancer cell types, including breast,[34-37] leukemia,[38-40] colon,[41-43] ovary,[44-46] squamous cell,[47,48] endometrial,[34] gastric,[49] and non-small-cell lung.[50,51] It may also increase the effectiveness of chemotherapeutic agents.[44,45] Phase one clinical trials show evidence of *in vivo* lymphocyte tyrosine kinase inhibition and anti-tumor activity of parenteral quercetin.[52] More clinically oriented research needs to be done in this area to discover effective dosage ranges and protocols.

Diabetic Complications

Quercetin's antioxidant activity and aldose reductase-inhibiting properties make it a useful addition to diabetic nutritional supplementation, to prevent cataracts and neurovascular complications.

Side Effects and Toxicity

Early studies on quercetin reported that its administration to rats caused an increased incidence of urinary bladder tumors. Subsequent studies on rats, mice, and hamsters have been unable to confirm this finding.[53,54]

Dosage

An oral dose of 400-500 mg three times per day is typically used in clinical practice. Since solubility is an issue in quercetin absorption,[4] a new, water-soluble quercetin molecule, quercetin chalcone, might be used in smaller doses; typically 250 mg three times per day.

References

1. Gugler R, Leschik M, Dengler HJ. Disposition of quercetin in man after single oral and intravenous doses. *Eur J Clin Pharmacol* 1975;9:229-234.
2. Hollman PC, de Vries JH, van Leeuwen SD, et al. Absorption of dietary quercetin glycosides and quercetin in healthy ileostomy volunteers. *Am J Clin Nutr* 1995;62:1276-1282.
3. Boulton DW, Walle UK, Walle T. Extensive binding of the bioflavonoid quercetin to human plasma proteins. *J Pharm Pharmacol* 1998;50:243-249.
4. Manach C, Regerat F, Texier O, et al. Bioavailability, metabolism and physiological impact of 4-oxo-flavonoids. *Nutrition Research* 1996;16:517-534.
5. Saija A, Scalese M, Lanza M, et al. Flavonoids as antioxidant agents: importance of their interaction with biomembranes. *Free Radic Biol Med* 1995;19:481-486.
6. Miller AL. Antioxidant flavonoids: structure, function and clinical usage. *Altern Med Rev* 1996;1:103-111.
7. Chang WS, Lee YJ, Lu FJ, Chiang HC. Inhibitory effects of flavonoids on xanthine oxidase. *Anticancer Res* 1993;13:2165-2170.
8. Nagao A, Seki M, Kobayashi H. Inhibition of xanthine oxidase by flavonoids. *Biosci Biotechnol Biochem* 1999;63:1787-1790.
9. Chen YT, Zheng RL, Jia ZJ, Ju Y. Flavonoids as superoxide scavengers and antioxidants. *Free Radic Biol Med* 1990;9:19-21.
10. Kuhlmann MK, Burkhardt G, Horsch E, et al. Inhibition of oxidant-induced lipid peroxidation in cultured renal tubular epithelial cells (LLC-PK1) by quercetin. *Free Radic Res* 1998;29:451-460.
11. O'Reilly JD, Sanders TA, Wiseman H. Flavonoids protect against oxidative damage to LDL *in vitro*: use in selection of a flavonoid rich diet and relevance to LDL oxidation resistance *ex vivo*? *Free Radic Res* 2000;33:419-426.
12. da Silva EL, Abdalla DS, Terao J. Inhibitory effect of flavonoids on low-density lipoprotein peroxidation catalyzed by mammalian 15-lipoxygenase. *IUBMB Life* 2000;49:289-295.
13. DeWhalley CV, Rankin JF, Rankin SM, et al. Flavonoids inhibit the oxidative modification of low density lipoproteins. *Biochem Pharmacol* 1990;39:1743-1749.

14. Skaper SD, Fabris M, Ferrari V, et al. Quercetin protects cutaneous tissue-associated cell types including sensory neurons from oxidative stress induced by glutathione depletion: cooperative effects of ascorbic acid. *Free Radic Biol Med* 1997;22:669-678.

15. Noroozi M, Angerson WJ, Lean ME. Effects of flavonoids and vitamin C on oxidative DNA damage to human lymphocytes. *Am J Clin Nutr* 1998;67:1210-1218.

16. Della Loggia R, Ragazzi E, Tubaro A, et al. Anti-inflammatory activity of benzopyrones that are inhibitors of cyclo- and lipo-oxygenase. *Pharmacol Res Commun* 1988;20:S91-S94.

17. Kim HP, Mani I, Ziboh VA. Effects of naturally-occurring flavonoids and biflavonoids on epidermal cyclooxygenase from guinea pigs. *Prostaglandins Leukot Essent Fatty Acids* 1998;58:17-24.

18. Raso GM, Meli R, Di Carlo G, et al. Inhibition of inducible nitric oxide synthase and cyclooxygenase-2 expression by flavonoids in macrophage J774A.1. *Life Sci* 2001;68:921-931.

19. Fox CC, Wolf EJ, Kagey-Sobotka A, Lichtenstein LM. Comparison of human lung and intestinal mast cells. *J Allergy Clin Immunol* 1988;81:89-94.

20. Bronner C, Landry Y. Kinetics of the inhibitory effect of flavonoids on histamine secretion from mast cells. *Agents Actions* 1985;16:147-151.

21. Midddleton E Jr, Drzewiecki G. Flavonoid inhibition of human basophil histamine release stimulated by various agents. *Biochem Pharmacol* 1984;33:3333-3338.

22. Chaudry PS, Cabera J, Juliani HR, Varma SD. Inhibition of human lens aldose reductase by flavonoids, sulindac, and indomethacin. *Biochem Pharmacol* 1983;32:1995-1998.

23. Harada S, Haneda E, Maekawa T, et al. Casein kinase II (CK-II)-mediated stimulation of HIV-1 reverse transcriptase activity and characterization of selective inhibitors *in vitro*. *Biol Pharm Bull* 1999;22:1122-1126.

24. Kaul TN, Middleton E Jr, Ogra PL. Antiviral effect of flavonoids on human viruses. *J Med Virol* 1985;15:71-79.

25. Pace-Asciak CR, Hahn S, Diamandis EP, et al. The red wine phenolics trans-resveratrol and quercetin block human platelet aggregation and eicosanoid synthesis: implications for protection against coronary heart disease. *Clin Chim Acta* 1995;235:207-219.

26. Hertog MG, Feskens J, Hollman PC, et al. Dietary antioxidant flavonoids and risk of coronary heart disease: the Zutphen Elderly Study. *Lancet* 1993;342:1007-1011.

27. Keli SO, Hertog MG, Feskens EJ, Kromhout D. Dietary flavonoids, antioxidant vitamins, and incidence of stroke: the Zutphen study. *Arch Intern Med* 1996;156:637-642.

28. Conquer JA, Maiani G, Azzini E, et al. Supplementation with quercetin markedly increases plasma quercetin concentration without effect on selected risk factors for heart disease in healthy subjects. *J Nutr* 1998;128:593-597.

29. Shoskes DA, Zeitlin SI, Shahed A, et al. Quercetin in men with category III chronic prostatitis: a preliminary prospective, double-blind, placebo-controlled trial. *Urology* 1999;54:960-963.

30. Katske F, Shoskes DA, Sender M, et al. Treatment of interstitial cystitis with a quercetin supplement. *Tech Urol* 2001;7:44-46.

31. Alarcon de la Lastra C, Martin MJ, Motilva V. Antiulcer and gastroprotective effects of quercetin: a gross and histologic study. *Pharmacology* 1994;48:56-62.

32. Mizui T, Sato H, Hirose F, Doteuchi M. Effect of antiperoxidative drugs on gastric damage induced by ethanol in rats. *Life Sci* 1987;41:755-763.

33. Beil W, Birkholz C, Sewing KF. Effects of flavonoids on parietal cell acid secretion, gastric mucosal prostaglandin production and Helicobacter pylori growth. *Arzneimittelforschung* 1995;45:697-700.

34. Scambia G, Raneletti FO, Panici PB, et al. Quercetin induces type-II estrogen-binding sites in estrogen-receptor-negative (MDA-MB231) and estrogen-receptor-positive (MCF-7) human breast-cancer cell lines. *Int J Cancer* 1993;54:462-466.

35. Scambia G, Raneletti FO, Panici PB, et al. Quercetin inhibits the growth of a multidrug-resistant estrogen-receptor-negative MCF-7 human breast-cancer cell line expressing type II estrogen-binding sites. *Cancer Chemother Pharmacol* 1991;28:255-258.

36. Singhal RL, Yeh YA, Prajda N, et al. Quercetin down-regulates signal transduction in human breast carcinoma cells. *Biochem Biophys Res Comm* 1995;208:425-431.

37. Choi JA, Kim JY, Lee JY, et al. Induction of cell cycle arrest and apoptosis in human breast cancer cells by quercetin. *Int J Oncol* 2001;19:837-844.

38. Larocca LM, Teofili L, Sica S, et al. Quercetin inhibits the growth of leukemic progenitors and induces the expression of transforming growth factor-B1 in these cells. *Blood* 1995;85:3654-3661.

39. Larocca LM, Teofili L, Leone G, et al. Antiproliferative activity of quercetin on normal bone marrow and leukaemic progenitors. *Br J Haematol* 1991;79:562-566.

40. Kim SY, Gao JJ, Kang HK. Two flavonoids from the leaves of *Morus alba* induce differentiation of the human promyelocytic leukemia (HL-60) cell line. *Biol Pharm Bull* 2000;23:451-455.

41. Pereira MA, Grubbs CJ, Barnes LH, et al. Effects of the phytochemicals, curcumin and quercetin, upon azoxymethane-induced colon cancer and 7,12-dimethylbenzy[a]anthracene-induced mammary cancer in rats. *Carcinogenesis* 1996;17:1305-1311.

42. Hayashi A, Gillen AC, Lott JR. Effects of daily oral administration of quercetin chalcone and modified citrus pectin. *Altern Med Rev* 2000;5:546-552.

43. Ranelletti FO, Maggiano N, Serra FG, et al. Quercetin inhibits p21-RAS expression in human colon cancer cell lines and in primary colorectal tumors. *Int J Cancer* 2000;85:438-445.

44. Scambia G, Raneletti FO, Panici PB, et al. Inhibitory effect of quercetin on primary ovarian and endometrial cancers and synergistic activity with cis-diamminedichloroplatinum(II). *Gynecol Oncology* 1992;45:13-19.

45. Scambia G, Raneletti FO, Panici PB, et al. Synergistic antiproliferative activity of quercetin and cisplatin on ovarian cancer cell growth. *Anticancer Drugs* 1990;1:45-48.

46. Li W, Shen F, Weber G. Ribavirin and quercetin synergistically downregulate signal transduction and are cytotoxic in human ovarian carcinoma cells. *Oncol Res* 1999;11:243-247.

47. Castillo MH, Perkins E, Campbell JH. The effects of the bioflavonoid quercetin on squamous cell carcinoma of head and neck origin. *Am J Surg* 1989;158:351-355.

48. ElAttar TM, Virji AS. Modulating effect of resveratrol and quercetin on oral cancer cell growth and proliferation. *Anticancer Drugs* 1999;10:187-193.

49. Yoshida M, Sakai T, Hosokawa N, et al. The effect of quercetin on cell cycle progression and growth of human gastric cancer cells. *FEBS Letters* 1990;260:10-13.

50. Caltagirone S, Raneletti FO, Rinelli A, et al. Interaction with type II estrogen binding sites and antiproliferative activity of tamoxifen and quercetin in human non-small-cell lung cancer. *Am J Resp Cell Mol Biol* 1997;17:51-59.

51. Le Marchand L, Murphy SP, Hankin JH, et al. Intake of flavonoids and lung cancer. *J Natl Cancer Inst* 2000;92:154-160.

52. Ferry DR, Smith A, Malkhandi J, et al. Phase I clinical trial of the flavonoid quercetin: pharmacokinetics and evidence for *in vivo* tyrosine kinase inhibition. *Clin Cancer Res* 1996;2:659-668.

53. Stavric B. Quercetin in our diet: from potent mutagen to probable anticarcinogen. *Clin Biochem* 1994;27:245-248.

54. Hertog MGL, Hollman PCH. Potential health effects of the dietary flavonol quercetin. *Eur J Clin Nutr* 1996;50:63-71.

Rhodiola rosea

Description

Rhodiola rosea (also known as golden root and Arctic root) has been categorized as an adaptogen by Russian researchers due to its observed ability to increase resistance to a variety of chemical, biological, and physical stressors. It is a popular plant in traditional medical systems in Eastern Europe and Asia, with a reputation for stimulating the nervous system, improving depression, enhancing work performance, improving sleep, eliminating fatigue, and preventing high altitude sickness.[1]

Active Constituents

Rhodiola species contain a range of antioxidant compounds, including p-tyrosol, organic acids (gallic acid, caffeic acid, and chlorogenic acid), and flavonoids (catechins and proanthocyanidins).[2,3]

The stimulating and adaptogenic properties of *Rhodiola rosea* are attributed to p-tyrosol, salidroside (synonym: rhodioloside and rhodosin), rhodioniside, rhodiolin, rosin, rosavin, rosarin, and rosiridin.[1,4] Rosavin is the constituent currently selected for standardization of extracts.[5]

p-Tyrosol has been shown to be readily and dose-dependently absorbed after an oral dose;[6,7] however, pharmacokinetic data on the other adaptogenic compounds found in *Rhodiola rosea* is unavailable.

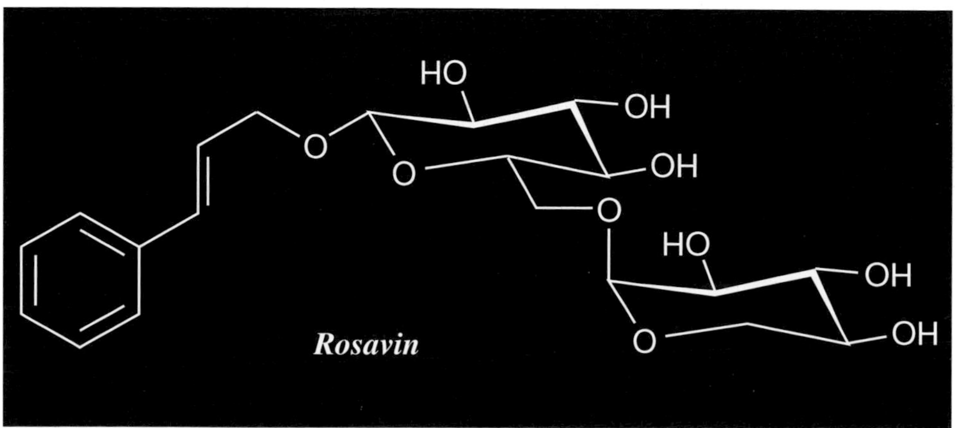

Rosavin

Mechanisms of Action

The adaptogenic properties, cardiopulmonary protective effects, and central nervous system activities of *Rhodiola rosea* have been attributed primarily to its ability to influence levels and activity of biogenic monoamines such as serotonin, dopamine, and norepinephrine in the cerebral cortex, brain stem, and hypothalamus. It is believed the changes in monoamine levels are due to inhibition of the activity of enzymes responsible for monoamine degradation and facilitation of neurotransmitter transport within the brain.[8]

In addition to these central effects, Rhodiola has been reported to prevent both catecholamine release and subsequent cyclic AMP elevation in the myocardium, and the depletion of adrenal catecholamines induced by acute stress.[9]

Rhodiola's adaptogenic activity might also be secondary to induction of opioid peptide biosynthesis and through the activation of both central and peripheral opioid receptors.[10-13]

Clinical Indications

Chronic Stress

In a physical endurance test, Rhodiola administration increased rat swimming time 135-159 percent.[14] When Rhodiola-treated rats were subjected to a four-hour period of non-specific stress, the expected elevation in beta-endorphin was either not observed or substantially decreased, leading researchers to the conclusion that the characteristic stress-induced perturbations of the hypothalamic-pituitary-adrenal axis can be decreased or totally prevented by Rhodiola supplementation.[10]

It is suggested that this plant has great utility as a therapy in asthenic conditions (decline in work performance, sleep disturbances, poor appetite, irritability, hypertension, headaches, and fatigue) developing subsequent to intense physical or intellectual strain, influenza and other viral exposures, and other illness.[15] Supplementation favorably influenced fatigue and mental performance in physicians during the first two weeks on night duty.[16]

Students receiving a standardized extract of *Rhodiola rosea* demonstrated significant improvements in physical fitness, psychomotor function, mental performance, and general well-being. Subjects receiving the Rhodiola extract also reported statistically significant reductions in mental fatigue, improved sleep patterns, a reduced need for sleep, greater mood stability, and a greater motivation to study. The average exam scores between students receiving the Rhodiola extract and placebo were 3.47 and 3.20, respectively.[17]

Cancer

All of the anti-cancer research on Rhodiola has been conducted in animal models. In these models, administration has resulted in inhibition of tumor growth and decreased metastasis in rats with transplanted solid Ehrlich adenocarcinoma and metastasizing rat Pliss lymphosarcoma[18] and transplanted Lewis lung carcinomas.[19]

Combining *Rhodiola rosea* extract with the anti-tumor agent cyclophosphamide in animal tumor models resulted in enhanced anti-tumor and anti-metastatic efficacy of drug treatment, as well as reduced drug-induced totoxicity.[19] Animal experimental data notes the addition of *Rhodiola rosea* extract to a protocol with Adriamycin results in improved inhibition of tumor dissemination (as compared to that found with Adriamycin alone). The combined protocol also prevented liver toxicity.[20]

Side Effects and Toxicity

Clinical feedback indicates at doses of 1.5-2.0 grams and above, *Rhodiola rosea* extract standardized for 2% rosavin might cause some individuals to experience an increase in irritability and insomnia within several days.

Evidence on the safety and appropriateness of *Rhodiola rosea* supplementation during pregnancy and lactation is currently unavailable.

Dosage

Dosage varies depending upon standardization. For chronic administration, a daily dose of 360-600 mg Rhodiola extract standardized for 1% rosavin, 180-300 mg of an extract standardized for 2% rosavin, or 100-170 mg of an extract standardized for 3.6% rosavin is suggested. Administration is normally begun several weeks prior to a period of expected increased physiological, chemical, or biological stress, and continued throughout the duration of the challenging event or activity.

When using *Rhodiola rosea* as a single dose for acute purposes (e.g., for an exam or athletic competition), the suggested dose is three times the dose used for chronic supplementation.

Rhodiola rosea has been administered for periods ranging from as little as one day (acute administration) up to four months. Until more specific information is available, a dosing regime following the established patterns used with other plant adaptogens – with periodic intervals of abstinence – seems warranted when *Rhodiola rosea* is being used chronically.

References

1. Petkov VD, Yonkov D, Mosharoff A, et al. Effects of alcohol aqueous extract from *Rhodiola rosea* L. roots on learning and memory. *Acta Physiol Pharmacol Bulg* 1986;12:3-16.
2. Lee MW, Lee YA, Park HM, et al. Antioxidative phenolic compounds from the roots of *Rhodiola sachalinensis* A. Bor. *Arch Pharm Res* 2000;23:455-458.
3. Ohsugi M, Fan W, Hase K, et al. Active-oxygen scavenging activity of traditional nourishing-tonic herbal medicines and active constituents of *Rhodiola sacra*. *J Ethnopharmacol* 1999;67:111-119.

4. Linh PT, Kim YH, Hong SP, et al. Quantitative determination of salidroside and tyrosol from the underground part of *Rhodiola rosea* by high performance liquid chromatography. *Arch Pharm Res* 2000;23:349-352.

5. Boon-Niermeijer EK, van den Berg A, Wikman G, Wiegant FA. Phyto-adaptogens protect against environmental stress-induced death of embryos from the freshwater snail *Lymnaea stagnalis*. *Phytomedicine* 2000;7:389-399.

6. Visioli F, Galli C, Bornet F, et al. Olive oil phenolics are dose-dependently absorbed in humans. *FEBS Lett* 2000;468:159-160.

7. Bonanome A, Pagnan A, Caruso D, et al. Evidence of postprandial absorption of olive oil phenols in humans. *Nutr Metab Cardiovasc Dis* 2000;10:111-120.

8. Stancheva SL, Mosharrof A. Effect of the extract of *Rhodiola rosea* L. on the content of the brain biogenic monamines. *Med Physiol* 1987;40:85-87.

9. Maslova LV, Kondrat'ev BI, Maslov LN, Lishmanov IB. The cardioprotective and antiadrenergic activity of an extract of *Rhodiola rosea* in stress. *Eksp Klin Farmakol* 1994;57:61-63. [Article in Russian]

10. Lishmanov IB, Trifonova ZV, Tsibin AN, et al. Plasma beta-endorphin and stress hormones in stress and adaptation. *Biull Eksp Biol Med* 1987;103:422-424. [Article in Russian]

11. Lishmanov IB, Maslova LV, Maslov LN, Dan'shina EN. The anti-arrhythmia effect of *Rhodiola rosea* and its possible mechanism. *Biull Eksp Biol Med* 1993;116:175-176. [Article in Russian]

12. Maimeskulova LA, Maslov LN, Lishmanov IB, Krasnov EA. The participation of the mu-, delta- and kappa-opioid receptors in the realization of the anti-arrhythmia effect of *Rhodiola rosea*. *Eksp Klin Farmakol* 1997;60:38-39. [Article in Russian]

13. Lishmanov IB, Naumova AV, Afanas'ev SA, Maslov LN. Contribution of the opioid system to realization of inotropic effects of *Rhodiola rosea* extracts in ischemic and reperfusion heart damage *in vitro*. *Eksp Klin Farmakol* 1997;60:34-36. [Article in Russian]

14. Azizov AP, Seifulla RD. The effect of elton, leveton, fitoton and adapton on the work capacity of experimental animals. *Eksp Klin Farmakol* 1998;61:61-63. [Article in Russian]

15. Germano C, Ramazanov Z, Bernal Suarez M. *Arctic Root (Rhodiola rosea): The Powerful New Ginseng Alternative*. New York, NY: Kensington Publishing Corp; 1999.

16. Darbinyan V, Kteyan A, Panossian A, et al. *Rhodiola rosea* in stress induced fatigue – a double blind cross-over study of a standardized extract SHR-5 with a repeated low-dose regimen on the mental performance of healthy physicians during night duty. *Phytomedicine* 2000;7:365-371.

17. Spasov AA, Wikman GK, Mandrikov VB, et al. A double-blind, placebo-controlled pilot study of the stimulating and adaptogenic effect of *Rhodiola rosea* SHR-5 extract on the fatigue of students caused by stress during an examination period with a repeated low-dose regimen. *Phytomedicine* 2000;7:85-89.

18. Udintsev SN, Shakhov VP. The role of humoral factors of regenerating liver in the development of experimental tumors and the effect of *Rhodiola rosea* extract on this process. *Neoplasma* 1991;38:323-331.

19. Udintsev SN, Schakhov VP. Decrease of cyclophosphamide haematotoxicity by *Rhodiola rosea* root extract in mice with Ehrlich and Lewis transplantable tumors. *Eur J Cancer* 1991;27:1182.

20. Udintsev SN, Krylova SG, Fomina TI. The enhancement of the efficacy of adriamycin by using hepatoprotectors of plant origin in metastases of Ehrlich's adenocarcinoma to the liver in mice. *Vopr Onkol* 1992;38:1217-1222. [Article in Russian]

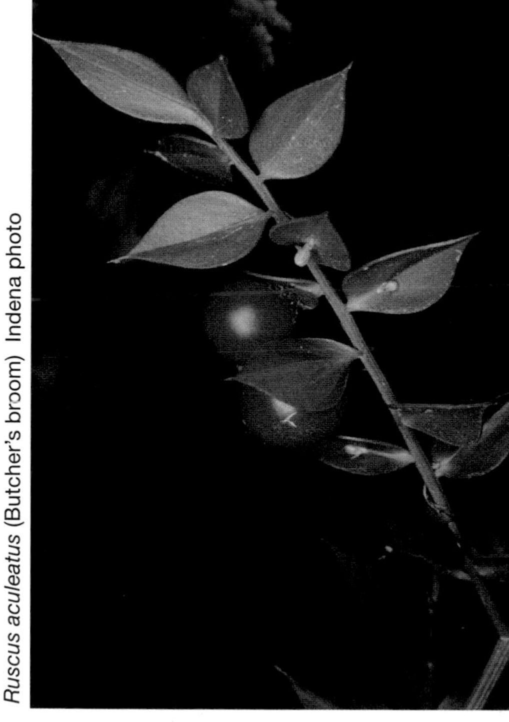
Ruscus aculeatus (Butcher's broom) Indena photo

Ruscus aculeatus

Description

Ruscus aculeatus (butcher's broom) is a member of the Liliaceae family and is native to Mediterranean Europe and Africa. It has tough, green, erect, striated stems that send out numerous short branches and very rigid leaves that are actually extensions of the stem and terminate in a single sharp spine. The small greenish-white flowers grow from the center of the leaves and bloom in the early spring. The thick root, typically collected in autumn, is used medicinally. The root has no odor, but has an initially sweetish taste that then turns slightly acrid.

Active Constituents

The primary active ingredients are the steroidal saponins ruscogenin and neoruscogenin, but other constituents have been isolated, including steroidal sapogenins and saponins, sterols, triterpenes, flavonoids, coumarins, sparteine, tyramine, and glycolic acid.[1-5] Although both the above- and below-ground parts of the plant contain ruscogenins, the concentration is higher in the root,[6] the part traditionally used medicinally.

Mechanisms of Action

One animal study[7] and numerous *in vitro* studies[8-13] indicate butcher's broom reduces vascular permeability. The ruscogenins from butcher's broom showed remarkable anti-elastase activity *in vitro* but were inactive against hyaluronidase.[14] These actions help explain the herb's apparent utility in patients with chronic venous insufficiency.

Animal and *in vitro* studies show butcher's broom to have a vasoconstrictive effect. The mechanism of this effect remains somewhat unclear. Some studies indicate direct postjunctional alpha-1 and alpha-2 adrenergic receptor activation by its steroidal saponins;[7] others indicate vasoconstriction is due to alpha-adrenergic blockade.[8] Hamster cheek pouch studies show that prazosin and diltiazem block butcher's broom's inhibition of histamine-induced permeability increase while rauwolscine does not, indicating that butcher's broom's venoconstrictive effect is mediated by calcium and alpha 1-adrenergic receptors at the microcirculatory level.[15,16]

Clinical Indications

The best-researched indications for butcher's broom are venous insufficiency, edema, premenstrual syndrome (PMS), and hemorrhoids. A single trial indicates butcher's broom may be useful in preventing diabetic retinopathy.

Venous Insufficiency/Varicosities

Four double-blind, placebo-controlled trials, and five open trials demonstrated an improvement in venous insufficiency symptoms such as itching, ankle diameter, tension of the leg, cramping, and malleolar edema.[17-24] One open, randomized clinical trial showed butcher's broom to be safe and more effective than rutoside in the treatment of patients with chronic venous insufficiency.[25] Most of these studies have insufficient sample sizes and other design flaws.

Edema

Butcher's broom may be beneficial for patients with edema of various types. One double-blind, placebo-controlled[26] and one open trial[27] showed butcher's broom to have a significant, positive effect in patients with lymph edema. In a small, uncontrolled trial, butcher's broom significantly improved symptoms in patients with edema secondary to calcium antagonist treatment (nifedipine and nicardipine) for hypertension.[10] In a randomized, double-blind, multi-center study of healthy volunteers (20 volunteers) and patients with chronic venous insufficiency (80 patients) or post-thrombotic syndrome (60 patients), butcher's broom alone appeared to increase lymphatic drainage and capillary sealing action.[12] Patients on butcher's broom showed a continuous decrease in ankle and leg volume over the course of the study, and the authors concluded this indicated a slow, reparative process that was not complete at the end of the study. Finally, a meta-analysis of three randomized, double-blind, cross-over studies of various products concluded butcher's broom both increases venous tone and reduces capillary filtration, resulting in an increase in lymph flow in patients with edema.[13] This action may explain the results of a small, double-blind, randomized study of butcher's broom's ability to speed healing of sprains and contusions.[28] In this study, using a butcher's broom/ sweet clover cream, the swelling of the injured leg measured against the uninjured leg was significantly reduced. The cream also significantly reduced the subjective perception of pain.

Premenstrual Syndrome

In a randomized, double-blind trial involving women with PMS, butcher's broom rapidly reduced symptoms of mastalgia and mood disorders, and showed a trend toward improving ankle edema.[11]

Hemorrhoids

Butcher's broom has been shown to have a significant effect on patients with hemorrhoids in an open trial, with 75 percent of participating physicians rating butcher's broom's efficacy as good or excellent.[29]

Diabetic Retinopathy

Butcher's broom was shown to be as or more effective than troxerutin for microangiopathic complications, including retinopathy, in 60 patients with type 2 diabetes.[30]

Orthostatic Hypotension

Researchers have theorized that Ruscus, because of its proven venotonic effects may be helpful as a treatment for chronic orthostatic hypotension.[31] Unlike many of the drug therapies for orthostatic hypotension, butcher's broom does not cause supine hypertension.

Butcher's Broom in Combination with other Botanicals

Many of the clinical trials on butcher's broom use commercial products that combine butcher's broom with trimethylhesperidine chalcone and ascorbic acid. Some studies combine butcher's broom with *Melilotus officinalis* (sweet clover, melilot) extract. This, of course, confuses the scientific evidence of butcher's broom's actual effect. While studies indicate butcher's broom has an action independent of these added compounds, and some studies indicate butcher's broom alone may have a stronger effect,[32] other studies indicate the combinations may have a positive synergistic effect.[33]

Side Effects and Toxicity

Most reviewers consider butcher's broom to be safe and list no contraindications.[34,35] Contact dermatitis has occasionally been reported in patients topically exposed to butcher's broom.[36,37] Nausea is uncommon with butcher's broom.[35] In one study of Cyclo 3 Fort (3 capsules three times daily), patients experienced edema, nausea, and abdominal pain significant enough to prompt volunteers to discontinue Cyclo 3 Fort in 3.5 percent of the patients.[24]

There may be theoretical reasons to avoid combining butcher's broom with alpha-adrenergic antagonist antihypertensive/spasmolytic drugs such as prazosin and terazosin.[1] Tyramine from butcher's broom could theoretically precipitate a hypertensive crisis when combined with these drugs. Similarly, tyramine-containing herbs should theoretically not be combined with monoamine oxidase inhibitors to avoid hypertensive crises. Preclinical information about butcher's broom's pharmacodynamics also suggests the possibility of interference with the efficacy of alpha-blockers. No clinical trials have directly addressed this issue.

There is insufficient data on the use of butcher's broom in pregnancy, although one uncontrolled trial of 20 pregnant women taking butcher's broom daily for venous insufficiency followed both fetal and post-birth indices and found no embryotoxic or other adverse effects.[19]

Dosage

Dosage for the alcoholic extract of the whole plant is 0.5-1.5 mL three times daily.[38] Dosage for capsules standardized for ruscogenins (as determined by the total of neoruscogenin and ruscogenin) is 7-11 mg,[34] although some experts recommend a higher dose of 16.5-33 mg of total rucogenins three times daily.[39] Commercial butcher's broom capsules (known variously as Cyclo 3 Fort®, Phlebodril® or Fabroven® and containing butcher's broom root combined with trimethylhesperidine chalcone and ascorbic acid) are used in many of the clinical studies. These products contain between 30-150 mg of butcher's broom per capsule, and a typical dose is 2 to 3 capsules three times daily.

References

1. Fetrow CW, Avila JR. *Professional's Handbook of Complementary and Alternative Medicines*. Springhouse, PA: Springhouse Corp.; 1999.
2. Rauwald HW, Grunwidi J. *Ruscus aculeatus* extract: unambiguous proof of the absorption of spirostanol glycosides in human plasma after oral administration. *Planta Med* 1991;57:A75-A76.
3. Dunouau C, Belle R, Oulad-Ali A, et al. Triterpenes and sterols from *Ruscus aculeatus*. *Planta Med* 1996;62:189-190.
4. Duke J. Dr. Duke's phytochemical and ethnobotanical databases. http://www.ars-grin.gov/cgi-bin/duke/farmacy2.pl; 2001.
5. Mimaki Y, Kuroda M, Kameyama A, et al. New steroidal constituents of the underground parts of *Ruscus aculeatus* and their cytostatic activity on HL-60 cells. *Phytochemistry* 1998;48:485-493.
6. St. Nikolov, Joneidi M, Panova D. Quantitative determination of ruscogenin in Ruscus species by densitometric thin-layer chromatography. *Pharmazie* 1976;31:611-612.
7. Svensjo E, Bouskela E, Cyrino FZ, et al. Antipermeability effects of Cyclo 3 Fort® in hamsters with moderate diabetes. *Clin Hemorheol Microcirc* 1997;17:385-388.
8. Bouskela E, Cyrino FZGA, Marcelon G. Effects of Ruscus extract on the internal diameter of arterioles and venules of the hamster cheek pouch microcirculation. *J Cardiovasc Pharmacol* 1993;22:221-222.
9. Miller VM, Marcelon G, Vanhoutte PM. Ruscus extract releases endothelin derived relaxing factor in arteries and veins. In: Vanhoute PM, ed. *Return Circulation and Norepinephrine: An Update*. Paris, France: John Libbey Eurotext; 1991:31-42.
10. Lagrue G, Behar A, Chaabane A, Laurent J. Edema induced by calcium antagonists. Effects of Ruscus extract on clinical and biological parameters. In: Vanhoute PM, ed. *Return Circulation and Norepinephrine: An Update*. Paris, France: John Libbey Eurotext; 1991:105-109.
11. Monteil-Seurin J, Ladure PH. Efficacy of Ruscus extract in the treatment of the premenstrual syndrome. In: Vanhoute PM, ed. *Return Circulation and Norepinephrine: An Update*. Paris, France: John Libbey Eurotext; 1991:43-53.
12. Rudofsky G. Efficacy of Ruscus extract in venolymphatic edema using foot volumetry. In: Vanhoute PM, ed. *Return Circulation and Norepinephrine: An Update*. Paris, France: John Libbey Eurotext; 1991:121-130.
13. Rudofsky G. Effect of Ruscus extract on the capillary filtration rate. In: Vanhoute PM, ed. *Return Circulation and Norepinephrine: An Update*. Paris, France: John Libbey Eurotext; 1991:219-224.
14. Facino RM, Carini M, Stefani R, et al. Anti-elastase and anti-hyaluronidase activities of saponins and sapogenins from *Hedera helix*, *Aesculus hippocastanum*, and *Ruscus aculeatus*: factors contributing to their efficacy in the treatment of venous insufficiency. *Arch Pharm (Weinheim)* 1995;328:721-724.

15. Bouskela E, Cyrino FZGA. Possible mechanisms for the effects of Ruscus extract on microvascular permeability and diameter. *Clin Hemorh* 1994;14:S23-S36.

16. Bouskela E, Cyrino FZGA, Marcelon G. Possible mechanisms for the inhibitory effect of Ruscus extract on increased microvascular permeability induced by histamine in hamster cheek pouch. *J Cardiovasc Pharmcol* 1994;24:281-285.

17. Parrado F, Buzzi A. A study of the efficacy and tolerability of a preparation containing *Ruscus aculeatus* in the treatment of chronic venous insufficiency of the lower limbs. *Clin Drug Invest* 1999;18:255-261.

18. Cappelli R, Nicora M, Di Perri T. Use of extract of *Ruscus aculeatus* in venous disease of the lower limb. *Drugs Exp Clin Res* 1988;14:277-283.

19. Rudofsky VG. Venentonisierung und kapillarabdichtung. *Fortschr Med* 1989;107:430-434. [Article in German]

20. Jaeger K, Eichlisberger CH, Lobs J, et al. Pharmacodynamic effects of Ruscus extract (Cyclo 3 Fort ®) on superficial and deep veins in patients with primary varicose veins. Assessment by duplexsonography. *Clin Drug Invest* 1999;111-119.

21. Baudet HJ, Collet D, Aubard Y, Renaudie P. Therapeutic test of Ruscus extract in pregnant women: evaluation of the fetal tolerance applying the pulse Doppler's method of the cord. In: Vanhoutte PM, ed. *Return Circulation and Norepinephrine: An Update*. Paris, France: John Libbey Eurotext; 1991:63-71.

22. Berg D. First results with Ruscus extract in the treatment of pregnancy related varicose veins. In: Vanhoutte PM, ed. *Return Circulation and Norepinephrine: An Update*. Paris, France: John Libbey Eurotext; 1991:55-61.

23. Kiesewetter H, Scheffler P, Jung F, et al. Effect of Ruscus extract in chronic venous insufficiency state I, II, and III. In: Vanhoutte PM, ed. *Return Circulation and Norepinephrine: An Update*. Paris, France: John Libbey Eurotext; 1991:163-169.

24. Weindorf N, Schultz-Ehrenburg U. Controlled study of increasing venous tone in primary varicose veins by oral administration of *Ruscus aculeatus* and trimethylhesperidinchalcone. *Z Hautkr* 1987;62:28-38. [Article in German]

25. Beltramino R, Penenory A, Buceta AM. An open-label, randomised multicentre study comparing the efficacy and safety of Cyclo 3 Fort versus hydroxyethyl rutoside in chronic venous lymphatic insufficiency. *Angiology* 2000;51:535-544.

26. Cluzan RV, Alliotl F, Ghabboun S, et al. Treatment of lymphedema of the upper arm after previous treatment for breast cancer. *Lymphology* 1996;29:29-35.

27. Jimenez Cossio JA, Magallon Ortin PJ, Capilla Montes MT, Coya Vina J. Therapeutic effect of Ruscus extract in lymphedemas of the extremities. In: Vanhoutte PM, ed. *Return Circulation and Norepinephrine: An Update*. Paris, France: John Libbey Eurotext; 1991:111-119.

28. Bohmer D. Action of Ruscus extract cream in the treatment of sports injuries. In: Vanhoutte PM, ed. *Return Circulation and Norepinephrine: An Update*. Paris, France: John Libbey Eurotext; 1991:171-179.

29. Bennani A, Biadillah MC, Cherkaoui A, et al. Acute attack of hemorrhoids: efficacy of Cyclo 3 Forte® based on results in124 cases reported by specialists. *Phlebologie* 1999;52:89-93.

30. Archimowicz-Cyrylowska B, Adamek B, Drozdżik M, et al. Clinical effect of buckwheat herb, Ruscus extract and troxerutin on retinopathy and lipids in diabetic patients. *Phytotherapy Res* 1996;10:659-662.

31. Redman DA. *Ruscus aculeatus* (butcher's broom) as a potential treatment for orthostatic hypotension, with a case report. *J Altern Complement Med* 2000;6:539-549.

32. Rudofsky G. Efficacy of Ruscus extract in venolymphatic edema using foot volumetry. In: Vanhoutte PM, ed. *Return Circulation and Norepinephrine: An Update*. Paris, France: John Libbey Eurotext; 1991:121-130.

33. Baurain R, Dom G, Trouet A. Protecting effect of Cyclo 3 Fort and its constituents for human endothelial cells under hypoxia. *Clin Hemorh* 1994;14:S14-S21.

34. Blumenthal M, Goldberg A, Brinckmann J, et al. *Herbal Medicine, Expanded Commission E Monographs*. Austin, TX: 2000.

35. McGuffin M, Hobbs C, Upton R, et al. *American Herbal Products Association's Botanical Safety Handbook*. Boca Raton, LA: CRC Press; 1997:100.

36. Landa N, Aguirre A, Goday J, et al. Allergic contact dermatitis from a vasoconstrictor cream. *Contact Dermatitis* 1990;22:290-291.

37. Elbadir S, El Ayed F, Renaud F, et al. L'allergie de contact aux ruscogenines. *Rev Fr Allergol* 1998;38:37-40. [Article in French]

38. Moore M. *Herbal Materia Medica*, 5th ed. Bisbee, AZ: Southwest School of Botanical Medicine.

39. Murray MT. *The Healing Power of Herbs*. Rocklin, CA: Prima Publishing Co.; 1983:35.

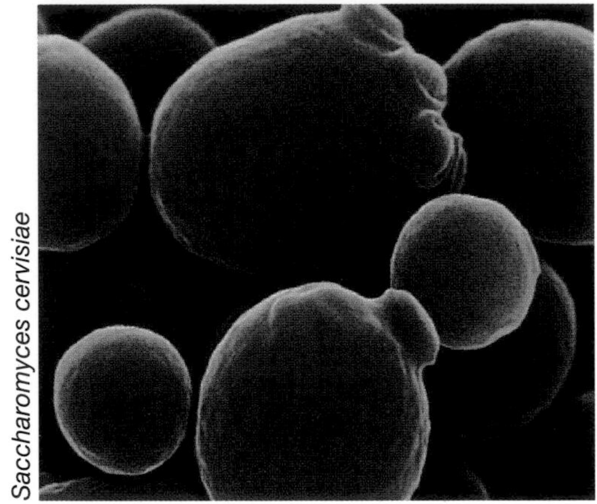
Saccharomyces cervisiae

Saccharomyces boulardii

Introduction

Saccharomyces boulardii, a nonpathogenic yeast, is a subspecies of *Saccharomyces cervisiae* (Brewer's yeast) and has a similar structure. *S. boulardii* has been shown to be effective in the treatment of antibiotic-associated diarrhea, recurrent *Clostridium difficile*-associated disease, Crohn's Disease, and HIV/AIDS-associated diarrhea.

Pharmacokinetics

Subsequent to oral administration and transport to the gastrointestinal tract, *S. boulardii* cells undergo irreversible degradation. In the large intestine, live cells are exposed to saccharolytic enzymes produced by the normal intestinal flora that hydrolyze polysaccharides in the cell wall. These same enzymes act to further degrade dead cells as well. Ultimately, *S. boulardii* appears in the bowel and feces.[1,2] Research indicates *S. boulardii* does not appear to colonize the intestinal tract, and a single oral dose is rapidly eliminated in the feces.[2] When *S. boulardii* was monitored in stools of patients given a dose of one gram daily, only one percent of the ingested dose was present and the organism was cleared completely from the stool within three days.[2] Conversely, when *S. boulardii* is administered to animals continuously (in drinking water), the fecal concentration of live cells is increased 50-100-fold, suggesting frequent dosing may be more effective.[3] In studies of patients taking ampicillin, *S. boulardii* recovery in the stool was increased 2.4 times, indicating when normal intestinal flora is altered, the level of *S. boulardii* in the intestine is elevated.[4]

Mechanisms of Action

S. boulardii appears to be taken up by the intestinal villa and to adhere to cells in the jejunum,[5,6] increasing brush border enzyme activity of lactase, alpha-glucosidase, and alkaline phosphatase, and increasing normal enterocyte maturation.[7] *S. boulardii* also exerts a protective effect on epithelial cells infected with *E. coli* by decreasing the level of intracellular infection and reducing the apoptotic effect of *E. coli* on intestinal epithelium.[8] *S. boulardii* has also been shown to increase intestinal secretory IgA production[9] and, in one human study, to activate the reticuloendothelial system, probably via a non-specific response.[10] In addition, *S. boulardii* neutralizes toxins produced by *Vibrio cholera* in epithelial cells of rat jejunum,[11] and prevents *Entamoeba histolytica* from adhering to human erythrocytes, a model of the first step in amoebic infection in humans.[12]

In *C. difficile*-related diarrhea and pseudomembranous colitis, Clostridium toxins bind to membrane receptors, causing intestinal fluid secretion and increased permeability of intestinal mucosa. *S. boulardii* contains a protease that neutralizes *C. difficile* toxins A and B, and also digests membrane receptors that bind to *C. difficile* toxin in the brush border epithelium of the ileum, thus exerting a protective effect on the gut lining.[13]

Clinical Indications

Antibiotic-associated Diarrhea

Antibiotic-associated diarrhea (AAD) occurs in 5-25 percent of patients receiving antibiotic therapy, and in cases of nosocomial epidemics the incidence has reached as high as 29 percent in hospitalized populations.[14] AAD is due primarily to infection with *Clostridium difficile* (20% of all cases) and less frequently to *Klebsiella oxytoca, Clostridium perfringens, Staphylococcus aureus, Candida sp., and Salmonella sp.*[15] The total incidence of gut-related disease caused by *C. difficile* ranges from 5-21 percent in hospitalized patients.[16,17] *C. difficile* diarrhea may manifest anywhere on the spectrum of AAD, acutely or 2-6 weeks post-antibiotic cessation. Twenty percent of patients with *C. difficile* diarrhea acquire pseudomembranous colitis, and fatality rates for recurrent pseudomembranous colitis may be as high as 10 percent in some populations.[14] After treatment with vancomycin or metronidazole, 20 percent of patients with *C. difficile*-associated diarrhea will continue to have diarrhea or colitis after medications are discontinued. Continued antibiotic treatment usually worsens the situation, resulting in prolonged symptomology.[16] Because *S. boulardii* is resistant to most antibiotics, it can be given simultaneously to prevent antibiotic-associated diarrhea.[18]

Studies of *S. boulardii* during and beyond the course of antibiotics in *C. difficile* diarrhea have shown it to be effective in preventing the return of *C. difficile,* as well as eliminating symptoms of infection.[19-22]

In one such case, the persistent nature of *C. difficile* infection is presented. Over an eight-month period, a patient with six documented cases of recurrent *C. difficile* colitis experienced repeated relapses, despite antibiotic treatment with four different antibiotics. Four episodes required hospitalization and rehydration.[19] Initial stool cultures showed high titers of *C. difficile* toxin that dropped rapidly during treatment with *S. boulardii* at a dosage of one gram daily for 28 days. Within seven days of *S. boulardii* administration the *C. difficile* toxin titer was zero. Diarrhea went into remission during the treatment period and on follow-up 18 months later, no further symptoms had occurred.[19]

Studies with documented recurrent *C. difficile* infection treated by standard antibiotic therapy along with *S. boulardii* have shown significant decreases in recurrence rates.[20-22] One double-blind, randomized, eight-week trial of 124 patients involved standard antibiotic therapy (metronidazole or vancomycin) for an average of 16 days in addition to *S. boulardii* one gram daily for 28 days (with overlap of antibiotic and *S. boulardii* for eight days).[20] Individuals who had a history of recurrent *C. difficile* infections were given high-dose vancomycin (two grams daily) and *S. boulardii,* and had a recurrence rate of zero. Those on vancomycin and placebo had a recurrence rate of 50 percent. Patients on low-dose vancomycin and *S. boulardii* had a 21 percent recurrence rate, compared to a rate of 62 percent recurrence with low-dose vancomycin and placebo. Even when all patients in the study (regardless of antibiotic type) with recurrent *C. difficile* were taken into account, the addition of *S. boulardii* significantly decreased the risk of recurrence (34.6% vs. 64.7% on placebo). There was, however, no beneficial effect of *S. boulardii* administration for those experiencing an initial episode of *C. difficile*-related diarrhea.[20] In a follow-up study using only high-dose vancomycin for 10 days and *S. boulardii* for 28 days (with an overlap of four days), 16.7 percent of patients on *S. boulardii* treatment had a repeated infection, while 50 percent on vancomycin and placebo had a recurrence.[21]

S. boulardii has also been used in infants and children with *C. difficile* enteropathies.[22] In 19 children (median age eight months), all of whom received a course of antibiotics for at least three days prior to enrollment, symptoms of diarrhea, malabsorption, or failure to thrive occurred as a result of *C. difficile* infection. The children were given *S. boulardii* in the following age-adjusted doses: 250 mg twice daily for those younger than one year; three times daily for those one to four years of age; and four times daily for those older than four years of age. The dosing regimens were continued for 15 days. In all but one child, symptoms resolved within seven days of treatment. Clearing of *C. difficile* toxin B occurred in 85 percent of the children after 15 days and in 73 percent of the children 30 days after treatment began. Most significantly, two months after initiation of treatment the pathologic changes (sparse and shortened microvilli) that had occurred in the colons of those most affected returned to normal on biopsy sampling. Two patients who experienced relapses were retreated with a two-week trial of *S. boulardii* and responded within seven days without further recurrences.[22]

In three placebo-controlled studies of AAD in adults (without benefit of stool cultures), *S. boulardii* was given in doses of one gram daily for 14 days. Treatment resulted in significant symptom reduction compared to placebo in all three studies. Those left unimproved on *S. boulardii* versus unimproved on placebo were: 9.5 percent versus 22 percent,[23] 7.2 percent versus 14.6 percent,[24] and 4.5 percent versus 17.5 percent.[25]

Irritable Bowel Syndrome

In a controlled trial of 34 patients with prior diagnosis of irritable bowel syndrome, the administration of *S. boulardii* was effective in decreasing diarrhea but did not affect abdominal pain and bloating.[26]

Crohn's Disease

In a placebo-controlled trial, 20 patients with established Crohn's disease and chronic diarrhea were given 250 mg *S. boulardii* three times daily for two weeks in addition to the basic treatment.[27] A significant reduction in frequency of bowel movements occurred, along with a reduction of scores in an index of disease activity (BEST index) when compared to baseline. At the end of two weeks, seven patients were placed in the control group and received placebo for an additional seven weeks. Ten of the 20 patients remained in the treatment group and continued to receive *S. boulardii*, 250 mg three times daily for seven weeks. The treatment group continued to show a significant reduction in bowel movement frequency and BEST index scores. Conversely, the placebo group had an increase in bowel movement frequency, and BEST index scores rose again until reaching initial values in the tenth week.[27]

In another trial, 32 patients with stabilized Crohn's disease were treated with either mesalamine or mesalamine and *S. boulardii* (one gram daily). After six months, 37.5 percent of the patients on mesalamine alone experienced relapse, while only 6.25 percent of patients on both therapies relapsed.[28]

HIV/AIDS

Although studies of *S. boulardii* in HIV patients have been limited, they are noteworthy. Three small trials were conducted in HIV-positive and AIDS-diagnosed individuals with diarrhea of unknown etiology. In one trial utilizing three grams daily of *S. boulardii*, fecal stool weights decreased significantly and stools became fully formed.[29] In another small trial, stool frequency decreased from nine to two stools per day and average body weight gain was 17.7 pounds.[30] In a placebo-controlled trial with 36 AIDS patients in which antibiotic treatment had been unsuccessful, 55 percent of patients given *S. boulardii* became diarrhea-free and only six percent of the placebo group regained normal stool function.[31]

Side Effects and Toxicity

While few side effects have been reported, Saccharomyces fungemia has been documented in immunosuppressed infants,[32] in hospitalized infants on *S. boulardii* therapy,[33] and in patients with in-dwelling vascular catheters.[34] Ingestion of therapeutic dosages of *S. boulardii* may cause flatulence.

Dosage

In most of the literature *S. boulardii* dosages are expressed in mg or gram amounts per day. However, the number of live organisms per gram is not listed in most literature. Clinically, it appears 10-20 billion organisms per day is an effective adult dosage range. Because *S. boulardii* is resistant to most antibiotics, it can be given simultaneously to prevent antibiotic-associated diarrhea.[18]

Warnings and Contraindications

Individuals with a yeast allergy should avoid *Saccharomyces boulardii* as it may cause itching, rash, and other common allergic symptoms. Immunosuppressed individuals should use *S. boulardii* with caution.

References

1. Lewis SJ, Freedman AR. Review article: the use of biotherapeutic agents in the prevention and treatment of gastrointestinal disease. *Aliment Pharmacol Ther* 1998;12:807-822.
2. Blehaut H, Massot J, Elmer GW, Levy RH. Disposition kinetics of *Saccharomyces boulardii* in man and rat. *Biopharm Drug Dispos* 1989;10:353-364.
3. Klein SM, Elmer GW, McFarland LV, et al. Recovery and elimination of the biotherapeutic agent, *Saccharomyces boulardii*, in healthy human volunteers. *Pharm Res* 1993;10:1615-1619.
4. Corthier G, Dubos F, Ducluzeau R. Prevention of *Clostridium difficile* induced mortality in gnotobiotic mice by *Saccharomyces boulardii*. *Can J Microbiol* 1986;32:894-896.
5. Cartwright-Shamoon J, Dickson GR, Dodge J, Carr KE. Uptake of yeast (*Saccharomyces boulardii*) in normal and rotavirus treated intestine. *Gut* 1996;39:204-209.
6. Chapoy P. Intestinal mode of action of *Saccharomyces boulardii*. *Gastroenterol Clin Biol* 1986;10:860-861. [Article in French]
7. Jahn HU, Ullrich R, Schneider T, et al. Immunological and trophical effects of *Saccharomyces boulardii* on the small intestine in healthy human volunteers. *Digestion* 1996;57:95-104.
8. Czerucka D, Dahan S, Mograbi B, et al. *Saccharomyces boulardii* preserves the barrier function and modulates the signal transduction pathway induced in enteropathogenic *Escherichia coli*-infected T84 cells. *Infect Immun* 2000;68:5998-6004.
9. Buts JP, Bernasconi P, Vaerman JP, Dive C. Stimulation of secretory IgA and secretory component of immunoglobulins in small intestine of rats treated with *Saccharomyces boulardii*. *Dig Dis Sci* 1990;35:251-256.
10. Caetano JA, Parames MT, Babo MJ, et al. Immunopharmacological effects of *Sacchaomyces boulardii* in healthy human volunteers. *Int J Immunopharmacol* 1986;8:245-259.
11. Czerucka D, Roux I, Rampal P. *Saccharomyces boulardii* inhibits secretagogue-mediated adenosine 3',5'-cyclic monophosphate induction in intestinal cells. *Gastroenterology* 1994;106:65-72.
12. Rigothier MC, Maccario J, Gayral P. Inhibitory activity of saccharomyces yeasts on the adhesion of *Entamoeba histolytica* trophozoites to human erythrocytes *in vitro*. *Parasitol Res* 1994;80:10-15.
13. Castagliuolo I, Riegler MF, Valenick L, et al. *Saccharomyces boulardii* protease inhibits the effects of *Clostridium difficile* toxins A and B in human colonic mucosa. *Infect Immun* 1999;67:302-307.
14. Bergogne-Berezin E. Treatment and prevention of antibiotic associated diarrhea. *Int J Antimicrob Agents* 2000;16:521-526.
15. Hogenauer C, Hammer HF, Krejs GJ, Reisinger EC. Mechanisms and management of antibiotic-associated diarrhea. *Clin Infect Dis* 1998;27:702-710.
16. Fekety R, Shah AB. Diagnosis and treatment of *Clostridium difficile* colitis. *JAMA* 1993;269:71-75.
17. Clabots CR, Johnson S, Olson MM, et al. Acquisition of *Clostridium difficile* by hospitalized patients: evidence for colonized new admissions as a source of infection. *J Infect Dis* 1992;166:561-567.
18. Bergogne-Berezin E. Ecologic impact of antibiotherapy. Role of substitution microorganisms in the control of antibiotic-related diarrhea and colitis. *Presse Med* 1995;24:145-148,151-152,155-156. [Article in French]

19. Kimmey MB, Elmer GW, Surawicz CM, McFarland LV. Prevention of further recurrences of *Clostridium difficile* colitis with *Saccharomyces boulardii*. *Dig Dis Sci* 1990;35:897-901.

20. McFarland LV, Surawicz CM, Greenberg RN, et al. A randomized placebo-controlled trial of *Saccharomyces boulardii* in combination with standard antibiotics for *Clostridium difficile* disease. *JAMA* 1994;271:1913-1918.

21. Surawicz CM, McFarland LV, Greenberg RN, et al. The search for a better treatment for recurrent *Clostridium difficile* disease: use of high-dose vancomycin combined with *Saccharomyces boulardii*. *Clin Infect Dis* 2000;31:1012-1017.

22. Buts JP, Corthier G, Delmee M. *Saccharomyces boulardii* for *Clostridium difficile*-associated enteropathies in infants. *J Pediatr Gastroenterol Nutr* 1993;16:419-425.

23. Surawicz CM, Elmer GW, Speelman P, et al. Prevention of antibiotic-associated diarrhea by *Saccharomyces boulardii*: a prospective study. *Gastroenterology* 1989;96:981-988.

24. McFarland LV, Surawicz CM, Greenberg RN, et al. Prevention of beta-lactam-associated diarrhea by *Saccharomyces boulardii* compared with placebo. *Am J Gastroenterol* 1995;90:439-448.

25. Adam J, Barret A, Barret-Bellet L, et al. A controlled clinical trial with lyophilized Ultra-Levure. A multicenter trial with 25 physicians and 388 cases. *Gaz Med Fr* 1977;84:2072-2078.

26. Maupas JL, Champemont P, Delforge M. Treatment of irritable bowel syndrome with *Saccharomyces boulardii* – a double-blind, placebo-controlled study. *Med Chir Dig* 1983;12:77-79.

27. Plein K, Hotz J. Therapeutic effects of *Saccharomyces boulardii* on mild residual symptoms in a stable phase of Crohn's disease with special respect to chronic diarrhea – a pilot study. *Z Gastroenterol* 1993;31:129-134.

28. Guslandi M, Mezzi G, Sorghi M, Testoni PA. *Saccharomyces boulardii* in maintenance treatment of Crohn's disease. *Dig Dis Sci* 2000;45:1462-1464.

29. Saint-Marc T, Sellem C, Rosello L, et al. Treatment of chronic diarrhea with *Saccharomyces boulardii*. *Sixth International Conference on AIDS,* San Francisco, CA: June 20-24, 1990 [abstract #Th.B. 363].

30. Saint-Marc T, Rossello-Prats L, Touraine JL. Efficacy of *Saccharomyces boulardii* in the treatment of diarrhea in AIDS. *Ann Med Interne* 1991;142:64-65. [Article in French]

31. Blehaut H, Saint-Marc T, Touraine JL. Double blind trial of *Saccharomyces boulardii* in AIDS related diarrhea. Submitted to *Eighth International Conference on AIDS* 1992.

32. Cesaro S, Chinello P, Rossi L, Zanesco L. *Saccharomyces cerevisiae* fungemia in a neutropenic patient treated with *Saccharomyces boulardii*. *Support Care Cancer* 2000;8:504-505.

33. Perapoch J, Planes AM, Querol A, et al. Fungemia with *Saccharomyces cerevisiae* in two newborns, only one of whom had been treated with Ultra-Levura. *Eur J Clin Microbiol Infect Dis* 2000;19:468-470.

34. Hennequin C, Kauffman-Lacroix C, Jobert A, et al. Possible role of catheters in *Saccharomyces boulardii* fungemia. *Eur J Clin Microbiol Infect Dis* 2000;19:16-20.

Schizandrae chinensis

Description

Schizandrae chinensis, a member of the Magnoliaceae family, has an extensive history of medical use in China. It is considered astringent in nature and is indicated in cases of chronic cough and dyspnea, diarrhea, night sweats, wasting disorders, irritability, palpitations, dream-disturbed sleep, and insomnia.[1] This herb's adaptogenic properties increase resistance to a wide range of physical, chemical, and emotional stressors, while promoting improved overall regulation of physiological processes. Experimental evidence suggests Schizandrae functions as a potent antioxidant and has hepatoprotective abilities. Research of the active ingredients is primarily focused on the various lignans and essential oils contained in the dried fruits of Schizandrae.

Clinical Indications

Hepatitis

Recent studies from China have found Schizandrae and its active components to be effective against viral and chemically-induced hepatitis.[2] Schizandrae was shown to lower SGPT levels in patients with chronic viral hepatitis and decrease the hepatotoxicity of carbon tetrachloride in animals.[3] Dimethyl-4, 4'-dimethoxy-5, 6, 5'-6'-dimethylenedioxybiphenyl-2, 2'-dicarboxylate (DDB), a synthetic analogue of schizandrin, is widely used in China as a hepatoprotective drug. While being highly effective at normalizing liver function, it has very few side effects.[4] Pharmacological studies on the bioactive lignans in Schizandrae found they increased liver protein and glycogen synthesis, inhibited carbon tetrachloride-induced lipid peroxidation, and had an inducing effect on the cytochrome P-450 enzyme system.[4]

In one study, powdered Schizandrae was administered to 102 patients with hepatitis. The overall success rate for normalizing liver enzymes was 76 percent, and in cases where SGPT levels were over 300 IU, the success rate was 72 percent. The average time in which liver enzymes returned to normal was 25 days, and no adverse side effects from the treatment were observed.[1]

Antioxidant Activity

Seven of the nine lignans from Schizandrae were found to inhibit vitamin C/NADPH-induced lipid peroxidation in rat liver microsomes. Of these compounds, schisanhenol and schizandrin were shown to be more effective than vitamin E at the same concentration.

Schizandrins B and C were found to have strongest scavenging effect against active oxygen radicals.[5] When these compounds were given orally to mice at 15 ml/kg, there was significant reduction in ethanol-induced malondialdehyde formation, with increased superoxide dismutase and catalase activity.[6]

Anti-Bacterial Effect

Decoctions of Schizandrae were found to possess strong *in vitro* inhibitory action on *Bacillus subtilis, Bacillus dysenteraie, Bacillus typhi,* and *Staphylococcus aureus.*[7]

Dosage and Toxicity

Therapeutic dosages are 400-450 mg powdered herb in capsules three times daily or 1-2 mL of a 1:3 ethanol tincture of Schizandrae three times daily. Toxic doses when orally administered to mice were approximately 10-15g/kg. Overdose symptoms include restlessness, insomnia and dyspnea.[1]

References

1. Bensky D, Gamble A. *Chinese Herbal Medicine: Materia Medica, Revised Edition.* Seattle, WA: Eastland Press; 1993.
2. Liu GT. Pharmacological actions and clinical use of fructus Schizandrae. *Chin Med J (Engl)* 1989;102:740-749.
3. Liu KT, Lesca P. Pharmacological properties of dibenzo[a,c]cycloctene derivatives isolated from fructus *Schizandrae chinsesis* III. Inhibitory effects on carbon tetrachloride induced lipid peroxidation, metabolism and covalent binding of CCl4 to lipids. *Chem Biol Interact* 1982;41:39-47.
4. Li XY. Bioactivity of neolignans from fructus Schizandrae. *Mem Inst Oswaldo Cruz* 1991;86:31-37.
5. Li XJ, Zhao BL, Liu GT, Xin WJ. Scavenging effects on active oxygen radicals by schizandrins with different structures and configurations. *Free Radic Biol Med* 1990;9:99-104.
6. Lu H, Liu GT. Effect of dibenzo[a,c]cyclootene lignans isolated from fructus Schizandrae on lipid peroxidation and anti-oxidative enzyme activity. *Chem Biol Interact* 1991;78:77-84.
7. Hong YH. *Oriental Materia Medica: A Concise Guide.* Long Beach, CA: Oriental Healing Arts Institute; 1986.

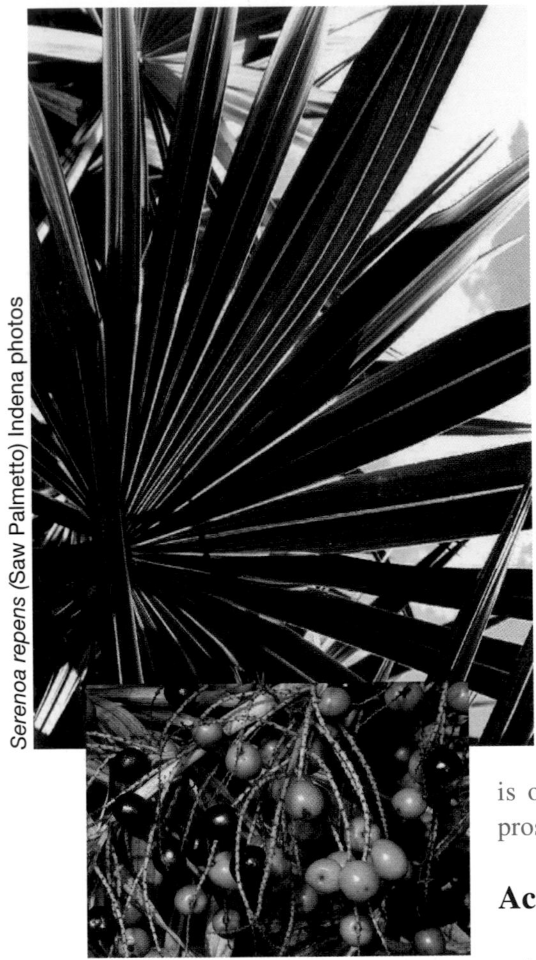
Serenoa repens (Saw Palmetto) Indena photos

Serenoa repens

Description

Serenoa repens (also known as *Sabal serrulata*, Saw Palmetto or Dwarf palm) is native to the U. S. South Atlantic coast, as well as Southern Europe and North Africa. This small palm tree grows to a height of six to ten feet, and has a fan-shaped crown of leaves and dark red berries approximately the size of olives.

Traditional indications for the use of Saw palmetto include cystitis, chronic bronchitis, asthma, diabetes, dysentery, indigestion, and "underdeveloped breasts." The berries have also been thought to be an aphrodisiac.[1] Modern usage of Saw palmetto is overwhelmingly for the treatment of benign prostatic hyperplasia (BPH).

Active Constituents

The berries contain approximately 1.5 percent volatile oil, comprised of 63 percent free fatty acids and 37 percent ethyl esters of those fatty acids. The fatty acids include caproic, caprylic, capric, lauric, palmitic, and oleic acids, and ethyl esters of these. In addition, the berries contain beta-sitosterol and its glucoside, beta sitosterol D-glucoside, as well as ferulic acid.[1] Myristoleic acid has recently been identified as a cytotoxic component in *Serenoa repens* extract, which raises the possibility that usage of Saw palmetto may be extended to the treatment of prostatic cancer.[2]

Mechanisms of Action

Testosterone is converted in prostatic cells to dihydrotestosterone (DHT), catalyzed by the enzyme steroid 5-alpha-reductase (5-AR). DHT binds to androgen receptors in the nucleus of prostate cells, stimulating cellular growth and division.[3-5] In benign prostatic hyperplasia (BPH) tissue, 5-AR levels are higher than in tissue not affected by BPH.[4,5] The presence of

DHT may also stimulate 5-AR activity, causing a positive feedback loop, and more DHT.[6] The standardized liposterolic Serenoa extract has been found to be a potent inhibitor of 5-AR, resulting in decreased tissue DHT. Serenoa also competitively inhibits binding of testosterone and DHT to cytosolic and nuclear androgen receptors.[7-9] As a 5-alpha-reductase inhibitor, the liposterolic extract of *Serenoa repens* demonstrates selectivity and specificity to prostatic cells when compared to epididymis, testes, kidney, skin, and breast cells.[10]

Another component of BPH is inflammation within the prostate gland. A standardized Serenoa extract has been shown to inhibit 5-lipoxygenase, and thus the downstream pro-inflammatory arachidonic acid metabolites leukotriene B4 (LTB4) and 5-hydroxyeicosatetraenoic acid (5-HETE).[11]

Clinical Indications

Benign Prostatic Hyperplasia

The liposterolic extract of the fruit, standardized to contain at least 85 percent fatty acids and sterols, is currently used in the treatment of BPH. Benign prostatic hyperplasia is one of the most common medical conditions in middle-aged and elderly males, with an incidence of 50-60 percent in men ages 40-60, and greater than 90 percent in men over 80. The disease process leading to symptomatology in older males probably begins as early as the late 20s, and may have an incidence rate of 10 percent at that age. Rarely a fatal disease, BPH affects lifestyle and comfort.[12]

A non-malignant hypertrophy of the prostate caused by hormonal processes and/or imbalances within the prostate, BPH begins in the periurethral region and includes the stromal, epithelial, and smooth muscle tissues of the gland. The fibrous capsule surrounding the gland forces most of the growth inward, compressing the urethra and causing the typical urinary symptoms characteristic of the disease. Primary symptoms include decreased force and caliber of the urine stream; urinary hesitancy, urgency, and frequency; post-void dribbling; incomplete emptying of the bladder; dysuria; and nocturia.[12]

In a double-blind, placebo-controlled study of 110 BPH patients, 160 mg twice per day of a standardized Serenoa extract significantly improved nocturia, dysuria, post-voiding residual urine, flow rate, patient self-rating, and the physician's overall assessment.[13] In another double-blind clinical study, urinary symptoms and flow rates were significantly improved in 42.9 percent of patients taking a Serenoa extract, compared to 15.4 percent of patients given placebo.[14] In an open trial, 67 percent of patients on Serenoa described their subjective symptom relief as "excellent," while 25 percent characterized their relief as "good."[15] No side effects or toxicity were noted.

An impressive review of randomized trials found via MEDLINE (1966 to 1997 search) compared treatment results of six phytotherapeutic agents: *Serenoa repens*, *Hypoxis rooperi*, *Secale cereale*, *Pygeum africanum*, *Urtica dioica*, and *Curcubita pepo*. Studies were included if men had BPH symptoms, phytotherapeutic agents were used singularly or in combination, a control group received placebo or pharmaceutical therapy for BPH, and treatment duration was a minimum of 30 days. This comprehensive study concluded that, when compared to the other phytotherapies, *Serenoa repens* provided the strongest therapeutic evidence for BPH.[16] Unlike other 5-alpha-reductase inhibitors, *Serenoa repens* creates this effect without inhibition of cellular prostate specific antigen (PSA) secretion. This allows for the continued use of PSA values for prostate cancer screening.[17]

The standard pharmaceutical therapy for BPH is the drug Proscar® (finasteride), a 5-AR inhibitor. A six-month, double-blind study of 1,098 BPH patients over 50 years of age compared Proscar (5 mg per day) with a standardized Serenoa extract (160 mg twice per day). Both treatments decreased BPH symptoms equally and improved quality of life. Although both treatments significantly improved symptomatology, it is interesting to note Proscar reduced prostate size by 18 percent and the Serenoa extract reduced it six percent.[18]

Prostate Cancer

In vitro studies have also demonstrated that myristoleic acid, found in the extract of *Serenoa repens*, induces apoptosis and necrosis in prostatic tumor cells,[2,19] posing the potential for Serenoa in the prevention and treatment of prostate cancer.

Polycystic Ovary Syndrome (PCOS)

Because of its antiandrogenic effects, Serenoa has been used clinically for polycystic ovary syndrome. Although formal studies have not been conducted to confirm the efficacy of Serenoa in PCOS, anecdotal clinical evidence points to its use in a protocol for this condition.[20]

Side Effects and Toxicity

There are no known cases of toxicity. Occasionally patients experience minor gastrointestinal symptoms including nausea and/or abdominal pain.[21]

Dosage

The dose of the standardized liposterolic Serenoa extract (85-95% fatty acids and sterols) used in the majority of clinical studies on BPH is 160 mg twice per day. Clinical results may be seen in six to eight weeks, although a six-month trial is the minimum to assess clinical efficacy. A three-month, double-blind comparison study of two dosage regimens – 160 mg once daily versus 160 mg twice daily – showed no significant differences between the dosages. This study of 100 outpatients with BPH symptoms noted improvements in maximum and mean urinary flow rates as well as a decrease in residual urine volume. Both dosage regimens significantly reduced the International Prostate Symptom Score (I-PSS) mean total compared to patient baseline.[22]

References

1. Duke JA. *Handbook of Medicinal Herbs*. Boca Raton, FL: CRC Press; 1985:443.
2. Iguchi K, Okumura N, Usui S, et al. Myristoleic acid, a cytotoxic component in the extract from *Serenoa repens*, induces apoptosis and necrosis in human prostatic LNCaP cells. *Prostate* 2001;47:59-65.
3. McConnell JD, Barry MJ, Bruskewitz RC, et al. *Benign Prostatic Hyperplasia: Diagnosis and Treatment.* Clinical practice guideline #8. AHCPR Publication no. 94-0582. Rockville, MD: Agency For Health Policy and Research, Public Health Service, U.S. Department of Health and Human Services; February 1994.
4. Metcalf BW, Levy MA, Holt DA. Inhibitors of steroid 5 alpha-reductase in benign prostatic hyperplasia, male pattern baldness and acne. *Trends Pharmacol Sci* 1989;10:491-495.
5. Tenover J. Prostates, pates, and pimples. The potential medical uses of steroid 5-alpha-reductase inhibitors. *Endocrinol Metab Clin North Amer* 1991;20:893-909.
6. George FW, Russell DW, Wilson JD. Feed-forward control of prostate growth: Dihydrotestosterone induces expression of its own biosynthetic enzyme, steroid 5-alpha-reductase. *Proc Natl Acad Sci* 1991;88:8044-8047.
7. Sultan C, Terraza A, Devillier C, et al. Inhibition of androgen metabolism and binding by a liposterolic extract of "*Serenoa repens* B" in human foreskin fibroblasts. *J Steroid Biochem* 1984;20:515-519.
8. Carilla E, Briley M, Fauran F, et al. Binding of Permixon, a new treatment for prostatic benign hyperplasia, to the cytosolic receptor in the rat prostate. *J Steroid Biochem* 1984;20:521-523.
9. Magdy El-Sheikh M, Dakkak MR, Saddique A. The effect of Permixon on androgen receptors. *Acta Obstet Gynecol Scand* 1988;67:397-399.
10. Paubert-Braquet M, Mencia Huerta JM, Cousse H, Braquet P. Effect of the lipidosterolic extract of *Serenoa repens* (Permixon) on the ionophore A23187-stimulated production of leukotriene B4 (LTB4) from human polymorphonuclear neutrophils. *Prostaglandins Leukot Essent Fatty Acids* 1997;57:299-304.
11. Bayne CW, Ross M, Donnelly F, Habib FK. The selectivity and specificity of the actions of the lipido-sterolic extract of *Serenoa repens* (Permixon) on the prostate. *J Urol* 2000;164:876-881.
12. Miller AL. Benign prostatic hyperplasia: nutritional and botanical therapeutic options. *Altern Med Rev* 1996;1:18-25.
13. Champault G, Patel JC, Bonnard AM. A double-blind trial of an extract of the plant *Serenoa repens* in benign prostatic hyperplasia. *Br J Pharmac* 1984:461-462.
14. Tasca A, Brulli M, Cavazzana A, et al. Treatment of the obstructive symptomatology of prostatic adenoma using an extract of *Serenoa repens*: a double-blind clinical study vs. placebo. *Min Urol Nefrol* 1985;37:87-91.
15. Carreras JO. Novel treatment with a hexane extract of *Serenoa repens* in the treatment of benign prostatic hypertrophy. *Arch Esp de Urol* 1987;40:310-313.
16. Wilt TJ, Ishani A, Rutks I, MacDonald R. Phytotherapy for benign prostatic hyperplasia. *Public Health Nutr* 2000;3:459-472.
17. Bayne CW, Donnelly F, Ross M, Habib FK. *Serenoa repens* (Permixon): a 5alpha-reductase types I and II inhibitor – new evidence in a coculture model of BPH. *Prostate* 1999;40:232-241.
18. Carraro JC, Raynaud JP, Koch G, et al. Comparison of phytotherapy (Permixon®) with finasteride in the treatment of benign prostatic hyperplasia; a randomized international study of 1,098 patients. *Prostate* 1996;29:231-240.
19. Vacherot F, Azzouz M, Gil-Diez-De-Medina S, et al. Induction of apoptosis and inhibition of cell proliferation by the lipido-sterolic extract of *Serenoa repens* (LSESr, Permixon) in benign prostatic hyperplasia. *Prostate* 2000;45:259-266.
20. Marshall K. Polycystic ovary syndrome: clinical considerations. *Altern Med Rev* 2001;6:272-292.
21. McGuffin M, Hobbs C, Upton R, Goldberg A, eds. *American Herbal Product Association's Botanical Safety Handbook.* Boca Raton, FL: CRC Press; 1997:107.
22. Stepanov VN, Siniakova LA, Sarrazin B, Raynaud JP. Efficacy and tolerability of the lipidosterolic extract of *Serenoa repens* (Permixon) in benign prostatic hyperplasia: a double-blind comparison of two dosage regimens. *Adv Ther* 1999;16:231-241.

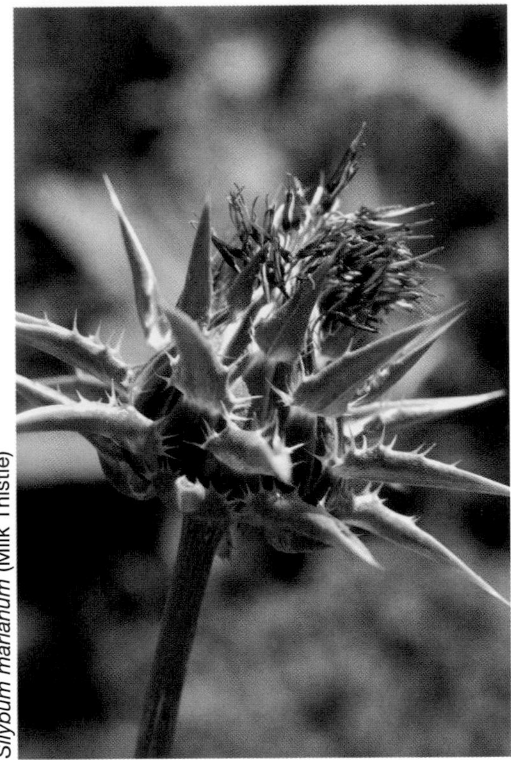
Silybum marianum (Milk Thistle)

Silybum marianum

Description

Silybum marianum (milk thistle) has been used for centuries as an herbal medicine for the treatment of liver disease. Its use for liver disorders dates back to Pliny the Elder, a Roman naturalist, who described milk thistle as being "excellent for carrying off bile." Milk thistle is an annual or biennial plant indigenous to Europe and is also found in some parts of the United States. It grows in rocky soils to a height of three to ten feet with an erect stem that bears large, alternating, prickly-edged leaves. The common name, milk thistle, is derived from the "milky white" veins on the leaves, which, when broken open, yield a milky sap. Flowering season is from June to August, and each stem bears a single, large, purple flower ending in sharp spines. The fruit portion of the plant is glossy brown or gray with spots.[1] Modern extracts of the plant are produced from the small hard fruits (often incorrectly referred to as seeds) that have the feathery tuft (known as the pappus) removed. These are referred to as achenes.

Active Constituents

In 1968, a flavonolignan complex in milk thistle fruit was identified and isolated. Named silymarin, this complex was found to be responsible for the medicinal benefits of the plant.[2] The silymarin complex is made up of three parts: silibinin (also called silybin), silydianin, and silychristin. Silibinin is the most active of the three, and is largely responsible for the hepatoprotective benefits attributed to silymarin.[3,4] Milk thistle fruit contains 1.5-3.0 percent flavonolignans. Modern extracts are typically standardized to 70-80 percent silymarin.[5]

Pharmacokinetics

Silymarin is not water soluble, making tea preparations ineffective; therefore it is usually administered orally in encapsulated form. Because absorption of silymarin from the gastrointestinal tract is only moderate (23-47%), it is best administered as a standardized extract of 70-80 percent silymarin. In animals and humans, peak plasma levels are reached in four to six hours after an oral dose. Silymarin is excreted primarily via the bile but some clearance is also achieved via the kidneys. The clearance half-life of silymarin is six to eight hours.[6]

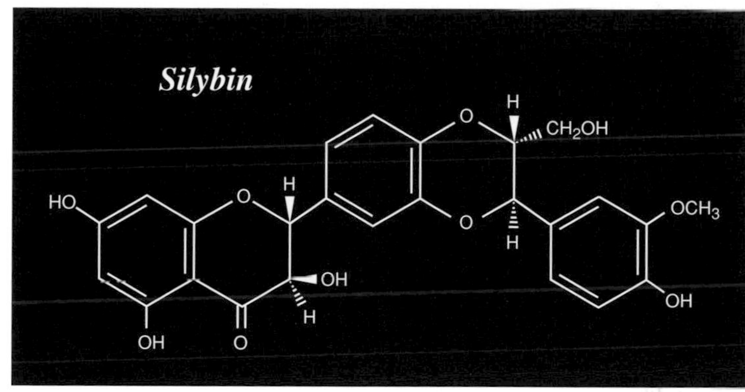

Mechanisms of Action

Silymarin's hepatoprotective effects are accomplished both directly and indirectly. The primary actions are as follows:

Hepatocellular Protection

Silymarin, and more specifically silibinin, directly aids hepatocytes by binding to the outside of the cells and blocking the binding of potential hepatocellular toxins. This was first noted in experimental studies investigating toxins from *Amanita phalloides* (death cap mushroom).[7,8] Ingesting this mushroom causes swift and severe damage to hepatocytes. Silymarin blocks the receptor sites by which the mushroom toxins enter the cells. In addition, toxins that have already penetrated hepatocytes are neutralized by silibinin. In animal studies, silymarin given within 10 minutes after Amanita toxin ingestion completely counteracted the toxic effects, and if given within 24 hours of toxin ingestion silymarin prevented death and greatly reduced liver damage.[9] Similar hepatoprotective effects have been shown in *in vitro* and animal studies against ethanol and acetaminophen.[10,11]

Antioxidant Activity

Silymarin is a potent free radical scavenger and has been noted to increase production of glutathione in hepatocytes.[12,13] Silymarin has been shown in one animal study to raise intracellular glutathione level by as much as 50 percent.[14] Silymarin also increases the activity of superoxide dismutase in erythrocytes.[15]

Regenerative Properties

Silymarin stimulates the regenerative ability of the liver to form new hepatocytes by stimulating the activity of DNA-dependent RNA-polymerase I.[16,17] This results in an increase in rRNA synthesis and increased protein synthesis. *In vitro* studies suggest this action extends only to normal hepatocytes and not cancerous cells.[18]

Antifibrotic Activity

The ability of silymarin to block fibrosis in the liver was first shown in a study with rats subjected to complete bile duct occlusion.[19] This action was later demonstrated in an open-label, uncontrolled study of 998 patients with liver disease due to a variety of factors, including alcohol abuse, chronic active hepatitis B or C, drugs, and chemical exposure.[20] Use of 140 mg of silymarin (equivalent to approximately 60 mg of silibinin) three times daily for three months led to a significant reduction in amino terminal procollagen III peptide (PIIINP), a marker of fibrosis. In 19 percent of the patients, this measure had dropped to the normal range expected for a healthy person.

Clinical Indications

Alcohol-Related Liver Disease and Cirrhosis

Standardized milk thistle extracts (containing 70–80% silymarin) are approved by the German Commission E for the treatment of "toxic liver damage and for supportive treatment in chronic inflammatory liver disease and hepatic cirrhosis."[21] Clinical support to date has been most significant in the treatment of alcohol-related liver disease as well as cirrhosis (particularly due to alcohol abuse).

Several European randomized, placebo-controlled clinical trials have found that serum bilirubin, AST, and ALT levels were decreased in patients with alcohol-related liver disease who took a standardized milk thistle extract delivering 420 mg of silymarin per day.[22-24] These clinical trials ranged from one to six months in length. In one trial, liver biopsy indicated positive changes in liver histology[23] while another noted a decrease in serum procollagen III peptide levels.[24]

Three double-blind, placebo-controlled trials have examined the effect of milk thistle extract on patients with cirrhosis, with mixed results. One trial found four-year survival rates were improved (58% in silymarin group vs. 39% for placebo group) in cirrhosis patients taking 420 mg of silymarin per day for an average of 41 months.[25] Results were best in patients with alcohol-related cirrhosis and those designated Child A. Similar results were seen in a 12-month trial of adult diabetics with alcoholic cirrhosis.[26] However, a two-year clinical trial found no influence on hepatic health or survival rates in adults with liver cirrhosis.[27]

A small pilot study on patients with primary biliary cirrhosis with a sub-optimal response to ursodeoxycholic acid also found no benefits from the use of milk thistle extract.[28]

Hepatitis

Several small clinical trials in Europe have suggested that milk thistle extract may be beneficial in the management of chronic viral hepatitis. Studies using 420 mg of silymarin per day for as long as nine months found a significant decrease in AST and ALT levels in patients with hepatitis B.[29,30] Histological improvements were also noted in patients undergoing liver biopsy. Similar results have been noted with a product that combines silymarin and phosphatidylcholine.[31,32] However, these results must be viewed as preliminary. Future clinical trials must focus on what role milk thistle extract may play in the treatment of viral hepatitis – particularly hepatitis C.

Hepatoprotection During Drug Therapy

Preliminary results suggest milk thistle extract may serve as a hepatoprotective agent for persons taking potentially hepatotoxic drugs such as psychotropics[33] and anthracycline during treatment for leukemia.[34] However, one clinical trial found no protective effects for milk thistle extract in patients taking tacrine.[35]

Drug-Botanical Interactions

Although no drug interactions are listed for milk thistle, a new *in vitro* study suggests it may inhibit CYP3A4 activity.[36] The ramifications of these findings for humans are unknown.

Side Effects and Toxicity

Milk thistle extract is virtually devoid of any side effects and may be used by a wide range of people, including pregnant and lactating women. Since silymarin does have some choleretic activity, it may have a mild, transient laxative effect in some individuals. This will usually cease within two or three days.

Dosage

The standard dosage of milk thistle extract, standardized to 70-80 percent silymarin, is 140 milligrams of silymarin three times daily. In persons with liver disease, it is recommended that this dose be used until clinical improvement is verified by laboratory tests. According to research and clinical experience, improvement should be noted in about eight weeks. However, in persons with chronic liver disease due to hepatitis or cirrhosis, ongoing use of silymarin may be necessary.

References

1. Bisset N. *Herbal Drugs and Pharmaceuticals*. London, England: CRC Press; 1994:121-123.
2. Wagner H, Horhammer L, Munster R. On the chemistry of silymarin (silybin), the active principle of the fruits of *Silybum marianum* (L.) Gaertn. (*Carduus marianus* L.) *Arzneimittelforschung* 1968;18:688-696. [Article in German]
3. Pelter A, Hansel R. The structure of silibinin (Silybum substance E6)–the first flavonolignan. *Tetrahedron Let* 1968;25:2911-2916.

4. Hikino H, Kiso Y, Wagner H, Fiebig M. Antihepatotoxic actions of flavonolignans from *Silybum marianum* fruits. *Planta Med* 1984;50:248-250.

5. Blumenthal M, Goldberg A, Brinckmann J, eds. *Herbal Medicine: Expanded Commission E Monographs.* Newton, MA: Integrative Medicine Communications; 2000:257-263.

6. Faulstich H, Jahn W, Wieland T. Silybin inhibition of amatoxin uptake in the perfused rat liver. *Arzneimittelforschung* 1980;30:452-454.

7. Tuchweber B, Sieck R, Trost W. Prevention by silibinin of phalloidin induced hepatotoxicity. *Toxicol Appl Pharmacol* 1979;51:265-275.

8. Vogel G, Tuchweber B, Trost W. Protection by silibinin against Amanita phalloides intoxication in beagles. *Toxicol Appl Pharmacol* 1984;73:355-362.

9. Valenzuela A, Videla LA. Silymarin protection against hepatic lipid peroxidation induced by acute ethanol intoxication in the rat. *Biochem Pharmacol* 1985;34:2209-2212.

10. Muriel P, Garciapina T, Perez-Alvarez V, Mourelle M. Silymarin protects against paracetamol-induced lipid peroxidation and liver damage. *J Appl Toxicol* 1992;12:439-442.

11. Campos R, Garrido A, Guerra R, Valenzuela A. Silibinin dihemisuccinate protects against glutathione depletion and lipid peroxidation induced by acetaminophen on rat liver. *Planta Med* 1989;55:417-419.

12. Feher J, Lang I, Deak G, et al. Free radicals in tissue damage in liver diseases and therapeutic approach. *Tokai J Exp Clin Med* 1986;11:123-134.

13. Valenzuela A, Aspillaga M, Vial S, Guerra R. Selectivity of silymarin on the increase of glutathione content in different tissues of the rat. *Planta Med* 1989;55:420-422.

14. Muzes G, Deak G, Lang I, et al. Effect of the bioflavonoid silymarin on the *in vitro* activity and expression of superoxide dismutase (SOD) enzyme. *Acta Physiol Hung* 1991;78:3-9.

15. Magliulo E, Carosi PG, Minoli L, Gorini S. Studies on the regenerative capacity of the liver in rats subjected to partial hepatectomy and treated with silymarin. *Arzneimittelforschung* 1973;23:161-167.

16. Sonnenbichler J, Zetl I. Stimulating influence of a flavonolignan derivative on proliferation, RNA synthesis and protein synthesis in liver cells. In: Okolocsanyi L, Csomos G, Crepaldi G, eds. *Assessment and Management of Hepatobiliary Disease*. Berlin: Springer-Verlag; 1987:265-272.

17. Sonnenbichler J, Goldberg M, Hane I, et al. Stimulating effects of silibinin on the DNA-synthesis in partially hepatectomized rat livers: non-response in hepatoma and other malignant cell lines. *Biochem Pharmacol* 1986;35:538-541.

18. Boigk G, Stroedter L, Herbst H, et al. Silymarin retards collagen accumulation in early and advanced biliary fibrosis secondary to complete bile duct obliteration in rats. *Hepatology* 1997;26:643-649.

19. Schuppan D, Strusser W. Legalon® lessens fibrosing activity in patients with chronic liver disease. *Z Allgemeinmed* 1998;74:577-584.

20. Schandalik R, Gatti G, Perucca E. Pharmacokinetics of silybin in bile following administration of silipide and silymarin in cholecystectomy patients. *Arzneimittelforschung* 1992;42:964-968.

21. Blumenthal M, Busse W, Goldberg A, et al, eds. *The Complete German Commission E Monographs.* Newton, MA: Integrative Medicine Communications; 1998:169-170.

22. Salmi HA, Sama S. Effects of silymarin on chemical, functional and morphological actions of the liver. *Scand J Gastroenterol* 1982;17:517-521.

23. DiMario FR, Farni L, Okolicsanyi L, Naccarato R. The effects of silymarin on the liver function parameters of patients with alcohol-induced liver disease: a double-blind study. In: De Ritis F, Csomos G, Bratz R, eds. *Der Toxish-metabolische Leberschaden*. Lubeck, Germany: Hans Verl-Kontor; 1981:54-58.

24. Feher J, Deak G, M¸zes G, et al. Liver-protective action of silymarin therapy in chronic alcoholic liver diseases. *Orv Hetil* 1989;130:2723-2727. [Article in Hungarian]

25. Ferenci R, Dragosics B, Dittrich H, et al. Randomized controlled trial of silymarin in patients with cirrhosis of the liver. *J Hepatol* 1989;9:105-113.

26. Velussi M, Cernogoi AM, DeMonte A, et al. Long-term (12 months) treatment with an antioxidant drug (silymarin) is effective on hyperinsulinemia, exogenous insulin need and malondialdehyde levels in cirrhotic diabetic patients. *J Hepatol* 1997;26:871-879.

27. Pares A, Planas R, Torres M, et al. Effects of silymarin in alcoholic patients with cirrhosis of the liver: results of a controlled, double-blind, randomized and multicenter trial. *J Hepatol* 1998;28:615-621.

28. Angulo P, Patel T, Jorgensen RA, et al. Silymarin in the treatment of patients with primary biliary cirrhosis with a suboptimal response to ursodeoxycholic acid. *Hepatology* 2000;32:897-900.

29. Berenguer J, Carrasco D. Double-blind trial of silymarin versus placebo in the treatment of chronic hepatitis. *Muench Med Wochenschr* 1997;119:240-260.

30. Poser G. Experience in the treatment of chronic hepatopathies with silymarin. *Arzneimittelforschung* 1971;21:1209-1212. [Article in German]

31. Vailati A, Aristia L. Randomized open study of the dose-effect relationship of a short course of IdB 1016 in patients with viral or alcoholic hepatitis. *Fitoterapia* 1993;64:219-227.

32. Buzzelli G, Moscarella S, Giusti A, et al. A pilot study on the liver protective effect of silybin-phosphatidylcholine complex (IdB 1016) in chronic active hepatitis. *Int J Clin Pharmacol Ther Toxicol* 1993;31:456-460.

33. Palasicano G, Portinasca P, Palmieri V, et al. The effect of silymarin on plasma levels of malondialdehyde in patients receiving long-term treatment with psychotropic drugs. *Curr Ther Res* 1994;55:537-545.

34. Invernizzi R, Bernuzzi S, Ciani D, Ascari E. Silymarin during maintenance therapy of acute promyelocytic leukemia. *Haematologica* 1993;78:340-341. [Letter]

35. Allain H, Sch¸ck S, Lebreton S, et al. Aminotransferase levels and silymarin in *de novo* tacrine-treated patients with Alzheimer's disease. *Dement Geriatr Cogn Disord* 1999;10:181-185.

36. Venkataramanan R, Ramachandran V, Komoroski BJ, et al. Milk thistle, a herbal supplement, decreases the activity of CYP3A4 and uridine disphosphoglucuronosyl transferase in human hepatocyte cultures. *Drug Metab Dispos* 2000;28:1270-1273.

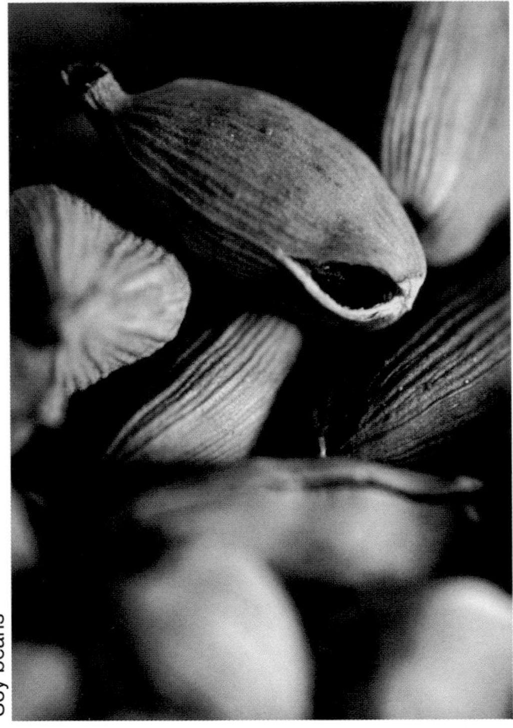

Soy beans

Soy Isoflavones

Introduction

Isoflavones are a class of phytochemicals found in soybeans, chickpeas, and other legumes. Soybeans have the highest concentration of isoflavones, as well as the highest concentration of the individual isoflavones thought to contain medicinal properties – genistein and daidzein. Isoflavones have antioxidant properties that protect the cardiovascular system from LDL oxidation. Isoflavones are also a type of phytoestrogen that have been studied for their role in the prevention of osteoporosis and symptoms of menopause, as well as breast and prostate cancer.

Biochemistry

The principal isoflavones in soy are genistein, daidzein, and their metabolites. Genistein has a hydroxyl group in the 5-position, giving it three hydroxyl groups, while daidzein has two. Isoflavones are members of the flavonoid family of plant compounds, which is in turn a member of the group of plant constituents known as polyphenols. Isoflavones are not as ubiquitous in nature as other flavonoids such as flavones and flavonols, being found primarily in one subfamily of Leguminosae, the Pailionoideae family.[1] Genistein is formed from biochanin A, and daidzein from formononetin.[2] Genistein and daidzein also occur in soy products in the form of their glycosides, genistin and daidzin.

Pharmacokinetics

Isoflavones undergo extensive metabolism in the intestinal tract prior to absorption. In the case of soy isoflavone glycosides, intestinal bacterial glucosidases cleave the sugar moieties, releasing the biologically active isoflavones, genistein and daidzein. In adults, genistein and daidzein are further transformed by bacteria to the metabolites equol, O-desmethylangolensis, dihydrogenistein, and p-ethylphenol. Because of soy intake by livestock,

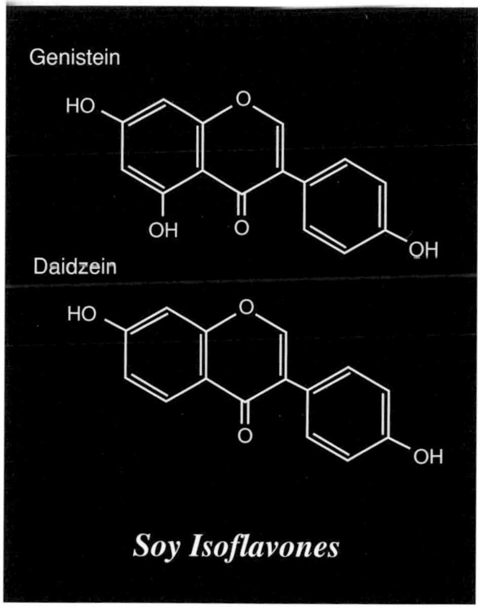

Soy Isoflavones

isoflavone metabolites are also consumed in dairy products and meat.[3] In at least one study, genistein was well absorbed in the small intestine by human subjects fed a soy beverage.[4] After absorption, isoflavones are transported to the liver; the effectiveness of this hepatic first-pass clearance influences the amount that reaches peripheral tissues.[4] Isoflavones and their metabolites are eliminated primarily via the kidneys.[5]

Mechanisms of Action

There are many proposed mechanisms for the therapeutic effects of isoflavones, including inhibition of protein tyrosine kinase (PTK), binding to estrogen receptors (although soy's inhibition of cancer cell growth does not seem to be entirely estrogen dependent),[6] inhibition of production of reactive oxygen species,[6] induction of DNA strand breakage resulting in apoptosis or cell death,[7] inhibition of angiogenesis,[8] modulation of sex steroid binding protein,[9] inhibition of 5 alpha-reductase,[10] inhibition of P-form phenolsulfotransferase (PST) -mediated sulfation,[11] inhibition of thrombin formation and platelet activation,[12] and increased LDL receptor activity.[13]

Clinical Indications

Cancer

There is considerable epidemiological evidence, including a review of 21 studies on 26 different cancer sites,[14] that soy isoflavones might provide protection from several types of cancer. These same researchers examined 26 different animal studies and found 17 of them demonstrated soy's protective effect from experimental carcinogenesis. *In vitro* studies found genistein to be a very potent inhibitor of angiogenesis.[8] Case-control, epidemiological, animal, and *in vitro* studies all point to the effectiveness of soy isoflavones for the prevention of breast cancer.[15-18] Epidemiological, animal, and *in vitro* evidence suggest soy isoflavones could help prevent prostate cancer.[19-22]

Cardiovascular Disease

Soy isoflavones inhibit atherosclerotic plaque formation by intervening at several steps in thrombus formation. Arterial thrombus formation is generally initiated by an injury to the endothelial cells lining the blood vessels. One of the first events after an injury is thrombin formation. This leads to a cascade of events, including platelet activation, resulting in thrombus formation. Genistein has been found to inhibit thrombin formation and platelet activation.[23] The pathogenesis of atherosclerotic plaque formation also involves, in addition to lipid accumulation, the infiltration of monocytes and T-lymphocytes into the artery wall, contributing to the thickening of the wall and occlusion of the vessel. Monocytes and lymphocytes adhere to endothelial cell surfaces via expression of certain "adhesion molecules." Infiltration and proliferation appear to be controlled by peptide growth factors. Increased levels of isoflavones, genistein in particular, appear to alter growth factor activity and inhibit cell adhesion and proliferation, all activities necessary for lesion formation in the intima of blood vessels.[24]

Soy protein supplementation also has a positive effect on lipid profiles in humans. A double-blind trial found soy supplementation, in amounts as low as 20 grams per day, effectively improved the blood lipid profile after just six weeks.[25] In another double-blind trial, 21 severely hypercholesterolemic patients – all with a history of resistance to HMG CoA reductase inhibitor therapy – ingested a soy protein drink (providing 35 grams protein per day) or placebo daily for four weeks.[26] The treatment group experienced a 6.5-7.4-percent reduction in total cholesterol levels. Although one meta-analysis suggested the isoflavone component of soy might account for up to 70 percent of its hypocholesterolemic effect,[27] there is also evidence of cholesterol-lowering effects from isoflavone-free products as well, suggesting the principal effect of soy on blood lipids may be mediated by its protein component.[28]

Osteoporosis

Animal studies have found soy protein isolates appear to enhance bone density,[29] and epidemiological evidence points to diets high in soy as a possible protection against osteoporosis.[30] A clinical study found 45 grams per day soy grits increased bone mineral density and improved vaginal cytology maturation index when compared to those given 45 grams per day wheat.[31] In a randomized, double-blind trial, supplementation with a soy protein isolate providing 90 mg soy isoflavones per day for six months produced significant increases in bone mineral content and density in the lumbar spine (but not elsewhere) of postmenopausal women compared with controls. A soy protein supplement with lower isoflavone content (56 mg per day) failed to produce this effect, suggesting an important role of isoflavones in protection of bone mineral density.[32] It is not clear what part soy isoflavones play in this protection, thus further investigation is warranted.

Menopause

Observational data indicate Japanese women, who have a dietary intake of soy isoflavones 50-100 times greater than that of Western diets, have a nearly 10-fold lower incidence of vasomotor symptoms than in U.S. or other Western women.[33] Soy isoflavones may help alleviate the physical symptoms of menopause. A two-month study compared the effect of a soy drink containing 80 mg isoflavones with a casein drink. Those taking the soy drink experienced a significant decline in hot flashes.[34] The soy group also experienced a decrease in LH and cholesterol and an increase in prolactin and growth hormone. A randomized, double-blind, multi-center trial found 60 grams soy protein per day for 12 weeks reduced the frequency of hot flashes by 45 percent in postmenopausal women, compared with a 30-percent reduction from placebo.[35] However, soy did not alter other menopausal complaints in the study. Similar results have been reported in other double-blind trials.[36,37]

Drug-Nutrient Interactions

Administration of levothyroxine concurrently with a soy protein dietary supplement results in decreased absorption of levothyroxine and the need for higher oral doses of levothyroxine to attain therapeutic serum thyroid hormone levels.[38]

In vitro and animal studies suggest genistein negates the inhibitory effect of tamoxifen on the growth of estrogen-dependent breast tumors.[39,40] Caution is warranted for postmenopausal women consuming genistein while on tamoxifen therapy for estrogen-responsive breast cancer.

Side Effects and Toxicity

Concern has been raised regarding the safety of using soy products with infants and young children because of the phytoestrogenic constituents, including the isoflavones. However, a long-term follow-up study of over 800 women and men who had been fed either soy formula or cow's milk formula during infancy found no significant differences between the soy and cow's milk groups for more than 30 outcomes, including height, weight, age of onset of puberty, breast size, or proportion of women who had had at least one pregnancy.[41]

Another concern regarding soy isoflavone supplementation is the potential that high doses might inhibit thyroid function, resulting in dietary-induced goiter. *In vitro* analysis found the isoflavones genestein and daidzein have the potential to block iodinization of tyrosine.[42] A study from Cornell University's Department of Pediatrics found the frequency of feedings with soy-based formulas early in life was significantly higher in children with autoimmune thyroid disease (31%) when compared to siblings (12%) or unrelated controls (13%).[43] Soy isoflavones have been reported to reduce thyroid function.[44] Soybean supplementation among 37 healthy Japanese adults (30 g per day for three months) led to a slight increase in TSH.[45] However, soy products have also been shown to cause an increase in thyroid function[46] or produce no change in thyroid function.[47]

Dosage

For osteoporosis prevention, 90 mg per day of soy isoflavones is recommended. For menopausal hot flashes, 60-80 mg of soy isoflavones per day appears to be effective. The amount of soy isoflavones in Asian diets is estimated to be in the range of 20-80 mg daily. Until more studies have been conducted on soy isoflavone extracts, the optimal dosage necessary to provide protection against cardiovascular disease and cancer remains unknown.

References

1. Harbone JB, Baxter H, eds. *Phytochemical Dictionary*. Basingstoke, England: Burgess Science Press; 1995.
2. Knight DC, Eden JA. A review of the clinical effects of phytoestrogens. *Obstet Gynecol* 1996;87:897-904.
3. Adlercreutz H, Mazur W. Phyto-estrogens and Western diseases. *Ann Med* 1997;29:95-120.
4. Barnes S, Sfakianos J, Coward L, Kirk M. Soy isoflavonoids and cancer prevention. Underlying biochemical and pharmacological issues. *Adv Exp Med Biol* 1996;401:87-100.
5. Setchell KD, Zimmer-Nechemias L, Cai J, Heubi JE. Exposure of infants to phyto-oestrogens from soy-based infant formula. *Lancet* 1997;350:23-27.
6. Wei H, Bowen R, Cai Q, et al. Antioxidant and antipromotional effects of the soybean isoflavone genistein. *Proc Soc Exp Biol Med* 1995;208:124-130.
7. Barnes S, Peterson TG, Coward L. Rationale for the use of genistein-containing soy matrices in chemoprevention trials for breast and prostate cancer. *J Cell Biochem Suppl* 1995;22:181-187.
8. Fotsis T, Pepper M, Adlercreutz H, et al. Genistein, a dietary-derived inhibitor of *in vitro* angiogenesis. *Proc Natl Acad Sci U S A* 1993;90:2690-2694.
9. Martin ME, Haourigui M, Pelissero C, et al. Interactions between phytoestrogens and human sex steroid binding protein. *Life Sci* 1996;58:429-436.
10. Evans BA, Griffiths K, Morton MS. Inhibition of 5 alpha-reductase in genital skin fibroblasts and prostate tissue by dietary lignans and isoflavonoids. *J Endocrinol* 1995;147:295-302.
11. Eaton EA, Walle UK, Lewis AJ, et al. Flavonoids, potent inhibitors of the human P-form phenolsulfotransferase. Potential role in drug metabolism and chemoprevention. *Drug Metab Dispos* 1996;24:232-237.
12. Wilcox JN, Blumenthal BF. Thrombotic mechanisms in atherosclerosis: potential impact of soy proteins. *J Nutr* 1995;125:631S-638S.
13. Potter SM. Soy protein and serum lipids. *Curr Opin Lipidol* 1996;7:260-264.
14. Messina MJ, Persky V, Setchell KD, Barnes S. Soy intake and cancer risk: a review of the *in vitro* and *in vivo* data. *Nutr Cancer* 1994;21:113-131.
15. Ingram D, Sanders K, Kolybaba M, Lopez D. Case-control study of phyto-oestrogens and breast cancer. *Lancet* 1997;350:990-994.
16. Wu AH, Ziegler RG, Horn-Ross PL. Tofu and risk of breast cancer in Asian-Americans. *Cancer Epidemiol Biomarkers Prev* 1996;5:901-906.
17. Peterson G, Barnes S. Genistein inhibition of the growth of human breast cancer cells: independence from estrogen receptors and the multi-drug resistance gene. *Biochem Biophys Res Commun* 1991;179:661-667.
18. Lamartiniere CA, Moore J, Holland M, Barnes S. Neonatal genistein chemoprevents mammary cancer. *Proc Soc Exp Biol Med* 1995;208:120-123.
19. Adlercreutz H, Markkanen H, Watanabe S. Plasma concentrations of phyto-oestrogens in Japanese men. *Lancet* 1993;342:1209-1210.
20. Pollard M, Luckert PH. Influence of isoflavones in soy protein isolates on development of induced prostate-related cancers in L-W rats. *Nutr Cancer* 1997;28:41-45.
21. Peterson G, Barnes S. Genistein and biochanin A inhibit the growth of human prostate cancer cells but not epidermal growth factor receptor tyrosine autophosphorylation. *Prostate* 1993;22:335-345.
22. Hempstock J, Kavanagh JP, George NJR. Growth inhibition of prostate cell lines *in vitro* by phyto-estrogens. *Br J Urol* 1998;82:560-563.

23. Wilcox JN, Blumenthal BF. Thrombotic mechanisms in atherosclerosis: potential impact of soy proteins. *J Nutr* 1995;125:631S-638S.

24. Raines EW, Ross R. Biology of atherosclerotic plaque formation: possible role of growth factors in lesion development and the potential impact of soy. *J Nutr* 1995;125:624S-630S.

25. Teixeira SR, Potter SM, Weigel R, et al. Effects of feeding 4 levels of soy protein for 3 and 6 wk on blood lipids and apolipoproteins in moderately hypercholesterolemic men. *Am J Clin Nutr* 2000;71:1077-1084.

26. Sirtori CR, Pazzucconi F, Colombo L, et al. Double-blind study of the addition of high-protein soya milk v. cows' milk to the diet of patients with severe hypercholesterolemia and resistance to or intolcrance of statins. *Br J Nutr* 1999;82:91-96.

27. Anderson JW, Johnstone BM, Cook-Newell ME. Meta-analysis of the effects of soy protein intake on serum lipids. *New Engl J Med* 1995;333:276-282.

28. Sirtori CR. Risks and benefits of soy phytoestrogens in cardiovascular diseases, cancer, climacteric symptoms and osteoporosis. *Drug Saf* 2001;24:665-682.

29. Arjmandi BH, Alekel L, Hollis BW, et al. Dietary soybean protein prevents bone loss in ovariectomized rat model of osteoporosis. *J Nutr* 1996;126:161-167.

30. Barnes S. Evolution of the health benefits of soy isoflavones. *Proc Soc Exp Biol Med* 1998;217:386-392.

31. Dalais FS, Rice GE, Bell RJ, et al. Dietary soy supplementation increases vaginal cytology maturation index and bone mineral density in postmenopausal women. *Am J Clin Nutr* 1998;68:S1519.

32. Potter SM, Baum JA, Teng H, et al. Soy protein and isoflavones: their effects on blood lipids and bone density in postmenopausal women. *Am J Clin Nutr* 1998;68:1375S-1379S.

33. Brzezinski A, Adlercreutz H, Shaoul R, et al. Short term effects of phytoestrogens-rich diet on postmenopausal women. *Menopause* 1997;4:89-94.

34. Harding C, Morton M, Gould V, et al. Dietary soy supplementation is estrogenic in menopausal women. *Am J Clin Nutr* 1998;68:S1532.

35. Albertazzi P, Pansini F, Bonaccorsi G, et al. The effect of dietary soy supplementation on hot flushes. *Obstet Gynecol* 1998;91:6-11.

36. Upmalis DH, Lobo R, Bradley L, et al. Vasomotor symptom relief by soy isoflavone extract tablets in postmenopausal women: a multicenter, double-blind, randomized, placebo-controlled study. *Menopause* 2000;7:236-242. Erratum in: *Menopause* 2000;7:422.

37. Scambia G, Mango D, Signorile PG, et al. Clinical effects of a standardized soy extract in postmenopausal women: a pilot study. *Menopause* 2000;7:105-111.

38. Bell DS, Ovalle F. Use of soy protein supplement and resultant need for increased dose of levothyroxine. *Endocr Pract* 2001;7:193-194.

39. Jones JL, Daley BJ, Enderson BL, et al. Genistein inhibits tamoxifen effects on cell proliferation and cell cycle arrest in T47D breast cancer cells. *Am Surg* 2002;68:575-577.

40. Ju YH, Doerge DR, Allred KF, et al. Dietary genistein negates the inhibitory effect of tamoxifen on growth of estrogen-dependent human breast cancer (MCF-7) cells implanted in athymic mice. *Cancer Res* 2002;62:2474-2477.

41. Strom BL, Schinnar R, Ziegler EE, et al. Exposure to soy-based formula in infancy and endocrinological and reproductive outcomes in young adulthood. *JAMA* 2001;286:807-814.

42. Divi RL, Chang HC, Doerge DR. Anti-thyroid isoflavones from soybean: isolation, characterization, and mechanisms of action. *Biochem Pharmacol* 1997;54:1087-1096.

43. Fort P, Moses N, Fasano M, et al. Breast and soy-formula feedings in early infancy and the prevalence of autoimmune thyroid disease in children. *J Am Coll Nutr* 1990;9:164-167.

44. Doerge Dr, Sheehan DM. Goitrogenic and estrogenic activity of soy isoflavones. Environ Health Perspect 2002;110:S349-S353.

45. Ishizuki Y, Hirooka Y, Murata Y, Togashi K. The effects on the thyroid gland of soybeans administered experimentally in healthy subjects. *Nippon Naibunpi Gakkai Zasshi* 1991;67:622-629. [Article in Japanese]

46. Forsythe WA. Soy protein, thyroid regulation and cholesterol metabolism. *J Nutr* 1995;125:619S-623S.

47. Bennink MR, Mayle JE, Bourquin LD, Thiagarajan D. Evaluation of soy protein in risk reduction for colon cancer and cardiovascular disease: Preliminary results. Second International Symposium on the Role of Soy in Preventing and Treating Chronic Disease. September 15-18, 1996. Brussels, Belgium.

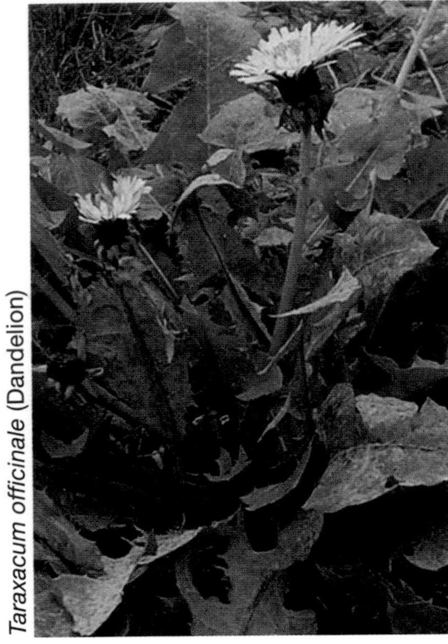
Taraxacum officinale (Dandelion)

Taraxacum officinale

Description

Taraxacum officinale (dandelion), a member of the Asteraceae family, grows to a height of about 12 inches, producing spatula-like leaves and yellow flowers that bloom year-round.[1] Upon maturation, the flower turns into the characteristic seed-containing puffball. Dandelion is grown commercially in the United States and Europe, and the leaves and root are used in herbal medicine. Commercial grade dandelion is typically harvested during the autumn when the inulin content is highest.

Dandelion is commonly used as a food. The leaves are used in salads and teas, while the roots are sometimes used as a coffee substitute. Dandelion leaves and roots have been used for hundreds of years to treat liver, gallbladder, kidney, and joint problems. Dandelion is traditionally considered an alterative and is used for conditions as varied as eczema and cancer.[2] In North America, the Iroquois people prepared infusions and decoctions of the root and whole herb to treat kidney disease, dropsy, and dermatological conditions. As is the case today, dandelion leaves have also been used historically as a diuretic.

Active Constituents

Dandelion root contains an abundance of sesquiterpene lactones, also known as bitter elements (principally taraxacin and taraxacerin).[3] Other related compounds include beta-amyrin, taraxasterol, and taraxerol, as well as free sterols (sitosterin, stigmasterin, and phytosterin). Other constituents include polysaccharides (primarily fructosans and inulin), smaller amounts of pectin, resin, and mucilage, and various flavonoids. Three flavonoid glycosides – luteolin 7-glucoside and two luteolin 7-diglucosides – have been isolated from the flowers and leaves. Hydroxycinnamic acids, chicoric acid, monocaffeyltartaric acid, and chlorogenic acid are found throughout the plant, and the coumarins, cichoriin, and aesculin have been identified in the leaf extracts.[4] Dandelion leaves are a rich source of a variety of vitamins and minerals, including beta carotene, non-provitamin A carotenoids, xanthophylls, chlorophyll, vitamins C and D, many of the B-complex vitamins, choline, iron, silicon, magnesium, sodium, potassium, zinc, manganese, copper, and phosphorous.

Mechanisms of Action

Digestive Effects

Bitter herbs such as dandelion have been used traditionally to stimulate digestion;[5] however, no pharmacological or clinical studies have been performed to date on this action.

Hepatobiliary Effects

Oral administration of dandelion root extracts has been shown to increase bile release from the gallbladder (cholagogue effect).[6] The bitter principals responsible for this cholagogue effect are also thought to increase bile production in the liver (choleretic effect).[7] A recent rat study found Taraxacum inhibits activity of hepatic phase I detoxification enzymes CYP1A2 (by 15%) and CYP2E (by 48%). Conversely, Taraxacum increased the activity of the phase II enzyme UDP-glucuronosyl transferase.[8]

Diuretic Activity

In experimental research on mice, high amounts of an aqueous extract of dandelion leaf (2 g per 1 kg body weight) has been shown to have diuretic activity comparable to furosemide.[9] Since dandelion is also a rich source of potassium, some think it is capable of replacing potassium lost through diuresis.

Hypoglycemic Effects

An animal study suggests dandelion might possess hypoglycemic activity.[10] This finding is probably in part a result of the high inulin content of the plant. Dandelion's effects on glucose metabolism have not been studied in humans to date.

Other Actions

Evidence suggests dandelion may influence nitric oxide production.[11] Nitric oxide is important for immune regulation and defense; however, this molecule can be inhibited by cadmium. An aqueous extract of dandelion has been shown to overcome this inhibitory effect of cadmium and work in a dose-dependent manner to restore nitric oxide production by mouse peritoneal macrophages.

Antitumor activity of the aqueous extract of dandelion root in mice has also been reported in the scientific literature.[12]

Clinical Indications

Classically listed as a cholagogue, dandelion root is approved by the German Commission E for the treatment of disturbances in bile flow, stimulation of diuresis, loss of appetite, and dyspepsia.[13] Although there are no published clinical trials on either dandelion root or leaf alone, it has a long history of use by natural health-care practitioners.

Liver/Gallbladder Stasis

Because of dandelion root's cholagogue[6] and choleretic effects,[7] it has been traditionally recommended for people with sluggish liver function due to alcohol abuse or poor diet. The increase in bile flow may help improve fat (including cholesterol) metabolism in the body; however, there are no clinical studies to support these uses. Patients with increased phase I metabolism coupled with impaired phase II activity may especially benefit from Taraxacum supplementation.[8]

Edema

Dandelion leaf is a diuretic[9] and thus may be considered in cases of edema from such conditions as congestive heart failure or premenstrual syndrome. As a diuretic it may also benefit those with hypertension. Although it is suggested dandelion spares potassium, attention to electrolyte balance may be warranted.

Colitis

A small Bulgarian clinical trial found dandelion root in combination with other herbs might be an effective intervention in chronic colitis.[14] Twenty-four patients with chronic non-specific colitis were treated with an herbal combination consisting of dandelion root, St. John's wort (*Hypericum perforatum*), lemon balm (*Melissa officinalis*), calendula flower (*Calendula officinalis*), and fennel seed (*Foeniculum vulgare*). Spontaneous and palpable pains along the large intestine disappeared in 96 percent of the patients by the 15th day of treatment.

Botanical-Drug Interactions

In an animal study, administration of a dandelion extract (actually *Taraxacum mongolicum*, a close relative of the more common western dandelion) concomitantly with ciprofloxacin decreased absorption of the drug.[15] This was found to be due to the high mineral content of the dandelion herb. Ciprofloxacin should not be taken within two hours of any dandelion preparation. Due to the potential diuretic effect of the leaves, they should be used with caution by those taking prescription diuretic drugs.

Side Effects and Toxicity

Because of its choleretic and cholegogue activity, dandelion leaf and root should not be used by people with gallstones or bile duct obstruction unless closely supervised by a health-care practitioner.[13] In cases of gastric ulcer or gastritis, dandelion should be used cautiously, as it may cause over-production of stomach acid. Although Taraxacum is high in potassium, it may not be high enough to offset possible potassium loss by long-term use of the leaves as a diuretic.

Constituents of dandelion may cause allergic reactions. The latex of fresh dandelion stems may cause an allergic rash in some people. Dandelion root contains a high amount of inulin, so persons with sensitivity to inulin should probably avoid dandelion. Although reports in the scientific literature refer only to the pollen as being a potential source of photoallergic contact dermatitis,[16,17] and an allergen capable of cross-reactivity in individuals with pollen allergy to other plants of the Compositae family,[18] a report documenting an anaphylactic reaction in an atopic patient following the oral ingestion of an herbal combination containing dandelion indicates a possible need for caution. In this case, the herbal compound was found to have trace amounts of pollen from dandelion and several other medicinal plants, which resulted in this systemic reaction.[19]

Dosage

As a general liver/gallbladder tonic and to stimulate digestion, 3-5 g of dried root or 5-10 ml of tincture made from the root can be taken three times per day.[11] As a mild diuretic or appetite stimulant, 4-10 g of dried leaves can be added to 1 cup (250 ml) of boiling water and drunk as a decoction. Alternatively, 2-5 ml of tincture made from the leaves can be taken three times per day.

References

1. Wichtl M. *Herbal Drugs and Phytopharmaceuticals*. Boca Raton, FL: CRC Press; 1994:486-489.
2. Blumenthal M, Goldberg A, Brinckmann J, eds. *Herbal Medicine: Expanded Commission E Monographs*. Newton, MA: Integrative Medicine Communications; 2000:78-83.
3. Leung AY, Foster S. *Encyclopedia of Common Natural Ingredients Used in Food, Drugs, and Cosmetics*. New York: John Wiley and Sons; 1996:205-207.
4. Williams CA, Goldstone F, Greenham J. Flavonoids, cinnamic acids and coumarins from the different tissues and medicinal preparations of Taraxacum officinale. *Phytochemistry* 1996;42:121-127.
5. Pizzorno JE, Murray MT. *Textbook of Natural Medicine*. London: Churchill Livingstone; 1999:979-982.
6. Vogel G. Natural substances with effects on the liver. In: Wagner H, Wolff P, eds. *New Natural Products and Plant Drugs with Pharmacological, Biological or Therapeutic Activity*. Heidelberg: Springer-Verlag; 1977.
7. Bohm K. Choleretic action of some medicinal plants. *Arzneimittelforschung* 1959;9:376-378.
8. Maliakal PP, Wanwimolruk S. Effect of herbal teas on hepatic drug metabolizing enzymes in rats. *J Pharm Pharmacol* 2001;53:1323-1329.

9. Racz-Kotilla E, Racz G, Solomon A. The action of *Taraxacum officinale* extracts on the body weight and diuresis of laboratory animals. *Planta Med* 1974;26:212-217.

10. Akhtar MS, Khan QM, Khaliq T. Effects of *Portulaca oleracae* (Kulfa) and *Taraxacum officinale* (Dhudhal) in normoglycaemic and alloxan-treated hyperglycaemic rabbits. *J Pak Med Assoc* 1985;35:207-210.

11. Kim HM, Lee EH, Shin TY, et al. *Taraxacum officinale* restores inhibition of nitric oxide production by cadmium in mouse peritoneal macrophages. *Immunopharmacol Immunotoxicol* 1998;20:283-297.

12. Kotobuki KK. Taraxacum extracts as antitumor agents. *Chem Abst* 1979;14:530.

13. Blumenthal M, Busse WR, Goldberg A, et al, eds. *The Complete Commission E Monographs: Therapeutic Guide to Herbal Medicines.* Boston, MA: Integrative Medicine Communications; 1998:118-120.

14. Chakurski I, Matev M, Koichev A, et al. Treatment of chronic colitis with an herbal combination of *Taraxacum officinale*, *Hipericum perforatum*, *Melissa officinaliss*, *Calendula officinalis* and *Foeniculum vulgare*. *Vutr Boles* 1981;20:51-54. [Article in Bulgarian]

15. Mark KA, Brancaccio RR, Soter NA, Cohen DE. Allergic contact and photoallergic contact dermatitis to plant and pesticide allergens. *Arch Dermatol* 1999;135:67-70.

16. Lovell CR, Rowan M. Dandelion dermatitis. *Contact Dermatitis* 1991;25:185-188.

17. Fernandez C, Martin-Esteban M, Fiandor A, et al. Analysis of cross-reactivity between sunflower pollen and other pollens of the Compositae family. *J Allergy Clin Immunol* 1993;92:660-667.

18. Chivato T, Juan F, Montoro A, Laguna R. Anaphylaxis induced by ingestion of a pollen compound. *J Investig Allergol Clin Immunol* 1996;6:208-209.

19. Zhu M, Wong PY, Li RC. Effects of *Taraxacum mongolicum* on the bioavailability and disposition of ciprofloxacin in rats. *J Pharm Sci* 1999;88:632-634.

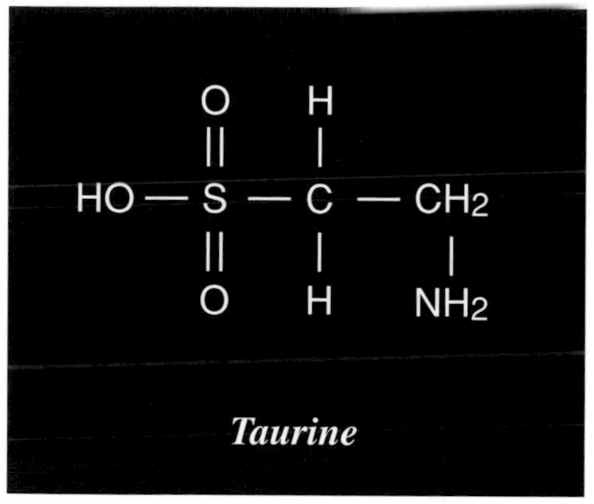

Taurine

Taurine

Introduction

Taurine is a conditionally essential amino acid found in the tissues of most animal species. It is not incorporated into proteins, but is found free in many tissues. Taurine is involved in a number of physiological processes including bile acid conjugation, osmoregulation, detoxification of xenobiotics, cell membrane stabilization, modulation of cellular calcium flux, and modulation of neuronal excitability. Low levels of taurine have been associated with retinal degeneration, growth retardation, and cardiomyopathy. Taurine has been used clinically in the treatment of cardiovascular diseases, hypercholesterolemia, seizure disorders, ocular disorders, diabetes, Alzheimer's disease, hepatic disorders, cystic fibrosis, and alcoholism.

Pharmacokinetics

Taurine (2-aminoethanesulfonic acid) is different from other amino acids in that it contains a sulfonic acid group in place of the carboxylic acid group, and it is not incorporated into proteins. Therefore, it is not an amino acid in the true sense of the word.[1] It is synthesized in human liver tissue from cysteine and methionine via three known pathways, all of which require pyridoxal-5'-phosphate, the active coenzyme form of vitamin B6.[2] The highest concentrations of taurine are found in the neutrophil and the retina, and the largest pools of taurine are found in skeletal and cardiac muscles.[3] Taurine excretion is via the urine or in the bile as bile salts.[4]

Mechanisms of Action

Bile Acid Conjugation

Bile acids, primarily cholic acid and chenodeoxycholic acid, result from cholesterol metabolism in the liver and are involved in emulsification and absorption of lipids and fat-soluble vitamins. In order for this to occur, bile acids must be bound to either glycine or taurine, forming bile salt conjugates. The conjugation of bile acids by taurine results in increased cholesterol solubility and excretion.[5,6]

Detoxification

Research has demonstrated that taurine reacts with and neutralizes hypochlorous acid, which is generated during oxidative neutrophil burst. The result is a stable taurochloramine compound, as opposed to unstable aldehyde compounds formed in states of taurine deficiency. Individuals who are taurine deficient may become more susceptible to tissue damage by xenobiotic agents such as aldehydes, chlorine, and certain amines.[3] Animal studies have also demonstrated taurine's ability to neutralize the potential hepatotoxic effects of carbon tetrachloride and retinol.[7,8] Research also suggests that translocation of bacterial endotoxins can be a factor in determining a person's response to xenobiotic insult. Even small amounts of endotoxin markedly enhance liver injury from hepatotoxic substances such as carbon tetrachloride, ethanol, and cadmium. Taurine was found to significantly inhibit intestinal endotoxin translocation and subsequently decrease hepatic injury from these substances.[9,10]

Membrane Stabilization

Taurine's ability to stabilize cell membranes may be attributed to several events. Taurine has been shown to regulate osmotic pressure in the cell, maintain homeostasis of intracellular ions, inhibit phosphorylation of membrane proteins, and prevent lipid peroxidation. As an osmotic regulator, it has been suggested that taurine, along with glutamic acid, is instrumental in the transport of metabolically generated water from the brain.[11]

Calcium Flux

Taurine is both an intra- and extracellular calcium regulator. Excessive accumulation of intracellular calcium ultimately leads to cell death. Excessive influx of calcium into cells has been demonstrated in various types of myocardial injury, as well as migraines and prolonged epileptic episodes. Taurine supplementation has been shown to be cardioprotective, and of benefit in patients predisposed to epilepsy or migraine.[4,12]

Clinical Indications

Cardiovascular Disease

Several studies indicate taurine is a safe, effective therapeutic tool in the management of various types of cardiovascular disease. Research indicates supplementation with taurine at three to six grams daily for two to three weeks results in reduced serum cholesterol levels in human subjects when compared to placebo.[5,6] In addition, taurine aids in the regulation of intracellular calcium levels, thereby protecting heart muscle from intracellular calcium imbalances, which can lead to cell death and subsequent myocardial damage.[11] Taurine's use in preventing cardiac arrhythmia is well documented and it is thought it may act by modulating potassium flux in and out of cardiac muscle cells.[13] Research has also shown taurine to be capable of lowering blood pressure, due to its positive inotropic effects,[14,15]

Taurine's antioxidant properties are seen in its ability to inhibit neutrophil burst and subsequent oxidative stress, which can result in reperfusion injury to heart tissue.[16] It is also capable of improving the clinical manifestations of congestive heart failure. A Japanese study revealed taurine was significantly more effective than placebo at decreasing the severity of dyspnea, palpitation, crackles, and edema in congestive heart failure patients, while increasing their capacity for exercise.[17]

Seizure Disorders

A number of studies have been conducted on taurine's role in alleviating seizure conditions. Unfortunately, many had design flaws, dosages varied greatly, and no firm conclusions can be drawn. Some patients with epilepsy have an aberration in taurine and glutamic acid metabolism. It is believed that taurine's anti-epileptic activity is due to its ability to maintain a normal glutamic acid concentration in the central nervous system.[2] As mentioned above, benefits may also be due to taurine's effect on intracellular calcium.[12] It appears however, that taurine's anti-epileptic action is transient and disappears rapidly over a period of a few weeks.[18]

Retinal Degeneration

Taurine is very abundant in the vertebrate retina, and taurine deficiency in cats has been shown to cause damage to the cone photoreceptor cells, resulting in permanent retinal degeneration. It is also thought that abnormalities in taurine metabolism might be associated with retinitis pigmentosa in humans.[1] Retinal taurine appears to regulate osmotic pressure, stabilize cell membranes as well as calcium ion concentrations, inhibit lipid peroxidation after oxidant exposure, and act as an antioxidant by scavenging damaging free radicals.[1,4]

Growth and Development

The research on retinal degeneration in taurine-deficient kittens[1] prompted further studies of taurine deficiency in formula-fed pre-term and full-term infants. Taurine is present in high concentrations in human milk, but significantly decreases over the first few months of the infant's life. Because humans have limited ability to synthesize taurine and infants have decreased capacity to store it, a dietary source of taurine is essential for normal development during the neonatal period.[19]

Research on taurine's effects on growth and development in humans shows it may act as a "growth modulator" and that taurine deficiency is responsible for neurological defects involving motor dysfunction and cerebral activity, growth retardation, and retinal degeneration.[4] Animal and *in vitro* studies also support the theory that taurine is essential for proper growth and development.[20,21] As a result, taurine has been added to most commercially available infant formulas.

Diabetes

Animal and human studies indicate that taurine supplementation is effective in alleviating some of the complications of insulin-dependent diabetes. Taurine has been found to influence blood glucose and insulin levels, as well as increasing glycogen synthesis, and it may also be involved in the functioning and integrity of pancreatic beta cells.[3] In insulin-dependent diabetic patients, both plasma and platelet taurine levels were decreased but were corrected by oral taurine supplementation.[22]

Cystic Fibrosis

Cystic fibrosis is usually characterized by nutrient malabsorption in the ileum, impaired bile acid conjugation, and steatorrhea.[23] Human studies using 30 mg/kg taurine daily for four months resulted in a significant decrease in fecal fatty acids.[23]

Alzheimer's Disease

Low levels of the neurotransmitter acetylcholine and altered taurine metabolism have been found in patients with Alzheimer's disease, and it is thought these abnormalities might contribute to the characteristic memory loss.[4] Also, taurine levels in cerebrospinal fluid were decreased in patients with advanced Alzheimer's disease.[24] To date, no clinical trials of taurine supplementation in patients with Alzheimer's disease have been conducted, but in animal models supplementation increased acetylcholine levels in brain tissue.[25]

Hepatic Disorders

In a double-blind, randomized study, acute hepatitis patients with significantly elevated bilirubin levels were given oral taurine - four grams three times daily after meals. Taurine-supplemented patients exhibited notable decreases in bilirubin, total bile acids, and biliary glycine:taurine ratios within one week when compared to control subjects. The icteric period was also decreased.[26]

In patients undergoing ursodeoxycholic acid (UDC) treatment for cholesterol gallstones, taurine therapy may also be beneficial. The taurine conjugate of UDC is better able to solubilize cholesterol than the glycine conjugate, thereby effecting a greater decrease in the bile acid pool size.[27]

Alcoholism

Both taurine and acamprosate (a synthetic taurine analog) have been shown to be clinically useful in treating patients with alcohol dependence. In patients undergoing alcohol withdrawal, taurine given at one gram three times daily for seven days resulted in significantly fewer psychotic episodes when compared to control subjects.[28] A pooled analysis of 11 studies involving over 3,000 patients given oral acamprosate at similar doses revealed it was more effective than placebo at preventing alcohol relapse. The efficacy appeared to be dose dependent and was enhanced by the addition of disulfiram.[29]

Side Effects and Toxicity

With few exceptions, animal and human studies have shown taurine administration to be safe, even at higher doses. Intense, temporary itching has been noted to occur in psoriasis patients at dosages of 2 g taurine daily[1] and some epileptic patients reported dosages of 1.5 g daily resulted in nausea, headache, dizziness, and gait disturbances.[30] One study found that taurine administration to patients with uncompensated adrenocortical insufficiency could induce hypothermia and hyperkalemia.[2]

Dosage

Taurine is usually administered orally, with the adult dosage being 500 mg to 3 g daily in divided doses. Pediatric dosages vary according to the size and age of the child, but range from 250 mg to 1 g daily in divided doses.

References

1. Kendler BS. Taurine: an overview of its role in preventative medicine. *Prev Med* 1989;18:79-100.
2. Shin HK, Linkswiler HM. Tryptophan and methionine metabolism of adult females as affected by vitamin B6 deficiency. *J Nutr* 1874;104:1348-1355.
3. Timbrell JA, Seabra V, Waterfield CJ. The *in vivo* and *in vitro* protective properties of taurine. *Gen Pharmac* 1995;26:453-462.
4. Bradford RW, Allen HW. Taurine in health and disease. *J Adv Med* 1996;9:179-199.
5. Hardison WGM, Grundy SM. Effect of bile acid conjugation patterns on bile acid metabolism in normal humans. *Gastroenterology* 1983:84:617-620.
6. Mizushima S, Nara Y, Sawamura M, Yamori Y. Effects of oral taurine supplementation on lipids and sympathetic nerve tone. *Adv Exp Med Biol* 1996;403:615-622.
7. Nakashima T, Taniko T, Kuriyama K. Therapeutic effect of taurine administration on carbon tetrachloride-induced hepatic injury. *Jpn J Pharmacol* 1982;32:583-589.
8. Gaull GE, Pasantes-Morales H, Wright CE. Taurine in human nutrition. In: *Taurine: Biological Actions and Clinical Perspectives*. New York, NY: Alan R. Liss, Inc.; 1985:3-21.
9. Roth RA, Harkema JR, Pestka JP, Ganey PE. Is exposure to bacterial endotoxin a determinant of susceptibility to intoxication from xenobiotic agents? *Toxicol Appl Pharmacol* 1997;147:300-311.
10. Wang WY. Intestinal endotoxin translocation in endotoxemic rats. *Sheng Li Ke Xue Jin Zhan* 1995;26:41-44. [Article in Chinese]
11. Van Gelder NM. Neuronal discharge hypersynchrony and the intracranial water balance in relation to glutamic acid and taurine redistribution: migraine and epilepsy. In: Pasantes-Morales H, Martin DL, Shain W, et al, eds. *Taurine: Functional Neurochemistry, Physiology, and Cardiology*. New York, NY: Wiley-Liss; 1990:Vol. 351.
12. Satoh H, Sperelakis N. Review of some actions of taurine on ion channels of cardiac muscle cells and others. *Gen Pharmac* 1998;30:451-463.

13. Chazov EI, Malchikova NV, Lipina GB, et al. Taurine and electrical activity of the heart. *Circ Res* 1974;35:S3-S11.

14. Fujita T, Ando K, Noda H, et al. Effects of increased adrenomedullary activity and taurine in young patients with borderline hypertension. *Circulation* 1987;75:525-532.

15. Bousquet P, Feldman J, Bloch R, Schwartz J. Central cardiovascular effects of taurine: comparison with homotaurine and muscimol. *J Pharmacol Exp Ther* 1981:219:213-218.

16. Raschke P, Massoudy P, Becker BF. Taurine protects the heart from neutrophil-induced reperfusion injury. *Free Radic Biol Med* 1995;19:461-467.

17. Azuma J, Sawamura A, Awata N, et al. Double-blind randomized crossover trial of taurine in congestive heart failure. *Curr Ther Res* 1983;34:543-557.

18. Konig P, Kriechbaum G, Presslich O, et al. Orally administered taurine in therapy-resistant epilepsy (author's transl). *Wien Klin Wochenschr* 1977;89:111-113. [Article in German]

19. Rassin DK, Sturman JA, Gaull GE. Taurine and other free amino acids in milk of man and other mammals. *Early Human Dev* 1978;2:1-13.

20. Hayes KC, Stephan ZF, Sturman JA. Growth depression in taurine-depleted infant monkeys. *J Nutr* 1980;110:2058-2064.

21. Gaull GE, Wright GE, Tallen JJ. Taurine in human lymphoblastoid cells: uptake and role in proliferation. In: Kuriyama J, Huxtable RJ, eds. *Sulfur Amino Acids: Biochemical and Clinical Aspects*. New York, NY: Alan R. Liss; 1983:297-303.

22. Franconi F, Bennardini F, Mattana A, et al. Plasma and platelet taurine are reduced in subjects with insulin-dependent diabetes mellitus: effects of taurine supplementation. *Am J Clin Nutr* 1995;61:1115-1119.

23. Smith U, Lacaille F, Pepage G, et al. Taurine decreases fecal fatty acid and sterol excretion in cystic fibrosis. A randomized double-blind study. *Am J Dis Child* 1991;145:1401-1404.

24. Csernansky JG, Bardgett ME, Sheline YI, et al. CSF excitatory amino acids and severity of illness in Alzheimer's disease. *Neurology* 1996;46:1715-1720.

25. Tomaszewski A, Kleinrok A, Zackiewicz A, et al. Effect of various amino acids on acetylcholine metabolism in brain tissue. *Ann Univ Mariae Curie Sklodowska* 1982;37:61-70. [Article in Polish]

26. Matsuyama Y, Morita T, Higuchi M, Tsujii T. The effect of taurine administration on patients with acute hepatitis. *Prog Clin Biol Res* 1983;125:461-468.

27. Igimi H, Carey MC. Cholesterol gallstone dissolution kinetics of crystalline (anhydrate monohydrate) cholesterol with chenodeoxycholate, ursodeoxycholate and their glycine and taurine conjugates. *J Lipid Res* 1981;22:254-271.

28. Ikeda H. Effects of taurine on alcohol withdrawal. *Lancet* 1977;2:509.

29. Wilde MI, Wagstaff AJ. Acamprosate. A review of its pharmacology and clinical potential in the management of alcohol dependence after detoxification. *Drugs* 1997;53:1038-1053.

30. Van Gelder NM, Sherwin AL, Sacks C, Andermann F. Biochemical observations following administration of taurine to patients with epilepsy. *Brain Res* 1975;94:297-306.

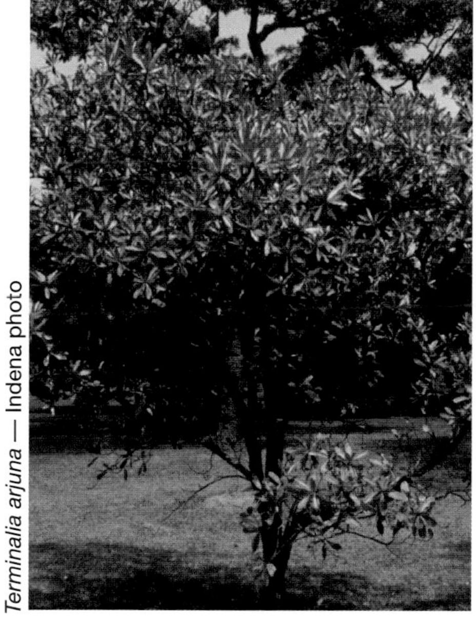

Terminalia arjuna — Indena photo

Terminalia arjuna

Description

Terminalia arjuna is a deciduous tree found throughout India growing to a height of 60-90 feet. The thick, white-to-pinkish-gray bark has been used in India's native Ayurvedic medicine for over three centuries, primarily as a cardiac tonic. Clinical evaluation of this botanical medicine indicates it can be of benefit in the treatment of coronary artery disease, heart failure, and possibly hypercholesterolemia. It has also been found to be antiviral and antimutagenic.

Active Constituents

Terminalia's active constituents include tannins, cardenolide, triterpenoid saponins (arjunic acid, arjunolic acid, arjungenin, arjunglycosides), flavonoids (arjunone, arjunolone, luteolin), gallic acid, ellagic acid, oligomeric proanthocyanidins (OPCs), phytosterols, calcium, magnesium, zinc, and copper.[1,2]

Mechanisms of Action

Improvement of cardiac muscle function and subsequent improved pumping activity of the heart seems to be the primary benefit of Terminalia. It is thought the saponin glycosides might be responsible for the inotropic effect of Terminalia, while the flavonoids and OPCs provide free radical antioxidant activity and vascular strengthening.[3] A dose-dependent decrease in heart rate and blood pressure was noted in dogs given Terminalia intravenously.[4] Recently, two new cardenolide cardiac glycosides were isolated from the root and seed of Terminalia.[5,6] The main action of these cardenolides is to increase the force of cardiac contraction by means of a rise in both intracellular sodium and calcium.

Clinical Indications

Angina Pectoris

An open study of Terminalia use in stable and unstable angina demonstrated a 50-percent reduction of angina in the stable angina group after three months ($p<0.01$). A significant reduction was also found in systolic blood pressure in these patients ($p<0.05$). During treadmill testing, both the onset of angina and the appearance of ST-T changes on ECG were significantly delayed in the stable angina group ($p<0.001$), indicating an improvement in exercise tolerance. The unstable angina group did not experience significant reductions in angina or systolic blood pressure. Both groups showed improvements in left ventricular ejection fraction. Evaluation of overall clinical condition, treadmill results, and ejection fraction showed improvement in 66 percent of stable angina patients and 20 percent of unstable angina patients after three months.[7] In this study Terminalia was also associated with a lowering of systolic blood pressure.

Two clinical studies found similar results when *Terminalia arjuna* was compared to isosorbide mononitrate in stable angina patients.[8,9] Both studies showed a similar reduction in the number of anginal episodes, as well as improvements in stress tests. In one study 58 males with chronic stable angina with evidence of ischemia on treadmill testing received *Terminalia arjuna* (500 mg every eight hours), isosorbide mononitrate (40 mg daily), or a matching placebo for one week each, separated by a wash-out period of at least three days in a randomized, double-blind, crossover design. Terminalia therapy was associated with a significant decrease in the frequency of angina and need for isosorbide dinitrate. Treadmill parameters improved significantly during therapy with Terminalia compared to those with placebo. Similar improvement in clinical and treadmill parameters were observed with isosorbide mononitrate compared to placebo therapy. No significant differences were observed in clinical or treadmill parameters when *Terminalia arjuna* and isosorbide mononitrate therapies were compared.[8]

Congestive Heart Failure

A double-blind, placebo-controlled, two-phase trial of Terminalia extract in 12 patients with severe refractory heart failure (NYHA Class IV) was conducted, in which either 500 mg Terminalia bark extract or placebo was given every eight hours for two weeks, in addition to the patients' current pharmaceutical medications (digoxin, diuretics, angiotensin-converting-enzyme inhibitors, vasodilators, and potassium supplementation). All patients experienced dyspnea at rest or after minimal activity at the start of the trial. Dyspnea, fatigue, edema, and walking tolerance all improved while patients were on Terminalia therapy. Treatment with Terminalia was also associated with significant improvements in stroke volume and left ventricular ejection fraction, as well as decreases in end-diastolic and end-systolic left ventricular volumes compared to placebo. In the second phase of the study, patients from phase I continued on Terminalia extract for two years. Improvements were noted in the ensuing 2-3 months, and were maintained through the balance of the study. After four months' treatment, nine patients improved to NYHA Class II and three improved to NYHA Class III.[10]

Cardiomyopathy/Post-Myocardial Infarction

A study was conducted on 10 post-myocardial-infarction patients and two ischemic cardiomyopathy patients, utilizing 500 mg Terminalia extract every eight hours for three months, along with conventional treatment. Significant reductions in angina and left ventricular mass, in addition to improved left ventricular ejection fraction, were noted in the Terminalia group; whereas, the control group taking only conventional drugs experienced decreased angina only. The two patients with cardiomyopathy improved from NYHA Class III to NYHA Class I during the study.[11]

Hyperlipidemia

Animal studies suggest Terminalia might reduce blood lipids. Rabbits made hyperlipidemic on an atherogenic diet were given an oral Terminalia extract, and had a significant, dose-related decrease in total- and LDL-cholesterol, compared to placebo ($p<0.01$)[12] However, the amounts used (100 mg/kg and 500 mg/kg body weight) were very large, and it remains to be seen if similar changes will be observed in humans taking relatively smaller oral doses. In a similar study of rats fed cholesterol (25 mg/kg body weight) alone or along with Terminalia bark powder (100 mg/kg) for 30 days, Terminalia feeding caused a smaller increase in blood lipids and an increase in HDL cholesterol, compared to the cholesterol-only group. The researchers concluded that inhibition of hepatic cholesterol biosynthesis, increased fecal bile acid excretion, and stimulation of receptor-mediated catabolism of LDL cholesterol were responsible for Terminalia's lipid-lowering effects.[13]

In another study, rabbits were fed a cholesterol-rich diet in combination with three indigenous Terminalia species; *Terminalia arjuna*, *T. belerica*, and *T. chebula*. Upon histological examination, the rabbits fed the diet and *T. arjuna* exhibited the most potent hypolipidemic effect, with partial inhibition of atheroma.[14]

In a randomized, controlled trial, Terminalia bark was compared to vitamin E. One-hundred-and-five patients with coronary heart disease (CHD) were matched for age, lifestyle, and diet variables, as well as drug treatment status. None of the patients were previously on lipid-lowering medications. Placebo, vitamin E (400 IU), and Terminalia (500 mg) were administered. Results showed no significant changes in the placebo group or the vitamin E group. The Terminalia group had a significant decrease in total cholesterol and LDL cholesterol. Lipid peroxidase levels decreased significantly in both vitamin E and Terminalia groups; however, there was a greater decrease in the vitamin E group.[15]

Other Clinical Indications

Terminalia bark harbors constituents with promising antimutagenic and anticarcinogenic potential that should be investigated further.[16-19] *In vitro* studies have also shown Terminalia to possess anti-herpes virus activity.[20]

Botanical-Drug Interactions

Terminalia arjuna extracts have been used in clinical studies concomitantly with standard heart medications, including digoxin, diuretics, angiotensin-converting-enzyme inhibitors, and vasodilators, with no reported adverse effects. Simultaneous use of Terminalia with other cardiac medications should be undertaken with caution.

Dosage and Toxicity

A typical dose of dried bark is 1-3 grams daily, while 500 mg bark extract four times per day has been used in congestive heart failure. No toxicity has been documented.

References

1. Bone K. *Clinical Applications of Ayurvedic and Chinese Herbs*. Warwick, Queensland, Australia. Phytotherapy Press; 1996:131-133.
2. Kapoor LD. *Handbook of Ayurvedic Medicinal Plants*. Boca Raton, FL. CRC Press; 1990:319-320.
3. Munasinghe TC, Seneviratne CK, Thabrew MI, Abeysekera AM. Antiradical and anilipoperoxidative effects of some plant extracts used by Sri Lanken traditional medical practitioners for cardioprotection. *Phytother Res* 2001;15:519-523.
4. Singh N, Kapur KK, Singh SP, et al. Mechanism of cardiovascular action of *Terminalia arjuna*. *Planta Med* 1982;45:102-104.
5. Yadav R.N., Rathore K. A new cardenolide from the roots of *Terminalia arjuna*. *Fitoterapia* 2001;72:459-461.
6. Yadav RN, Rathore K. A new cardenolide from the seeds of *Terminalia arjuna*. *J Asian Nat Prod Res* 2000;2:97-101.
7. Dwivedi S, Agarwal MP. Antianginal and cardioprotective effects of *Terminalia arjuna*, an indigenous drug, in coronary artery disease. *J Assoc Physicians India* 1994;42:287-289.
8. Bharani A, Ganguli A, Mathur LK, et al. Efficacy of *Terminalia arjuna* in chronic stable angina: a double-blind, placebo-controlled, crossover study comparing *Terminalia arjuna* with isosorbide mononitrate. *Indian Heart J* 2002;54:170-175.
9. Kumar PU, Adhikari P, Pereira P, Bhat P. Safety and efficacy of 'Hartone'-a proprietary herbal product primarily containing *Terminalia arjuna* in stable angina pectoris patients. *J Assoc Physicians India* 1999;47:685-689.
10. Bharani A, Ganguly A, Bhargave KD. Salutary effect of *Terminalia arjuna* in patients with severe refractory heart failure. *Int J Cardiol* 1995;49:191-199.
11. Dwivedi S, Jauhari R. Beneficial effects of *Terminalia arjuna* in coronary artery disease. *Indian Heart J* 1997;49:507-510.
12. Ram A, Lauria P, Gupta R, et al. Hypocholesterolaemic effects of *Terminalia arjuna* tree bark. *J Ethnopharmacol* 1997;55:165-169.
13. Khanna AK, Ramesh C, Kapoor NK. *Terminalia arjuna*: an Ayurvedic cardiotonic regulates lipid metabolism in hyperlipidaemic rats. *Phytotherapy Res* 1996;10:663-665.
14. Shaila HP, Udupa SL, Udupa AL. Hypolipidemic activity of three indigenous drugs in experimentally induced atheroclerosis. *Int J Cardiology* 1998;67:119-124.

15. Gupta R, Singhal S, Goyle A, Sharma VN. Antioxidant and hypocholesterolaemic effects of *Terminalia arjuna* tree-bark: a randomized placebo-controlled trial. *J Assoc Physicians India* 2001;49:231-235.

16. Kaur S, Grover IS, Kumar S. Antimutagenic potential of extracts isolated from *Terminalia arjuna*. *J Environ Pathol Toxicol Oncol* 2001;20:9-14.

17. Nagpal A, Meena LS, Kaur S, et al. Growth suppression of human transformed cells by treatment with bark extracts from a medicinal plant, *Terminalia arjuna*. *In Vitro Cell Dev Biol Anim* 2000;36:544-547.

18. Kaur K, Arora S, Kumar S, Nagpal A. Modulatory effect of phenolic fractions of *Terminalia arjuna* on the mutagenicity in Ames assay. *J Environ Pathol Toxicol Oncol* 2002;21:45-56.

19. Pasquini R, Scassellati-Sforzolini G, Villarini M, et al. In vitro protective effects of *Terminalia arjuna* bark extracts against the 4-nitroquinoline-N-oxide genotoxicity. *J Environ Pathol Toxicol Oncol* 2002;21:33-44.

20. Cheng HY, Lin CC, Lin TC. Antiherpes simplex virus type 2 activity of casuarinin from the bark of *Terminalia arjuna*. *Antiviral Res* 2002;55:447-455.

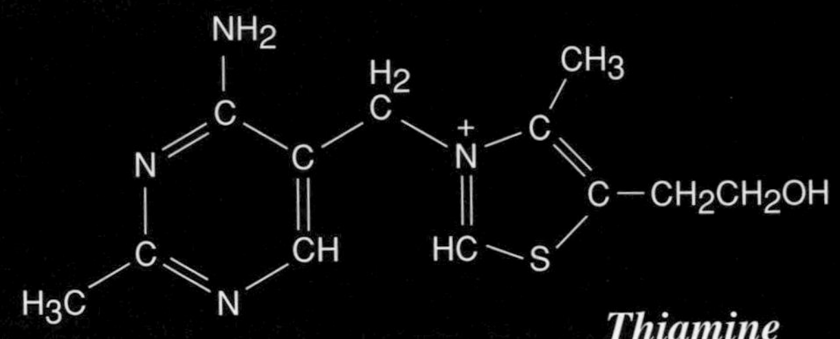

Thiamine

Thiamine

Introduction

Thiamine, also known as vitamin B1, is a water-soluble, B-complex vitamin necessary to metabolize proteins, carbohydrates, and fats. Thiamine is involved as a cofactor in numerous enzymes, and is essential in every cell for ATP production via the Krebs cycle.

Biochemistry and Pharmacokinetics

Thiamine functions as a coenzyme in more than 24 enzymes, the primary enzymes being pyruvate dehydrogenase (for energy production in the Krebs cycle), transketolase (lipid and glucose metabolism, production of branched chain amino acids, and production and maintenance of myelin sheath), and 2-oxo-glucarate dehydrogenase (synthesis of acetylcholine, GABA, and glutamate).[1] Thiamine is necessary in the functioning of the hexose monophosphate shunt, an anabolic pathway used proportionately more in adrenal cortex, leukocytes, erythrocytes and mammary gland tissue. Thiamine is crucial in glucose energy-utilizing pathways, particularly in the central nervous system, which needs a continuous supply of glucose. Thiamine has also been shown to mimic acetylcholine in the brain,[2] which may explain its possible action in Alzheimer's disease and other dementias.[3,4]

The body stores approximately 25-30 mg of thiamine, mainly in skeletal muscle, heart, brain, liver and kidneys – organs with high metabolic need. In a deficient state, body stores can be depleted in 2-3 weeks.[5] As early as one week after thiamine stores are depleted the blood-brain barrier is disrupted and local cerebral hypoperfusion results, leading to the classic signs of Wernicke's encephalopathy.[6]

Deficiency States and Symptoms

Thiamine deficiency, manifesting as beriberi or Wernicke-Korsakoff psychosis, has been considered to be a problem only in non-developed countries where white rice is a staple of the diet or in advanced alcoholics. However, the work of Lonsdale[7] and others have shown that thiamine deficiency occurs in a variety of situations, including a diet high in simple carbohydrates consisting mainly of processed food (sulfites destroy thiamine),[7] complications of alcohol misuse,[8] total parenteral nutrition (TPN),[9] gastrointestinal surgery,[10] severe infection,[11] eating disorders,[12] hyperemesis gravidarium,[13] renal dialysis,[14] in cancer patients (especially those treated with chemotherapy),[15] long-term diuretic use,[16] and in AIDS.[17]

Lonsdale has also reported clinical evidence of increased thiamine need in major depressive disorder, inborn errors of metabolism, hyperactivity and autonomic dysfunction.[1]

Symptoms of thiamine deficiency are diverse and vary with the degree of severity of the deficiency. Symptoms include depression, weakness, dizziness, insomnia, back pain, myalgia, muscular atrophy, palpitations, anorexia, nausea, vomiting, weight loss, hypotension, hypothermia, bradycardia at rest, tachycardia with sinus arrhythmia on exertion,[18] constipation, digestive disturbances, memory loss, peripheral neuropathy, pain sensitivity, dyspnea, and sonophobia.[19] Emotional instability, mood lability, uncooperative behavior, and fearfulness with agitation have also been seen in adolescents with documented thiamine deficiency.[20] Signs of severe thiamine deficiency seen in Wernicke's encephalopathy include ataxia, opthalmoplegia, nystagmus, and delirium.[8]

Thiamine deficiency, diagnosed by plasma levels, red cell transketolase, or thiamine pyrophosphate percentage effect, has been documented in adolescents eating an average American diet,[20] in 38 percent of a group of non-alcoholic psychiatric patients,[21] 33-55 percent of geriatric populations,[22] and 30-80 percent of alcoholic populations.[23,24] Thiamine is also depleted in those exposed to formaldehyde, and by long-term use of the following prescription drugs: phenytoin, penicillins, cephalosporins, aminoglycosides, tetracycline derivatives, loop diuretics, fluoroquinolones, sulfonamide derivatives, and trimethoprim.[25]

Clinical Indications

Alcoholism

Thiamine deficiency in alcoholism stems from a variety of causes. In addition to low intake, absorption is inhibited and hepatic activation of thiamine coenzymes is decreased.[26] Psychosis resulting from chronic alcohol use is believed to be primarily a result of thiamine deficiency, and appears to be on the rise worldwide.[2]

Wernicke's encephalopathy, the condition leading to sensory, motor, and cognitive deficits and the long-term consequence of Korsakoff's psychosis in alcoholics, occurs primarily as a consequence of thiamine deficiency.[27] Treatment of Wernicke's encephalopathy necessitates intravenous thiamine for at least 3-10 days followed by a high potency B vitamin complex for as long as improvement continues.[8]

HIV/AIDS

Moderate to severe thiamine deficiency has been seen in up to 23 percent of HIV-positive or AIDS-diagnosed non-alcoholic individuals.[17] In prospective epidemiologic studies, thiamine intakes above 7.5 mg (the RDA is 1.5 mg) were associated with increased survival. The highest levels of vitamin B1 and vitamin C intake were associated with significantly decreased progression from HIV to AIDS.[28] Thiamine-deficiency encephalopathy has been seen in HIV/AIDS patients with no alcohol abuse history.[11]

Congestive Heart Failure (CHF)

The etiology of heart failure is complex, but evidence for the role of micronutrients, particularly thiamine, is clear.[29] Thiamine deficiency leads to impaired oxidative metabolism. Subsequently, pyruvate and lactate levels increase, leading to vasodilation and possible metabolic acidosis, retention of water and sodium leading to edema, and biventricular heart failure, known as "wet beriberi." Reversal occurs with thiamine repletion. Iatrogenic contributions may include the use of cardiac medications (specifically furosemide and digoxin), which both decrease thiamine uptake in myocytes. Low whole blood levels of thiamine are evident in CHF patients who have been treated with loop diuretics.[30]

Thiamine supplementation in patients with CHF has been shown to significantly improve left ventricular ejection fraction and raise blood pressure 10 mm Hg, an indication of reversal of the pathological vasodilation seen in cardiac beriberi.[31]

Pregnancy, Hyperemesis Gravidarum, and Gestational Diabetes

Thiamine deficiency is common in pregnancy; in one study 25-30 percent of pregnant women had low red-cell transketolase levels, compared to controls.[32] Pregnant women with hyperemesis gravidarum have a greater risk of thiamine deficiency, and may need to be supplemented with high doses of thiamine.[13]

Women with gestational diabetes are even more likely to become thiamine deficient; 50 percent of study populations have been shown to have low transketolase levels.[33] In one study, 19 percent of gestational diabetics on standard prenatal thiamine supplementation were thiamine deficient.[35] A significant correlation exists between maternal thiamine deficiency and macrosomia (abnormally high body weight) in infants; however, an even stronger correlation was seen in macrosomic neonates from gestational diabetic mothers when the infants were born thiamine deficient.[34]

Mood and Cognitive Performance

A controlled, one-year trial with 127 young adults given 15 mg thiamine, along with other B vitamins at dosages 10 times the RDA,[4] found the most significant association was improved cognitive function and improved thiamine status in females.

Another controlled trial of thiamine and mood investigated 80 older females on 10 mg thiamine daily for 10 weeks.[35] Compared to baseline assessment and placebo, those on thiamine experienced significant increases in appetite, body weight, energy intake, general well-being, reduced daytime sleep, improved sleep patterns, decreased fatigue, and increased activity levels.

Drug-Nutrient Interactions

Thiamine can be depleted by long-term use of the following prescription drugs: phenytoin, penicillins, cephalosporins, aminoglycosides, tetracycline derivatives, loop diuretics, fluoroquinolones, sulfonamide derivatives, and trimethoprim.[25]

Side Effects and Toxicity

Thiamine toxicity in the oral form is nonexistent.[7]

Dosage

Dosages of thiamine are condition-specific. To treat Wernicke's encephalopathy, parenteral thiamine is necessary.[8] Oral doses of 50 mg thiamine daily have been used in alcoholics without encephalopathy to raise RBC transketolase levels.[36] Research by Cheraskin and Ringsdorf of "recommended optimal nutrient levels" found individuals taking 9 mg thiamine daily had fewer symptoms associated with illness and chronic degenerative disease than their peers.[37,38] They also suggested a wider range of supplemental intake may be necessary for those on diets high in refined carbohydrate (5-15 mg day). Lonsdale[7] has published case studies indicating 150 mg thiamine in divided daily doses may be needed to treat individuals with thiamine deficiency symptoms resulting from increased individual requirements.

References

1. Thomson AD, Pratt OE. Interaction of nutrients and alcohol: absorption, transport, utilization and metabolism. Watson RR, Watzl B, eds. *Nutrition and Alcohol*. Boca Raton, FL: CRC Press;1992:75-99.
2. Meador K, Nichols ME, Franke P, et al. Evidence for a central cholinergic effect of high dose thiamine. *Ann Neurol* 1993;34:724-726.
3. Meador K, Loring D, Nichols M, et al. Preliminary findings of high-dose thiamine in dementia of Alzheimer's type. *J Geriatr Psychiatry Neurol* 1993;6:222-229.
4. Benton D, Fordy J, Haller J. The impact of long-term vitamin supplementation on cognitive functioning. *Psychopharmacol* 1995;117:298-305.
5. Velez RJ, Myers B, Guber MS. Severe acute metabolic acidosis (acute beriberi): an avoidable complication of total parenteral nutrition. *JPEN J Parenter Enteral Nutr* 1985;9:216-219.
6. Heye N, Terstegge K, Sirtl C, et al. Wernicke's encephalopathy – causes to consider. *Intensive Care Med* 1994;20:282-286.
7. Lonsdale D. *The Nutritionist's Guide to the Clinical Use of Vitamin B-1*. Tacoma, WA: Life Sciences Press: 44-77.
8. Cook C, Hallwood PM, Thomson AD. B vitamin deficiency and neuropsychiatric syndromes in alcohol misuse. *Alcohol Alcohol* 1998;33:317-336.
9. Kitamura K, Yamaguchi T, Tanaka H, et al. TPN-induced fulminant beriberi: a report on our experience and a review of the literature. *Surg Today* 1996;26:769-776.
10. Seehra H, MacDermott N, Lascelles RG, Taylor TV. Wernicke's encephalopathy after vertical banded gastroplasty for morbid obesity. *BMJ* 1996;312:434.
11. Lindboe CF, Loberg EM. Wernicke's encephalopathy in non-alcoholics. An autopsy study. *J Neurol Sci* 1989;90:125-129.

12. Winston AP, Jamieson CP, Madira W, et al. Prevalence of thiamin deficiency in anorexia nervosa. *Int J Eat Disord* 2000;28:451-454.
13. Togay-Isikay C, Yigit A, Mutluer N. Wernicke's encephalopathy due to hyperemesis gravidarum: an under-recognised condition. *Aust N Z J Obstet Gynaecol* 2001;41:453-456.
14. Reuler JB, Girard DE, Cooney TG. Wernicke's encephalopathy. *N Engl J Med* 1985;312:1035-1039.
15. Bleggi-Torres LF, de Medeiros BC, Ogasawara VS, et al. Iatrogenic Wernicke's encephalopathy in allogeneic bone marrow transplantation: a study of eight cases. *Bone Marrow Transplant* 1997;20:391-395.
16. Wilcox CS. Do diuretics cause thiamine deficiency? *J Lab Clin Med* 1999;134:192-193.
17. Butterworth RF, Gaudreau C, Vincelette J, et al. Thiamine deficiency and Wernicke's encephalopathy in AIDS. *Metab Brain Dis* 1991;6:207-212.
18. Williams RD, Mason HL, Power MH, et al. Induced thiamine deficiency in man; relation of depletion of thiamine to development of biochemical defect and of polyneuropathy. *Arch Int Med* 1943;71:2176-2177.
19. Werbach MR. *Nutritional Influences on Illness, 2nd Ed*. Tarzana, CA: Third Line Press; 1993:676-677.
20. Lonsdale D, Schamberger RJ. Red cell transketolase as indicator of nutritional deficiency. *Am J Clin Nutr* 1980;33:205-211.
21. Schwartz RA, Gross M, Lonsdale D, Schamberger RJ. Transketolase activity in psychiatric patients. *J Clin Psychiatry* 1979;40:427-429.
22. Chen MF, Chen LT, Gold M, Boyce HW Jr. Plasma and erythrocyte thiamin concentration in geriatric outpatients. *J Am Coll Nutr* 1996;15:231-236.
23. Baines M. Detection and incidence of B and C vitamin deficiency in alcohol-related illness. *Ann Clin Biochem* 1978;15:307-312.
24. Thomson AD, Jeyasingham M, Pratt O, Shaw GK. Nutrition and alcoholic encephaolpathies. *Acta Med Scand Suppl* 1987;717:55-65.
25. Pelton R, LaValle JB, Hawkins E, Krinsky DL, eds. *Drug-Induced Nutrient Depletion Handbook*. Hudson, OH: Lexi-Comp; 1999:258.
26. Leevy CM. Thiamin deficiency and alcoholism. *Ann NY Acad Sci* 1982;378:316-326.
27. Lishman WA. Cerebral disorder in alcoholism. *Brain* 1981;104:1-20.
28. Tang AM, Graham NM, Kirby AJ, et al. Dietary micronutrient intake and risk of progression to acquired immunodeficiency syndrome (AIDS) in human immunodeficiency virus type-1 (HIV-1)-infected homosexual men. *Am J Epidemiol* 1993;138:937-951.
29. Witte KK, Clark AL, Cleland JG. Chronic heart failure and micronutrients. *J Am Coll Cardiol* 2001;37:1765-1774.
30. Brady JA, Rock CL, Horneffer MR. Thiamine status, diuretic medications and the management of congestive heart failure. *J Am Diet Assoc* 1995;95:541-544.
31. Seligmann H, Halkin H, Raucfleisch S, et al. Thiamine deficiency in patients with congestive heart failure receiving long-term furosemide therapy: a pilot study. *Am J Med* 1991;91:151-155.
32. Heller S, Salkeld RM, Korner WF. Vitamin B1 status in pregnancy. *Am J Clin Nutr* 1974;27:1221-1224.
33. Bakker SJ, ter Maaten JC, Gans RO. Thiamine supplementation to prevent induction of low birth weight by conventional therapy for gestational diabetes mellitus. *Med Hypotheses* 2000;55:88-90.
34. Baker H, Hockstein S, DeAngelis B, Holland BK. Thiamin status of gravidas treated for gestational diabetes mellitus compared to their neonates at parturition. *Int J Vit Nutr Res* 2000;70:317-320.
35. Smidt LJ, Cremin FM, Clifford AJ. Influence of thiamin supplementation on the health and general well-being of an elderly Irish population with marginal thiamin deficiency. *J Gerontol* 1991;46:M180.
36. Baines M, Bligh JG, Madden JS. Tissue thiamine levels of hospitalized alcoholics before and after oral or parenteral vitamins. *Alcohol Alcohol* 1988;23:49-52.
37. Cheraskin E, Ringsdorf WM, Medford FH, Hicks BS. The "ideal" daily vitamin B1 intake. *J Oral Med* 1978;33:77-79.
38. Cheraskin E, Ringsdorf WM. How much carbohydrate should we eat? *Am Lab* 1974;6:31-35.

Mixed Tocopherols

Introduction

Vitamin E is a generic term used to describe all tocopherol and tocotrienol derivatives that exhibit the biological activity of alpha-tocopherol. While alpha-tocopherol is considered to be responsible for the majority of the biological action of vitamin E, beta-, gamma-, and delta-tocopherol also occur naturally in food. Tocopherols are oily, yellow liquids found in the seeds, leaves, and other lipid-containing parts of plants. Alpha-tocopherol is found largely in the chloroplasts of plant cells, while other tocopherols are found primarily outside of the chloroplasts. This compartmentalization implies different activities for the various tocopherol molecules in plants.

Vitamin E is known for its antioxidant, immune-enhancing, anti-inflammatory, and anti-platelet aggregation effects. Vitamin E is used clinically to prevent cardiovascular disease, cancer, cataracts, complications of diabetes, and to improve immune function. Although the majority of research has been on alpha-tocopherol, investigations are being performed on the contributions of beta-, gamma-, and delta-tocopherol to the action of vitamin E.

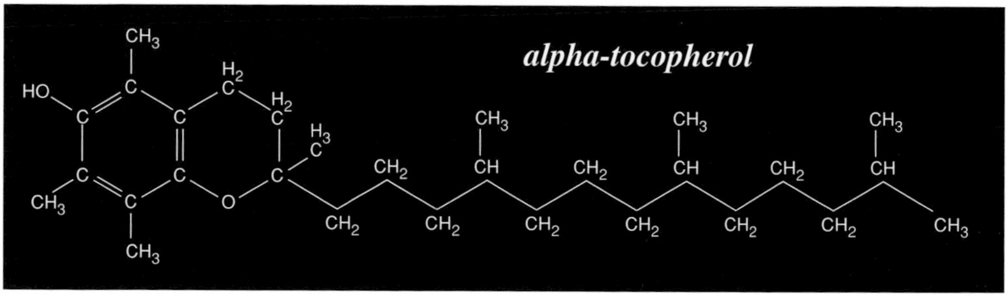

alpha-tocopherol

Pharmacokinetics

Tocopherols are absorbed in the small intestine (primarily the jejunum) by passive diffusion. After absorption, tocopherols enter the lymphatic system and are subsequently transported to the liver in chylomicrons. In the liver, they are bound to tocopherol transfer protein for distribution to other tissues. Tocopherols concentrate in adipose compartments of various tissues such as the liver, heart, adrenal glands, brain, and nervous system. Tocopherols are excreted through the feces, skin, and urine.

Although gamma-tocopherol is the most abundant tocopherol in the American diet, alpha-tocopherol is found in the serum and red blood cells of healthy volunteers in the highest concentration.[1] Gamma-tocopherol is also found in both plasma and red cells, while beta- and delta-tocopherol are found in the plasma only in minute amounts.

The predominance of alpha-tocopherol in the serum appears to be due to its preferential binding to tocopherol transfer protein.[2] Because of this binding affinity, most of the absorbed beta-, gamma-, and delta-tocopherol is secreted into bile and excreted in the feces. Alpha-tocopherol is largely excreted in the urine. Supplementation with high doses of alpha-tocopherol has been shown to deplete the plasma levels of gamma-tocopherol,[3] and may do the same with other tocopherols.

Mechanisms of Action

A major biochemical activity of tocopherols is protection from free radicals and products of oxygenation. Specifically, tocopherols appear to detoxify lipid peroxy radicals, as well as block the reactivity of singlet oxygen radicals.[4] Vitamin E works in conjunction with other antioxidant nutrients to quench free radicals. Vitamin E also inhibits lipoxygenase, an enzyme responsible for the formation of pro-inflammatory leukotrienes. Tocopherols appear to inhibit platelet aggregation through inhibition of protein kinase C[5] and increased action of nitric oxide synthase.[6]

Anti-cancer actions of vitamin E have demonstrated a difference in activity for individual tocopherols. Alpha-tocopherol inhibits production of protein kinase C and collagenase,[7] two enzymes that facilitate cancer cell growth. Gamma-tocopherol has been shown to have superior growth inhibitory effect on human prostate cancer cell lines when compared to alpha-tocopherol.[8] Delta-tocopherol has exhibited growth inhibitory activity against mouse mammary cancer cell lines, while alpha- and gamma-tocopherol has not.[9]

Clinical Indications

Cardiovascular Disease

Epidemiological studies have demonstrated an inverse relationship between vitamin E intake and cardiovascular disease risk.[10,11] However, randomized and controlled trials have reported conflicting results as to whether vitamin E supplementation reduces atherosclerosis progression and cardiovascular disease events.[12,13] Recent studies looking at mixed tocopherols for the prevention of cardiovascular disease have indicated mixed tocopherols may have a stronger inhibitory effect on lipid peroxidation than alpha-tocopherol alone.[14] Mixed tocopherols were also superior to alpha-tocopherol in protecting rat myocytes from hypoxia-reoxygenation damage.[15] Another study showed the combination of alpha-, gamma-, and delta-tocopherol inhibited human platelet aggregation and lipid peroxidation more than the three tocopherols in isolation, suggesting a synergistic platelet-inhibitory effect.[6]

In the Cambridge Heart Antioxidant Study (CHAOS), 202 patients with angiographically proven atherosclerosis were given d-alpha-tocopherol (800 IU per day, 400 IU per day, or placebo) While vitamin E (alpha-tocopherol) reduced the risk of nonfatal myocardial infarction by 77 percent, there was a non-significant excess of cardiovascular deaths in the vitamin E group. Most deaths, however, occurred in the early period after diagnosis; when early deaths were excluded there were fewer deaths among vitamin E-supplemented individuals. All causes of mortality were also not significantly higher in the vitamin E group.[16] In a follow-up trial, no beneficial preventive effect was seen with supplementation of 400 IU per day vitamin E for 4.5 years.[12]

Treatment of patients with intermittent claudication with 300 IU d-alpha-tocopherol acetate for 2-5 years improved walking distance compared to vasodilating or anticoagulant medications.[17]

Cancer Prevention

Supplementation of male smokers for 5-8 years with 50 IU d,l-alpha-tocopherol led to a 32-percent reduction in prostate cancer incidence and a 41-percent reduction in prostate cancer mortality compared to placebo.[18] A non-significant, 22-percent reduction in colon cancer incidence was also seen in the treatment group in this trial.[19] Vitamin E, in combination with other antioxidant vitamins, has been shown to reduce the recurrence rate of bladder cancer[20] and colorectal adenomas[21] compared to placebo. A number of animal and *in vitro* studies have outlined the anti-cancer potential of vitamin E.[22,23] Several mechanisms of vitamin E are considered important in this regard, including stimulation of wild-type p53 tumor suppressor gene, down-regulation of mutant p53, activation of heat shock proteins, and an anti-angiogenic effect mediated by blockage of transforming growth factor-alpha.[22]

Gynecological Conditions

In women with dysmenorrhea, supplementation with 50 mg alpha-tocopherol three times per day for two menstrual cycles reduced symptoms in 68 percent of women, compared with 18 percent of those taking placebo.[24] Another double-blind trial found supplementation with 400 IU vitamin E per day improved symptoms of premenstrual syndrome.[25] In breast cancer survivors, supplementation with 800 IU per day led to a significant reduction in hot flash symptoms compared to women taking placebo.[26]

HIV/AIDS

Research in murine AIDS using a 15-fold increase in dietary vitamin E (160 IU/L liquid diet) demonstrated normalization of immune parameters that are altered in HIV/AIDS.[27] Vitamin E has also been shown to protect against bone marrow toxicity, a well established side effect of AZT.[28] A study of the effects of d-alpha-tocopherol on bone marrow cultures from stage IV AIDS patients revealed similar findings.[29]

Immunity

Vitamin E may enhance certain clinically-relevant *in vivo* indexes of T-cell-mediated function in healthy elderly persons. In 88 free-living, healthy subjects at least 65 years of age, 200 mg per day vitamin E improved antibody response to various vaccines. No adverse effects were observed with vitamin E supplementation.[30] Vitamin E may enhance resistance to viral diseases, as was shown in a study of 209 elderly subjects. Higher plasma vitamin E levels correlated with a reduced number of infections over a three-year period.[31]

Diabetes

Fuller et al found vitamin E, at a dosage of 1,200 IU daily in the form of tocopheryl acetate, elicited significant reductions in LDL oxidation, but had no significant effect on lowering plasma glycosylated protein or glycosylated hemoglobin in diabetes.[32] Kuznetsov et al found normalization of lipid peroxidation in hypertensive diabetics with alpha-tocopherol acetate.[33] Douilet et al found a significant protective effect of vitamin E and selenium on the kidneys of diabetic rats. Plasma lipid peroxides, glucose, and triglycerides were also decreased.[34] Cary and McCarty report on 19/20 diabetic patients who had improvement or no progression of retinopathy when supplemented with 500 mcg selenium, 800 IU vitamin E, 10,000 IU vitamin A, and 1 g vitamin C daily for several years.[35]

Researchers divided 80 diabetics suffering from complications into four groups. One group served as the control group; one received lipoic acid 600 mg daily; one received 1,200 IU d-alpha-tocopherol; and the fourth received 100 mcg selenium. All groups treated with antioxidants showed significant diminution of urinary albumin and thiobarbituric acid (a reactive species and indicator of oxidative processes). Neuropathy symptoms regarding thermal and vibratory senses were significantly improved.[36]

Drug-Nutrient Interactions

High doses of vitamin E might potentiate the effects of drugs that interfere with platelet aggregation or blood clotting, such as warfarin. It may be advisable to reduce the dosage of supplemental vitamin E when taking these medications, or adjust the dosage of both warfarin and vitamin E for optimal therapeutic effect.

Side Effects and Toxicity

The toxicity of oral vitamin E supplementation is understood to be quite low. Supplementation with 3,200 IU vitamin E for nine weeks was well tolerated in one double-blind trial, with the only adverse effects reported being intestinal cramps and diarrhea.[37] Patients who self-administered 100-800 IU vitamin E for an average of three years were found to have no significant toxic effects, including no abnormalities of the liver, kidneys, blood sugar, or coagulation pathways.[38]

One published case report from 1974 described a patient taking warfarin who developed prolonged bleeding times on self-administration of 1,200 IU vitamin E per day.[39] This abnormality resolved on discontinuation of vitamin E. However, two clinical trials, one double-blind, did not find any reduction of warfarin effect with vitamin E administration at doses up to 1,200 IU.[40,41] A complete review of the toxicity of vitamin E supplementation can be found in Bendich and Machlin.[42]

Dosage

The optimal supplementation dosage of mixed tocopherols is undetermined, and no specific recommendations have been made; however, 200 - 1,200 IU is the most commonly prescribed dosage. The recommended daily intake of vitamin E (d-alpha tocopherol) is 22.4 IU, and the suggested upper limit is 1,490 IU daily.[43] The synthetic form of vitamin E, d,l-alpha tocopherol, is one-half the potency of natural d-alpha-tocopherol; therefore, the dosage of synthetic vitamin E should be adjusted accordingly.

References

1. Chow CK. Distribution of tocopherols in human plasma and red blood cells. *Am J Clin Nutr* 1975;28:756-760.
2. Brigelius-Flohe R, Traber MG. Vitamin E: function and metabolism. *FASEB J* 1999;13:1145-1155.
3. Handelman GJ, Machlin LJ, Fitch K, et al. Oral alpha-tocopherol supplements decrease plasma gamma-tocopherol levels in humans. *J Nutr* 1985;115:807-813.
4. Kamal-Eldin A, Appelqvist LA. The chemistry and antioxidant properties of tocopherols and tocotrienols. *Lipids* 1996;31:671-701.
5. Freedman JE, Farhat JH, Loscalzo J, Keaney JF Jr. Alpha-tocopherol inhibits aggregation of human platelets by a protein kinase C-dependent mechanism. *Circulation* 1996;94:2434-2440.
6. Li D, Saldeen T, Romeo F, Mehta JL. Different isoforms of tocopherols enhance nitric oxide synthase phosphorylation and inhibit human platelet aggregation and lipid peroxidation: implications in therapy with vitamin E. *J Cardiovasc Pharmacol Ther* 2001;6:155-161.
7. Azzi A, Stocker A. Vitamin E: non-antioxidant roles. *Prog Lipid Res* 2000;39:231-255.
8. Moyad MA, Brumfield SK, Pienta KJ. Vitamin E, alpha- and gamma-tocopherol, and prostate cancer. *Sem Urol Oncol* 1999;17:85-90.
9. McIntyre BS, Briski KP, Gapor A, et al. Antiproliferative and apoptotic effects of tocopherols and tocotrienols on preneoplastic and neoplastic mouse mammary epithelial cells. *Proc Soc Exp Biol Med* 2000;224:292-301.
10. Stampfer MJ, Hennekens CH, Manson JE, et al. Vitamin E consumption and the risk of coronary disease in women. *N Engl J Med* 1993;328:1444-1449.
11. Rimm EB, Stampfer MJ, Ascherio A, et al. Vitamin E consumption and the risk of coronary heart disease in men. *N Engl J Med* 1993;328:1450-1456.
12. Blumberg JB. An update: vitamin E supplementation and heart disease. *Nutr Clin Care* 2002;5:50-55.
13. Hodis HN, Mack WJ, LaBree L, et al. Alpha-tocopherol supplementation in healthy individuals reduces low-density lipoprotein oxidation but not atherosclerosis: the Vitamin E Atherosclerosis Prevention Study (VEAPS). *Circulation* 2002;106:1453-1459.

14. Liu M, Wallin R, Wallmon A, Saldeen T. Mixed tocopherols have a stronger inhibitory effect on lipid peroxidation than alpha-tocopherol alone. *J Cardiovasc Pharmacol* 2002;39:714-721.

15. Chen H, Li D, Saldeen T, et al. Mixed tocopherol preparation is superior to alpha-tocopherol alone against hypoxia-reoxygenation injury. *Biochem Biophys Res Commun* 2002;291:349-353.

16. Stephens NG, Parsons A, Schofield PM, et al. Randomised controlled trial of vitamin E in patients with coronary disease: Cambridge Heart Antioxidant Study (CHAOS). *Lancet* 1996;347:781-786.

17. Haeger K. Long-time treatment of intermittent claudication with vitamin E. *Am J Clin Nutr* 1974;27:1179-1181.

18. Heinonen OP, Albanes D, Virtamo J, et al. Prostate cancer and supplementation with alpha-tocopherol and beta-carotene: incidence and mortality in a controlled trial. *J Natl Cancer Inst* 1998;90:440-446.

19. Albanes D, Malila N, Taylor PR, et al. Effects of supplemental alpha-tocopherol and beta-carotene on colorectal cancer: results from a controlled trial (Finland). *Cancer Causes Control* 2000;11:197-205.

20. Lamm DL, Riggs DR, Shriver JS, et al. Megadose vitamins in bladder cancer: a double-blind clinical trial. *J Urol* 1994;151:21-26.

21. Roncucci L, DiDonato P, Carati L, et al. Antioxidant vitamins or lactulose for the prevention of the recurrence of colorectal adenomas. Colorectal Cancer Study Group of Modena and the Health Care District 16. *Dis Colon Rectum* 1993;36:227-234.

22. Shklar G, Oh SK. Experimental basis for cancer prevention by vitamin E. *Cancer Invest* 2000;18:214-222.

23. Prasad KN, Edwards-Prasad J. Vitamin E and cancer prevention: recent advances and future potentials. *J Am Coll Nutr* 1992;11:487-500.

24. Butler EB, McKnight E. Vitamin E in the treatment of dysmenorrhea. *Lancet* 1955;i:844-847.

25. London RS, Murphy L, Kitlowski KE, et al. Efficacy of alpha-tocopherol in the treatment of the premenstrual syndrome. *J Reprod Med* 1987;32:400-404.

26. Barton DL, Loprinzi CL, Quella SK, et al. Prospective evaluation of vitamin E for hot flashes in breast cancer survivors. *J Clin Oncol* 1998;16:495-500.

27. Wang Y, Huang DS, Eskelson CD, et al. Normalization and restoration of nutritional status and immune functions by vitamin E supplementation in murine AIDS. *J Nutr* 1994;124:2024-2032.

28. Ganser A, Greher J, Volkers B, et al. Azidothymidine in the treatment of AIDS. *N Engl J Med* 1988;318:250-251.

29. Geissler RG, Ganser A, Ottmann OG, et al. In vitro improvement of bone marrow-derived hematopoietic colony formation in HIV-positive patients by alpha-D-tocopherol and erythropoietin. *Eur J Haematol* 1994;53:201-206.

30. Meydani SN, Meydani M, Blumberg JB, et al. Vitamin E supplementation and in vivo immune response in healthy elderly subjects. A randomized controlled trial. *JAMA* 1997;277:1380-1386.

31. Chavance M, Herbeth B, Fournier C, et al. Vitamin status, immunity and infections in an elderly population. *Eur J Clin Nutr* 1989;43:827-835.

32. Fuller CJ, Chandalia M, Garg A, et al. RRR-alpha-tocopheryl acetate supplementation at pharmacologic doses decreases low-density-lipoprotein oxidative susceptibility but not protein glycation in patients with diabetes mellitus. *Am J Clin Nutr* 1996;63:753-759.

33. Kuznetsov NS, Abulela AM, Neskromnyi VN. The comparative evaluation of the efficacy of tocopherol acetate in the combined treatment of patients with hypertension and diabetes mellitus. *Vrach Delo* 1994;12:133-136.

34. Douillet C, Tabib A, Bost M, et al. A selenium supplement associated or not with vitamin E delays early renal lesions in experimental diabetes in rats. *Proc Soc Exp Biol Med* 1996;211:323-331.

35. Crary EJ, McCarthy MF. Potential clinical applications for high-dose nutritional antioxidants. *Med Hypotheses* 1984;13:77-98.

36. Kahler W, Kuklinski B, Ruhlmann C, Plotz C. Diabetes mellitus – a free radical-associated disease. Results of adjuvant antioxidant supplementation. *Z Gesamte Inn Med* 1993;48:223-232.

37. Anderson TW, Reid DB. A double blind trial of vitamin E in angina pectoris. *Am J Clin Nutr* 1974;27:1174-1178.

38. Farrell PM, Bieri JG. Megavitamin E supplementation in man. *Am J Clin Nutr* 1975;28:1381-1386.

39. Corrigan JJ, Marcus FI. Coagulopathy associated with vitamin E ingestion. *JAMA* 1974;230:1300-1301.

40. Corrigan JJ, Ulfers LL. Effect of vitamin E on prothrombin levels in warfarin-induced vitamin K deficiency. *Am J Clin Nutr* 1981;34:1701-1705.

41. Kim JM, White RH. Effect of vitamin E on the anticoagulant response to warfarin. *Am J Cardiol* 1996;77:545-546.

42. Bendich A, Machlin LJ. Safety of oral intake of vitamin E. *Am J Clin Nutr* 1988;48:612-619.

43. Hendler SS, Rorvik D. *PDR for Nutritional Supplements*, 1st ed. Des Moines, IA: Medical Economics – Thompson Healthcare; 2001:517-520.

$$CH_2 = CH(CH_2)_8 CO_2 H$$

Undecylenic Acid

Undecylenic Acid

Introduction

Most organic fatty acids are fungicidal and have been used for centuries as antimicrobial agents, originally in the manufacture of soaps. In the last 50 years, however, they have found use both *in vitro* as yeast and mold inhibitors in food stuffs, and as topical and systemic antifungals. Undecylenic acid (10-undecenoic acid) is an eleven-carbon monounsaturated fatty acid, $C_{11}H_{20}O_2$. A substance found naturally in the body (occurring in sweat), undecylenic acid is produced commercially by the vacuum distillation of castor bean oil, via the pyrolysis of ricinoleic acid. It is an economical antifungal agent and is the active ingredient in many topical over-the-counter antifungal preparations.[1] Undecylenic acid has been shown to be approximately six times more effective as an antifungal than caprylic acid.[2]

Biochemistry and Pharmacokinetics

Wyss et al demonstrated more than 50 years ago that the greater the number of carbon atoms in the fatty acid chain, the greater the fungicidal activity, up to the point exceeding eleven carbon atoms, where solubility becomes the limiting factor.[3]

Although the fungistatic and fungicidal effects of fatty acids have been well documented, they can be somewhat irritating to mucous membranes in certain people, and commonly used fatty acids such as caprylic and undecylenic acid have an objectionable taste and odor. Consequently, the calcium, magnesium, and sodium salts of these fatty acids have been offered as reasonable alternatives. Undecylenate salts have been shown to possess as much as four times the fungicidal effect of undecylenic acid, and may be over 30 times more effective than caprylic acid.[4] Unfortunately, the antifungal effects of these fatty acid salts are more sensitive to pH than the free fatty acids. When tested over a pH range from 4.5 to 6.0, the antifungal activities of both undecylenic acid and calcium undecylenate are quite pronounced; the minimal inhibitory concentration of calcium undecylenate against *Candida albicans* is 200 ppm at pH 6.0. However, above pH 6.0, the calcium salt is less active than the free acid, perhaps due to the suppression of ionization of the salt at higher pH levels.[5]

Alkaline pH levels in the intestinal tract can be caused by intestinal flora imbalance, especially by *C. albicans*.[6] Therefore, for fatty acid salts to be effective in vivo, they must be delivered to the site of fungal overgrowth in the intestinal tract at an acid pH, thus avoiding both the release of excess bicarbonate from the pancreas (which would alkalinize the pH) and damage to the sensitive intestinal mucosa.[7] This can most efficiently be accomplished with a nominal amount of a substance in a time-release form, such as betaine HCl, that gradually liberates small quantities of the acid throughout the intestinal tract, simultaneously releasing the fatty acid salt.

Mechanism of Action

Undecylenic acid has long been known to have antifungal properties. At least one of the mechanisms underlying its antifungal effect is its inhibition of morphogenesis of *Candida albicans*. In a study on denture liners, undecylenic acid in the liners was found to inhibit conversion of yeast to the hyphal form.[8] Hyphae were associated with active infection. The authors speculated on possible mechanisms including interference with fatty acid biosynthesis, which can inhibit germ tube (hyphae) formation. Medium-chain fatty acids (a category of fatty acids in which undecylenic acid is included) have also been shown to disrupt the pH of the cell cytoplasm by being proton carriers.[9]

Clinical Indications

Vaginal/Gastrointestinal Candidiasis

Undecylenic acid has been shown to be effective in preventing fungal overgrowth associated with vaginal and gastrointestinal candidiasis via its fungicidal activity. A study published in the Journal of the American Medical Association found a direct correlation between vaginal yeast infections and simultaneous overgrowth of Candida in the digestive tract.[10] Undecylenic acid has long been known to be fungicidal against *Candida albicans*, thus helping achieve a healthy balance of normal vaginal and intestinal flora.[2]

Thrush

Since undecylenic acid acts systemically, oral administration can inhibit or even prevent oral candidiasis, or thrush. While large-scale clinical studies have not been conducted, many case reports confirm undecylenic acid's efficacy in thrush. During lactation, oral administration of undecylenic acid to nursing mothers can prevent thrush in babies. The milk, however, may taste slightly different to the infant.

Dermatomycoses

Undecylenic acid is the active ingredient in Desinex® cream and a number of other over-the-counter topical antifungals. It is responsible for the antifungal effect of these medications against such organisms as *Candida albicans*, *Trychophyton species*, *Epidermophyton inguinale*, and *Microsporum audouini*.[1]

A double-blind study of 151 patients with tinea pedis demonstrated that a powder containing 2-percent undecylenic acid and 20-percent zinc undecylenate resulted in a remarkable decrease in infection rate and symptomology, when compared to patients given a placebo powder. Eighty-five patients who were culture positive for *Trychophyton rubrum* or *Trychophyton mentagrophytes* were assigned to receive the active powder, and of these, 88 percent had negative cultures after four weeks, compared to 17 percent of those treated with placebo powder. There were no side effects or adverse reactions to the powder containing undecylenic acid and its zinc salt.[5]

Herpes Simplex Infection

Undecylenic acid has been shown to have antibacterial and antiviral properties *in vitro* and is effective topically against the *Herpes simplex* virus in both animals and humans. Two studies, one using a 20-percent solution[11] and the other a 15-percent cream,[12] demonstrated a decrease in the incidence and duration of viral shedding in subjects inoculated with herpes simplex virus. Patients also experienced a significant decrease in pain and tenderness at the lesion site. The antiviral activity was, however, of relatively short duration and most pronounced when undecylenic acid was applied during the prodromal stage of outbreak. Slight local skin irriation and dysgeusia (altered sense of taste) were experience by some subjects.[9,10]

Denture Stomatitis

Candida albicans is a major cause of denture stomatitis, an inflammation of the tissues underlying dentures. The organism exists in two cellular morphologies – the round yeast form found in asymptomatic carrier states and the branching hyphal form found in active infections. Resilient liners are frequently used to treat denture stomatitis, and McLain et al demonstrated that liners containing undecylenic acid completely inhibited the conversion of the yeast form of *Candida albicans* to the hyphal form, thereby inhibiting proliferation of the yeast.[8]

Side Effects and Toxicity

Relatively small doses of undecylenic acid and its salts have been shown to have powerful antifungal properties, and the dosages necessary to achieve therapeutic benefit appear to be safe. Capsules or gelcaps of undecylenic acid should not be opened and mixed with food or drink as the taste and odor is objectionable and it may also be irritating to mucous membranes. Additionally, undecylenic acid should not be applied directly to the skin, unless diluted in oil or a cream base to a dilution of at least 15-20 percent or less, as it may otherwise result in skin irritation.

Dosage

Undecylenic acid given orally is typically in an oil-based gelcap or as powder (in the case of its salts) in a two-part capsule. Adult dosage is usually 450-750 mg undecylenic acid daily in three divided doses.

References

1. Shapiro AL, Rothman S. Undecylenic acid in the treatment of dermatomycoses. *Arch Dermatol Syphilol* 1945;52:166-171.
2. Neuhauser I. Successful treatment of intestinal moniliasis with fatty acid-resin complex. *Arch Intern Med* 1954;93:53-60.
3. Wyss BJ. The fungistatic and fungicidal action of fatty acids and related compounds. *Arch Biochem* 1945;7:415.
4. Peck SM, Rosenfeld H. The effects of hydrogen ion concentration, fatty acids and vitamin C on the growth of fungi. *J Invest Dermatol* 1938;1:237-265.
5. Chretien JH, Esswein JG, Sharpe LM, et al. Efficacy of undecylenic acid-zinc undecylenate powder in culture positive tinea pedis. *Int J Dermatol* 1980;19:51-54.
6. Barrie SA. Comprehensive digestive stool analysis. In: Pizzorno JE, Murray MT, eds. *A Textbook of Natural Medicine.* Seattle, WA: JBC Press; 1986:II: CDSA-1-4.
7. Prince HN. Effect of pH on the antifungal activity of undecylenic acid and its calcium salt. *J Bacteriol* 1959;78:788-791.
8. McLain N, Ascanio R, Baker C, et al. Undecylenic acid inhibits morphogenesis of *Candida albicans*. *Antimicrob Agents Chemother* 2000;44:2873-2875.
9. Steven S, Hofemyer JHS. Effects of ethanol, octanoic and decanoic acids on fermentation and the passive influx of protons throught the plasma membrane of *Saccharomyces cerevisiae. Appl Microbiol Biotechnol* 1993;38:356-363.
10. Miles MR, Olsen L, Rogers A. Recurrent vaginal candidiasis. *JAMA* 1977;238:1836-1837.
11. Bourne N, Ireland J, Stanberry LR, Bernstein DI. Effect of undecylenic acid as a topical microbicide against genital herpes infection in mice and guinea pigs. *Antiviral Res* 1999;40:139-144.
12. Shafran SD, Sacks SL, Aoki FY, et al. Topical undecylenic acid for herpes simplex labialis: a multicenter, placebo-controlled trial. *J Infect Dis* 1997;176:78-83.

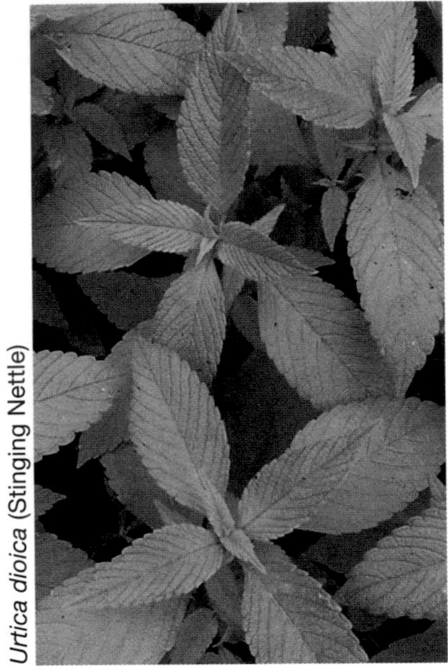
Urtica dioica (Stinging Nettle)

Urtica dioica *Urtica urens*

Description

Urtica dioica (stinging nettle) and *Urtica urens* (dwarf nettle) are members of the Urticaceae family native to Eurasia, and are considered therapeutically interchangeable.[1] The term nettle will be used here to refer simultaneously to stinging and dwarf nettle.

Nettles are ruderal, preferring wet, waste spaces. Stinging nettle is taller than dwarf nettle and is perennial; dwarf nettle is an annual. Both plants have fleshy, drooping, serrated, roughly heart-shaped leaves. The leaves and stems are covered with stinging hairs (dwarf nettle leaves are smooth and more delicate). Both produce inconspicuous green-white flowers in late spring or summer. The leaf, flower, seed, and root of nettle are used differently and probably contain different chemical constituents.

Active Constituents and Mechanisms of Actions

Like all green vegetables, nettle leaf is a micronutrient dense, nutritious food; however, it should be steamed or cooked before ingesting to destroy the stinging hairs, which contain histamine, formic acid, acetylcholine, acetic acid, butyric acid, leukotrienes, 5-hydroxytryptamine, and other irritants.[2,3] Contact with the hairs leads to a mildly painful sting, development of an erythematous macule, and itching or numbness for a period lasting from minutes to days. Medicinal extracts of nettle do not cause this reaction, as the hairs are destroyed in processing.

It appears the hydrophilic components of nettles, including lectins and polysaccharides, are important, particularly in prostate disease;[4] however, hydrophobic constituents have not been ruled entirely unimportant.[5] Each constituent may have individual effects, with the combination acting differently than any one constituent in isolation.

Nettle root lignans such as (--)-3,4-divanillyltetrahydrofuran may be important in benign prostatic hyperplasia (BPH) and other androgen- and estrogen-sensitive conditions because they may interfere with binding of sex hormone binding globulin (SHBG) to testosterone, the testosterone receptor, and/or the SHBG receptor.[6,7] Nettle lectins and sterols did not show anti-SHBG effects in these studies.

The steroidal compounds stigmasterol, stimast-4-en-3-one, and campesterol have been shown to inhibit the prostatic sodium/potassium pump, which might contribute to nettle's effects in BPH.[5] The small quantity of beta-sitosterol in nettle root (<0.01% of total mass) is unlikely to have an effect on BPH, given that 60 mg of beta-sitosterol daily is the usual amount necessary to reduce symptoms.[8]

Urtica dioica agglutinin (UDA) is a heat- and acid-resistant lectin found in stinging nettle, primarily the root. UDA induces a pattern of T-lymphocyte activity not seen with any other known plant lectin.[9] UDA appears to prevent formation of a systemic lupus erythematosus-like condition in mice and has diverse antiviral effects *in vitro*.[10,11] UDA antagonizes the epidermal growth factor receptor, an effect that may be of benefit in interfering with the pathogenesis of BPH.[12]

9-hydroxy-10-trans-12-cis-octadecadienic acid (HOA) from nettle root inhibits aromatase in prostate tissue.[13] A whole plant extract combined with *Prunus africanum* (pygeum) bark also inhibits aromatase.[14]

Polysaccharides and caffeic malic acid (CMA) are both found to some extent in all parts of nettle. Polysaccharides stimulate T-lymphocyte activity and complement activation *in vitro*.[2] Urtica polysaccharides and CMA demonstrated anti-inflammatory activity *in vitro* and in animal studies, via cyclooxygenase and lipoxygenase inhibition.[2,15] Isolated polysaccharides promoted tumor necrosis factor (TNF) production *in vitro*, while whole plant extracts inhibited TNF.[2,16]

Clinical Indications

Benign Prostatic Hyperplasia

The best researched indication for nettle is the use of the root in men with symptomatic BPH, something nettle is not known for traditionally. The leaves of nettle have never been assessed for this indication. At least four double-blind clinical trials confirm the efficacy of nettle root for BPH symptoms alone or in combination. A combination with pygeum extract at two dose levels, a combination with alpha adrenergic antagonists, and a combination with *Serenoa repens* (saw palmetto) fruit extracts have all shown the benefits of nettle root.[17-19] In perhaps the best trial, a combination of nettle and saw palmetto was just as effective as finasteride (Proscar®) in improving symptoms of BPH over 48 weeks in a double-blind trial, with fewer and milder adverse effects in the herbal group than the drug group.[20] Uncontrolled trials have also demonstrated nettle's effectiveness.[21]

Arthritis, Neuralgia, and Related Conditions

Topical application of fresh nettle leaves as a counterirritant for patients with various pain syndromes has a long history. Weiss mentions this approach for lumbalgia, sciatica, chronic tendinitis and sprains, and osteoarthritis.[22] As long as individuals are not allergic to nettle, this approach is safe. Two case studies suggest topically applied Urtica can help reduce osteoarthritis pain.[23] In a unique double-blind study, topical Urtica was compared to application of *Lamium album* (white nettle), a plant that has evolved to look like nettle but does not have stinging hairs.[24] Only Urtica was associated with relief of arthritic symptoms in this trial. Oral dosing of nettle leaf preparations has also been investigated in rheumatic conditions. In one open trial, a leaf extract was associated with symptom reduction comparable to that achieved with non-steroidal anti-inflammatory drugs (NSAIDS).[25] Nettle leaf (50 g of stewed leaves daily with food) was shown to potentiate the efficacy of sub-therapeutic doses of the NSAID diclofenac in another open study.[26]

Urinary Tract Conditions

The German Commission E approves the use of nettle leaf as supportive therapy in patients with lower urinary tract infections (combined with immune and antimicrobial therapy) and to prevent and treat formation of urinary gravel.[1]

Allergic Rhinitis

One open trial found nettle leaf was helpful for patients with allergic rhinitis.[27] More rigorous trials have not been conducted to confirm this finding. The anti-inflammatory effects of nettle leaf mentioned above suggest nettle may be useful for allergic diseases of all types.

Other Traditional Uses

Nettle leaf has traditionally been used for numerous other conditions, although clinical trials have not been conducted to confirm the efficacy of this approach. Anaphylactic shock, gout, hair loss, mild bleeding (particularly mild menorrhagia), and insufficient lactation are some of the traditional indications for nettle leaf.

Side Effects and Toxicity

Internal use of nettle is not associated with any significant adverse effects. Fresh nettle causes stings as discussed above, and may rarely lead to severe allergic reactions in susceptible individuals. Fresh nettle is not recommended to be eaten, as it can cause pain and inflammation in the upper digestive tract.

Dosage

The typical dose of nettle juice is 1 tablespoon (15 ml) in 4-6 oz water three times per day. Steamed (for 10-15 minutes) leaves can be eaten or added to soup. Vinegar or lemon improve flavor and may improve absorption of minerals. Tincture of the leaf or root is taken at a dose of 1/2-1 tsp (2-5 ml) three times per day, or as part of a formula with other herbs. Nettle leaf tea can be made by steeping 2-3 tsp herb in 1 pint of boiled water for 10-15 minutes – three cups or more per day should be used. Freeze-dried herb in capsules generally come in 240-300 mg amounts, and typically 1-2 capsules three times per day are used. For BPH a decoction of the root (2-3 tsp of root boiled for 10-15 minutes, 3 cups per day) or concentrated root extracts (5-10:1 weight:volume, 300-400 mg tid) are used.

References

1. Blumenthal M, Busse WR, Goldberg A, et al, eds. *The Complete German Commission E Monographs: Therapeutic Guide to Herbal Medicines*. Austin: American Botanical Council and Boston: Integrative Medicine Communications, 1998:216.
2. Wagner H, Willer F, Samtleben R, Boos G. Search for the antiprostatic principle of stinging nettle (*Urtica dioica*) roots. *Phytomedicine* 1994;1:213-224.
3. Emmelin N, Feldberg W. Distribution of acetylcholine and histamine in nettle plants. *New Phytologist* 1949;48:143-148.
4. Collier HOJ, Chesher GB. Identification of 5-hydroxytryptamine in the sting of the nettle. *Br J Pharmacol* 1956;11:186-189.
5. Hirano T, Homma M, Oka K. Effects of stinging nettle root extracts and their steroidal components on the Na+, K(+)-ATPase of the benign prostatic hyperplasia. *Planta Med* 1994;60:30-33.
6. Schuttner M, Gansser D, Spiteller G. Lignans from the roots of *Urtica dioica* and their metabolites bind to human sex hormone binding globulin (SHBG). *Planta Med* 1997;63:529-532.
7. Hryb DJ, Khan MS, Romas NA, Rosner W. The effect of extracts of the roots of the stinging nettle (*Urtica dioica*) on the interaction of SHBG with its receptor on human prostatic membranes. *Planta Med* 1995;61:31-32.
8. Berges RR, Windeler J, Trampisch HJ, Senge T. Randomised, placebo-controlled, double-blind clinical trial of beta-sitosterol in patients with benign prostatic hyperplasia. *Lancet* 1995;345:1529-1532.
9. Galelli A, Truffa-Bachi P. *Urtica dioica* agglutinin. A superantigenic lectin from stinging nettle rhizome. *J Immunol* 1993;151:1821-1831.
10. Musette P, Galelli A, Chabre H, et al. *Urtica dioica* agglutinin, a V beta 8.3-specific superantigen, prevents the development of the systemic lupus erythematosus-like pathology of MRL lpr/lpr mice. *Eur J Immunol* 1996;26:1707-1711.
11. Balzarini J, Neyts J, Schols D, et al. The mannose-specific plant lectins from Cymbidium hybrid and *Epipactis helleborine* and the (N-acetylglucosamine)n-specific plant lectin from *Urtica dioica* are potent and selective inhibitors of human immunodeficiency virus and cytomegalovirus replication *in vitro*. *Antiviral Res* 1992;18:191-207.
12. Wagner H, Geiger WN, Boos G, Samtleben R. Studies on the binding of *Urtica dioica* agglutinin (UDA) and other lectins in an *in vitro* epidermal growth factor receptor test. *Phytomedicine* 1995;2:287-290.
13. Kraus R, Spitelleer G, Bartsch W. (10-E, 12Z)-9-hydroxy-10,12-octadecadienic acid, an aromatase-inhibiting substance from the root extract of *Urtica dioica*. *Liebigs Ann Chem* 1991;19:335-339. [Article in German]

14. Hartman RW, Mark M, Soldati F. Inhibition of 5-alpha reductase and aromatase by PHL-00801 (Prostatonin), a combination of PY 102 (*Pygeum africanum*) and UR 102 (*Urtica dioica*) extracts. *Phytomedicine* 1996;3:121-128.

15. Obertreis B, Giller K, Teucher T, et al. Anti-inflammatory effect of *Urtica dioica* folia extract in comparison to caffeic malic acid. *Arzneimittelforschung* 1996;46:52-56. [Article in German]

16. Obertreis B, Ruttkowski T, Teucher T, et al. *Ex-vivo in-vitro* inhibition of lipopolysaccharide stimulated tumor necrosis factor-alpha and interleukin-1 beta secretion in human whole blood by extractum *Urticae dioicae* foliorum. *Arzneimittelforschung* 1996;46:389-394.

17. Krzeski T, Kazon M, Borkowski A, et al. Combined extracts of *Urtica dioica* and *Pygeum africanum* in the treatment of benign prostatic hyperplasia: double-blind comparison of two doses. *Clin Ther* 1993;15:1011-1020.

18. Neumann HG. Combination therapy of benign prostatic hyperplasia (BPH) with phytotherapy and selective alpha1-blockade. *Urologe B* 1993;33:384-385. [Article in German]

19. Vontobel HP, Herzog R, Rutishauser G, Kres H. Results of a double-blind study on the effectiveness of ERU capsules in the conservative treatment of benign prostatic hyperplasia. *Urologe A* 1985;24:49-51. [Article in German]

20. Sokeland J, Albrecht J. Combination of Sabal and Urtica extract vs. finasteride in benign prostatic hyperplasia (Aiken stages I to II). Comparison of therapeutic effectiveness in a one year double-blind study. *Urologe A* 1997;36:327-333. [Article in German]

21. Belaiche P, Lievoux O. Clinical studies on the palliative treatment of prostatic adenoma with extract of Urtica root. *Phytother Res* 1991;5:267-269.

22. Weiss RF. *Herbal Medicine,* 6th ed. Gothenburg, Sweden: Ab Arcanum and Beaconsfield; UK: Beaconsfield Publishers Ltd; 1988:261-262.

23. Randall CF. Stinging nettles for osteoarthritis pain of the hip. *Br J Gen Pract* 1994;44:533-534.

24. Randall C, Randall H, Dobbs F, et al. Randomized controlled trial of nettle sting for treatment of base-of-thumb pain. *J R Soc Med* 2000;93:305-309.

25. Sommer RG, Sinner B. IDS 23 in the therapy of rheumatic disease. Do you know the new cytokine antagonists? *Therapiewoche* 1996;46:44-49. [Article in German]

26. Chrubasik S, Enderlein W, Bauer R, Grabner W. Evidence for the antirheumatic effectiveness of herba *Urticae dioicae* in acute arthritis: a pilot study. *Phytomedicine* 1997;4:105-108.

27. Mittman P. Randomized, double-blind study of freeze-dried *Urtica dioica* in the treatment of allergic rhinitis. *Planta Med* 1990;56:44-47.

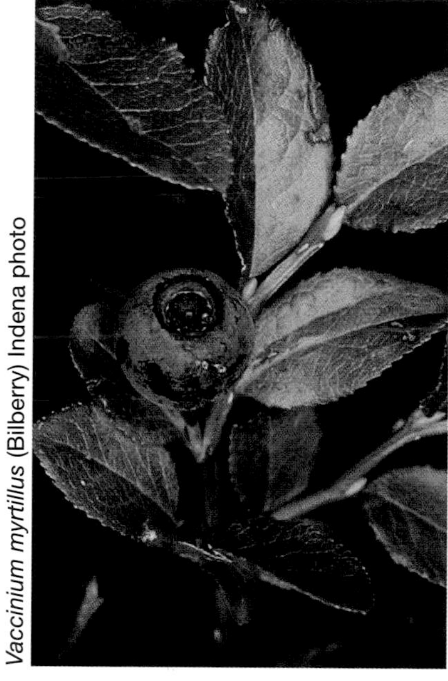

Vaccinium myrtillus (Bilberry) Indena photo

Vaccinium myrtillus

Description

Vaccinium myrtillus (bilberry) is a member of the Ericaceae family, and is also known as European blueberry, huckleberry, or blueberry. It is a shrubby perennial plant one to two feet in height and can be found in the mountains and forests of Europe and the northern United States. Its branches contain alternating, elliptical, bright green leaves, and its flowers, which appear from April to June, are reddish or pink, and bell-shaped. The fruit of the bilberry plant is blue-black or purple and differs from the American blueberry in that the meat of the fruit is purple, rather than cream or white. Fruit is harvested July through September, and time of ripeness is somewhat dependent on plant elevation. Plants growing at higher elevations generally ripen later than those at lower elevations. Bilberry has been used as food for centuries due to its high nutritive value, and today represents a precious wild delicacy. Bilberry's history of medicinal use dates back to the Middle Ages, but it did not become widely known to herbalists until the 16th century when its use was documented for treating bladder stones, biliary disorders, scurvy, coughs, and lung tuberculosis. More recently, bilberry fruit extracts have been used for the treatment of diarrhea, dysentery, and mouth and throat inflammations. Bilberry leaf decoctions have been used to lower blood sugar in diabetes.[1] Currently, bilberry research is focused on the treatment of ocular disorders, vascular disorders, and diabetes mellitus.

Active Constituents

Several active constituents have been isolated from the berries and leaves of the bilberry plant, including anthocyanoside flavonoids (anthocyanins), vitamins, sugars, and pectins, which are found in the berries, and quercetin, catechins, tannins, iridoids, and acids, which are found in the leaves.[2,3] The anthocyanosides are considered the most important of the pharmacologically active components. Anthocyanoside concentration in the fresh fruit is approximately 0.1 to 0.25 percent, while concentrated bilberry extracts are usually standardized to 25-percent anthocyanosides.[3] The berry's anthocyanoside content increases as the fruit ripens, while the reverse is true of its leaf constituents.[4]

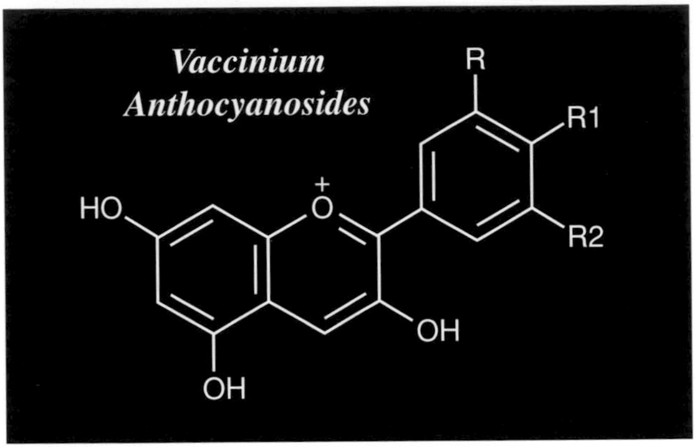

Vaccinium Anthocyanosides

R, R1, R2, HO, OH, OH, $\overset{+}{O}$

Mechanisms of Action

Although bilberry constituents have multiple pharmacological actions, most of the research has focused on the anthocyanosides. Extracts containing anthocyanosides have been shown to possess strong antioxidant properties,[5] stabilize collagen fibers and promote collagen biosynthesis,[6-8] decrease capillary permeability and fragility,[9] and inhibit platelet aggregation.[10] Anthocyanosides and other bilberry leaf constituents prevent the release and synthesis of pro-inflammatory compounds such as histamine, prostaglandins, and leukotrienes.[6-8,11] In addition, bilberry leaf decoctions administered orally have been shown to lower blood glucose levels.[12]

Clinical Applications

Ophthalmologic Disorders

The mechanisms of action behind bilberry's beneficial effect on the eye are not completely understood. They include the ability to improve oxygen and blood delivery to the eye and to scavenge free radicals that can disrupt collagen structures and contribute to conditions such as cataracts and macular degeneration. In addition, the anthocyanosides have an affinity for the pigmented epithelium (visual purple) area of the retina, the portion of the retina responsible for vision and adjustments to light and dark.[13,14]

Vision Improvement

Bilberry extract's visual enhancement properties were first studied by French researchers on Royal Air Force pilots during World War II. Administration of bilberry extract resulted in improved nighttime visual acuity, faster adjustment to darkness, and faster restoration of visual acuity after exposure to glare.[15,16] Later studies confirmed this effect,[17,18] although a subsequent double-blind, placebo-controlled, crossover study conducted on U.S. Navy SEAL personnel did not. Fifteen male subjects given 160 mg bilberry extract (standardized to 25-percent anthocyanosides) three times daily for three weeks, showed no significant improvement in either night visual acuity or night contrast sensitivity compared to placebo.[19] Conversely, studies of bilberry extract on individuals with retinitis pigmentosa and hemeralopia (inability to see distinctly in bright light) demonstrated a significant improvement in visual performance.[18,20] It may be the most significant effects will be observed in those with impaired visual acuity.

Glaucoma

Consumption of bilberry extracts may offer significant protection against the development of glaucoma due to its collagen-enhancing and antioxidant properties. The reduced tensile strength and integrity of aging eye tissue may result in the increased intraocular pressure and loss of peripheral vision seen in glaucoma. In one study, eight patients with glaucoma were given a single oral dose of 200 mg *Vaccinium myrtillus* anthocyanosides and demonstrated improvement based on electroretinography.[13] A collagen-stabilizing effect on the trabecular meshwork, facilitating aqueous outflow, may provide a potential mechanism.

Cataracts

Bilberry anthocyanosides may offer therapeutic benefit in prevention of cataracts. Animal studies show diets high in anthocyanoside flavonoids retard the development of cataracts in rats.[21,22] A clinical study, in which bilberry extract (180 mg twice daily of a 25-percent anthocyanoside extract) was given with vitamin E, demonstrated arrested cataract formation in 48 of 50 patients with senile cortical cataracts.[23]

Diabetic Retinopathy

In Europe, bilberry anthocyanoside extracts are recognized as highly effective in preventing diabetic retinopathy, with several clinical studies supporting its use.[24-28] In a double-blind study, 14 patients with diabetic and/or hypertensive retinopathy were supplemented with bilberry extract equivalent to 115 mg anthocyanosides daily (or placebo) for one month. Significant improvements were observed in the ophthalmoscopic parameters of 11 subjects receiving bilberry, and 12 patients showed improvement in angiographic parameters.[27] Additional clinical studies of bilberry's positive effects in treating retinopathy have been conducted in Europe but are not available in English.

Vascular Disorders

Bilberry extracts improve microcirculation. Animal studies have shown it to be of benefit in decreasing vascular permeability and improving vascular tone and blood flow.[28,29] Clinical trials in humans have yielded similar results. Fifteen patients with polyneuritis due to peripheral vascular insufficiency were given 480 mg/day of bilberry extract and significant improvement was noted in microcirculation.[30] In another study, the same dosage of bilberry extract given to 47 patients with various venous diseases resulted in reduced capillary flow as well as an elimination of microstagnation and blood stasis of the foot.[31] A review of uncontrolled trials from 1979 to 1985 on a total of 568 patients with venous insufficiency of the lower limbs showed bilberry extract was effective in rapidly decreasing symptomology and improving both venous microcirculation and lymph drainage.[32]

Diabetes Mellitus

Bilberry leaf decoctions have a long history of folk use as a hypoglycemic agent. Research demonstrates that oral administration of bilberry leaf decoctions reduce hyperglycemia in dogs, even in the presence of concurrently injected glucose.[33,34] This effect is attributed to the myrtillin anthocyanoside, apparently the most active hypoglycemic component.[34]

In addition, bilberry anthocyanosides enhance collagen integrity, stabilize capillary permeability, and inhibit sorbitol accumulation, thus providing protection against vascular and neurological sequelae of diabetes.

Other Effects

Bilberry extracts have demonstrated anti-inflammatory properties in animals, and thus may be useful in the treatment of conditions such as rheumatoid arthritis.[35] Additionally, women with dysmenorrhea were given bilberry extract (115 mg anthocyanosides per day) for three days before and during menstruation. A significant improvement in pelvic/lumbosacral pain, mammary tension, nausea, and lower-limb heaviness was noted.[36] Bilberry extracts have also been shown to have strong antiplatelet aggregating activity in humans when given at doses of 480 mg daily for 30-60 days.[37] The antiulcer activity of one of bilberry's anthocyanosides (IdB 1027) has been demonstrated in various experimental models. Magistretti et al demonstrated that IdB 1027 decreased the incidence and severity of numerous forms of experimentally induced ulcers in Sprague Dawley and Wistar rats.[38] Another significant property of bilberry extracts is the capability to exert potent protective action on LDL particles during copper-mediated oxidation. This was accomplished using only trace amounts of *V. myrtillus* extract (15 to 20 mcg/mL); therefore, the extract may be even more potent than ascorbic acid in protecting LDL from oxidative stress.[39]

Side Effects and Toxicity

As might be expected with a food, bilberry consumption is very safe. Dosages as high as 400 mg/kg body weight have been administered to rats without toxicity. Long-term oral administration in humans of doses equivalent to 180 mg/kg anthocyanosides per day for six months produced no toxic effects. No mutagenic or carcinogenic effects were observed.[40] Since bilberry extracts have antiplatelet aggregating properties, very high doses should be used cautiously in patients with hemorrhagic disorders and those taking anticoagulant or antiplatelet drugs. A review of studies comprising over 2,000 subjects taking bilberry extract reported only mild side effects affecting the gastrointestinal, cutaneous, or nervous system.[40]

Dosage

Recommended dosages of bilberry depend on what form of the fruit is being consumed. If consuming fresh berries, 55-115 grams three times daily is recommended. Most bilberry is in the form of aqueous extract standardized to 25-percent anthocyanosides at a dose of 80-160 mg three times daily. The actual dosage of anthocyanosides is 20-40 mg three times daily.

References

1. Grieve M. *A Modern Herbal.* Vol.1. New York, NY: Dover Publications; 1971:385-386.
2. Benigni R, Capra C, Cattorini PE. *Plante Medicinali – Chimica Farmacologia E Terapia*. Vol.II. Milano, Italia: Inverni della Beffa; 1962:951-958.
3. Baj A, Bombardelli E, Gabetta B, Martinelli EM. Qualitative and quantitative evaluation of *Vaccinium myrtillus* anthocyanins by high-resolution gas chromatography and high-performance liquid chromatography. *J Chromatography* 1983;279:365-372.
4. Morazzoni P, Bombardelli E. *Vaccinium myrtillus I. Fitoterapia* 1996;67:3-29.
5. Salvayre R, Braquet P, Perruchot T. Douste-Blazy L. *Flavonoids and Bioflavonoids 1981.* Amsterdam-Oxford-New York: Elsevier Press; 1982:437-442.
6. Kuhnau J. The flavonoids. A class of semi-essential food components. Their role in human nutrition. *Wld Rev Nutr Diet* 1976;24:117-191.
7. Harvsteen B. Flavonoids, a class of natural products of high pharmacological potency. *Biochem Pharmacol* 1983;32:1141-1148.
8. Gabor M. Pharmacologic effects of flavonoids on blood vessels. *Angiologica* 1972;9:355-374.
9. Mian E, Curri SB, Lietti A, Bombardelli E. Anthocyanosides and the walls of the microvessels: further aspects of the mechanism of action of their protective effect in syndromes due to abnormal capillary fragility. *Minerva Med* 1977:68:3565-3581.
10. Bottecchia D, et al. Preliminary reports on the inhibitory effect of *Vaccinium myrtillus* anthocyanosides on platelet aggregation and clot retraction. *Fitoterapia* 1987;48:3-8.
11. Amella M, Bronner C, Briancon F, et al. Inhibition of mast cell histamine release by flavonoids and bioflavonoids. *Planta Medica* 1985;51:16-20.
12. Bever B, Zahnd G. Plants with oral hypoglycemic action. *Quart J Crude Drug Res* 1979;17:13996.
13. Caselli L. Clinical and electroretinographic study on activity of anthocyanosides. *Arch Med Int* 1985;37:29-35.
14. Wegmann R, Maeda K, Tronch P, Bastide P. Effects of anthocyanosides on photoreceptors. Cytoenzymatic aspects. *Ann Histochim* 1969;14:237-256.
15. Jayle GE, Aubert L. Action des glucosides d'anthocyanes sur la vision scotopique et mesopique du sujet normal. *Therapie* 1964:19:171-185. [Article in French]
16. Terrasse J, Moinade S. Premiers resultats obtenus avec un nouveau facteur vitamininique P "les anthocyanosides" extraits du *Vaccinium myrtillus. Presse Med* 1964;72:397-400. [Article in French]
17. Sala D, Rolando M, Rossi PL, Pissarello L. Effect of anthocyanosides on visual performances at low illumination. *Minerva Oftalmol* 1979;21:283-285.
18. Gloria E, Peria A. Effect of anthocyanosides on the absolute visual threshold. *Ann Ottalmol Clin Ocul* 1966;92:595-607. [Article in Italian]

19. Muth ER, Laurent JM, Jasper P. The effect of bilberry nutritional supplementation on night visual acuity and contrast sensitivity. *Altern Med Rev* 2000;5:164-173.

20. Junemann G. On the effect of anthocyanosides on hemeralopia following quinine poisoning. *Klin Monatsbl Augenheilkd* 1967;151:891-896. [Article in German]

21. Pautler EL, Ennis SR. The effect of diet on inherited retinal dystrophy in the rat. *Curr Eye Res* 1984;3:1221-1224.

22. Hess H, Knapka JJ, Newsome DA, et al. Dietary prevention of cataracts in the pink-eyed RCS rat. *Lag Anim Sci* 1985;35:47-53.

23. Bravetti G. Preventive medical treatment of senile cataract with vitamin E and anthocyanosides: clinical evaluation. *Ann Ottalmol Clin Ocul* 1989;115:109. [Article in Italian]

24. Scharrer A, Ober M. Anthocyanosides in the treatment of retinopathies. *Klin Monatabl Augenheilkd* 1981;178:386-389. [Article in German]

25. Chaundry PS, Cambera J, Juliana HR, Varma SD. Inhibition of human lens aldose reductase by flavonoids, sulindac and indomethacin. *Biochem Pharmacol* 1983;32:1995-1998.

26. Varma SD, Mizuno A, Kinoshita JH. Diabetic cataracts and flavonoids. *Science* 1977;195:87-89.

27. Perossini M, et al. Diabetic and hypertensive retinopathy therapy with *Vaccinium myrtillus* anthocyanosides (Tegens): Double-blind placebo controlled clinical trial. *Ann Ottalmol Clin Ocul* 1987;113:1173. [Article in Italian]

28. Lietti A, Cristoni A, Picci M. Studies on *Vaccinium myrtillus* anthocyanosides. I. Vasoprotective and anti-inflammatory activity. *Arzneimittelforschung* 1976;26:829-832.

29. Colantuoni A, Bertuglia S, Magistretti MJ, Donato L. Effects of *Vaccinium myrtillus* anthocyanosides on arterial vasomotion. *Arzneimittelforschung* 1991;41:905-909.

30. Pennarola R, et al. The therapeutic action of the anthocyanosides in microcirculatory changes due to adhesive-induced polyneuritis. *Gazz Med Ital* 1980;139:485-491. [Article in Italian]

31. Ghiringhelli C, Gregoratti L, Marastoni F. Capillarotropic activity of anthocyanosides in high doses in phlebopathic stasis. *Minerva Cardioangiol* 1978;25:255-276.

32. Bratman S, Kroll D. *The Natural Pharmacist: Clinical Evaluation of Medicinal Herbs and Other Therapeutic Natural Products*. Roseville, CA: Prima Publishing; 1999:Bilberry 1-5.

33. Allen FM. Blueberry leaf extract. Physiologic and clinical properties in relation to carbohydrate metabolism. *JAMA* 1927;89:1577-1581.

34. Bever B, Zahnd G. Plants with oral hypoglycemic action. *Quart J Crude Drug Res* 1979;17:139-196.

35. Rao CN, Rao VH, Steinman B. Influence of bioflavonoids on the collagen metabolism in rats with adjuvant induced arthritis. *Ital J Biochem* 1981;30:54-62.

36. Colombo D, Vescovini R. Controlled trial of anthocyanosides from *Vaccinium myrtillus* in primary dysmenorrhea. *G Ital Ost Ginecol* 1985;7:1033-1038.

37. Puilleiro G, et al. *Ex vivo* study of the inhibitory effects of *Vaccinium myrtillus* anthocyanosides on human platelet aggregation. *Fitoterapia* 1989;60:69-75.

38. Magistretti MJ, Conti M, Cristoni A. Antiulcer activity of anthocyanidin from *Vaccinium myrtillus. Arzneimittelforschung* 1988;38:686-690.

39. Laplaud PM, Lelubre A, Chapman MJ. Antioxidant action of *Vaccinium myrtillus* extract on human low density lipoproteins *in vitro*: initial observations. *Fundam Clin Pharmacol* 1997;11:35-40.

40. Eandi M. Post-marketing investigation on Tegens“ preparation with respect to side effects. 1987. Cited in Morazzoni P, Bombardelli E. *Vaccinium myrtillus I. Fitoterapia* 1996;67:3-29.

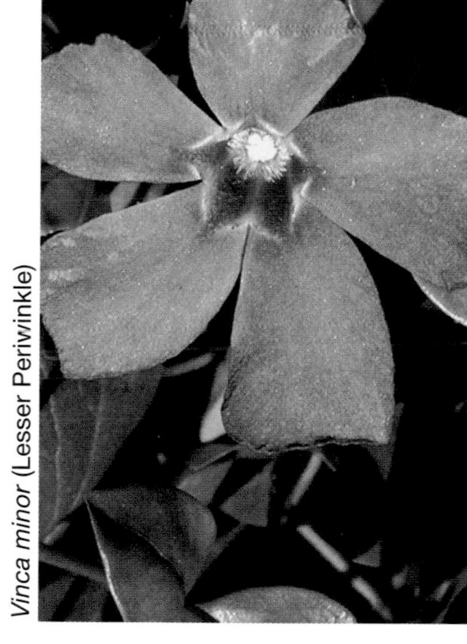
Vinca minor (Lesser Periwinkle)

Vinpocetine

Description

Vinpocetine (vinpocetine-ethyl apovincaminate) was synthesized in the late 1960s from the alkaloid vincamine, extracted from the leaf of the lesser periwinkle plant (*Vinca minor*).[1] Vinpocetine was made available under the trade name Cavinton in 1978 and has since been used widely in Japan, Hungary, Germany, Poland, and Russia for the treatment of cerebrovascular-related pathologies.[2] Several clinical studies have confirmed the neuroprotective effects of this compound.

Pharmacokinetics

Vinpocetine, when taken on an empty stomach, has an absorption rate of 6.7 percent.[3] When taken with food, absorption increases 60-100 percent. Vinpocetine reaches the bloodstream approximately one hour after administration, whether taken with food or on an empty stomach.[4] The elimination half-life of the oral form is one to two hours and the majority of vinpocetine is eliminated from the body within eight hours [3]

Recent studies, either following i.v. infusion of vinpocetine in patients with cerebrovascular disorders or using positron emission tomography (PET) scans in animals, have shown that vinpocetine crosses the blood-brain barrier and is taken up by cerebral tissue.[5,6] PET studies have also clearly shown in human subjects vinpocetine is preferentially absorbed in the central nervous system at twice the level that would be expected according to total body distribution.[7] The highest uptake of vinpocetine was seen in the thalamus, putamen, and neocortical regions.

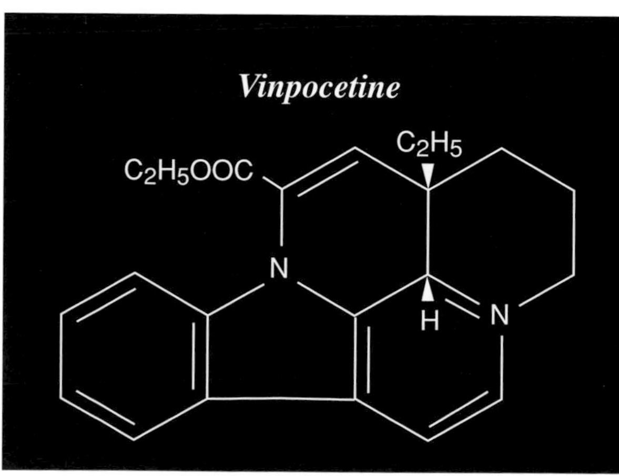

Mechanisms of Action

Vinpocetine appears to have several different mechanisms of action that allow for its antioxidant, vasodilating, and neuroprotective activities.

Voltage-dependent Sodium Channel Inhibition

It has been hypothesized that vinpocetine's application in ischemic stroke is secondary to its effect on voltage-dependant sodium channels in the brain.[8] Inhibition of sodium channels in neural tissue is the primary mechanism of several different drugs reported to have neuroprotective effects in experimental ischemia.[9] This action, effectively blocking accumulation of sodium in neurons, decreases the damage of reperfusion injury and may be beneficial in lessening the toxic effects of oxidative stress resulting from anoxia.[10]

Phosphodiesterase-1 Inhibition

Vinpocetine inhibits Ca^{+2}/calmodulin-dependent phosphodiesterase (PDE) type 1.[11] This effect would theoretically lead to an increase of cyclic AMP over cyclic GMP and may be responsible for the benefits in cerebral circulation and decreased platelet aggregation observed after vinpocetine administration.[12]

Antioxidant Effects

Like vitamin E, vinpocetine is an effective scavenger of hydroxyl radicals.[13] It has also been shown to inhibit lipid peroxidation in synaptosomes of murine brain tissue and to protect against global anoxia and hypoxia in animals. Vinpocetine has decreased areas of neuronal necrosis in animal models up to 60 percent in experimentally-induced ischemia.[10]

Other Neuroprotective Effects

Vinpocetine has been shown to protect neurons from the toxicity of glutamate and N-methyl-d-aspartate (NMDA).[14] Vinpocetine lowers blood viscosity in patients with cerebrovascular disease,[15] has significant vasodilating properties,[16] decreases platelet aggregation,[17] and increases and maintains erythrocyte flexibility under oxidative stress,[18] all of which are potentially beneficial in cerebrovascular disease. Vinpocetine causes a selective increase in cerebral blood flow and increases cerebral metabolic rate.[19,20]

Clinical Indications

Chronic Cerebral Vascular Ischemia

Two PET studies in chronic stroke patients have shown that vinpocetine has a significant effect in increasing glucose uptake and metabolism in the healthy cortical and subcortical regions of the brain, particularly in the area surrounding the region of the stroke.[21] A study in

15 chronic ischemic stroke patients found that a two-week vinpocetine trial significantly increased cerebral blood flow in the non-symptomatic hemisphere.[10] Recent studies using Doppler sonography and near infrared spectroscopy have shown increased perfusion of the middle cerebral artery in patients with chronic cerebrovascular disease given a single infusion of vinpocetine.[10]

Acute Ischemic Stroke

Although small studies have shown that vinpocetine has an immediate vasodilating effect in cerebrovascular circulation,[10] a meta-analysis of the existing studies examining short- and long-term fatality rates with vinpocetine was unable to assess efficacy.[2] In the analysis of eight studies in acute stroke patients (vinpocetine was administered within two weeks of event), only one study met the meta-analysis criteria. In the selected trial, three weeks after onset of i.v. vinpocetine therapy, 8 of 17 vinpocetine patients and 12 of 16 placebo patients were determined "dependent" (unable to live without assistance), and all were still alive. The meta-analysis authors were unable to determine a beneficial effect of vinpocetine, but did state that considering the *in vitro* studies and animal data, vinpocetine has potential to be effective in acute stroke. Properly designed studies have not yet been conducted.

Degenerative Senile Cerebral Dysfunction

A meta-analysis of six randomized, controlled trials involving 731 patients with degenerative senile cerebral dysfunction showed that vinpocetine was highly effective in the treatment of senile cerebral dysfunction. Using several psychometric testing scales in addition to physical symptoms (speech and movement capacity, muscular coordination and strength, sensory-perceptual ability) the researchers were able to show a highly significant effect of vinpocetine on both cognitive and motor functions.[22]

Alzheimer's Disease

Although evidence has been limited to one small study, the results suggest that vinpocetine supplementation may not be effective as a therapy for Alzheimer's disease. A double-blind, placebo-controlled study of vinpocetine in 15 Alzheimer patients, treated with increasing doses of vinpocetine (30, 45, and 60 mg per day) in an open-label pilot trial during a one-year period, resulted in no improvement.[23]

Tinnitus/ Meniere's Disease/Visual Impairment

Vinpocetine has been used in the treatment of acoustic trauma with subsequent hearing loss and tinnitus.[24] Disappearance of tinnitus occurred in 50 percent of those who started vinpocetine within one week of the trauma. Regardless of the time since the incident, 79 percent of patients had improved hearing and 66 percent had a significant decrease in the severity of the tinnitus.

Vinpocetine has also been found to be effective in treating Meniere's disease and in visual impairment secondary to arteriosclerosis.[25,26]

Drug Interactions

Because vinpocetine decreases platelet aggregation it should be avoided in patients on blood thinning medications.

Side Effects and Toxicity

Some studies have noted flushing, rashes, or minor gastrointestinal problems in some subjects; however, these side effects did not warrant discontinuation of the medication.[22]

In one study no significant side effects were reported, even in larger doses of 20 mg three times daily.[23]

Dosage

All of the above studies used either 10 mg vinpocetine 3 times daily orally or i.v. vinpocetine. Patients with chronic cerebrovascular disorders that were included in the meta-analysis[22] had been on an oral dosage of 10 mg three times daily.

References

1. Lorincz C, Szasz K, Kisfaludy L. The synthesis of ethyl apovincaminate. *Arzneimittelforschung* 1976;26:1907.
2. Bereczki D, Fekete I. A systematic review of vinpocetine therapy in acute ischaemic stroke. *Eur J Clin Pharmacol* 1999;55:349-352.
3. Miskolczi P, Kozma K, Polgar M, Vereczkey L. Pharmacokinetics of vinpocetine and its main metabolite apovincaminic acid before and after the chronic oral administration of vinpocetine to humans. *Eur J Drug Metab Pharmacokinet* 1990;15:1-5.
4. Lohmann A, Dingler E, Sommer W, et al. Bioavailability of vinpocetine and interference of the time of application with food intake. *Arzneimittelforschung* 1992;42:914-917.
5. Polgar M, Vereczkey L, Nyary I. Pharmacokinetics of vinpocetine and its metabolite, apovincaminic acid, in plasma and cerebrospinal fluid after intravenous infusion. *J Pharm Biomed Anal* 1985;3:131-139.
6. Gulyas B, Halldin M, Karlsson P, et al. Brain uptake and plasma metabolism of [11C]vinpocetine: a preliminary PET study in a cynomolgus monkey. *J Neuroimaging* 1999;9:217-222.
7. Guylas B, Halldin C, Farde L. PET studies on the uptake and regional distribution of [11C]vinpocetine in human subjects. *Arch Neurol*. In press.
8. Molnar P, Erdo SL. Vinpocetine is as potent as phenytoin to block voltage-gated Na^+ channels in rat cortical neurons. *Eur J Pharmacol* 1995;273:303-306.
9. Urenjak J, Obrenovitch TP. Pharmacological modulation of voltage-gated Na^+ channels: a rational and effective strategy against ischemic brain damage. *Pharmacol Rev* 1996;48:21-67.
10. Bonoczk P, Gulyas B, Adam-Vizi V, et al. Role of sodium channel inhibition in neuroprotection: effect of vinpocetine. *Brain Res Bull* 2000;53:245-254.
11. Beavo JA. Cyclic nucleotide phosphodiesterases: functional implications of multiple isoforms. *Physiol Rev* 1995:75:725-748.

12. Chiu PJ, Tetzloff G, Ahn HS, Sybertz EJ. Comparative effects of vinpocetine and 8-Br-cyclic GMP on the contraction and ^{45}Ca-fluxes in the rabbit aorta. *Am J Hypertens* 1988;1:262-268.

13. Stolc S. Indole derivatives as neuroprotectants. *Life Sci* 1999;65:1943-1950.

14. Miyamoto M, Murphy TH, Schnaar RL, Coyle JT. Antioxidants protect against glutamate-induced cytotoxicity in a neuronal cell line. *J Pharmacol Exp Ther* 1989;250:1132-1140.

15. Osawa M, Maruyama S. Effects of TCV-3B (vinpocetine) on blood viscosity in ischemic cerebrovascular diseases. *Ther Hung* 1985;33:7-12.

16. Tamaki N, Kusunoki T, Matsumoto S. The effect of vinpocetine on cerebral blood flow in patients with cerebrovascular disorders. *Ther Hung* 1985;33:13-21.

17. Kuzuya F. Effects of vinpocetine on platelet aggregability and erythrocyte deformability. *Ther Hung* 1985;33:22-34.

18. Hayakawa M. Comparative efficacy of vinpocetine, pentoxifylline and nicergoline on red blood cell deformability. *Arzneimittelforschung* 1992;42:108-110.

19. Imamoto T, Tanabe M, Shimamoto N, et al. Cerebral circulatory and cardiac effects of vinpocetine and its metabolite, apovincaminic acid, in anaesthetized dogs. *Arzneimittelforschung* 1984;34:161-169.

20. Shibota M, Kakihana M, Nagaoka A. The effect of vinpocetine on brain glucose uptake in mice. *Nippon Yakurigaku Zasshi* 1982;80:221-224. [Article in Japanese]

21. Szakall S, Boros I, Balkay L, et al. Cerebral effects of a single dose of intravenous vinpocetine in chronic stroke patients: a PET study. *J Neuroimaging* 1998;8:197-204.

22. Nagy Z, Vargha P, Kovacs L, et al. Meta-analysis of Cavinton. *Praxis* 1998;7:63-68.

23. Thal LJ, Salmon DP, Lasker B, et al. The safety and lack of efficacy of vinpocetine in Alzheimer's disease. *J Am Geriatr Soc* 1989;37:515-520.

24. Konopka W, Zalweski P, Olszewski J, et al. Treatment results of acoustic trauma. *Otolaryngol Pol* 1997;51:281S-284S. [Article in Polish]

25. Ribari O, Zelen B, Kollar B. Ethyl apovincaminate in the treatment of sensorineural impairment of hearing. *Arzneimittelforschung* 1976;26:1977-1980.

26. Kahan A, Olah M. Use of ethyl apovincaminate in ophthalmological therapy. *Arzneimittelforschung* 1976;26:1969-1972.

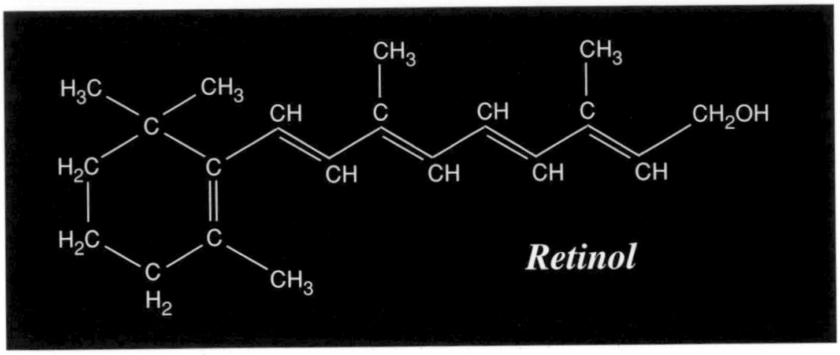

Retinol

Vitamin A

Introduction

Vitamin A is both a fat-soluble vitamin and a hormone, contributing to the visual pigment rhodopsin and controlling gene transcription that allows for the normal proliferation and differentiation of epithelial cells. Vitamin A also modulates the immune response through lymphopoesis, apoptosis, cytokine production, the function of neutrophils, and lymphocytes, and immunoglobin production.[1] Therapeutically, retinoids, the active metabolites of retinoic acid (naturally occurring vitamin A) are effective chemopreventive agents in the treatment of skin, head and neck, breast, and liver cancers and certain forms of leukemia.

Biochemistry and Mechanisms of Action

Vitamin A exists in animal products as retinyl esters and in plant foods as the precursor carotenoid family. Beta-carotene is cleaved to retinyl esters and retinoic acid in the enterocyte of the small intestine and packaged into chylomicrons along with retinol from preformed vitamin A for transport to the liver for storage as retinol in hepatic stellate cells.[2] When needed, retinol is transported to tissues bound to retinol binding protein (a zinc-dependent protein). Zinc deficiency disturbs normal retinol metabolism, and supplementation with zinc has been shown to treat retinol-resistant night-blindness.[3] In the eye, retinol is oxidized to retinaldehyde, the basis of the visual pigments rhodopsin and iodopson. It is also oxidized to retinoic acid, the parent compound of natural retinoids.[4] Two specific isomers, all-trans-retinoic acid and 9-cis-retinoic acid, have been found to bind to specific receptors in the nucleus of target cells and assist in regulating the cell replication cycle through transcription factors-tumor suppressor proteins p53 and p105, which are both strong inhibitors of uncontrolled cell growth.[5]

Retinoids, through their interaction with nuclear retinoic acid receptors in tissue, control gene expression and promote normal proliferation and differentiation of epithelial tissue, particularly mucous membrane epithelium.

Vitamin A functions in the immune system in the modulation of diverse pathways: in the expression of mucins and keratins, lymphopoesis, cytokine production, neutrophil maturation and function, the functional expression of natural killer cells, monocytes and macrophages, T and B lymphocytes, and immunoglobin production.[6]

Deficiency States and Symptoms

Vitamin A deficiency is internationally profound and widespread, and responsible for one third of all mortality in infants and preschool-age children worldwide.[6] Although morbidity and mortality are usually referred to as a problem only in developing countries, it has also been documented in children and adults in the United States. In low income young women aged 19-34, over half consume less than 70 percent of the RDA for vitamin A and one-third consume less than 50 percent of the RDA.[7]

Low serum retinol levels are found in Crohn's disease patients,[8] in alcoholics,[9] diabetics,[10] and in juvenile arthritics.[11] Lowered vitamin A levels may also occur with overuse of laxatives, chronic intake of mineral oil, chronic cortisone usage, cigarette smoking, zinc deficiency, vitamin D deficiency, excessive iron consumption, organophosphate (DDT and PCB) exposure, cold exposure, nitrate ingestion, and excessive consumption of refined carbohydrates.[12] Vitamin A deficiency is related to increased susceptibility to measles, malaria, tuberculosis, and other respiratory and intestinal infectious diseases.[6]

Clinical Applications

Diseases of the Eye

Vitamin A deficiency has been linked to ocular disorders that result from oxidative damage to the photoreceptor cells and the pigmented epithelium of the retina. Night blindness, age-related macular degeneration, retinitis pigmentosa, retinopathy, and xeropthalmia are related to either vitamin A deficiency or impaired vitamin A metabolism.[13-15] Retinitis pigmentosa occurs as a result of altered vitamin A metabolism without lowered blood retinol levels; however, Vitamin A supplementation can be helpful in individuals with this condition. A long-term study utilizing 15,000 IU supplemental vitamin A daily slowed the rate of decline of retinal function in these patients.[15]

Cervical Dysplasia

Vitamin A regulates genes that control squamous proliferation. Vitamin A deficiency in animal models caused squamous metaplasia of columnar cervical cells.[16] Low levels of vitamin A are also very common in smokers with cervical dysplasia.[17] When compared to controls, women with cervical dysplasia have been found to have significantly lower levels of serum retinol and serum beta-carotene.[18,19] Women infected with HIV have a higher prevalence of vitamin A deficiency than the general population. In a study of 1,314 HIV-positive women, this deficiency was significantly associated with cancerous cervical squamous intraepithelial lesions (SILs).[20] The association remained independent of markers of HIV disease stage, status of human papilloma virus infection, and overall nutritional status. Vitamin A deficiency status was also independent of CD4 count or viral load. Cervical SILs were almost twice as likely in women with abnormally low vitamin A levels (15 percent of the study population).

Retinoic acid was used topically and intravenously to reverse mild-to-severe cervical dysplasia in 96.29 percent of a study population.[21] Topical treatment with all-trans retinoic acid alone has been equally effective in moderate dysplasia.[22]

Cancer

Vitamin A has been used in the prevention and treatment of specific pre-malignant, malignant, and recurrent neoplasms.[23] Retinoic acid has been found to be effective in suppressing pre-malignant cells in oral leukoplakia, laryngeal dysplasia, bronchial metaplasia and dysplasia, and cervical dysplasia.[24] Retinoids prevent the development of second primary cancers in head and neck and lung cancer patients who have been treated for a primary tumor.[25] Retinoids, in combination with interferons, have been used to treat cutaneous squamous cell carcinoma, with a 50-68 percent response rate.[26] Retinoic acid therapy has also been shown to significantly improve the survival of children with neuroblastoma by suppressing residual disease after chemotherapy.[27]

A three-year clinical study using retinoic acid in patients with xeroderma pigmentosum resulted in a significant reduction in the number of new and recurrent skin tumors (basal cell and squamous cell carcinoma).[28] The tumor frequency increased 8.5-fold after retinoic acid was discontinued. Acute promyelocytic leukemia has been shown to respond to all-trans retinoic acid added to chemotherapy. Survival rates in two randomized studies of 1,000 patients treated with all-trans retinoic acid (45 mg/m^2 per day) in addition to chemotherapy showed complete remission rates of 93 and 94 percent.[29,30]

Because levels of retinoic acid used in oncology are very high, (average dose 45-50 mg/m^2 body surface area per day, up to 330,000 IU daily) trials have used synthetic retinoids in an attempt to moderate toxicity symptoms.[31]

Combination trials of vitamin A and interferon have been used in human studies on squamous cell cancer, cervical cancer, renal cell carcinoma, chronic myelogenous leukemia, and laryngeal dysplasia.[32] A recent study in patients with head and neck squamous cell tumors used alpha-tocopherol in an attempt to moderate toxicity of both alpha-interferon and 13-cis-retinoic acid.[33] Antioxidants, specifically vitamin E, have been theorized to limit vitamin A toxicity symptoms. In a trial that attempted to prevent recurrence of advanced head and neck tumors or second primary tumors, patients were given 167,000 IU/m^2 body surface area of 13-cis-retinol (approximately 300,000 IU per day) and 1,200 IU alpha-tocopherol, in addition to interferon-alpha daily for 12 months. Thirty-eight of 44 patients completed the 12 months of treatment with only mild-to-moderate side effects. Median 1-and 2-year disease-free survival rates were 91 percent and 84 percent, respectively.

Menorrhagia

In a South African study of 71 women with menorrhagia, low serum retinol levels were found in the majority of those studied.[34] Treatment of 40 patients with 25,000 IU vitamin A twice daily for 15 days completely alleviated symptoms in 58 percent and significantly reduced blood loss in 35 percent.

Infectious Diseases

Because vitamin A maintains the integrity of mucous membranes, increases surface glycoproteins, is integral to the production of secretory IgA, and is involved in humoral and cellular immunity, its application in infectious diseases logically follows.[6]

In a U.S. study, 50 percent of children diagnosed with acute measles virus were vitamin A deficient.[35] Therapeutic use of vitamin A in measles has been confirmed in multiple studies where it has reduced mortality by at least 50 percent.[36] Infection with respiratory syncytial virus has been correlated with low vitamin A levels in children whose blood levels of vitamin A were normalized with the administration of 25,000 IU.[37] Intramuscular injections of 2,000 IU daily for the first month of life in very-low-birth-weight pre-term infants have been used to effectively decrease risk for bronchopulmonary dysplasia.[38]

Children with no indication of vitamin A deficiency (normal serum retinol levels), but susceptibility to respiratory infections, were given 3,800 IU vitamin A three times weekly for 11 months, resulting in a 20-percent lower incidence of respiratory infections.[39]

HIV Infection

Vitamin A deficiency occurs commonly in HIV infection and worsens as the disease progresses.[40] Low levels are specifically problematic in pregnant women and are directly linked to infant mortality and vertical transmission. Vitamin A-deficient mothers are 3.7 times more likely to transmit the virus to their children.[41] Seventy percent of children born to HIV-positive mothers are vitamin A deficient.[42] The use of supplemental vitamin A prior to and at the time of birth has reduced the likelihood of transmission in pre-term infants by almost 50 percent.[43]

Drug-Nutrient Interactions

There is a risk of hypervitaminosis if vitamin A supplements are taken with retinoid drugs (used for skin disorders). Cholestyramine, colestipol hydrochloride, (both cholesterol lowering drugs) and mineral oil (as a laxative) may reduce absorption of vitamin A. People taking these drugs over a long period should consider taking a vitamin A supplement.[44]

Side Effects and Toxicity

Vitamin A is a teratogen; however supplementation of oil-soluble vitamin A in excess of 10,000 IU daily during pregnancy has been associated with a low incidence (less than 20 in the past 30 years) of documented birth defects.[45] The recommended dose for pregnant women in the U.S. is up to 8,000 IU daily, even though most studies have shown at least 20,000 IU daily is necessary to increase teratogenic risk.[46] One study in which women took daily oral doses of 30,000 IU did not significantly increase blood retinoic acid levels above physiologic normal ranges.[47] The main toxicity symptoms in chronic supplementation are headache, alopecia, chelosis, pruritis, hepatomegaly, bone and joint pain. After termination of intake, the majority of cases remit without permanent damage.[48] Toxicity symptoms after single pediatric doses of 165,000-330,000 IU of vitamin A are self-limited and non-life threatening (headaches, nausea, vomiting) and studies looking at toxicity of single doses of 100,000-200,000 IU in preschool children found minimal risk.[49]

The vast majority of chronic toxicity cases have occurred at levels of daily supplementation of 12,000 to 600,000 IU in children and 50,000 to1,000,000 IU in adults over a period of weeks to years. Vitamin A intolerance-toxicity symptoms occurring after chronic intakes at levels of 6,000 to 53,000 IU is less common and thought to be related to a genetic or metabolic defect in vitamin A handling.[50]

Dosage

Dosages in treatment of chronic pediatric respiratory infections range from 3,800 IU three times weekly in vitamin A nourished children to 200,000 IU single dose in suspected vitamin A deficiency.[39] In measles, with suspicion of vitamin A deficiency, the recommended protocol is 200,000 IU upon diagnosis and 200,000 IU two weeks later.[49] Recommended single doses in suspicion of vitamin A deficiency in pediatric chronic diarrhea or pediatric lower respiratory infection are 200,000 IU.

Adult RDA for vitamin A is 3,000 IU for men, 2,300 IU for women, and 2,500 IU for pregnant or reproductive age women. The Tolerable Upper Intake Levels (highest level of daily vitamin A intake that is likely to pose no risk of adverse health effects in almost all individuals) are 10,000 IU for men and women, and 9,300 IU for pregnant or reproductive age women.[51] Dosages for disease states are individualized and referenced in the clinical indications above.

References

1. Semba RD. The role of vitamin A and related retinoids in immune function. *Nutr Rev* 1998;56:S38-S48.
2. Patrick L. Beta-carotene: the controversy continues. *Altern Med Rev* 2000;5:530-545.
3. Christian P, West KP Jr. Interactions between zinc and vitamin A: an update. *Am J Clin Nutr* 1998;68:S435-S441.

4. Hansen LA, Sigman CC, Andreola F, et al. Retinoids in chemoprevention and differentiation therapy. *Carcinogenesis* 2000;21:1271-1279.

5. DiSepio D, Ghosn C, Eckert RL, et al. Identification and characterization of a retinoid-induced class II tumor suppressor/growth regulatory gene. *Proc Natl Acad Sci* USA 1998;95:14811-14815.

6. Semba RD. Vitamin A and immunity to viral, bacterial, and protozoan infections. *Proc Nutr Soc* 1999;58:719-727.

7. Humphrey JH, West KP. Vitamin A deficiency: role in childhood infection and mortality. In:*Micronutrients in Health and in Disease Prevention*. Bendich A, Butterworth CE, eds. New York: Marcel Dekker; 1991:307-329.

8. Rosenberg IH, Bengoa JM, Sitrin MD. Nutritional aspects of inflammatory bowel disease. *Annu Rev Nutr* 1985;5:463-484.

9. Leiber CS. Alcohol, liver, and nutrition. *J Am Coll Nutr* 1991;10:602-632.

10. Abahusain MA, Wright J, Dickerson JW, de Vol EB. Retinol, alpha-tocopherol and carotenoids in diabetes. *Eur J Clin Nutr* 1999;53:630-635.

11. Helgeland M, Svendsen E, Forre O, Haugen M. Dietary intake and serum concentrations of antioxidants in children with juvenile arthritis. *Clin Exp Rheumatol* 2000;18:637-641.

12. Crinnion WJ. Environmental medicine. In: Pizzorno JE, Murray M, eds. *Textbook of Natural Medicine, 2nd Ed.* New York, NY: Churchill Livingstone; 1999:287-300.

13. McLaren DS. Vitamin A deficiency disorders. *J Indian Med Assoc* 1999;97:320-323.

14. Head KA. Natural therapies for ocular disorders, part one: diseases of the retina. *Altern Med Rev* 1999;4:342-359.

15. Berson EL, Rosner B, Sandberg MA, et al. A randomized trial of vitamin A and vitamin E supplementation for retinitis pigmentosa. *Arch Ophthalmol* 1993;111:761-772.

16. Jetten AM, De Luca LM, NelsonK, et al. Regulation of cornfin alpha expression in the vaginal and uterine epithelium by estrogen and retinoic acid. *Mol Cell Endocrinol* 1996;123:7-15.

17. Palan PR, Mikhail MS, Goldberg GL, et al. Plasma levels of beta-carotene, lycopene, canthaxanthin, retinol, and alpha- and tau-tocopherol in cervical intraepithelial neoplasia and cancer. *Clin Cancer Res* 1996;2:181-185.

18. Dawson E, Nosovitch H, Hannigan E. Serum vitamin and selenium changes in cervical dysplasia. *Fed Proc* 1984;43:612.

19. Romney SL, Palan BR, Basu J, et al. Nutrients antioxidants in the pathogenesis and prevention of cervical dysplasias and cancer. *J Cell Biochem Suppl* 1995;23:96-103.

20. French AL, Kirstein LM, Massad LS, et al. Association of vitamin A deficiency with cervical squamous intraepitheroial lesions in human immunodeficiency virus-infected women. *J Infect Dis* 2000;182:1084-1089.

21. Ruidi C, Aihua D, Peiyu B, et al. Chemoprevention of cancer of uterine cervix: a study on chemoprevention of retinamide II from cervical precancerous lesions. *J Cell Biochem Suppl* 1997;28:140-143.

22. Meyskens FL JR, Surwit E, Moon TE, et al. Enhancement of regression of cervical intraepithelial neoplasia (moderate dysplasia) with topically applied all-trans retinoic acid: A randomized trial. *J Natl Cancer Inst* 1994;86:539-543.

23. Niles RM. Recent advances in the use of vitamin A (retinoids) in the prevention and treatment of cancer. *Nutrition* 2000;16:1084-1089.

24. Lotan R. Retinoids in cancer chemoprevention. *FASEB J* 1996;10:1031-1039.

25. Contreras Vidaurre EG, Bagan Sabastian JV, Gavalda C, Torres Cifuentes EF. Retinoids: application in premalignant lesions and oral cancer. *Med Oral* 2001;6:114-123.

26. Lippman SM, Parkinson DR, Itri LM, et al. 13-cis retinoic acid and interferon-2a. Effective combination therapy for advanced squamous cell carcinoma of the skin. *J Natl Cancer Inst* 1992;84:235-240.

27. Lovat PE, Ranalli M, Bernassola F, et al. Synergistic indiction of apoptosis of neuroblastoma by fenretinide or CD437 in combination with chemotherapeutic drugs. *Int J Cancer* 2000;88:977-985.

28. Kraemer KH, DiGiovanna JJ, Peck GL. Chemoprevention of skin cancer in xeroderma pigmentosum. *J Dermatol* 1992;19:715-718.

29. Degos L, Dombret H, Chomienne C, et al. allptrans-retinoic acid as a differentiating agent in the treatment of acute promyelocitic leukemia. *Blood* 1995;85:2643-2653.

30. Avvisati G, Baccarini M, Ferrara F, et al. AIDA protocol (all-trans retinoic acid + idarubicin) in newly diagnosed acute promyelocytic leukemia (APL): a pilot study of Italian cooperative group GIMENA. *Blood* 1996;88:1390.

31. Hansen LA, Sigman CC, Andreola F, et al. Retinoids in chemoprevention and differentiation therapy. *Carcinogenesis* 2000;21:1271-1279.

32. Lotan R, Clifford JL, Lippman SM. Retinoids and interferons: combination studies in human cancer. In: *Vitamin A and Retinoids: An Update of Biological Aspects and Clinical Applications.* Livrea MA, ed. Boston, MA: Birkhauser Verlag; 2000:221-230.

33. Shin DM, Khuri FR, Murphy B, et al. Combined interferon-alfa, 13-cis-retinoic acid, and alpha-tocopherol in locally advanced head and neck squamous cell carcinoma: novel bioadjuvant phase II trial. *J Clin Oncol* 2001;19:3010-3017.

34. Lithgow DM, Politzer WM. Vitamin A in the treatment of menorrhagia. *S Afr Med J* 1977;51:191-193.

35. Arrieta AC, Zaleska M, Stutman MI. Vitamin A in children with severe measles in Long Beach, CA. *J Pediatr* 1992;121:75-78.

36. Hussey GD, Klein M. A randomized, controlled trial of vitamin A in children with severe measles. *N Engl J Med* 1990;323:160-164.

37. Neuzil KM, Gruber WC, Chytil F, et al. Safety and pharmacokinetics of vitamin A therapy for infants with respiratory syncytial infections. *Antimicrob Agents Chemother* 1995;39:1191-1193.

38. Shenai JP, Kennedy KA, Chytil F, et al. Clinical trial of vitamin A supplementation in infants susceptible to bronchopulmonary dysplasia. *J Pediatr* 1987;111:269-277.

39. Pinnock CB, Douglas RM, Badcock NR. Vitamin A status of children who are prone to respiratory tract infections. *Aust Paediatr J* 1986;22:95-99.

40. Baum MK, Shor-Posner G, Lu Y, et al. Micronutrients and HIV-1 progression. *AIDS* 1995;9:1051-1056.

41. Semba RD, Miotti PG, Chiphangwi JD, et al. Infant mortality and maternal vitamin A deficiency during human immunodeficiency virus infection. *Clin Infect Dis* 1995;21:966-972.

42. Cunningham-Rundles S, Kim SH, Dnistrian A, et al. Micronutrient and cytokine interaction in congenital pediatric HIV infection. *J Nutr* 1996;126:S2674-S2679.

43. Coutsoudis A, Pillay K, Spooner E, et al. Randomized trial testing the effect of vitamin A supplementation on pregnanacy outcomes and early mother-to-child HIV-1 transmission in Durban, South Africa. *AIDS* 1999;13:1517-1524.

44. Morton I, Hall J. Vitamins, Minerals and Supplements. In: Glenn J, Searcy J, eds. *The Avery Complete Guide to Medicine*. New York, NY: Penguin Putman Inc; 2001:922-923.

45. Azais-Braesco V, Pascal G. Vitamin A in pregnancy: requirements and safety limits. *Am J Clin Nutr* 2000;71:S1325-S3133.

46. Teratology Society Position Paper: recommendations for vitamin A use during pregnancy. *Teratology* 1987;35:269-275.

47. Miller RK, Hendrickx AG, Mills JL, et al. Periconceptual vitamin A use: How much is teratogenic? *Reprod Toxicol* 1998;12:75-78.

48. Olson JA. Requirements and safety of vitamin A in humans. In: *Vitamin A and Retinoids: An Update of Biological Aspects and Clinical Applications.* Livrea MA, ed. Boston, MA: Birkhauser Verlag; 2000:29-44.

49. World Health Organization. *Indicators for assessing vitamin A deficiency and their application in monitoring and evaluating intervention programs.* Micronutrient series 96-10. Geneva: World Health Organization: 1-66.

50. Olson JA Upper limits of vitamin A in infant formulas, with some comments on vitamin K. *J Nutr* 1989;119:S1820-S1824.

51. Food and Nutrition Board, Institute of Medicine. Vitamin A. In: *Dietary Reference Intakes*. Washington DC: National Academy Press; 2001:82-161.

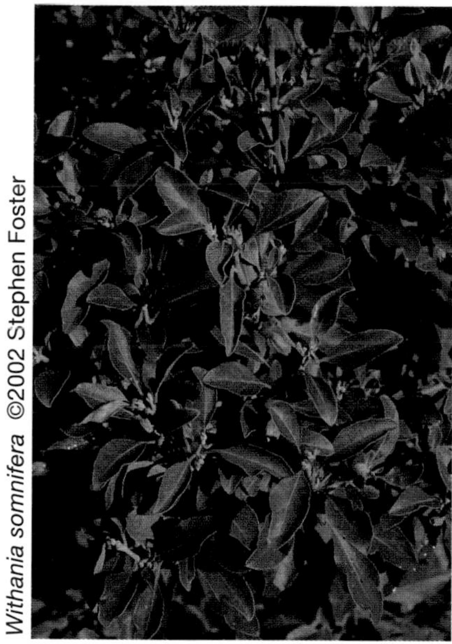
Withania somnifera ©2002 Stephen Foster

Withania somnifera

Description

Withania somnifera, also known as ashwagandha or winter cherry, is regarded as a primary herbal tonic of the Ayurvedic medical system. Ashwagandha is a small, woody shrub in the Solanaceae family that grows about two feet in height. It is found in Africa, the Mediterranean, and India. Because of the wide growing range, there are considerable morphological and chemotypical variations in terms of local species. However, the primary alkaloids of both the wild and the cultivated species appear to be the same.

Active Constituents

The major biochemical constituents of ashwagandha are steroidal alkaloids and steroidal lactones in a class of constituents called withanolides, that are extracted from the root.[1] At present, 11 alkaloids, 35 withanolides, and several sitoindosides from this plant have been isolated and studied. A sitoindoside is a withanolide containing a glucose molecule at carbon 27. Ashwagandha is also rich in iron.

Mechanisms of Action

The withanolides serve as important hormone precursors that can convert into human physiologic hormones as needed. Ashwagandha is thought to be amphoteric; i.e., it can help regulate important physiologic processes. The theory is that when there is an excess of a certain hormone, the plant-based hormone precursor occupies cell membrane receptor sites so the actual hormone cannot attach and exert its effect. If the hormone level is low, the plant-based hormone exerts a small effect. Ashwagandha is also considered to be an adaptogen, a substance that can increase a person's ability to withstand stressors.

Clinical Indications

Anti-Aging

In a double-blind clinical trial, ashwagandha (3 g daily for one year) was tested in a group of 101 healthy males, 50-59 years old. A significant improvement in hemoglobin, red blood cell count, hair melanin, and seated stature was observed. Serum cholesterol decreased and nail calcium was preserved. Erythrocyte sedimentation rate decreased significantly and 71.4 percent reported improvement in sexual performance.[2]

Immunomodulation and Hematopoiesis

A series of animal studies show ashwagandha to have profound effects on the hematopoietic system, acting as an immunoregulator and a chemoprotective agent.[3,4] In a mouse study, administration of a powdered root extract from ashwagandha was found to enhance total white blood cell count. In addition, this extract inhibited delayed-type hypersensitivity reactions and enhanced phagocytic activity of macrophages when compared to a control group.[5]

Ashwagandha exhibited stimulatory effects, both *in vitro* and *in vivo*, on the generation of cytotoxic T lymphocytes, and demonstrated the potential to reduce tumor growth.[6] The chemopreventive effect was demonstrated in a study of ashwagandha root extract on induced skin cancer in Swiss albino mice given ashwagandha before and during exposure to the skin cancer-causing agent 7,12-dimethylbenz(a)anthracene. A significant decrease in incidence and average number of skin lesions was demonstrated compared to the control group. Additionally, levels of reduced glutathione, superoxide dismutase, catalase, and glutathione peroxidase in the exposed tissue returned to near normal values following administration of the extract. The chemopreventive activity is thought to be due in part to the antioxidant/free radical scavenging activity of the extract.[7]

Anxiety and Depression

In a study performed to assess the anxiolytic and antidepressive actions of ashwagandha in rats compared to commonly prescribed pharmaceuticals. an extract of the root, containing bioactive glycowithanolides (WSG), was administered orally, once daily for five days. The results were compared to a group administered the benzodiazepine lorazepam for anxiolytic activity, and the tricyclic antidepressant imipramine for antidepressant investigation. Both the WSG group and the lorazepam group had reduced brain levels of tribulin, a marker of clinical anxiety following administration of the anxiogenic agent pentylenetetrazole. WSG also exhibited an antidepressant effect comparable to that induced by imipramine in the forced swim-induced "behavioral despair" and "learned helplessness" tests.[8] Other similar studies confirm these results, lending support to the use of WSG as an antistress adaptogen.[9-12]

Cardiovascular Protection

Hypoglycemic, diuretic, and hypocholesterolemic effects of ashwagandha root were assessed in human subjects. Six type 2 diabetes mellitus subjects and six mildly hypercholesterolemic subjects were treated with a powder extract for 30 days. A decrease in blood glucose comparable to that of an oral hypoglycemic drug was observed. Significant increases in urine sodium, urine volume, and decreases in serum cholesterol, triglycerides, and low-density lipoproteins were also seen.[13]

Other Therapeutic Considerations

Studies also show ashwagandha to be effective in the treatment of hypothyroidism,[14] osteoarthritis,[15] inflammation,[16,17] and tardive dyskinesia.[18] Studies also reveal ashwagandha to be a potential antimicrobial agent.[19,20]

Drug-Botanical Interactions

There are anecdotal reports that ashwagandha may potentiate the effects of barbiturates; therefore, caution should be used if taking this combination.

Side Effects and Toxicity

Ashwagandha is generally safe when taken in the prescribed dosage range.[21] Large doses have been shown to cause gastrointestinal upset, diarrhea, and vomiting.

Dosage

A typical dose of ashwagandha is 3-6 grams daily of the dried root, 300-500 mg of an extract standardized to contain 1.5 percent withanolides, or 6-12 ml of a 1:2 fluid extract per day.

Warnings and Contraindications

Large doses of ashwagandha may possess abortifacient properties; therefore, it should not be taken during pregnancy.

References

1. Elsakka M, Grigorescu E, Stanescu U, et al. New data referring to chemistry of *Withania somnifera* species. *Rev Med Chir Soc Med Nat Iasi* 1990;94:385-387.
2. Bone K. *Clinical Applications of Ayurvedic and Chinese Herbs. Monographs for the Western Herbal Practitioner.* Australia: Phytotherapy Press; 1996:137-141.
3. Kuttan G. Use of *Withania somnifera* Dunal as an adjuvant during radiation therapy. *Indian J Exp Biol* 1996;34:854-856.
4. Ziauddin M, Phansalkar N, Patki P, et al. Studies on the immunomodulatory effects of Ashwagandha. *J Ethnopharmacol* 1996;50:69-76.
5. Davis L, Kuttan G. Immunomodulatory activity of *Withania somnifera*. *J Ethnopharmacol* 2000;71:193-200.
6. Davis L, Kuttan G. Effect of *Withania somnifera* on CTL activity. *J Exp Clin Cancer Res* 2002;21:115-118.
7. Prakash J, Gupta SK, Dinda AK. *Withania somnifera* root extract prevents DMBA-induced squamous cell carcinoma of skin in Swiss albino mice. *Nutr Cancer* 2002;42:91-97.
8. Bhattacharya SK, Bhattacharya A, Sairam K, Ghosal S. Anxiolytic-antidepressant activity of *Withania somnifera* glycowithanolides: an experimental study. *Phytomedicine* 2000;7:463-469.

9. Bhattacharya A, Ghosal S, Bhattacharya SK. Antioxidant effect of *Withania somnifera* glycowithanolides in chronic footshock stress-induced perturbations of oxidative free radical scavenging enzymes and lipid peroxidation in rat frontal cortex and striatum. *J Ethnopharmacol* 2001;74:1-6.

10. Singh B, Saxena AK, Chandan BK, et al. Adaptogenic activity of a novel, withanolide-free aqueous fraction from the root of *Withania somnifera. Phytother Res* 2001;15:311-318.

11. Archana R, Namasivayam A. Antistressor effect of *Withania somnifera. J Ethnopharmacol* 1999;64:91-93.

12. Dhuley JN. Adaptogenic and cardioprotective action of ashwagandha in rats and frogs. *J Ethnopharmacol* 2000;70:57-63.

13. Andallu B, Radhika B. Hypoglycemic, diuretic and hypocholesterolemic effect of winter cherry (*Withania somnifera*) root. *Indian J Exp Biol* 2000;38:607-609.

14. Panda S, Kar A. *Withania somnifera* and *Bauhinia purpurea* in the regulation of circulating thyroid hormone concentrations in female mice. *J Ethnopharmacol* 1999;67:233-239.

15. Kulkarni RR, Patki PS, Jog VP, et al. Treatment of osteoarthritis with a herbomineral formulation: a double-blind, placebo-controlled, cross-over study. *J Ethnopharmacol* 1991;33:91-95.

16. Angalagan K, Sadique J. Influence of an Indian medicine (ashwagandha) on acute-phase reactants in inflammation. *Indian J Exp Biol* 1981;19:245-249.

17. Begum VH, Sadique J. Long-term effect of herbal drug *Withania somnifera* on adjuvant-induced arthritis in rats. *Indian J Exp Biol* 1988;26:877-882.

18. Bhattacharya SK, Bhattacharya D, Sairam K, Ghosal S. Effect of *Withania somnifera* glycowithanolides on a rat model of tardive dyskinesia. *Phytomedicine* 2002;9:167-170.

19. Abou-Douh AM. New withanolides and other constituents from the fruit of *Withania somnifera. Arch Pharm* 2002;335:267-276.

20. Choudhary MI, Dur-e-Shahwar, Parveen Z, et al. Antifungal steroidal lactones from *Withania coagulance. Phytochemistry* 1995;40:1243-1246.

21. Aphale AA, Chhibba AD, Kumbhaakarna NR, et al. Subacute toxicity study of the combination of ginseng (*Panex ginseng)* and ashwagandha (*Withania somnifera)* in rats: a safety assessment. *Indian J Physiol Pharmacol* 1998;42:299-302.

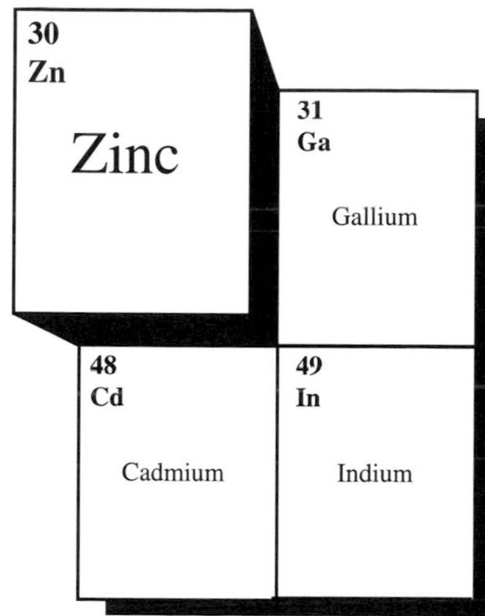

Zinc

Introduction

Zinc is a cofactor in over 300 metalloenzymes, and is able to directly affect gene expression, signal transduction, transcription, and cellular replication through nonenzymatic pathways.[1] Zinc plays a role in the synthesis of protein, fat, and cholesterol, as well serving as a cofactor for SOD, alcohol metabolism, and insulin function. Zinc is also important for its role in the immune system, cell growth and differentiation, prostate health, and taste perception.

Biochemistry and Mechanisms of Action

Zinc has anti-inflammatory action mediated through inhibition of nitric oxide formation.[2] There is a greater incidence of chronic diarrhea in zinc-deficient children,[3] and zinc supplementation has historically improved chronic diarrhea in malnourished children.[4]

Zinc acts as an antioxidant through mechanisms outside its role in the antioxidant enzyme superoxide dismutase. Zinc has been shown to protect vitamin E stores,[5] stabilize membrane structures,[6] prevent LDL and VLDL oxidation,[7] protect against carbon tetrachloride-induced hepatitis,[8] and maintain tissue levels of metallothionein, a potential free radical scavenger.[9]

Recent studies exploring the mechanisms of zinc deficiency and immune suppression have shown zinc deficiency (like protein-calorie malnutrition) elevates the production of glucocorticoids through up-regulation of the hypothalamic-pituitary-adrenocortical axis.[10] Emerging research in the mouse model has shown that zinc deficiency, through glucocorticoid release, actually causes a depletion of precursor T and B cells in the bone marrow and thymus, suppressing lymphocyte production.

Zinc has a regulatory role in apoptosis, as it both induces and blocks cellular apoptosis, depending on the cellular concentration.[11] At very high concentrations, zinc can induce apoptosis in immune cells, possibly the mechanism responsible for the immune suppression of high supplemental doses of zinc. Apoptosis plays a role in many disease states, including autoimmune diseases, Alzheimer's and Parkinson's disease, stroke, ischemia, cancer, and HIV infection.[11]

Pharmacokinetics

Zinc absorption occurs throughout the length of the small intestine, but in greater amount in the jejunum, by active transport and diffusion. Active transport into the bloodstream is mediated by binding to albumin, alpha-2-macroglobulin, or transferrin.[1] Iron, copper, and phytates inhibit zinc absorption.

Zinc is stored in the spleen, muscle, liver, and bone marrow. Other tissues with high concentrations of zinc include the prostate, skin, spermatozoa, and retina. Red and white blood cells also have high concentrations of zinc. Elimination of zinc is primarily through the feces and urine, with smaller amounts eliminated through the skin.

Deficiency States and Symptoms

Severe zinc deficiency is seen only in combination with protein-calorie malnutrition, long-term intravenous feeding, or in the inherited disorder acrodermatitis enteropathica.[12] Nutritional zinc deficiency, however, has been well documented in otherwise "well-nourished" infants and young children, children and adults with chronic diarrhea, infants and children with impaired physical growth,[13] children at risk for or with a history of pneumonia,[14] and in infants and children with impaired neuropsychological activity.[15,16] Zinc deficiency has also been documented in sickle cell anemia,[17] renal disease, alcoholism, teenage pregnancy,[18] anorexia nervosa, bulimia,[19] the elderly,[20] HIV infection,[21] burn patients, and those with chronic gastrointestinal disease.[12]

Because zinc is crucial in cellular growth and replication, rapidly replicating cells such as embryonic and fetal tissue, cells of the central nervous system, the gastrointestinal system, and the immune system are particularly vulnerable to zinc restriction. Infants, young children, and individuals with acute or chronic infections that necessitate mounting a continuous immune response, as well as people with injuries or illness that requires tissue repair, are most at risk for zinc deficiency.[12]

The immune system is particularly dependent on a steady supply of zinc. Studies in mice with 30 days of sub-optimal zinc intake have shown a 30-80 percent loss of immune function.[22] Alterations in the immune status of human subjects having only minimal zinc deficiencies include defective natural killer function, decreased interleukin-2 production, anergy,[23] and lymphopenia.[22]

Manifestations of severe zinc deficiency include diarrhea, dermatitis, alopecia, and poor wound healing. Signs of mild-to-moderate zinc deficiency include growth retardation (as related to protein metabolism) male hypogonadism, poor appetite, low immunity, rough skin, mental lethargy, and impaired taste acuity (hypogeusia). The symptoms of acrodermatitis enteropathica, an autosomal recessive disease with impaired zinc absorption, exhibit a classic manifestation of zinc deficiency: eczematoid skin lesions, alopecia, diarrhea, and concurrent bacterial and yeast infections.

Clinical Indications

Anorexia Nervosa and Bulimia Nervosa

Zinc deficiency symptoms, including anorexia, poor growth, weight loss, amenorrhea, and depression are common symptoms occurring in anorexia nervosa.[24] Altered gastrointestinal function that decreases zinc absorption, and high levels of exercise that increase zinc needs are factors that may predispose anorectics to zinc deficiency.[25] Zinc deficiency occurs in 50 percent of anorexia nervosa patients and 40 percent of bulimics.[19,26]

A controlled trial using zinc supplementation in anorectics found a significant increase in body mass index (BMI) in those on 14 mg elemental zinc from oral zinc gluconate.[27] Other trials have also found a significant increase in weight gain with zinc supplementation.[28-31]

Pediatric Diarrhea

In diarrhea, decreased transit time, as well as secretory fluid released in the small intestine, prevents nutrient absorption. Zinc is necessary for regeneration of the absorptive mucosa of the intestine. In infants less than one year old, diarrhea lasting longer than 10 days typically results in low serum zinc levels.[32] This appears to precipitate a cycle of zinc malabsorption and intestinal inflammation that, if unabated, can create chronic intestinal pathology and further lowering of tissue zinc stores.[32] A meta-analysis of studies of zinc supplementation in childhood diarrhea concluded zinc supplementation has a consistent, positive effect on the duration and severity of episodes of diarrhea.[33,34] The doses used in the studies ranged from 20-40 mg elemental zinc per day.

Age-Related Macular Degeneration

Clinical trials using zinc in age-related macular degeneration (AMD) have been based on the phenomenon of high zinc content in the retinal pigment epithelium, the tissue under the retina that nourishes the rods and cones. Using prior studies that provided evidence for pharmacological doses of zinc in prevention of vision loss in AMD,[35] the Age-Related Eye Disease Study (AREDS) assessed the effect of zinc in 3,640 patients with AMD. The study compared zinc alone, antioxidants alone, or zinc plus antioxidants against placebo.[36] The trial, lasting 6.3 years, assessed the effects of (1) antioxidants: vitamin C, 500 mg; vitamin E, 400 IU; and beta carotene, 15 mg; (2) zinc: 80 mg as zinc oxide; and copper, 2 mg as cupric oxide; (3) antioxidants plus zinc; or (4) placebo. Comparison with placebo showed a statistically significant decrease in the risk of developing advanced AMD in the antioxidants-plus-zinc group, i.e., the odds were reduced by 27 percent. The use of zinc (and copper) alone resulted in a 25-percent reduction. When those who had only a small probability of progressing were excluded, the odds for the rest of the participants dropped even more, with 33 percent less likely to progress with both zinc and antioxidants and 30 percent less likely to progress with zinc alone. Those on both antioxidants and zinc were able to reduce their risk of losing vision by one-third.

Epidemiological studies assessing zinc intake in those with AMD found moderate levels of dietary and supplemental zinc – a median intake of 40 mg per day in men and 25 mg per day in women – were not effective in decreasing risk for AMD.[37]

Diabetes

Diabetics have a significant risk for zinc deficiency. Low plasma and erythrocyte levels, abnormal taste acuity, and low levels of plasma thymulin activity have been found in significant proportions among type 1 and 2 diabetics.[38-40]

In murine models of diabetes, zinc supplementation has been shown to lower elevated serum glucose levels and to decrease risk for onset and severity of diabetes in diabetes-prone mice.[41,42] In zinc-deficient women with type 2 diabetes, 30 mg zinc glycinate was used to raise insufficient plasma zinc and 5'nucleotidase activities (a sensitive indicator of zinc status).[40] Zinc supplementation, at 30 mg per day, has also been shown to elevate selenium glutathione peroxidase levels in diabetics with retinopathy.[43] In another study with insulin-dependent diabetics, 660 mg of daily zinc salts were found to significantly improve peripheral neuropathy.[44]

HIV/AIDS

Zinc deficiency has been documented in HIV infection in multiple studies.[21,45] The utility of supplemental zinc in HIV infection has been documented in both pediatric and adult HIV infection. Zinc supplementation has improved CD4 counts, reduced viral load, and reduced risk of recurrent opportunistic infections (specifically Candidia esophaghitis and *Pneumocystis carinii* pneumonia) in CDC stage IV patients (CD4 cells under 50) on AZT.[46]

Caution has been expressed regarding supplemental zinc in HIV due to the fact that two HIV proteins in viral replication are zinc-dependent. Recent studies, however, have shown zinc finger proteins are also necessary for inactivation of the virus and evidence from feline HIV models implies low zinc levels contribute to the progression of the virus more than they offer protection against viral replication.[46]

Other Conditions

Zinc has been shown to be effective in a number of other disease states. Supplementation has been shown to reduce infectious bronchitis in children[15] and in Downs Syndrome patients.[47] Zinc supplementation has also been shown to decrease risk for infection from leprosy, malaria, and congenital herpes;[46] to slow the progression of Alzheimer's Disease;[48] to decrease prostatic swelling in benign prostatic hypertrophy;[49] to improve mean sperm counts in oligospermia;[50] and to increase the healing rate of gastric and lower limb ulcers.[51,52] Zinc also enhances exercise performance[53] and immune function in the elderly.[54]

Drug-Nutrient Interactions

Zinc reduces absorption of ciprofloxacin, penicillamine, and tetracyclines. Oral contraceptives and tetracyclines may reduce plasma zinc levels.[55] Zinc absorption is reduced with insufficient gastric acid production and with the use of H2-receptor antagonists.[56] It is suggested to take zinc supplements and acid-blocking drugs at separate times during the day.

Nutrient-Nutrient Interactions

Large doses of zinc may reduce copper absorption. Long-term doses of zinc required to deplete copper are reported to vary from 150 to 5,000 mg per day.[57] Studies in patients with sickle cell anemia who were given 150 mg zinc daily for 3-6 months, and were not supplemented with copper, became neutropenic and copper deficient.[58] As little as 2 mg copper per day can prevent copper deficiency with 150 mg zinc supplementation.[59]

Zinc reduces absorption of oral iron supplementation, and vice-versa.[60-62] This is clinically relevant when using supplemental iron in pregnancy. The inclusion of zinc in prenatal supplements may reduce the potential for iron supplements to adversely influence zinc status in pregnant women, subsequently reducing the risk of intrauterine zinc deficiency.[62]

Side Effects and Toxicity

Zinc at doses of 30 mg and above often causes stomach upset, nausea, and possible vomiting, an effect that is reduced when zinc is taken with food. Zinc toxicity with associated copper deficiency has been documented in a case of zinc gluconate supplementation at 850-1,000 mg per day for one year. Symptoms included fatigue and dyspnea on exertion. Objective findings included anemia, neutropenia, pallor, and orthostatic pulse changes.[63]

Dosage

Doses beyond the RDA of 15 mg/day have not been established. Other dosages are condition-specific. It may be important to note that 30 mg elemental zinc as glycinate chelate in studies with diabetics was unable to raise 5'nucleotidase levels to those of controls and was insufficient to normalize serum zinc levels in diabetics with neuropathy.[40] It appears certain populations of diabetics or individuals with malabsorption may need larger amounts of zinc. It is noteworthy that 660-mg doses of zinc salts were used in diabetics to successfully treat peripheral neuropathy symptoms.[44]

References

1. Vallee BL, Falchuk KH. The biochemical basis of zinc physiology. *Physiol Rev* 1993;73:79-118.
2. Abou-Mohamed G, Papapetropoulos A, Catravas JD, Caldwell RW. Zn2+ inhibits nitric oxide formation in response to lipopolysaccharides: implications in its anti-inflammatory activity. *Eur J Pharmacol* 1998;341:265-272.
3. Bahl R, Bhandari N, Hambidge KM, Bhan MK. Plasma zinc as a predictor of diarrheal and respiratory morbidity in children in an urban slum setting. *Am J Clin Nutr* 1998;68:S414-S417.
4. Bhutta ZA, Bird SM, Black RE, et al. Therapeutic effects of oral zinc in acute and persistent diarrhea in children in developing countries: pooled analysis of randomized controlled trials. *Am J Clin Nutr* 2000;72:1516-1522.
5. Bunk MJ, Dnistrian AM, Schwartz MK, Rivlin RS. Dietary zinc deficiency decreases plasma concentrations of vitamin E. *Proc Soc Exp Biol Med* 1989;190:379-384.
6. Bray TM, Bettger WJ. The physiological role of zinc as an antioxidant. *Free Radic Biol Med* 1990;8:281-291.
7. DiSilvestro RA, Blostein-Fujii A. Moderate zinc deficiency in rats enhances lipoprotein oxidation *in vitro*. *Free Radic Biol Med* 1997;22:739-742.
8. DiSilvestro RA, Carlson GP. Effects of mild zinc deficiency, plus or minus acute phase response, on CC14 hepatotoxicity. *Free Radic Biol Med* 1994;16:57-61.
9. Cousins RJ. Absorption, transport, and hepatic metabolism of copper and zinc: special reference to metallothionein and ceruloplasmin. *Physiol Rev* 1985;65:238-309.
10. Fraker PJ, King LE, Laakko T, Vollmer TL. The dynamic link between the integrity of the immune system and zinc status. *J Nutr* 2000;130:S1399-S1406.
11. Webb SJ, Harrison DJ, Wyllie AH. Apoptosis: an overview of the process and its relevence in disease. *Adv Pharmacol* 1997;41:1-34.
12. Hambidge M. Human zinc deficiency. *J Nutr* 2000;130:S1344-S1349.
13. Hambidge M, Krebs NF, Walravens A. Growth velocity of young children receiving a dietary zinc supplement. *Nutr Res* 1985;1:306-316.
14. Buttha ZA, Black RE, Brown KH, et al. Prevention of diarrhea and pneumonia by zinc supplementation in children in developing countries: pooled analysis of randomized controlled trials. *J Pediat* 1999;135:689-697.
15. Sazawal S, Bentley M, Black RE, et al. Effect of zinc supplementation on observed activity in low socioeconomic Indian preschool children. *PEDS* 1996;98:1132-1137.
16. Bentley ME, Caulfield LE, Ram M, et al. Zinc supplementation affects the activity patterns of rural Guatemalan infants. *J Nutr* 1997;127:1333-1338.
17. Prasad AS. Zinc deficiency in sickle cell disease. *Prog Clin Biol Res* 1984;165:49-58.
18. Endre L, Beck F, Prasad A. The role of zinc in human health. *J Trace Elem Exp Med* 1990;3:337.
19. Humphries LL, Vivian B, Stuart M, et al. Zinc deficiency and eating disorders. *J Clin Psychiatr* 1989;50:456-459.
20. Sandstead HH. Is zinc deficiency a public health problem? *Nutrition* 1995;11:87-92.
21. Baum MK, Shor-Posner G, Campa A. Zinc status in human immunodeficiency virus infection. *J Nutr* 2000;130:S1421-S1423.
22. Fraker P, King L. Changes in the regulation of lymphopoiesis and myelopoiesis in the zinc-deficient mouse. *Nutr Rev* 1998;56:S65-S69.
23. Kaplan J, Hess JW, Prasad AS. Impairment of immune function in the elderly: association with mild zinc deficiency. In: *Essential and Toxic Trace Elements in Human Health and Disease.* New York; Alan R. Liss: 1988:309-317.

24. Shay NF, Manigan HF. Neurobiology of zinc-influenced eating behavior. *J Nutr* 2000;130:S493-S1499.
25. Dinsmore WW, Alerdice JT, McMaster D, et al. Zinc absorption in anorexia nervosa. *Lancet* 1985;1:1041-1042.
26. McClain CJ, Stuart MA, Vivian B, et al. Zinc status before and after zinc supplementation of eating disorder patients. *J Am Coll Nutr* 1992;11:694-700.
27. Birmingham CL, Goldner EM, Bakan R. Controlled trial of zinc supplementation in anorexia nervosa. *Int J Eating Disord* 1994;15:251-255.
28. Safai-Kutti S. Oral zinc supplementation in anorexia nervosa. *Acta Psych Scand Supp* 1990;361:14-17.
29. Yamaguchi H, Arita Y, Hara Y, et al. Anorexia nervosa responding to zinc supplementation: a case report. *Gastroenterol Jap* 1992;27:554-558.
30. Bryce-Smith D, Simpson R. Case of anorexia nervosa responding to zinc sulphate. *Lancet* 1984;2:350.
31. Esca SA, Brenner W, Mach K, et al. Kwashiorkor-like zinc deficiency syndrome in anorexia nervosa. *Acta Derm-Venereol* 1979;361-364.
32. Wapnir RA. Zinc deficiency, malnutrition and the gastrointestinal tract. *J Nutr* 2000;130:S1388-S1392.
33. Brown KH, Peerson JM, Allen LH. Effect of zinc supplementation on children's growth: a meta-analysis of intervention trials. *Bibl Nutr Dieta* 1998;54:76-83.
34. Sazawal S, Black RE, Bhan MK, et al. Efficacy of zinc supplementation in reducing the incidence and prevalence of acute diarrhea – a community-based, double-blind, controlled trial. *Am J Clin Nutr* 1997;66:413-418.
35. Newsome DA, Swartz M, Leone NC, et al. Oral zinc in macular degeneration. *Arch Opthalmol* 1993;111:1200-1209.
36. Age-Related Eye Disease Study Research Group. A randomized, placebo-controlled, clinical trial of high-dose supplementation with vitamins C and E, beta carotene, and zinc for age-related macular degeneration and vision loss: AREDS Report No. 8. *Arch Opthalmology* 2001;119:1417-1436.
37. Cho E, Stampfer MJ, Seddon JM, et al. Prospective study of zinc intake and the risk of age-related macular degeneration. *Ann Epidemiol* 2001;11:328-336.
38. Mooradian AD, Morely JE. Mirconutrient status in diabetes mellitus. *Am J Clin Nutr* 1986;45:877-895.
39. Moutschen MP, Scheen AJ, Lefebvre PJ. Impaired immune responses in diabetes mellitus: anaylsis of the factors and mechanisms involved. Relevance to the increased susceptibility of diabetic patients to specific infections. *Diabete Metab* 1992;18:187-201.
40. DiSilvestro RA. Zinc in relation to diabetes and oxidative disease. *J Nutr* 2000;130:S1509-S1511.
41. Simon SF, Taylor CG. Dietary zinc supplementation attenuates hyperglycemia in db/db mice. *Exp Biol Med* 2001;226:43-51.
42. Tobia MH, Zdanowicz MM, Wingertzahn MA, et al. The role of dietary zinc in modifying the onset and severity of spontaneous diabetes in the BB Wistar rat. *Mol Genet Metab* 1998;63:205-213.
43. Faure P, Benhamou PY, Perard A, et al. Lipid peroxidation in insulin-dependent diabetic patients with early retina degenerative lesions: effects of an oral zinc supplementation. *Eur J Clin Nutr* 1995;49;282-288.
44. Gupta R, Garg VK, Mathur DK, Goyal RK. Oral zinc therapy in diabetic neuropathy. *J Assoc Physicians India* 1998;46:939-942.
45. Patrick L. Nutrients and HIV: Part 2 – Vitamins A and E, zinc, B-vitamins, and magnesium. *Altern Med Rev* 2000;5:39-51.
46. Mocchegiani E, Muzzioli M. Therapeutic application of zinc in human immunodeficiency virus against opportunistic infections. *J Nutr* 2000;130:S1424-S1431.
47. Licastro F, Chiricolo M, Mocchegiani E, et al. Oral zinc supplementation in Down's syndrome subjects decreased infections and normalized some humoral and cellular immune parameters. *J Intell Disabil Res* 1994;38:149-162.

48. Huang X, Cuajungco M, Atwood CS, et al. Alzheimer's disease, beta-amyloid protein, and zinc. *J Nutr* 2000;130:S1488-S1492.
49. Fahim M, Fahim Z, Der R, et al. Zinc treatment for the reduction of hyperplasia of the prostate. *Fed Proc* 1976;35:361.
50. Netter A, Hartoma R, Nakoul K. Effect of zinc administration on plasma testosterone, dihydrotestosterone and sperm count. *Arch Androl* 1981;7:69-73.
51. Formmer DJ. The healing of gastric ulcers by zinc sulphate. *Med J Austr* 1975;2:793.
52. Hallbrook T, Lanner E. Serum zinc and healing of various leg ulcers. *Lancet* 1972;2:780-782.
53. Krotiewski M, Gudmundson M, Backstrom P, et al. Zinc and muscle strength and endurance. *Acta Physiol Scand* 1982;116:309-311.
54. Bodgen JD, Oleske JM, Lavenhar MA, et al. Effects of one year supplementation with zinc and other micronutrients on cellular immunity in the elderly. *J Am Coll Nutr* 1990;9:214-215.
55. Mason P. *Dietary Supplements*. London, UK: Pharmaceutical Press; 2001:254.
56. Sterniolo GC, Montino MC, Rosetto L, et al. Inhibition of gastric acid secretion reduces zinc absorption in man. *J Am Coll Nutr* 1991;10:372-375.
57. Cunnane SC. *Zinc: Clinical and Biochemical Significance*. Boca Raton, FL: CRC Press; 1988:65-66.
58. Prasad AS. Zinc: the biology and therapeutics of an ion. *Ann Intern Med* 1996;125:142-144.
59. Prasad AS. Essentiality and toxicity of zinc. *Scand J Work Environ Health* 1993;19:134-136.
60. Sandstrom B. Micronutrient interactions: effects on absorption and bioavailability. *Br J Nutr* 2001;85:S181-S185.
61. Brzozowska A. Interaction of iron, zinc and copper in the body of animals and humans. *Rocz Panstw Zakl Hig* 1989;40:302-312. [article in Polish]
62. Solomons NW. Competitive interaction of iron and zinc in the diet: consequences for human nutrition. *J Nutr* 1986;116:927-935.
63. Walsh CT, Sandstead HH, Prasad AS, et al. Zinc: health effects and research priorities for the 1990s. *Environ Health Perspect* 1994;102:S5-S46.

B

C

D

E

H

T

U

V

W

X

Z